Tar
Adult Psychiatrica

From the publishers of the Tarascon Pocket Pharmacopoeia®

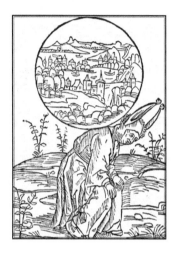

Josiane Cobert, MD, FACFE

Medical Director, Child/Adolescent In-Patient Psychiatric Service
Trinitas Regional Medical Center
Elizabeth, NJ

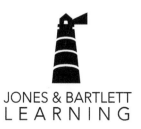

JONES & BARTLETT
L E A R N I N G

World Headquarters

Jones & Bartlett Learning
40 Tall Pine Drive
Sudbury, MA 01776
978-443-5000
info@jblearning.com
www.jblearning.com

Jones & Bartlett Learning Canada
6339 Ormindale Way
Mississauga, Ontario L5V 1J2
Canada

Jones & Bartlett Learning International
Barb House, Barb Mews
London W6 7PA
United Kingdom

Jones & Bartlett Learning books and products are available through most bookstores and online booksellers. To contact Jones & Bartlett Learning directly, call 800-832-0034, fax 978-443-8000, or visit our website, www.jblearning.com.

Substantial discounts on bulk quantities of Jones & Bartlett Learning publications are available to corporations, professional associations, and other qualified organizations. For details and specific discount information, contact the special sales department at Jones & Bartlett Learning via the above contact information or send an email to specialsales@jblearning.com.

The author, editors, and publisher have made every effort to provide accurate information. However, they are not responsible for errors, omissions, or for any outcomes related to the use of the contents of this book and take no responsibility for the use of the products and procedures described. Treatments and side effects described in this book may not be applicable to all people; likewise, some people may require a dose or experience a side effect that is not described herein. Drugs and medical devices are discussed that may have limited availability controlled by the Food and Drug Administration (FDA) for use only in a research study or clinical trial. Research, clinical practice, and government regulations often change the accepted standard in this field. When consideration is being given to use of any drug in the clinical setting, the healthcare provider or reader is responsible for determining FDA status of the drug, reading the package insert, and reviewing prescribing information for the most up-to-date recommendations on dose, precautions, and contraindications, and determining the appropriate usage for the product. This is especially important in the case of drugs that are new or seldom used.

Library of Congress Cataloging-in-Publication Data
Cobert, Josiane.
   Tarascon adult psychiatrica / Josiane Cobert.
     p. ; cm.
   Adult psychiatrica
   Includes bibliographical references and index.
   ISBN-13: 978-0-7637-7639-8
   ISBN-10: 0-7637-7639-4
1. Psychiatry—Handbooks, manuals, etc.   I. Title.   II. Title: Adult psychiatrica.
   [DNLM: 1. Mental Disorders—Handbooks.   2. Adult.   WM 34]
   RC456.C63 2010
   616.89—dc22   2010036989

6048

Printed in the United States of America
14 13 12 11 10   10 9 8 7 6 5 4 3 2 1

Production Credits

Senior Acquisitions Editor: Nancy Anastasi Duffy
Editorial Assistant: Sara Cameron
Associate Production Editor: Laura Almozara
Marketing Manager: Rebecca Rockel
V.P., Manufacturing and Inventory Control: Therese Connell
Composition: Newgen Imaging Systems Pvt Ltd
Cover Design: Kate Ternullo
Cover Image: Courtesy of Special Collections, University of Houston Libraries. Woodcut from Sebastian Brant's *The Ship of Fools*, 1494. Plate number XXIV titled 'Of Too Much Care', attributed to the Haintz-Nar-Meister.
Printing and Binding: Cenveo
Cover Printing: Cenveo

CONTENTS

ABBREVIATIONS

abnl: abnormal
AE: adverse event
alk phos: alkaline phosphatase
AM: in the morning
AMA: against medical advice

bid: twice a day

C/A: children and adolescents
CR: controlled release

DA: dopamine
DAergic: dopaminergic
DC: discontinue, discontinuation
DDI: drug–drug interactions
Dx, dx: diagnosis
DZ: dizygote (twins)

ER: extended release

FGA: first-generation antipsychotics (typical)

gl: general

hs: hour of sleep/bedtime
HTN: hypertension, high blood pressure
hx: history

IR: immediate release

MZ: monozygote (twins)

NE: norepinephrine
nl: normal
N/V: nausea/vomiting

OD: overdose

PM: in the evening
Pt, pt: patient

qd: every day
qid: four times a day

SE: side effect
SGA: second-generation antipsychotics (atypical)
SR: sustained release
Sx, sx: symptom
Sz, sz: schizophrenia

tid: three times a day
tx, Tx, rx, Rx: treatment

vs: versus

wk: week
wkly: weekly

ACKNOWLEDGMENTS

Many thanks to Drs. Romulo Aromin, Robert Bennett, Jaya Gavini, and Suma Srishaila for their assistance and review of the manuscripts.

The *Tarascon Adult Psychiatrica* arranges drugs by clinical class with a comprehensive index in the back. Trade names are italicized and capitalized. Drug doses shown in mg/kg are generally intended for children, while fixed doses represent typical adult recommendations. Each drug entry is divided as follows:

WARNING—Black-box warnings, if any, with lower level warnings in the "notes" section.

ADULT—Selected adult FDA-approved indications and doses listed in typical frequency of use.

PEDS—Selected peds FDA-approved indications and doses listed in typical frequency of use.

UNAPPROVED ADULT—Selected adult non-FDA-approved (i.e., "off-label") indications and doses listed in typical frequency of use.

UNAPPROVED PEDS—Selected pediatric non-FDA-approved (i.e., "off-label") indications and doses listed in typical frequency of use.

FORMS—Formulations available from manufacturers (e.g., tabs, caps, liquid, susp, cream, lotion, patches, etc.), including specification of trade, generic, and over-the-counter forms. Scored pills are designated as such. Not all pharmacies stock all items, of course.

NOTES—Selected notes, additional warnings, major adverse drug interactions, dosage adjustment in renal/hepatic insufficiency, therapeutic levels, etc.

Each drug entry contains the following codes:

> METABOLISM and EXCRETION: **L** = primarily liver; **K** = primarily kidney; **LK** = both, but liver > kidney; **KL** = both, but kidney > liver.

♀ **SAFETY IN PREGNANCY**: **A** = safety established using human studies; **B** = presumed safety based on animal studies; **C** = uncertain safety—no human studies and animal studies show an adverse effect; **D** = unsafe—evidence of risk that may in certain clinical circumstances be justifiable; **X** = highly unsafe—risk of use outweighs any possible benefit. For drugs that have not been assigned a category: **+** generally accepted as safe, **?** safety unknown or controversial, **–** generally regarded as unsafe.

▶ **SAFETY IN LACTATION**: **+** generally accepted as safe, **?** safety unknown or controversial, **–** generally regarded as unsafe. Many of our "+" listings are taken from the AAP policy "The Transfer of Drugs and Other Chemicals Into Human Milk" (see www.aap.org) and may differ from those recommended by manufacturers.

© **DEA-CONTROLLED SUBSTANCES**: **I** = high abuse potential, no accepted use (e.g., heroin, marijuana); **II** = high abuse potential and severe dependence liability (e.g., morphine, codeine, hydromorphone, cocaine, amphetamines, methylphenidate, secobarbital). Some states require triplicates; **III** = moderate dependence liability (e.g., *Tylenol #3, Vicodin*); **IV** = limited dependence liability (benzodiazepines, propoxyphene, phentermine); **V** = limited abuse potential (e.g., *Lomotil*).

$ RELATIVE COST: Cost codes used are "per month" of maintenance therapy (e.g., antihypertensives) or "per course" of short-term therapy (e.g., antibiotics). Codes are calculated using average wholesale prices (at press time in US$) for the most common indication and route of each drug at a typical adult dosage. For maintenance therapy, costs are calculated based upon a 30-day supply or the quantity that might typically be used in a given month. For short-term therapy (≤ 10 days), costs are calculated on a single treatment course. When multiple forms are available (e.g., generics), these codes reflect the least expensive generally available product. When drugs don't neatly fit into the classification scheme above, we have assigned codes based upon the relative cost of other similar drugs. *These codes should be used as a rough guide only*, because (1) they reflect cost, not charges; (2) pricing often varies substantially from location to location and time to time; and (3) HMOs, Medicaid, and buying groups often negotiate quite different pricing. Your mileage may vary. Check with your local pharmacy if you have any question.

♣ **CANADIAN TRADE NAMES**: Unique common Canadian trade names not used in the United States are listed after a club symbol. Trade names used in both nations or only in the United States are displayed without such notation.

Code cost:
$ < $25
$$ $25 to $49
$$$ $50 to $99
$$$$ $100 to $199
$$$$$ ≥$200

1 ■ INTRODUCTION: CLASSIFICATION, GUIDELINES, RATING SCALES, AND TESTING

Screening for mental health: www.mentalhealthscreening.org

Two classifications are used (both accepted by Medicare, Medicaid, and private insurance companies for reimbursement):

- the *Diagnostic and Statistical Manual of Mental Disorders*, 4th edition, Text Revision (2000; *DSM-IV-TR*)
- the *International Classification of Diseases*, 10th revision of the World Health Organization's ICD (2007; *ICD-10*)

THE *DSM-IV-TR*

(1) It **is a multiaxial system,** evaluating pts along five variables:
- **Axis I**: clinical disorders and conditions that may be a focus of clinical attention
- **Axis II**: personality disorders and mental retardation
- **Axis III**: gl medical conditions (present in addition to the mental disorder; may be causative or secondary or unrelated; if related or causative, should be put on Axis I and Axis III)
- **Axis IV**: psychosocial and environmental problems (contributing to the development or exacerbation of the current disorder; stressors may be + or −)
- **Axis V**: global assessment of functioning (GAF) scale during a particular time (at the time of evaluation and highest level of functioning for a few months during the preceding year; based on social, occupational, and psychologic functioning). GAF ranges from superior functioning (100) to some mild sx or mild difficulties in functioning (70) to serious sx such as suicidal ideations or any serious impairment in functioning (50), to some impairment in reality testing or major impairment in several areas (40), to presence of psychosis or serious impairment in judgment (30), to some danger of hurting self or others without clear expectation of death (20) to persistent danger for self or others (10).

(2) Severity: mild, moderate, severe; may be in partial or full remission.

(3) Multiple diagnoses may be given with the principal diagnosis listed first.

(4) A provisional diagnosis may be used if the full criteria cannot be produced (not enough information at the time of diagnosis).

(5) If a pt had a previous but not current diagnosis, write this as "prior history."

(6) The category of not otherwise specified (NOS) is used if the presentation does not meet the full criteria for any specific disorder but is close to it, if the sx pattern is not included in the *DSM* classification, or if the presentation is atypical.

DEFINITION OF MENTAL DISORDER

A clinically significant behavioral or psychologic pattern associated with present distress or disability in an individual; this pattern must not be an expectable or culturally sanctioned response to a particular event. It is due to a dysfunction in the individual and not just a deviance between the individual and the society.

Psychosis: loss of reality testing and impairment of mental functioning manifested by delusions, hallucinations, confusion, impaired memory, and possible grossly disorganized behavior. Psychotic disorders are pervasive developmental disorder (PDD), schizophrenia, schizophreniform disorders, schizoaffective disorders, delusional disorder, brief psychotic disorder, shared psychotic disorder, psychotic disorder due to a medical condition or substance-induced, psychotic disorder NOS. Psychotic features may exist in some mood disorders.

Neurosis: chronic or recurrent nonpsychotic disorder characterized by anxiety. The sx are distressing to the individual and recognized by the individual as alien (ego dystonic); reality testing is grossly intact; personality organization is intact. It is not a term used in the *DSM-IV-TR* but there is still a class called neurotic, stress-related, and somatoform disorders in the *ICD-10*; this includes anxiety disorders, somatoform disorders, dissociative disorders, sexual disorders, and dysthymic disorders.

GUIDELINES

As per the American Psychiatric Association (APA), *specific criteria in the DSM for each mental disorder are guidelines* and reflect a consensus of current formulation of evolving knowledge in the field; however, there are limitations such as loose boundaries between categories, heterogeneity in defining diagnostic features, and the like; the classification, used for clinical, educational, and research settings, must be employed with appropriate clinical training, experience, and exercise of clinical judgment, as a common language for communication; in forensic settings, there is a risk of misusing diagnostic information (legal vs clinical concerns).

PSYCHIATRIC RATING SCALES

- **Mostly used for schizophrenia and psychosis**:
  - BPRS (Brief Psychiatric Rating Scale)
  - SANS (Schedule for the Assessment of Negative Symptoms)
  - SADS (Schedule for Affective Disorders and Schizophrenia)
  - PANSS (Positive and Negative Syndrome Scale)
  - SAPS (Scale for the Assessment of Positive Symptoms)
- **Mostly used for mood disorders**:
  - MRS (Mania Rating Scale)
  - Beck Depression Inventory
  - HAM-D (Hamilton Rating Scale for Depression)
- **Mostly used for anxiety disorders**:
  - Y-BOCS (Yale-Brown Obsessive-Compulsive Scale)
  - HAM-A (Hamilton Anxiety Scale)
- **Mostly used for functioning assessment**:
  - GAF (Global Assessment of Functioning) Scale
  - SOFAS (Social and Occupational Functioning Assessment Scale)
  - CGI-S and CGI-I (Clinical Global Impression scales for Severity and Improvement)

PSYCHOLOGICAL TESTING

Provides specific information complementary to the psychiatric hx and the mental status exam.

- **Psychological tests** frequently used:
  - **Rorschach test**: ink blots are used for free associations. This test helps in the assessment of defense mechanisms and ego boundaries and in psychodynamic formulation.
  - **Thematic Apperception Test (TAT)**: the pt looks at pictures of people in a variety of situations and makes up a story for each picture. This test provides information about interpersonal relationships and internal preoccupations (needs, defenses, conflicts).
  - **Sentence Completion Test (SCT)**: the pt finishes incomplete sentences. This provides insight into defenses, fears, and thought processes.
  - **Minnesota Multiphasic Personality Inventory (MMPI)**: questions assess personality characteristics.
  - **Draw-a-Person Test (DPT)**: the pt is first asked to draw a person and then to draw another person of the opposite sex. This test shows how the pt relates to his or her environment and may show evidence of brain damage.
- **Neuropsychological tests** to assess specific functions of the brain:
  - **Bender Gestalt Test**: test of visual-motor and spatial abilities
  - **Halstead-Reitan Neuropsychological Battery**: evaluates (through 8 tests) visual, auditory, and tactual input; verbal communication; spatial and sequential perception; the ability to analyze information, form mental concepts, and make judgments; motor output; attention, concentration, and memory
  - **Luria-Nebraska Neuropsychological Battery (LNNB)**: measures functioning in multiple areas including motor skills, language abilities, intellectual abilities, nonverbal auditory skills, and visual-spatial skills
  - **Wechsler Adult Intelligence Scale (WAIS)**: measures verbal intelligence quotient (VIQ), performance IQ (PIQ), and full-scale IQ (FIQ)
  - **Wisconsin Card Sorting Test (WCST)**: prototype of abstract reasoning task; routinely used to assess frontal lobe function

Definition: study of the distribution, incidence, prevalence, and duration of diseases in populations.

TYPES OF STUDIES

- **Cohort study**: longitudinal study following a group of patients with a particular disease, exposure to a drug, or other factor to see how they do over time. They may be compared to another unexposed group.
- **Retrospective studies**: based on past data
- **Prospective studies**: longitudinal studies going forward in time based on observing events as they occur
- **Cross-sectional studies**: also called prevalence studies, these look at the prevalence and characteristics of a disease in the studied population at one particular point in time.
- **Case history study**: retrospective study examining persons with a particular disease
- **Case control study**: a retrospective study examining persons with a particular disease and comparing them with a group of patients from the same population without that disease.
- **Clinical trial**: a comparison study to determine the effects of a given rx in which selected pts will receive a course of the rx and another group (control group) will receive either no rx or an alternate one, but not the given rx:
  - **Double-blind study**: pts and clinicians do not know what is given (rx, placebo, or alternative rx).
  - **Cross-over study**: a study of two groups, one receiving an rx and the other a control for a certain period of time after which the two groups switch treatments. Each group serves as its own control as well as being compared to the other group.

Diagnostic reliability (also called interrater reliability): consistency in how different examiners give the same diagnosis in one pt and in how the same diagnosis is given to the same pt over time.

Diagnosis validity refers to the accuracy of a diagnosis:

- **Face validity**: gl consensus among experienced clinicians that a particular diagnosis exists.
- **Descriptive validity**: a disorder that has characteristic features enough to distinguish it from others (predictive validity: the diagnosis predicts accurately rx response and clinical course; construct validity: the diagnosis is based on understanding the underlying pathophysiology and confirming with biologic markers).

TABLE 2.1.   Validity of Diagnostic Tests

Test	Disease present	Disease absent
Test positive	TP (true positive)	FP (false positive)
Test negative	FN (false negative)	TN (true negative)

TEST SENSITIVITY

- **Shows a true positive rate**: diseased person with abnormal test results
- **False positive**: nondiseased person with abnormal test results suggesting disease = $1 -$ Specificity

TESTS SPECIFICITY

- **Shows a true negative rate**: nondiseased person with normal test results
- **False negative**: diseased person with normal test results (test missed the disease) = $1 -$ Sensitivity

PREDICTIVE VALUES

- **Of abnormal test results (PV+)**: proportion of abnormal test results that are true positive
- **Of normal test results (PV−)**: proportion of normal test results that are true negative

BIOSTATISTICS

Definition: mathematic science of describing, organizing, and interpreting medical data. Descriptive statistics are numerical values about observations (mean, median, standard deviation, variance); inferential statistics are numerical values used to draw conclusions about probabilities on the basis of a sample (analysis of variance, probability, probability value).

Analysis of variance (ANOVA): set of statistical procedures designed to compare different groups of observations, to determine if the differences are due to chance alone or experimental influence.

Control group: does not receive rx. May receive an alternate rx or no rx at all.

Correlation coefficient: measurement of the direction and strength of the relationship between two variables; indicates the degree of relationship but nothing about cause and effect:

- **Spearman rank order** (for ordinal data/data ranked in order) shows the relationship (if any) between two sets of data.
- **Pearson correlation coefficient** ρ for nominal data/data organized in categories: a positive correlation means that if one variable moves up, the other variable moves up too (in the same direction); a negative correlation means that the variables move in opposite directions; r is any value between -1 and $+1$ (if is 0, it means either a weak relationship or no relationship); if it is close to $+1$ or -1, it means a strong relationship)

Distribution: values that are organized according to the frequency of occurrence (frequency distribution); a normal distribution is the "bell curve." Also called the Gaussian distribution.

Incidence: number of **new cases** occurring over a specified time (usually 1 yr).

Measure of central tendency: a central value around which other values are distributed:

- **Mean**: adding a set of scores and then dividing by the number of scores; the mean is the average score
- **Median**: the value in the middle of a set of measurements such that half the values are greater than the median and half are less.
- **Mode**: the value that appears most frequently in a set of measurements.

Null hypothesis: the assumption that there is no significant difference between two samples of a population.

Odds ratio (OR): statistical measure comparing two groups to see the likelihood of a particular event or disease occurring. An OR of 1 suggests the event is equally likely in each group; >1 suggests one group will likely have it more than the other group.

Percentile rank: the percentage of scores in a distribution exceeded by any particular score.

Power: is the probability of identifying a true difference, the probability that the statistical test in question will reject a false null hypothesis.

Prevalence: The number of existing cases of a disorder (all pts with dis)

- **Point prevalence**: number of people who have a disorder at a specific point in time
- **Period prevalence**: number of people who have a disorder at any time during a specific period of time
- **Lifetime prevalence**: a measure at a point in time of the number of people who had a disorder at some point during their lives (based on subject recall and may be inaccurate)
- **Treated prevalence**: the number of people being treated for a disorder (point, or period prevalence).

Probability: likelihood that an event will happen (probability of 0 means that the event is certain not to occur; a probability of 1 means that the event will certainly occur).

p value: the probability of obtaining a result by chance alone (a p value of .01 means that the probability of obtaining a result by chance alone is 1 in 100).

- Likelihood ratio (pos. results) = Sensitivity + (1 – Specificity)
- Likelihood ratio (neg. results) = (1 – Sensitivity) + Specificity
- Pretest odd ratio = Pretest probability + (1 – Pretest probability)
- Posttest odds ratio = Pretest odds ratio × Likelihood ratio
- Posttest probability = Posttest odds ratio + (Posttest odds ratio + 1)

TABLE 2.2.   Probability

Likelihood ratio	Change from pretest to posttest probability
>10 or < 0.1	Large, often conclusive
5–10 or 0.1–0.2	Moderate
2–5 or 0.2–0.5	Small, sometimes important
0.5–2	Rarely important

Adapted from Jaeschke, R., Guyatt, G. H., & Sackett, D. L. (1994). Users' guides to the medical literature. III. How to use an article about a diagnostic test. B. What are the results and will they help me in caring for my patients? The Evidence-Based Medicine Working Group. *Journal of the American Medical Association, 271*, 703–707.

Randomization: in a clinical trial each pt is assigned to a control or the experimental rx group in a manner based purely on chance; done to eliminate biases (both known and unknown).

Regression analysis: method to predict the value of 1 variable (*x*) in relation to the value of another variable (*y*).

Risk factor: a factor that may support a causal connection in a disorder; it is shown by temporality if the factor precedes the disorder, can be repeated, is specific, and its elimination also eliminates the disorder.

- **Relative risk**: ratio of the incidence of the disease among people exposed to the incidence among people not exposed.
- **Attributable risk**: the absolute incidence of the disease in exposed people that can be attributed to the exposure (subtracting the incidence of the disease in nonexposed people from the total incidence of the disease among the people exposed).

Risk ratio (RR): The likelihood of one group developing the disease after exposure to a possible cause compared to another group not exposed to that possible cause.

Sensitivity: proportion of pts with the condition that the test can detect (true positives divided by sum of true positive + false negatives): $= TP/(TP + FN)$.

Specificity: proportion of pts without the condition that the test finds negative (number of true negatives divided by the sum of the number of true negatives +false positives) $= TP/(FP + TN)$.

Standard deviation (SD): represented by the Greek letter sigma (σ); in a normal distribution: ± 1 SD includes 68% of the population, ± 2 SD includes 95% of the population, and ± 3 SD includes 99% of the population.

Type I error: it is the false claim of a true difference when the observed difference is due entirely to chance.

Type II error: it is the false acceptance of the null hypothesis when in fact there is a true difference (not due to chance alone), but the difference is very small.

Variable: a characteristic that can assume different values in different experimental situations

- **Independent variables**: qualities that the experimenter systematically varies (e.g., time, sex, type of drug, age)
- **Dependent variables**: qualities measuring the influence of the independent variable or the outcome of the experiment (e.g., the measure of a specific reaction to a drug)

3 ■ DIAGNOSTIC EVALUATION

Clinical interview of the patient: ensure privacy, avoid interruptions, keep a comfortable distance with the pt, and allow for sufficient time (30 min for a cooperative pt, 90 min for a geriatric pt or someone with a complex hx).

METHODS

- Unstructured, open-ended interview.
- Structured format.

THREE TYPES OF CLINICAL PSYCHIATRIC EVALUATIONS

- **General psychiatric evaluation.** The goal is to:
  - Make a **diagnosis**.
  - Estimate the **severity** of the pt's condition.
  - Decide on an **initial course of action**.
  - Develop a relationship with the pt (**therapeutic alliance**).
  - Have a **dynamic understanding** of the pt.
  - **Engage the patient in treatment.**
- **Evaluation in the emergency department**: to decide on safety issues, make the diagnosis, assess the support system, the needed level of care, contact other involved agencies, family, or friends for information, medical evaluation needed for appropriate diagnosis and rx.
- **Clinical consultation** (requested by other physicians or others to assist in the diagnosis, rx, or management of a pt with a suspected or known mental disorder or behavioral problem).

The evaluation consists of psychiatric hx, mental status examination, complete physical examination, laboratory tests, and more specific psychologic or biologic tests if needed.

It is important to collect facts and information from the pt's interpretation style and nonverbal communications (allowing the pt to express concerns, finding the reasons for coming for help: **why now**?), to allay anxiety by being supportive, nonjudgmental, encouraging, not hurried. Start in a nonstructured way and transition to a more formal style to identify all important missed data. (R/O early on risk of aggression, suicide or the presence of an organic cause: **need to hospitalize**?)

Concluding the interview: allow time for questions, ask the pt for authorization to speak with collaterals, give appropriate comments about diagnostic impressions, proposed rx, length of rx.

Physical examination: done by an internist, family practitioner, or the psychiatrist.

Collateral information through phone or in person as needed (needs consent; if impossible, caution with **confidentiality**).

FORMAT FOR REPORTING THE PSYCHIATRIC EVALUATION

- **Identifying information** (age, sex, marital status, race)
- **Chief complaint**: reason for consultation as a direct quote from the pt.
- **Referral source**
- **Hx of present illness**
  - Current sx: date of onset, duration, and types of sx
  - Previous psychiatric sx and their rx
  - Recent contributing stressful life events
  - Why is this consultation asked for, just now?
- **Past psychiatric hx**
  - Previous diagnoses
  - Past psychiatric rx (inpatient and outpatient)
  - Past use of medications: effects, side effects (SEs), complications.

- Past suicidal attempts and violent behaviors, access to weapons.
- Current medications
- **Allergies** to drugs, foods, and other allergies
- **Past medical hx**:
  - Current and previous medical problems
  - Review all rx (prescriptions, over-the-counter, home remedies, complementary medicines, herbal)
- **Family hx of psychiatric and nonpsychiatric disorders**, suicide, alcohol and substance abuse, criminality.
- **Personal and social hx**: source of income, level of education (if children: regular or special education setting), relationships (marriages, sexual orientation, pregnancies and children, friends), current household situation, support network, church involvement, current use of alcohol or illicit drugs, legal problems, occupational hx.
- **Developmental hx**: birth problems, developmental milestones, school performances, family situation during childhood, foster placements, current relationships with family members.
- **Mental status examination at the time of the interview**

TABLE 3.1.   Mental Status Examination

Grooming
General description: behavior
Affect
Mood
Thought processes: formal and content (delusions)
Speech (logical or not)
Abnormal perceptions (hallucinations, illusions, misperceptions)
Level of consciousness (confusion, attention, concentration, alertness)
Orientation
Memory (immediate, short- and long term)
Suicidal and homicidal ideations
Intelligence
Judgment
Insight

- **Grooming and dress**, level of hygiene, clothing.
- **General description**: unusual physical characteristics, any abnormal movement, sense of relatedness, eye contact, attitude with interviewer, psychomotor agitation or retardation, restlessness, distractibility, impulse control. Describe motor behaviors:
  - **Echopraxia** (pathologic imitation of another person's movements)
  - **Catatonia**: postural abnormalities (**catalepsy**: immobile position constantly maintained; **catatonic excitement**: agitation with purposeless motor activity; **catatonic stupor**: very slowed motor activity with a seemingly unawareness of surroundings; **catatonic rigidity**: voluntary keeping a rigid posture; **catatonic posturing**: voluntary keeping an inappropriate or bizarre posture for long periods of time; **waxy flexibility**: where the position of the pt may be molded; **akinesia**: lack of physical movement).
  - **Negativism**: complete resistance to follow any directions.
  - **Cataplexy**: transient muscle weakness due to emotions.
  - **Stereotypy**: repetitive pattern of behavior or speech.
  - **Mannerism**: regular involuntary movement with a pattern.
  - **Automatism**: automatic performance of an act with a symbolic unconscious meaning.
  - **Mutism**: lack of speech (no structure abnormality).
  - **Overactivity**: psychomotor agitation (due to inner tension, unproductive), hyperactivity, tics, sleepwalking, **akathisia** (subjective feeling of muscular tension with restlessness, pacing, "ants in the pants" feelings), **compulsion** (uncontrollable impulse to perform an act repetitively), **ataxia** (lack of coordination), tremor (>1 beat/s, rhythmic, usually ↓ during sleep), **floccillation** (aimless picking at clothes or bedclothes), aggression.
  - **Hypoactivity**: **hypokinesis** (↓ motor activity with slowing of thoughts and speech), **abulia** (lowered impulse to act and think), **dyskinesia** (difficulty performing voluntary movements), **bradykinesia**

(slow motor activity, decreased spontaneous movement), **amimia** (inability to make gestures or comprehend those made by others).

Mimicry: imitative motor activity.

Acting out: direct expression of an unconscious impulse.

Anergia: lack of energy.

Astasia abasia: bizarre gait with inability to stand or walk (no specific organic lesion).

Twirling: continually rotating in the direction in which the head is turned.

Dystonia: slow, sustained contractions of some muscles.

Affect: observed expression of emotions

Appropriate: harmony between emotion tone and the accompanying idea, thought, and speech.

Inappropriate: disharmony between emotion tone and the accompanying idea, thought, and speech.

Blunted: severe reduction in the intensity of externalized emotions.

Restricted or constricted: reduction in the intensity of externalized emotions.

Flat: absence of any sx of affective expression (immobile face, monotonous voice).

Labile: rapid changes in emotions, unrelated to external stimuli.

Mood: internal, subjective, sustained emotional tone experienced and reported by the patient and observed by others.

Dysphoric: unpleasant.

Euthymic: normal, absence of depressed or elevated mood.

Expansive: the expression of feelings is without restraints with overestimation of their importance.

Irritable: the pt is easily annoyed or angered.

Labile: oscillations between euphoria and depression or anxiety.

Elevated: more cheerful than usual.

Euphoric: intense elation with grandiosity.

Ecstasic: feeling of intense rapture.

Depressed: feeling of sadness.

Anhedonic: loss of interest and enjoyment from pleasurable activities.

Hypomanic: mood state characteristic of mania but less intense.

Manic: elation, agitation (associated with hypersexuality, fast thinking, pressured speech)

Melancholic: severely depressed mood.

"La belle indifference": inappropriate attitude of lack of concern about one's disability.

Other emotions may be described: anxiety (caused by anticipation of a danger), free-floating anxiety (pervasive and unfocused), fear (caused by a realistic danger), agitation, tension, panic, apathy, ambivalence, abreaction (emotional discharge after recalling a painful experience), **shame (failure to live up to self-expectations), guilt (feeling attached to doing what is perceived as being wrong).**

Thought processes:

Use of language: quality, quantity of speech, tone, associations, fluency.

Formal thought disorder: loosened associations, neologisms, and illogical constructs. If the thought process is disordered and there is inability to distinguish reality from fantasy, the pt is psychotic.

Assess reality testing: ability to objectively evaluate the world outside the self.

Illogical thinking: contains errors in conclusions or marked internal contradictions.

Magical thinking: thinking in which thoughts, words, or actions can cause or prevent events (like in younger children).

Primary process thinking: thinking that is unrealistic, not concordant with logic or reality (like in dreams, psychosis).

Neologism: new word created for psychologic reasons.

Word salad: incoherent mixture of words and phrases.

Circumstantiality: speech is characterized by over inclusion of details, long to reach the point.

Tangentiality: association of thoughts that do not reach the point.

Incoherence: disorganized thought with no logic or grammatical connections, not understandable.

Perseveration: inability to change the subject of a conversation.

Verbigeration: meaningless repetitions of words or phrases.

Echolalia: repeats the words or phrases of another person.

Condensation: fusion of various concepts into one.

Derailment: deviation in the train of thought without thought blocking.

Flight of ideas: Rapid verbalizations with constant shifting from one idea to another; the ideas tend to stay connected.

Clang associations: association of words similar in sound (but not in meaning) with no logical connection.

Thought blocking: abrupt interruption in train of thought with no recall of what was going to be said or of what was said.

Loosening of associations: ideas shift from one subject to another in an unrelated way; speech may become incoherent.

Glossolalia: speaking in tongues (if not cultural).

Content thought disorder:

Poverty of content: vagueness, obscure phrases.

Overvalued idea: sustained false belief maintained less firmly than a delusion.

Delusion: false belief based on incorrect inference from reality, which cannot be corrected by reasoning (mood-congruent or mood-incongruent); may be bizarre, systematized; may be nihilistic, delusion of poverty, somatic delusion, paranoid delusions (delusion of persecution, delusion of grandeur, delusion of reference), delusion of self-accusation, delusion of control, of infidelity, erotomania, pseudologia fantastica (lying in which the pt appears to believe in the reality of his or her fantasies and to act on them).

Derealization: feelings of unrealness involving the outer environment.

Depersonalization: feelings of unrealness involving oneself.

Egomania: pathologic self-preoccupation.

Hypochondria: exaggerated concern about one's health based on unrealistic interpretations of physical sensations.

Obsession: persistence of thought that cannot be eliminated by logical effort and is associated with anxiety.

Compulsion: pathologic need to act on an impulse, frequently in response to an obsessive thought (to decrease anxiety).

Coprolalia: saying obscene words compulsively.

Phobia: persistent irrational pathologic fear of a specific stimulus or situation.

Noesis: a sudden revelation with a sense that a person has been chosen to be a leader.

Speech, language:

Disturbances in speech: pressure of speech, logorrhea (coherent, logical), poverty of speech, poverty of content, dysprosody (loss of normal speech melody), dysarthria (problems in articulation), abnormal volume of speech, stuttering, cluttering (rapid and jerky spurts of speech), acalulia (nonsense speech with impaired comprehension), bradylalia (abnormally slow speech), alexia (loss of reading ability), agraphia (disturbance in writing).

Aphasias: true language disturbance (disturbance in language output):

Motor aphasia: understanding remains but ability to speak is very impaired (e.g., Broca aphasia or expressive aphasia).

Sensory aphasia: loss of ability to comprehend the meaning of words with spontaneous speech that is nonsensical and incoherent (e.g., Wernicke aphasia or receptive aphasia).

Nominal aphasia: difficulty finding the correct name for an object.

Global aphasia: combination of expressive and receptive aphasias.

Alogia: inability to speak because of dementia or mental retardation.

Coprophasia: involuntary use of vulgarity.

Abnormal perceptions: hallucination (false sensory perception not associated with real external stimuli) may be hypnagogic (while falling asleep, nonpathologic); hypnopompic (while awakening from sleep, nonpathologic); auditory (mostly in psychiatric disorders); visual or olfactory or gustatory or tactile or somatic (mostly associated with medical disorders); may be mood-congruent or mood-incongruent; **synesthesias** (one type of stimulation evokes the sensation of another, e.g., the hearing of a sound giving a visual hallucination); **trailing phenomenon** (moving objects are seen as a series of discrete and discontinuous images); **illusions** (misperception or misinterpretation of real external stimuli).

Level of consciousness: confusion, attention, concentration.

Orientation: to person, time, and place.

Memory:

  Disturbance of memory: **amnesia** (partial or total inability to recall past experiences; may be **anterograde** when it affects events occurring after a point in time or **retrograde** if it affects events occurring before a point in time); **paramnesia** (falsification of a memory by distortion of recall: fausse reconnaissance, unconscious retrospective falsification, confabulation which is unconscious, "déjà vu" or "entendu" or "pense," false memory/the recollection of an event that never happened); **hypermnesia**; screen memory (a consciously tolerable memory covering a painful memory), blackout.

  Levels of memory: immediate (within seconds or minutes), recent (over the past few days), recent past (few months), remote (distant past).

Suicidal and homicidal ideations and plans.

Intelligence: includes ability to understand, recall, and constructively integrate past learning in addressing new situations. Assess if presence of mental retardation, dementia (global decline in intelligence without clouding of consciousness); fund of knowledge; concrete thinking (literal thinking without use of metaphor) or abstract thinking (multidimensional thinking with use of metaphor); calculating, reading abilities.

Judgment: (ability to assess a situation correctly and to act appropriately in that situation): critical or automatic or impaired judgment.

Insight: (ability to understand the true cause and meaning of a situation): intellectualized or true or impaired.

PHYSICAL NEUROLOGIC EXAMINATION

Handedness

Head, pupils, funduscopic exam

Cranial nerves:

  Mnemonic (for cranial nerves): On Old Olympus Towering Tops A Friendly Viking Grew Vines and Hops.

  I (olfactory): identify odors (soap, coffee, cloves); alcohol, ammonia, and other irritants test the nociceptive receptors of the 5th nerve (not used, except to detect malingering).

  For the visual system:

    II (optic): provides sensory input for vision

    III (oculomotor): raises eyelids, moves eyes, adjusts amount of light entering the eyes, focuses lenses.

    IV (trochlear): moves superior obliques.

    VI (abducens): moves lateral rectus.

  V (trigeminal): three sensory divisions (ophthalmic, maxillary, mandibular):

    Ophthalmic division: sensory input from cornea, tear glands, scalp, forehead, upper eyelids.

    Maxillary and mandibular division: motor function of the masseter muscles, sensory input from teeth, gums, lip, lining of palate, skin of face.

  VII (facial): moves muscles of facial expression, input to tear and salivary glands, sensory input for taste in anterior two-thirds of the tongue.

  VIII (vestibulocochlear, acoustic): sensory input for equilibrium and hearing.

  IX (glossopharyngeal): sensory input from pharynx, tonsils, posterior tongue, and carotid arteries; moves muscles of swallowing and salivary glands, helps regulate BP.

  X (vagus): moves muscles of speech and swallowing; transmits impulses to heart and smooth muscles of visceral organs.

  XI (spinal accessory): turns head, shrugs shoulders.

  XII (hypoglossal): moves tongue.

Elementary sensation: cortical sensory function (identifying an object in the palm or numbers written in the palm, distinguishing 2 points from one in the palm and on the fingers); temperature sense, sense of joint position, Romberg test (sense of postural position); sense of vibration. If sensation is disturbed: localization of the lesion necessary at peripheral nerve, nerve roots, spinal cord (a level below which sensation is reduced), brain stem (crossed face-body) or brain (hemi sensory loss).

Cerebellar testing: coordination (finger-to-nose or knee-to-shin maneuvers), stance, and gait.

Motor system: muscle strength (grading), atrophy, hypertrophy, fasciculations (brief, fine, irregular twitches of the muscle visible under the skin), myotonia (↓ relaxation of muscle after a sustained contraction or direct percussion of the muscle), increased resistance followed by relaxation (clasp-knife phenomenon), abnormal involuntary movements, asymmetric development, muscle tone, rigidity, apraxia (inability to execute a voluntary motor movement previously learned, despite normal muscle function), movement disorder (tremor, dyskinesias/myoclonus, tics, chorea, athetosis, dystonia), clonus.

Reflex testing:

- **DTRs**: biceps reflex (C5), radial reflex (C6), triceps (C7), quadriceps knee jerk (L4), ankle jerk (S1)
- **Superficial abdominal reflex**
- **Plantar response**: Babinski sign
- **Abnormal reflexes**: snout, sucking, grasp reflex (in diffuse cortical disease)

Cerebral functions: aphasia (receptive or expressive), apraxia, amnesia, agnosia, delirium, dementia, seizures, sleep disorders stupor, coma

Cerebrovascular examination: BP, auscultation of carotid arteries, peripheral pulses, temporal arteries, cerebrovascular diseases, head trauma, tumor

Autonomic system testing: postural hypotension, sweating + or −, Horner syndrome (ptosis + miosis + anhidrosis on one side); bowel, bladder, sexual dysfunctions.

TABLE 3.2. Distinguishing Upper from Lower Motor Neuron Disease

Signs	Upper motor neuron disease	Lower motor neuron disease
Reflexes	Hyperactive Babinski sign Possible sustained clonus	Diminished or absent
Atrophy	Absent, may appear later on	Present
Fasciculations	Absent	Present
Tone	Increased	Decreased or absent

TABLE 3.3. Disturbances of Higher Cortical Function

Aphasia: disorder of language due to brain dysfunction
Apraxia: inability to carry out motor activities despite intact comprehension and motor function
Agnosia: failure to recognize or identify objects despite intact sensory function
Constructional difficulties: inability to copy three-dimensional figures, assemble blocks, or arrange sticks in specific designs

TABLE 3.4. Hemispheric Specialization

Hemispheres	Left hemispheric syndromes	Right hemispheric syndromes
Role	Written and spoken language (such as in aphasias) Verbal memory Regulation of mood	Visual and spatial memory Temporal orientation Communication related to emotional experience (lack of capacity to express and/or recognize emotions such as aprosodia; or prosopagnosia: difficulty recognizing the faces of individuals previously known)
Symptoms if lesions	Primary progressive aphasia (usually expressive, then diffuse language impairment, memory loss, and dementia) Depression	Specific delusions (delusional jealousy, feelings of depersonalization, déjà vu experience)

LOCALIZED BRAIN PATHOLOGY

TABLE 3.5.   Symptoms in Frontal Lobe Lesions

- **Focal neurologic sx** may help to indicate a frontal lobe lesion.
- **Alterations**:
  - **of motor activities** (lack of spontaneity, ↓ rate and amount of mental/physical activity, akinetic mutism, inability to perform or reproduce complex movements generalized in time)
  - **of intellectual impairment** (poor concentration, inability to carry out plans, attention deficit, trouble sequencing tasks, slowed mental processing)
  - **of personality change** (placidity, lack of concern over consequences of action, social indifference esp. with bathing, dressing, bowel and bladder control, childish excitement [moria], inappropriate joking, punning, instability, and superficiality of emotion)
  - **of language dysfunction** (Broca aphasia, mutism)

- **Other types**:

TABLE 3.6.   Symptoms in Parietal Lobe Lesions

Dominant (usually left) parietal lobe disease	Right-left confusion Alexia with agraphia, with or without anomia Constructional difficulty Gerstmann syndrome (right-left disorientation, inability to localize fingers/finger agnosia, agraphia, acalculia) Ideomotor apraxia Astereognosis (inability to recognize objects in the hand) Difficulty with writing (agraphia) Difficulty with mathematics (acalculia) Disorders of language (fluent aphasia) Inability to perceive objects normally (agnosia)
Nondominant (right) parietal lobe disease	Neglecting part of the body or space (contralateral neglect) Difficulty in making things (constructional apraxia): drawing, copying, or manipulating spatial patterns Dressing apraxia Geographic disorientation Calculation or writing difficulties Astereognosis of the left side Denial or neglect of contralateral space (anosognosia) ↓ drawing ability
Bilateral damage in parietal lobes: "Balint syndrome"	Inability to voluntarily control the gaze (ocular apraxia) Inability to integrate components of a visual scene (simultanagnosia) Inability to accurately reach for an object with visual guidance (optic ataxia)

TABLE 3.7.   Psychiatric Manifestations of Temporal Lobe Disease

- **Unilateral temporal lobe lesions—dominant temporal lobe**
  - Wernicke aphasia: frequently mistaken for a psychotic break with neologisms
  - Dysfunctions in memory
  - Amusia: defect in ability to appreciate music
- **Nondominant temporal lobe**
  - Agnosia for sounds
  - Dysprosody: disturbed timing, stress, and melody of spoken speech
- **Bilateral temporal lobe lesion**
  - Korsakoff amnesia
  - Kluver-Bucy syndrome: visual agnosia, apathy and placidity, disturbance of sexual function, dementia, aphasia, amnesia
- **Ictal phenomenon**
  - Psychosensory
    - Hallucinations (visual, auditory, olfactory)
    - Illusions (visual, auditory)
  - Affective sx
  - Cognitive sx (déjà vu, jamais-vu, forced thinking)
  - Impaired consciousness
  - Automatism

TABLE 3.8.   Effects of Occipital Lobe Disorders

- **Anton syndrome**: denial of blindness
- **Balint syndrome**: inability to integrate complex visual scenes (simultanagnosia); inability to accurately direct hand or other movements by visual guidance (optic ataxia); inaccurate voluntary eye movements to visual stimuli (oculomotor apraxia)
- **Visual agnosias**: a normal percept stripped of meaning (prosopagnosia: inability to recognize faces; color agnosia: inability to distinguish colors)
- **Alexia**: inability to read
- **Hallucinations**

THE LIMBIC SYSTEM (SUBSTRATUM OF EMOTIONS)

The limbic system includes the hypothalamus, the hippocampus, the amygdala, and other nearby areas; primarily responsible for the emotional life; is involved with motivation, attention, emotion, and memory (it was said to mediate "the four Fs": fear, food, fight, and fornication, or more appropriately, gender role, territoriality, and bonding).

(1) **Hypothalamus**: concerned with *homeostasis*, regulating hunger, thirst, response to pain, levels of pleasure, sexual satisfaction, anger and aggressive behavior, the autonomic nervous system (pulse, blood pressure, breathing, arousal in response to emotional circumstances).

(2) **Hippocampus**: short-term and long-term *memory*

(3) **Amygdala**: *aggression*, reaction to things provoking fear or sexual response.

(4) **Other areas**:

- **Cingulate gyrus** (focusing attention on emotionally significant events; associating memories to smells and to pain).
- **Ventral tegmental area of the brain stem**: responsible for *pleasure*.
- **Basal ganglia**: responsible for repetitive behaviors, reward experiences, and focusing attention.
- **Prefrontal cortex**: thinking about the future, making plans, and taking action; plays a part in pleasure and addiction.

Psychiatric disturbances from diseases of the limbic system (substratum of emotions: "the visceral brain") **and hypothalamus** (controls body temperature, hunger, thirst, fatigue, and circadian cycles).

TABLE 3.9.   Psychiatric Symptoms in Limbic System Lesions

Emotional lability: pathological laugher and crying
Rage and aggression
Altered sexual behavior
Delusions
Anorexia nervosa, bulimia
Sleep disorders

CEREBELLUM

TABLE 3.10.   Signs of Cerebellar Disease

Motor symptoms:
    Ataxia: wide-based gait, reeling
    Decomposition of movement: inability to properly sequence fine, coordinated acts
    Dysarthria: inability to articulate words properly
    Difficulties swallowing
    Dysdiadochokinesia: inability to perform rapid alternating movements
    Dysmetria: inability to control range of a movement
    Hypotonia: decreased muscle tone
    Nystagmus: involuntary rapid oscillation of the eyeballs in a horizontal, vertical, or rotary direction
    Scanning speech: slow enunciation, hesitation at the beginning of a word
    Tremor: rhythmic, alternating, oscillatory movement of a limb as it approaches a target (intention tremor) or of proximal musculature when fixed posture (sustention tremor)

Nonmotor symptoms: It is becoming more evident that the cerebellum plays a role in cognition and emotion (mood and psychotic disorders, anxiety disorders, and personality changes)

TABLE 3.11. Basic Screening Tests

Complete blood count (CBC) with differential, hematocrit, hemoglobin
Renal function tests
Thyroid function tests
Liver function tests
Electrolytes
Blood sugar
Lipid profile

Any suspected medical or neurologic condition should be evaluated with appropriate tests.

NEUROENDOCRINE TESTS

Thyroid function tests:

- **Normal**: Total T4 (5–12 µg/dL or 64–142 nmol/L), **free T4** (varies with method, ng/dL), **free thyroxine index** (FT4I: 6.5–12.5), **total T3** (95–190 ng/dL), sensitive serum **TSH** (RIA) (0.3–10 µIU/mL or mU/L), resin T3 uptake (25–35%). **Antithyroid antibodies**: none
- **Diagnosing hypothyroidism**: Serum FT4 and TSH:
  - FT4 normal and TSH normal: euthyroid
  - FT4 low and TSH high: primary hypothyroidism
  - FT4 low and TSH normal or low: secondary hypothyroidism → TRH test (normal response = hypothalamic lesion; no response = pituitary lesion)
- **TRH stimulation test**: IV injection of 500 mg of TRH (protirelin 500 µg IV) produces a sharp ↑ in serum TSH measured at 15, 30, 60, and 90 min. Normal test shows an ↑ in TSH from 5 to 25 µIU/mL above the baseline. An ↑ of <7 µIU/mL is a blunted response.
- **Other possible tests**: thyroid scan (not during pregnancy), thyroid ultrasound, TRS stimulation, T4 suppression, biopsy.
- **Monitoring for pts on lithium**: before rx, repeat TSH level at 6 months, then repeat thyroid function tests q yr.

Dexamethasone-suppression test:

May be used to confirm diagnosis of major depression. The relation between DST and clinical symptomatology is very complex (research suggests it is a severity marker rather than directly related to the sx); it is rarely used (1 mg dexamethasone equals 25 mg of cortisol)

- **Test**: give 1 mg dexamethasone po at 11 PM, measure plasma cortisol at 8 AM, 4 PM, 11 PM. Suppression is seen when cortisol is <5 µg/dL (test is +, meaning that the hypothalamic–adrenal–pituitary axis functions well). Test becomes negative when depression responds to treatment.
- **False positive results** with: medications (anticonvulsants, high-dosage estrogen rx, tricyclic drug withdrawal), cardiac failure, high blood pressure, cancers, infections, unstable medical problems (major trauma, dehydration, Cushing disease, diabetes mellitus, malnutrition, dementia, old age, alcohol abuse), pregnancy.
- **False negative results** with: Addison disease, long-term steroid rx, hypopituitarism, indomethacin, and other medications.
- **Sensitivity**: 45% in major depressive disorder (MDD), 70% in MDD with psychotic features
- **Specificity**: 70–90%
- **Prognosis**: Pts who fail to suppress morning cortisol level (positive test: cortisol >10 µg/dL) may have a positive response to electroconvulsive therapy (ECT) or tricyclic antidepressants (TCAs).

Other endocrine tests:

Prolactin (normal: 5–25 ng/mL in women and 5–15 ng/mL in men; antipsychotics may raise the level up to 20 times, with the exception of clozapine and olanzapine; r/o pregnancy, other medications such as oral contraceptives, estrogens, TCAs, SSRIs, propanolol, hypothyroidism; if elevated may need an MRI to eliminate a prolactinoma), growth hormone, gonadotrophin-releasing hormone (GnRH), FSH, LH, testosterone, estrogen.

Catecholamines (mostly evaluated for research purpose)
- **5-HIAA** (5-hydroxyindolacetic acid):
  - ↑ in urine of pts with carcinoid tumors, pts on phenothiazines, pts eating foods high in serotonin (e.g., walnuts, bananas, avocados)
  - ↓ in cerebrospinal fluid (CSF) of pts who are suicidal or violent
- **VMA** (vanillylmandelic acid), **norepinephrine, epinephrine**:
  - Blood levels ↑ in pts with pheochromocytoma
  - Noerepinephrine metabolite MHPG (3-methoxy-4-hydroxyphenylglycol) ↓ in pts with MDD and suicide attempts.

RENAL FUNCTION TESTS
- **Tests: blood urea nitrogen (BUN), creatinine, creatinine-clearance (24-h urine), urine analysis.**
- **Monitoring for pts on lithium**: before rx, creatinine at 6 months, then repeat renal function tests q yr.

LIVER FUNCTION TESTS (LFTs)
- **Tests: Direct bilirubin** (0.1–0.3 mg/dL), **indirect bilirubin** (0.2–0.7 mg/dL), **urine bilirubin** (none), **serum albumin** (3.4–4.7 g/dL), **total protein** (6–8 g/dL), **alkaline phosphatase** (30–115 IU/L), **ALT** (SGPT: 5–35 IU/L), **AST** (SGOT: 5–40 IU/L), **PT** (prothrombine time): 11 to 13.5 s.

BLOOD TESTS FOR SEXUALLY TRANSMITTED DISEASES: VDRL, HIV
TESTS TO CONSIDER WHEN USING PSYCHOTROPIC DRUGS:
- **Benzodiazepines**: baseline LFT, check urine if suspicion of abuse.
- **Antipsychotics**: lipid panel, fasting blood glucose
  - CBC, LFTs. SMA12, lipid panel (possible metabolic syndrome), and ECG (check particularly QTc)(if pts have cardiac histories or using drugs that prolong QTc).
  - Caution with clozapine due to risk of agranulocytosis (1–2%): baseline CBC with differential, CBC q wk and CBC for 4 wk after discontinuation. **Need to register to Clozaril National Registry (1-800-448-5938)**. Registration and reporting forms may be downloaded from the Healthcare Professional section of the Clozaril Web site (www.clozaril.com) through the "Prescriber or Medical Director Registration Form". The pharmacy must be registered as well to dispense the drug; The prescriber is responsible for registering any patient for will receive the medication by registering the patient in two ways: (1) by visiting www.clozarilregistry.com and requesting registration on-line OR (2) by calling the CNR at 1-800-448-5938.
  - See clinical management in Chapter 6 (part: treatment with antipsychotics)
- **TCAS and tetracyclics**: ECG prior to rx and q yr; **blood levels** for: imipramine (**Tofranil: therapeutic level 200–250 ng/mL or total imipramine and its metabolite desmethylimipramine should exceed 120ng/mL**), desipramine (**Norpramine: therapeutic level usually >125 ng/mL**), nortriptyline (**Pamelor has a therapeutic window between 50 and 150 ng/mL**), amitriptyline (**Elavil: therapeutic levels 75–175 ng/mL**). Draw blood 10 to 14 hr after last dose. High levels ↑ risks for cardiotoxicity. Note: blood levels should include **the measure of active metabolites (imipramine → desipramine and amitriptyline → nortriptyline)**: this may change some of the ranges.
- **MAOIs**: baseline BP and monitor during rx. Avoid tyramine-containing food.
- **Lithium**: baseline thyroid function tests, renal function tests, CBC, ECG. Lithium levels are to be monitored (**maintenance level: 0.6–1.2 mEq/L**, more rarely 1.5–1.8 mEq/L). Some pts respond to lower levels (usually >0.4 mEq/L). Toxicity risks if >2 mEq/L. Draw lithium levels 8 to 12 hr after last dose, usually 2 times/wk at the beginning of rx, then q month. Pregnancy test to be done if appropriate.
- **Carbamazepine**: Prior to rx: CBC, platelet count, reticulocyte count, q wk in 1st 3 months of rx, then q month (risks of aplastic anemia, agranulocytosis, thrombocytopenia, leukopenia). LFTs q 3–6 months. **(Therapeutic levels: 8–12 ng/mL, toxicity if >15 ng/mL)**. ECG, serum electrolytes, pregnancy test need to be done.
- **Tacrine** (Cognex): risk of liver damage. LFTs at baseline and transaminase levels q wk for 5 months. Rarely used now.

LUMBAR PUNCTURE:
If sudden changes in cognition, neurologic signs, seizures.

TESTS FOR SUBSTANCE ABUSE:

TABLE 3.12.   Testing for Substance Abuse

Substances tested	Length of time detected in urine	In the hair	In the blood	Possible false positive results
Alcohol	6–24 hr	Up to 90 days	12–24 hr	
Amphetamine	1–3 days	Up to 90 days	12 hr	Amantadine, Bupropion, chlorpromazine, L-deprenyl, desipramine, dextroamphetamine, ephedrine, phenylephedrine, labetanol, MDMA, methamphetamine, phentermine, methylphenidate, phenylpropanolamine, promethazine, pseudoephedrine, ranitidine, ritodrine, selegiline, thioridazine, trazodone, trimipramine
Methamphetamine		Up to 90 days	1–3 days	
MDMA (Ecstasy)	24 hr	Up to 90 days	25 hr	
Barbiturate (except Phenobarbital)	2–4 days for short-acting	Up to 90 days	1–2 days	
Phenobarbital	2–3 months	Up to 90 days	4–7 days	
Benzodiazepine	Therapeutic use: up to 7 days Chronic use (>1 yr): 4–6 wk	Up to 90 days	6–48 hr	Oxaprozin, sertraline
LSD	24–72 hr	Up to 3 days	0–3 hr	
PCP	Occasional use: 3–7 days; chronic use: up to 30 days	Up to 90 days	1–3 days	Dextromethorphan, diphenydramine, ibuprofen, imipramine, ketamin, meperidine, mesoridazine, thioridazine, tramadol, venlafaxine, O-demethyl venlafaxine
Cannabis	3–5 days (occasional) to 4 wk (chronic use)	Up to 90 days	Up to 24 hr	Dronabinol, NSAIDs, elfavirenz, PPIs, Tolmetin
Cocaine	6–8 hr (metabolites 2–4 days)	Up to 90 days	2–5 days	Coca leaf tea, topical anesthetics containing cocaine
Codeine	2–3 days	Up to 90 days	2–3 days	
Morphine	48–72 hr	Up to 90 days	1–2 days	Dextromethorphan, diphenydramine, heroin, opiates, poppy seeds, quinine, quinolones, rifampicin, verapamil, and metabolites
Heroin	1–3 days	Up to 90 days	1–2 days	
Methadone	3 days	Up to 97 days	24 hr	

(1) Oral fluid or saliva testing results parallel to that of blood (except for THC and benzodiazepines). Oral fluid will detect THC from ingestion up to a maximum period of 18 to 24 hr. Low saliva: plasma ratio continues to cause difficulty in oral fluid detection of benzodiazepines.

(2) Urine cannot detect current drug use. It takes approximately 6 to 8 hr or more for drug to be metabolized and excreted in urine. Similarly, hair requires 2 wk, and sweat, 7 days.

SPECIAL TESTS

- **Sodium lactate test** (provocation of panic attacks): IV injection of sodium lactate may be used to confirm the diagnosis of panic disorder which may be stopped by alprazolam or TCAs but not β-blockers.
- **Amobarbital interview (Amytal)**: used sometimes in pts with catatonia, stupor, dissociative disorders, also to differentiate organic from functional disorders. Benzodiazepines may be used instead. Administer a total of 200 to 500 mg for adults and 25 to 50 mg for children (occasionally more) of sodium amobarbital IV at the rate of 25 to 50 mg/min, while the interviewer talks with the pt and halts the drug temporarily when the desired level of sedation is attained. (Lateral nystagmus for light sedation, slurred speech for a deeper state); contraindicated during pregnancy, pulmonary disease, porphyria.

EEG

Helps to rule out a variety of conditions:

- Epilepsy: (particularly temporal lobe epilepsy), also helps with the diagnosis of "pseudo-seizures" in psychiatric pts. To note: 30% of epileptics have a normal EEG between attacks.
- Pts with a delirium usually have diffuse EEG slowing (except delirium tremens from alcohol withdrawal, and confusion due to sedative-hypnotics)
- In dementia of Alzheimer disease, EEG is normal early on but abnormal in later stages
- In pseudo-dementia: EEG is normal
- In organic brain pathologies (brain tumor, cerebral infarcts, brain trauma), EEG may be normal or abnormal.

BRAIN IMAGING

- **Structural techniques**:

    CT scan: used to screen for organic brain disease (older pts with sudden psychiatric sx, pts with a hx of head trauma)

    MRI: differentiate better between white and gray matter, identify better demyelization disorders, dementias, infarctions, neoplasm.

- **Functional techniques**:

    PET scan: provides a direct measure of brain glucose metabolism.

    SPECT scans: reflect the blood flow and are a more indirect measure of metabolism, used in differential diagnosis of stroke, dementias, epilepsy, and maybe in the future for psychiatric disorders.

4 ■ HUMAN DEVELOPMENT

TABLE 4.1. The Stages in Child Development

Newborn: birth to 28 days
Infant: 1–12 months
Toddler: 1–3 yr
Preschooler: 3–5 yr
School-age: 5–11 yr
Preteen or tween: 11–12 yr
Teen: 13 and above

SIGMUND FREUD (THE FOUNDER OF PSYCHOANALYSIS)
Topographic model of the mind: three "regions" were first described.

TABLE 4.2. Freud's Topographic Model

The Conscious: in which all perceptions are brought into awareness, characterized by secondary process thinking (logical)
The Preconscious: its content can be brought into conscious awareness by focusing attention; helps to censor unacceptable wishes
The Unconscious: its content (instincts seeking fulfillment) is kept away from awareness by censorship; characterized by primary process thinking (led by the pleasure principle, aimed at instinctual discharge, characterized by lack of logic, contradictions, poor sense of time, high energy, "like in dreams")

The Instinct or Drive theory was then considered

TABLE 4.3. Instinct Theory

Each instinct has 4 components: its source, impetus, aim, and object
Libido (or libidinal energy): a force by which the sexual instinct or need for pleasure is represented in the mind
Ego instincts: containing the nonsexual components, dealing with self-preservation
Aggressive instincts: sexual and nonsexual; life and death instincts (Eros and Thanatos)

Description of pleasure and reality principles

TABLE 4.4. Pleasure and Reality Principles

Pleasure principle: inborn tendency to avoid pain and seek pleasure through the discharge of tension
Reality principle: learned function that delays immediate gratification and tied to the maturation of the ego

Developmental stages: the phases correspond to successive shifts in the investment of sexual energy by areas associated with eroticism (mouth, anus, genitalia). The successful resolution of these phases is essential to normal adult functioning.

TABLE 4.5. Freud's Developmental Stages

● **Oral phase**: (birth to 1 yo) the oral zone is dominant for need satisfaction and modes of expression
● **Anal phase**: (age 1–3 yr) the maturation of sphincters permits more voluntary control over retention or expulsion of feces
● **Urethral phase**: transition and overlapping phase between anal and phallic phases
● **Phallic phase**: (age 3–5 yr) with increased sexual interests and oedipal phase, castration anxiety, penis envy until resolution of the oedipal complex (institution of the superego)
● **Latency phase**: (age 5–6 until puberty) with its somewhat inactivity of the sexual drives (further maturation of ego functions)
● **Genital phase**: (age 11–13 up to young adulthood) with its intensification of libidinal drives, the end of dependence on the parents, and establishment of mature object relations

Carl Gustav Jung: external factors play a role in people's personal development. Libido involves all kinds of psychic energy (not only sexual).

Harry Stack Sullivan: each phase of development is influenced by interactions with people and the quality of the relationships.

ERIK ERIKSON: eight stages; 1–5 during childhood and 6–8 from young adulthood to old age; biology, culture, and society all interact. A crisis in each phase must be negotiated before a person moves on to the next phase.

TABLE 4.6.   Erikson's Developmental Stages

1.	**Trust vs mistrust** (oral sensory): birth to 1 yr
2.	**Autonomy vs shame** and doubt (muscular-anal): 1–3 yr
3.	**Initiative vs guilt** (locomotor genital): 3–5 yr
4.	**Industry vs inferiority** (latency): 6–11 yr
5.	**Ego identity vs role confusion**: 11 yr and through end of adolescence
6.	**Intimacy vs isolation**: young manhood
7.	**Generativity vs stagnation**: adulthood
8.	**Ego integrity vs despair**: maturity

JEAN PIAGET: theory of cognitive development; made of four stages. The sequence of stages depends on central nervous system (CNS) growth and life experiences.

TABLE 4.7.   Piaget's Cognitive Developmental Stages

- **Sensorimotor operations**: birth up to 2 yr (characterized by the attainment of object permanence, symbolization)
- **Preoperational thought**: 2–7 yr (characterized by sense that punishment for bad deeds is unavoidable, egocentrism, "animistic thinking"/thoughts that physical events and objects have feeling and intentions, "phenomenalistic causality"/ events that occur together are thought to cause one another)
- **Concrete operations**: 7–11 yr (ability to take other people's point of view, to group things according to some characteristics, sense of conservation of matter, sense of reversibility of matter)
- **Formal operations**: 11 yr to end of adolescence (ability to think abstractly, to reason in a deductive way)

Daniel Levinson: The life cycle is composed of four eras, each lasting about 25 yr, with identified 4–5 yr transitional periods between eras.

TEMPERAMENTAL DIFFERENCES

Work of Chess and Thomas (described inborn observed differences):

TABLE 4.8.   Temperamental Characteristics

- **Activity level**: motor component
- **Rythmicity**: feeding and elimination pattern, sleep–wake cycle
- **Approach or withdrawal** : nature of response to a new stimulus
- **Adaptability**: how a child adapts to a change in the environment
- **Intensity of reactions**: energy spent in mood expression
- **Threshold of responsiveness**: intensity level of stimulus needed to provoke any reaction
- **Quality of mood**: pleasant vs unpleasant
- **Distractibility**: in the presence of an outside stimulus
- **Attention span and persistence**: length of time spent on an activity and it's continuation in spite of obstacles

They also described a range of normal patterns, as well as a goodness of fit between the mother and the child:

- Difficult children: 10% who react intensely, sleep poorly are difficult to comfort
- Easy children: 40%, who have regular patterns, are flexible in adapting to changes and easily comforted
- The others: 50% present with a mixture of the two types

Work of Winnicott: described the holding environment in which infants are contained, the transitional object, mother providing a "good-enough" mothering (ability to respond to the infant's needs) which will help with the evolving sense of self.

ATTACHMENT

Harry Harlow: studied social learning in monkeys (newborns, isolated from a real monkey mother, placed with two types of surrogate mothers, one with a feeding bottle and one with a terry-cloth surrogate; monkeys were comforted only by the soft terry-cloth mannequin but showed clinging behaviors when frightened). Both types of reared monkeys were unable to adjust to the normal life of a monkey colony.

John Bowlby: Early separation of infants from their mothers has negative effects. Physical contact when hungry or distressed is necessary for attachment behavior.

Mary Ainsworth: Pattern of infant attachment affects future adult emotional relationships. Importance of mother's sensitive responsiveness to infant signals with bodily contact to ↓ anxiety and promote secure attachments.

Rene Spitz: severe developmental retardation due to maternal neglect (infants in institutions).

Margaret Mahler: children acquire a sense of identity separate from their mothers; theory of separation-individuation.

TABLE 4.9.   Mahler's Developmental Stages

Normal autism: birth up to 2 months (periods of sleep and arousal)
Symbiosis: 2–5 months (perceptual abilities to distinguish the inner from the outer world, but mother–infant is still perceived as a fused unity)
Differentiation: 5–10 months (neurologic development + ↑ alertness; progressive distinction of self and of mother)
Practicing: 10–18 months (the child becomes more autonomous and explores the outer world)
Rapprochement: 18–24 months (independence alternates with need for closeness and reassurance/refueling)
Object constancy: 2–5 yr (child recognizes gradually the permanence of mother even when not in her presence)

DEFINITIONS

- **Stranger anxiety**: starts at 26 wk, max at 32 wk (8 months); fear of strangers is due to the ability to distinguish caretakers from others
- **Separation anxiety**: happens between 10 and 18 months when the child is physically separated from his caretaker

DEVELOPMENT

PRIOR TO ADOLESCENCE

At birth: present are rooting reflex (puckering of the lips with perioral stimulation), grasp reflex, plantar reflex (Babinski), knee reflex, the abdominal reflexes, the startle reflex (Moro), tonic neck reflex. Normally, the grasp, the startle, and the tonic neck reflex disappear by the fourth month.

■ **Language and cognitive development**

- **Infancy period**: vocalization after 8 wk. By the end of the second year children begin to use symbolic play and language.
- **Toddler period (starts in the 2nd yr of life up to 3rd yr)**: is a language learning phase, negativism (independence development), beginning of reasoning, tolerating delays, engaging in symbolic activities
- **Preschool period (between 2½ and 6 yr)**: Language ↑, ↑ usage of sentences, symbolic thinking ↑, prelogic, intuitive and egocentric thinking are present
- **Middle years (elementary school)**: language expresses complex ideas, need for rules and order, logical thinking, development of abstract thinking, ability to write and draw, ↑ academic learning and accomplishments, ↑ gross motor coordination and muscle strength, ↑ independence, learning, socialization, ↑ identification with adults, ↑ gender identity, ↑ peer interactions, ↑ capacity for compassion and sharing, absence of overt sexual behaviors

■ **Emotional and social development**

- **Infancy**: imitative behavior by third and fourth months, spontaneous smile by age 2 months, smile related to an outsider by age 4 months. Complete dependence on adults for survival. Mood is first related to internal states (hunger), then to external cues. Risk of depression if separation from mother during second half of the first year.
- **Toddler period**: differentiates pleasure from displeasure, ↑ new games with others, ↑ demonstration of emotions (love, anger, anxiety, shyness), fear of the dark, and need for reassurance
- **Preschool period**: complex emotions are expressed (love, jealousy, envy, shame, guilt), ↑ cooperation and sharing, ↑ tolerance of anxiety, ↑ empathy and love, ↑ awareness of body parts (genitalia,

preoccupation with illnesses, injuries), obey to parental directions, ↑ conscience with a sense of right and wrong, sibling rivalry, distinction of reality and fantasy in pretend games, secrets, changes in drawings of human figures (from formal to more abstract and emotionally laden), use of imaginary friends

- **In middle years**: development of a close same-sex friendship by age 10

■ **Sexual development**

- Sexual differentiation exists from birth: parents' expectations and responses to the child sex. Curiosity about anatomic sex is healthy.
- **By age 2½; gender identity (conviction of being a boy or a girl) is fixed**. Role of culture and social trends in terms of gender plays.
- Control of daytime urination is complete by age 2½ and nighttime by age 4 (as well as bowel control).
- In preschool phase: awareness of anatomic differences between the sexes.
- In the middle years: prefers to interact with same-sex children (psychosexual "moratorium").
- Sex role development: parallels gender identity, involves identification with culturally acceptable male or female behaviors, seen in play activities (appears by age 2) (Taken from table in Kaplan, p. 35, 8th ed. See resources chapter for details of Kaplan. Data adapted from Joseph Campas at the University of Denver and from other researchers.)

■ **Sleep**

- During the first year: poor differentiation between reality and fantasy (dreams experienced as true); at age 3: children may believe that their dream is shared by others; at age 4: dreams are known to be unique to each individual
- By age 5: realization that dreams are not real; by age 7: children know that they created the dream
- The content parallels the cognitive and emotional development.
- Need for sleep: first few weeks of life: 60% of time (↑ if prematurity), sleep-wake cycle of a newborn is about 3-hr long

■ **Family factors in child development**

- **Family stability**: harmonious interactions or not, personal vulnerability to unstable homes (boys > girls; younger children > older, inborn characteristics), physical or sexual abuse, drug abuse
- **Type of parenting**: four types described (authoritarian, permissive, indifferent, and reciprocal). Need for consistency and reward for good behaviors and punishment for negative ones, in the context of a loving environment
- **Working mothers**: no negative impact if stable and good parenting
- **Spacing of children**: 10% of births have been unwanted, 20% have been wanted but not well timed. Average of two children per family. Repeated childbearing: more demands on the parents, with ↑ interactions and discipline
- **Birth order**: first born: possibly achieving the most, more authoritarian, more sibling rivalry, receive more attention from parents; middle child receiving the least attention; younger children learn from older siblings, receiving more attention, more spoiled?
- **Children and divorce, single parent families, stepparents**: usually not fully understood before age 7. Children 3–6 yo believe they are responsible. Fantasy about having the parents reunited is frequent. Recovery may take 3–5 yr. One-third of the children have lasting trauma effects (anger, sadness, depression, aggressivity, suicide attempts, anxiety); frequent poor adaptation to a new stepparent, stepsibling
- **Adoptions**: 2.5 millions of children are adopted each year, 50% by relatives or stepparents. ↑ Aggressivity, stealing, learning problems, preoccupations with natural parents, conflicts with adoptive parents
- **Death of a parent during childhood**: ↑ depression

ADOLESCENCE

Starts with puberty, variable in age of onset, length, rate of growth, sexual development, mental maturation, education and knowledge, characterized by biologic, psychologic, and social developmental changes.

TABLE 4.10.   Three Variable Periods

Early age: 11–14 yr
Middle age: 14–17 yr
Late age: 17–20 yr

■ **Psychosexual development**
Adolescents struggle with their sex drives (intellectualization, repression, sublimation). Experimentation with masturbation, heterosexual experiences, homosexual experiences may occur. 0.5–4% of adolescents may need counseling about dealing with sexual orientation. The average age for first sexual intercourse is about 16 yo in the United States.

Menarche: onset of the menstrual function; variable (earlier than in the past, around age 13, correlating frequently with mother's age of menarche)

■ **Neurologic changes:** dendritic connections change (↑ by environmental stimuli or pruned back)

■ **Cognitive and personality development:** Thought process becomes more abstract, future-oriented; Creativity ↑, interest in humanitarian issues, religion, ethics ↑; ↑ ability to negotiate demands of school, peers, parents with need for ↑ independent choices; role of the peer group accelerates the separation from the family.

■ **Parenting:** generation "gap"; balances the need to continue to set limits and be supportive; role of family harmony or disharmony on the adolescent.

■ **Development of morals:** internalization of ethic principles, regulation of conduct; ability to recognize what is good for the society at large (Kohlberg's 3rd level of morality).

■ **Choice of occupation:** ability to make choices, sustain motivation, acquire competency.

■ **Risk-taking behaviors:** use of drugs; pregnancy; abortion; prostitution; violence?

ADULTHOOD

The longest phase in Western societies; works of Erickson, of Colarusso, of Levinson, of Neugarten.

TABLE 4.11. Phases of Adulthood

Phases	Description	Tasks
Young adulthood (17–40 yo)	Early adult transition: 17–22 Building an entry life structure: 22–28 Transition: 28–33 Building a culminating life structure: 33–40	Develop a young-adult sense of self and others (3rd individuation) Develop adult friendships Develop capacity for intimacy and commitment to another person; marriage adjustments Become a biologic and psychologic parent Develop a relationship of mutuality and equality with own parents Establish an adult work identity Develop adult forms of play Develop a new attitude toward time
Middle adulthood (40–65 yo)	Midlife transition: 40–45 Building an entry life structure: 45–50 Transition: 50–55 Building a culminative life structure: 55–60	Process of reviewing the past (power, maturity, productivity, competitiveness); Considering the future (possibilities, commitments, direction); lifestyle Emotional and physical well-being; level of self-awareness; maturity, wisdom Sexuality (physical, psychologic components; climaterium); midlife crisis?; growth–death issues; Socialization, communication with family and friends, Separations: empty nest, divorce, custody problems, adultery
Late adulthood or old age (>65 yo)	Late-life transition: 60–65	Life expectancy is increasing (F > M) Leading causes of death: heart disease, cancer, stroke, in the elderly and accidents when >65 Adaptation to biologic, psychologic, and social losses Quality of life (productivity, affective status, functional status, cognitive status); sense of satisfaction or despair; sense of autonomy? Sexual activity? Retirement (positive and negative consequences) Socioeconomic status (Medicare, Social Security, private pensions); long-term care Psychiatric problems? Giving up position of authority; evaluating achievements

5 ■ PRINCIPLES OF PSYCHOPHARMACOLOGY

PHARMACOLOGIC ACTIONS

TABLE 5.1. Pharmacodynamics

Receptor mechanisms	The receptor of the drug is the cellular component to which the drug binds and initiates its effects. The drug may be an agonist or an antagonist of the receptor, full or partial
Dose–response curve	Measures the action of the drug against the dose
Potency	Refers to the relative dose needed to achieve certain effects
Clinical efficacy	The maximal clinical response achievable by the drug
Therapeutic index	Measures the toxicity or safety of the drug. The median toxic dose is the dose at which 50% of pts have a specific toxic effect. The median effective dose is the dose at which 50% of pts have a specific therapeutic effect Therapeutic index = median toxic dose/median effective dose Caution with interindividual and intraindividual variations, idiosyncratic drug responses
Tolerance	When a person becomes less responsive to a drug
Dependence	A physical need to receive the drug
Withdrawal	Sx that appear after discontinuing a drug

TABLE 5.2. Pharmacokinetics

- **Absorption**: drugs need to reach the brain through the bloodstream. Oral absorption depends on GI circumstances, lipid solubility. Stomach acidity ↓ with gastric ion pump inhibitors (Prilosec, Prevacid), histamine H2 receptor blockers (Tagamet, Pepcid, Zantac), and antacids. Anticholinergic drugs ↓ GI motility. Dopamine receptor antagonists (Reglan) ↑ GI motility. Parenteral administration may be given IV, IM (regular drugs or depot preparations), changing the speed of absorption
- **ADME**: absorption, distribution, metabolism, elimination—the key pharmacokinetic data to know for any drug
- **Distribution**: drugs may circulate free (can pass through the blood–brain barrier) or protein-bound (cannot). Good distribution of the drug relies on high cerebral blood flow, high lipid solubility, and high receptor affinity
- **Bioavailability**: the fraction of an administered dose of unchanged drug that reaches the systemic circulation and is available at the site of action
- **"Area under the curve" (AUC)**: refers to the total amount of drug that has been absorbed into the systemic circulation
- C_{max}: Maximum plasma concentration of a drug at a given time point
- T_{max}: time to attain C_{max}

METABOLISM AND EXCRETION

- **Metabolism**: By oxidation, reduction, hydrolysis (all being phase I reactions, dependent on hepatic function and the CYP system), conjugation (glucuronidation or phase II in the liver and other systems). The liver is the main site of metabolism. Drug metabolism is complex: presence of a drug transport mechanism **called P-glycoprotein (P-gp)** which is an ATP-dependent drug transporter present in the membranes of cells in the intestine, liver, kidney, blood–brain barrier and limits drug absorption and availability in the blood and CNS (calcium channel blockers, amitriptyline, chlorpromazine, fluphenazine, haloperidol, quinidine may inhibit action of P-gp; St John's wort, morphine, phenobarbital ↑ expression of P-gp).

- **The excretion (clearance) routes** are bile, feces, urine, and to a lesser degree sweat, saliva, tears, breast milk, respiration.

- **Important measures**:

    ◦ **Peak plasma concentration**: time between the administration of a drug and its peak conc. in the plasma (depends on route of administration and rate of absorption).

    ◦ **Drug's half-life** (time needed to reduce the plasma conc. by half). A drug needs usually 5 half-lives in time to achieve a steady plasma level (if the drug is given at intervals less than its half-life). The steady-state conc. is when the rate of drug availability equals the rate of drug elimination. Conversely, the patient needs a period of 5 half-lives to eliminate about 95% of the drug. Note that the reported half-life for a drug is usually the mean, and individual patients may vary considerably from the mean with a longer or shorter half-life.

    ◦ **Clearance**: the amount of drug excreted in a specific period of time.

HEPATIC CYTOCHROME P450 ENZYMES (CYP)

> **NOTE:**
> - CYP450 system: Proteins (enzymes) found in cells that metabolize many compounds including drugs. P450 refers to the wavelength of light absorbed by the pigment in the cytochromes
> - Example: for CYP 2 D 6: The number 2 refers to the enzyme family, D refers to the subfamily, and 6 refers to the individual gene coding for the enzyme
> - See Appendix on Inhibitors, Inducers, and Substrates of Cytochrome P450 Isozymes on page 326
> - **Inhibitors will ↓ metabolism of substrates and generally lead to ↑ drug effect (unless the substrate is a prodrug)**
> - **Inducers will ↑ metabolism of substrates and generally lead to ↓ drug effects (unless the substrate is a prodrug)**

Poor metabolizers have an inefficient version of CYP enzymes which are responsible for the inactivation of most psychotropic drugs. These enzymes are located in the hepatocytes and other tissues.

Three ways of working on the CYP system:

- **Induction**: ↑ metabolism and ↓ plasma conc. of the drug that is a substrate of that enzyme
- **Noncompetitive inhibition**: some drugs that are not substrates for a particular enzyme may still indirectly inhibit the enzyme and ↓ the metabolism of other drug substrates and ↑ the conc. of the other drug. If one CYP enzyme is inhibited, its substrate accumulates until metabolized by an alternate CYP enzyme.
- **Competitive inhibition**: two or more substrates for a particular enzyme administered together may produce a competitive inhibition (usually nonclinically important)

  This is a major source of adverse drug interactions, since changes in CYP enzyme activity may affect the metabolism and clearance of various drugs. For example, if one drug inhibits the CYP-mediated metabolism of another drug, the second drug may accumulate within the body to toxic levels, possibly causing an overdose. It seems also that there is NG3R2 overlap between substrates for P-gp and those for CYP3A4 system.

URIDINE DIPHOSPHATE GLUCURONOSYLTRANSFERASES

Uridine diphosphate glucuronosyltransferases (UGTs) have received less attention than CYP enzymes; responsible for metabolism of anxiolytics, antidepressants, mood stabilizers, and antipsychotics. Psychotropic inhibitors of UGTs are: amitriptyline, chlorpromazine, clomipramine, diazepam, lorazepam, valproic acid, verapamil; psychotropic inducers of UGTs are carbamazepine, phenobarbital, phenytoin. Inhibition of the metabolism of carbamazepine by valproic acid in part results from an effect on UGTs. Amitriptyline and clomipramine ↓ metabolism of morphine (may contribute to opioid toxicity). The psychopharmacologic significance of this type of interaction is not well understood.

Check also: www.drug-interactions.com.

Flockhart, D. A. (2007). *Drug interactions: Cytochrome P450 drug interaction table.* Indianapolis: Indiana University School of Medicine. http://medicine.iupui.edu/clinpharm/ddis/table.asp. Accessed August 19, 2010.

See also Appendix on Inhibitors, inducers, and substrates of cytochrome P450 isozymes.

DRUGS DEVELOPMENT

Phase I trials: to determine safety and tolerability of a new drug, assess pharmacokinetic effects and potential for SE; the drug is administered to about 100 normal persons.

Phase II trials: the new drug is used on 100–200 patients to assess efficacy, safety, dosage, AE.

Phase III trials: on 1,000–3,000 pts (occasionally more) to validate the previous studies and determine optimum dosage schedules and use on specific populations (study of emergence of adverse events). It is only after phase III that the pharmaceutical company can apply to the Food and Drug Administration (FDA) to market the drug. Note that uncommon AEs are not usually picked up from clinical trials and only emerge after the drug is on the market.

Once marketed, the drug enters **Phase IV** (postmarketing experience on a larger population).

DEA

RESOURCES

DEA's Diversion Control Program Web site: www.DEAdiversion.usdoj.gov

DEA homepage: www.dea.go

SCHEDULES OF CONTROLLED SUBSTANCES

The drugs and other substances that are considered controlled substances under the CSA are divided into five schedules:

All drugs listed in Schedule I have no currently accepted medical use in treatment in the United States and therefore may not be prescribed, administered, or dispensed for medical use. In contrast, drugs listed in Schedules II through V all have some accepted medical use and therefore may be prescribed, administered, or dispensed for medical use.

TABLE 5.3. Schedules of Controlled Substances

	Schedule I substances	Schedule II substances	Schedule III substances	Schedule IV substances	Schedule V substances
Characteristics	• Not currently accepted medical use in treatment in the United States, lack of accepted safety for use under medical supervision, high potential for abuse	• High potential for abuse with severe psychologic or physical dependence	• Potential for abuse less than substances in Schedules I or II	• Lower potential for abuse relative to substances in Schedule III	• Lower potential for abuse relative to substances listed in Schedule IV
Examples	• Heroin; lysergic acid diethylamide (LSD); marijuana (cannabis); peyote; methaqualone; and methylenedimethoxymethamphetamine ("Ecstasy")	• Morphine, codeine, opium, amphetamine (Dexedrine® or Adderall®), methamphetamine (Desoxyn®), and methylphenidate (Ritalin®), cocaine, amobarbital, glutethimide, and pentobarbital	• Products with <15 mg of hydrocodone/dosage unit (i.e., Vicodin®) and products with <90 mg of codeine/dosage unit (i.e., Tylenol with codeine®), benzphetamine (Didrex®), phendimetrazine, dronabinol (Marinol®), ketamine, anabolic steroids such as oxandrolone (Oxandrin®)	• Propoxyphene (Darvon® and Darvocet-N 100®), alprazolam (Xanax®), clonazepam (Klonopin®), clorazepate (Tranxene®), diazepam (Valium®), lorazepam (Ativan®), midazolam (Versed®), temazepam (Restoril®), and triazolam (Halcion®)	• Cough preparations containing not more than 200 mg of codeine per 100 mL or per 100 g (Robitussin AC®, and Phenergan with codeine)
Registration		• Required	• Required	• Required	• Required
Receiving records		• Order forms (DEA Form-222)	• Invoices, readily retrievable	• Invoices, readily retrievable	• Invoices, readily retrievable
Prescriptions		• Written prescription (see exceptions*)	• Written, oral, or fax	• Written, oral, or fax	• Written, oral, or fax, or over the counter**
Refills		• No	• No more than 5 within 6 months	• No more than 5 within 6 months	• As authorized when prescription is issued
Distribution between registrants		• Order forms (DEA Form-222)	• Invoices	• Invoices	• Invoices
Security		• Locked cabinet or other secure storage	• Locked cabinet or other secure storage	• Locked cabinet or other secure storage	• Locked cabinet or other secure storage
Theft or significant loss		• Report and complete DEA Form 106	• Report and complete DEA Form 106	• Report and complete DEA Form 106	• Report and complete DEA Form 106

Note: All records must be maintained for 2 yr, unless a state requires a longer period.

Note: prescribing requirements vary by state.

*Emergency prescriptions require a signed follow-up prescription

Exceptions: A facsimile prescription serves as the original prescription when issued to residents of Long Term Facilities, Hospice patients, or compounded IV narcotic medications

**Where authorized by state controlled substances authority.

Adapted from Rannazzisi, J. T., & Caverly, M. W. (2006). Practitioner's manual: An informational outline of the Controlled Substance Act. Retrieved October 27, 2010 from http://www.deadiversion.usdoj.gov/pubs/manuals/pract/

TREATMENT FAILURES

TABLE 5.4.   Treatment Failures

- Errors in diagnosis
- Drug's AEs and SEs
- Subtherapeutic dosage of the medicine, not given long enough, lack of beneficial effects
- Individual variations due to the pt's absorption, metabolism, and excretion of the drug or pharmacogenic variability
- DDIs
- **Noncompliance with rx**: due to discomfort with rx, expense of rx, religious and cultural beliefs about rx, maladaptive coping skills, presence of a severe mental disorder
- **Drug noncompliance**: poor education about the drug treatment, complex dosages, lack of insurance, no money
- **Psychopathology**: psychosis, dementia, mental retardation (MR), illiteracy, impaired hearing or vision, hopelessness, paranoia, personality disorder, substance abuse, other comorbidities
- **Poor clinician–patient relationship**: The physician must show that the medicine relieves distressing symptoms (daily benefit), will help achieve one's life goal, will prevent symptoms from coming back (relapse prevention); he will help pt to see that the rx is important for marital or family relationships, to understand that the drug is needed even though the pt feels better, to think that benefits are more than side effects, to help with the fear of stigma; need to recognize quickly when pt stops the medicine; include the family in the treatment; understand pt's point of view; agree to try alternative rx if too many SE.

SPECIAL CONSIDERATIONS

- **Children**: may need high doses; but start with small doses
- **Elderly**: Combine with behavioral interventions; treat underlying medical problems; choose on SEs profile; may metabolize slowly, take usually many different drugs (interactions?); more susceptible to toxicity (risk of falls if oversedated; R/O alcohol or substance abuse; start with smaller dose (½ the usual) starting dose), ↑ slowly.

  Dosing of antipsychotics for dementia is much lower than for schizophrenia (work on agitation, aggression, irritability, delusions): risperidone 0.25 bid, max 2 mg/d; olanzapine 2.5 qd, max 10 mg/d; quetiapine 0.25 qd, max 200 mg/d

  Anticholinergic effects of antipsychotics are a concern for the elderly (especially in Alzheimer's where there is already a cholinergic deficit) → worsening of cognition. If haloperidol is used: use very low doses (0.25–1 mg q 4–12 hr)

- **Pregnant and nursing women**: avoid any drug during the first trimester or during breast-feeding. Lithium and anticonvulsants are the most teratogenic psychopharmacologic drugs.

TABLE 5.5.   Pregnancy and Psychotropic Medications

- **Malformations** associated with maternal drug use depend on the properties of the drug and the point of exposure:
  - Up to 32 days postconception can affect neural tube development and closure
  - Days 21–56 after conception may affect normal heart formation
  - Days 42–63 may influence development of the lip and palate. Craniofacial anomalies can also occur after the first trimester

- **Lithium**:
  - 400-fold ↑ rate for CV malformations, most notably **Ebstein's anomaly**, associated with lithium exposure in utero; Ebstein's anomaly among lithium users: 1 per 1,000 (0.1%) to 2 per 1,000 (0.2%), or 20–40 times higher than rates in the general population
  - **Higher-weight babies, neonatal complications if rx with lithium in late pregnancy**: cardiac dysfunction, diabetes insipidus; hypothyroidism; low muscle tone; lethargy; hepatic abnormalities; respiratory difficulties
  - **Discontinuation of lithium proximate to delivery and reinstitution immediately after delivery** significantly ↓ neonatal complications while maintaining maternal euthymia

- **Carbamazepine**: neural tube defects are 0.5–1%; risks ↑ if given with valproate (due to ↑ toxic epoxide metabolites; oxcarbazepine may be less teratogenic as it does not produce the epoxide metabolite); is associated with lower birth weight and mean head circumference; causes fetal vitamin K deficiency (vitamin K is necessary for normal mid-facial growth and function of clotting factors). Give vitamin K 20 mg/d po throughout pregnancy and give 1 mg vitamin K IM to neonates after in utero carbamazepine exposure. Observe neonate for possible hyperbilirubinemia

Continued

TABLE 5.5.   Pregnancy and Psychotropic Medications   Continued

- **Lamotrigine**: major fetal anomalies (2.6% including 0.89% for midline cleft formations); risks ↑ if dosage >200 mg/d. No reports of obstetrical or neonatal complications associated with lamotrigine monotherapy. Potential for maintenance rx option (protects against bipolar depression, well tolerated, safer than other mood stabilizers)

- **Valproate**: teratogen (neural tube: 5–9%, lumbosacral > anencephalic; cardiovascular, craniofacial); acute and long-term adverse effects on infant development. Possible neonatal liver toxicity, hypoglycemia, withdrawal sx (irritability, jitteriness, feeding problems, abnormal muscle tone). ↑ Risk of MR, LD (reduce dose or change to another anticonvulsant prior to conception)

- **Atypical antipsychotic medications**: no pattern of defects in neonate but weight gain, insulin resistance, gestational diabetes, preeclampsia in mothers

- **Typical antipsychotic agents**: phenothiazines and butyrophenones are used to treat hyperemesis gravidarum, nausea, and psychotic disorders in pregnancy; may have fewer risks than mood stabilizers

- **Antidepressants, benzodiazepines and sedative-hypnotics**: rarely used and controversial

- **If ECT used**: < SE, not teratogenic. Minimize risk for fetal tachycardia and arrhythmias by avoiding atropine, ensuring adequate oxygenation. Monitor fetal heart during ECT

Adapted from Stowe, Z. N., & Newport, D. J. (2007). The management of bipolar disorder during pregnancy: Treatment options for women with bipolar disorder during pregnancy. Retrieved August 19, 2010 from: http://www.medscape.com/viewarticle/565128_4

TABLE 5.6.   FDA Use-in-Pregnancy Ratings

• **Category A**	• Adequate, well-controlled studies in pregnant ♀ have not shown an increased risk of fetal abnormalities to the fetus in any trimester of pregnancy
• **Category B**	• Animal studies have revealed no evidence of harm to the fetus; however, no adequate and well-controlled studies in pregnant ♀ or • Animal studies have shown an adverse effect, but adequate and well-controlled studies in pregnant ♀ have failed to demonstrate a risk to the fetus in any trimester
• **Category C**	• Animal studies have shown an adverse effect, and there are no adequate and well-controlled studies in pregnant ♀ or • No animal studies have been conducted, and there are no adequate and well-controlled studies in pregnant ♀
• **Category D**	• Adequate well-controlled or observational studies in pregnancy ♀ have demonstrated a risk to the fetus. However, the benefits of therapy may outweigh the potential risk
• **Category X**	• Adequate well-controlled or observational studies in animals or pregnant ♀ have demonstrated positive evidence of fetal abnormalities or risks. The use of the product is contraindicated in ♀ who are or who may become pregnant

Note: Few drugs have been studied in pregnant women and thus the effects on the mother and fetus are generally not known specifically. Contact: The California Teratogen Information service available at www.ctispregnancy.org which is kept up to date and the excellent center at the University of Toronto known as Motherisk (http://www.motherisk.org/women/index.jsp).

Source: Cobert, B. & Biron, P. (2009). Practical Drug Safety from A to Z. Sudbury, MA: Jones & Bartlett Learning. p. 285.

- **Pts with liver or renal insufficiency**: use reduced dosage (½), monitor carefully.

POTENTIAL ADVERSE EFFECTS DUE TO PSYCHOPHARMACOLOGIC DRUGS

TABLE 5.7.   Potential Adverse Effects due to Psychopharmacologic Drugs

Psychopharmacologic medication	Potential adverse effects
• **Serotonergic**: SSRI, SNRI	• Akathisia, sleep disturbance (somnolence, insomnia), anxiety, agitation, headache, weight gain, GI upset, diarrhea, nausea, vomiting, sexual dysfunction (decreased libido, anorgasmia, priapism), hyponatremia (in elderly, primarily with fluoxetine or paroxetine), possible serotonin syndrome (fever, sweating, confusion, myoclonus, hyperreflexia, muscle rigidity, agitation, autonomic dysfunction with ataxia, shivering, diarrhea, hypotension)

Continued

TABLE 5.7.   Potential Adverse Effects due to Psychopharmacologic Drugs   Continued

• **Antidopaminergic D2:** Antipsychotics (greater effects with higher potency neuroleptics)	• **Extrapyramidal sx** (EPS): akathisia (restlessness, constant moving, dysphoria); dystonia (sudden, involuntary sustained contraction of a group of muscles, lock jaw, oculogyric crisis, torticollis, opisthotonos); parkinsonism (slow, resting tremor, cogwheel rigidity, akinesia); tardive dyskinesia (slow choreiform movements/tongue, facial muscles, upper extremities, or whole body) • Sedation, cardiac effects, orthostatic hypotension, weight gain, agranulocytosis (clozapine) • **Endocrine sx**: increased prolactinemia, menstrual dysfunction, sexual dysfunction

• **Blockade of muscarinic acetylcholine receptors (Muscarinic M1):**
   TCAs (greater effects with amitriptyline, doxepin, trimipramine)
   Mirtazapine, alprazolam
   Antihistamines (Benadryl, Phenergan)
   Antiparkinsonian (Cogentin, Artane)
   Medicines containing scopolamine
   Antipsychotics (Thorazine, Stelazine)
	• Blurred vision (near vision), dilated pupils, constipation, ↓ salivation (dry mouth), ↓ sweating, delayed or retrograde ejaculation, depression, dysuria, nausea, vomiting, headache, diarrhea, drowsiness, delirium, ↑ asthma, fever, memory problems, narrow-angle glaucoma, photophobia, sinus tachycardia, urinary retention, anxiety, confusion, psychosis, delirium → seizures, stupor, coma (some sx more pronounced in elderly population)

• **β receptor antagonists**: (propranolol) • **α$_2$ agonists**: (clonidine, methyldopa) • **α$_1$ adrenergic receptor blockers action** (in thioridazine)	• Dizziness, postural hypotension, reflex tachycardia, nasal congestion, retrograde ejaculation, drowsiness, ↓ salivation (dry mouth), headache, weakness, nausea, constipation. Allergic reaction may occur (rash, hives, cardio effects)
• **Antihistaminic H1**: (Benadryl, Phenergan)	• Hypotension, sedation, weight gain
• **Multiple neurotransmitter systems**: (Antidepressants, multiple drugs used together)	• Sensitivity reaction, allergic reactions, anorexia, cardiac conduction abnormalities, nausea, vomiting, seizures, blood dyscrasias, restlessness, agitation, headache

Adapted from Sadock, B. J., & Sadock, V. A. (2002). *Kaplan and Sadock's Synopsis of Psychiatry: Behavioral Sciences/Clinical Psychiatry* (9th ed). Baltimore, MD: Lippincott Williams & Wilkins. p. 980.

TABLE 5.8.   Risk Factors Contributing to QTc Prolongation

• **Female**: QT is longer during the first half of the menstrual cycle
• **Elderly**: multiple medications, pharmacokinetic and pharmacodynamic differences
• **Electrolyte imbalance**: low K+ and low Mg++
• **Alcoholism**
• **Congenital long QT syndrome**: risk of torsade de pointe and sudden death
• **Cardiac disease (MI, arrhythmias, CHF)**: risk of arrhythmias
• **Medication OD with drugs prolonging QTc**: QTc prolongation may be dose dependent; Many drugs increase QT and adding them together increases risk
• **Concomitant medications(drug combinations)**: drug interaction leading to inhibition of CYP enzymes and ↑ drug level and risk of QT prolongation
• **Endocrine and metabolic problems**: diabetes, obesity, hypothyroidism (electrolytes imbalance, cardiovascular problems)
• **CNS dysfunctions (stroke, trauma, infections)**: leading to instable autonomic system

Normal range (women: 350–450 ms; men: 350–430 ms); QT length when corrected for heart rate is called QTc.

TABLE 5.9. Drug-Induced Central Hyperthermic Syndromes
All will need supportive measures, cooling, possible gastric lavage. See malignant hyperthermia association: http://medical.mhaus.org/

Common syndromes	Signs/symptoms	Related drugs	Treatment
• Neuroleptic malignant syndrome	• Hyperthermia, muscular rigidity, altered mental status, diaphoresis, leukocytosis, delirium, rhabdomyolysis, autonomic dysfunction, tachycardia, hypotension; ↑ CPK, EPS; rapid onset, death if untreated	• All neuroleptics and others: lithium, haloperidol, fluphenazine, prochlorperazine, promethazine, clozapine, risperidone, metoclopramide, methyldopa	• Stop antipsychotic drug; rapid cooling, sedation; correct volume depletion • Bromocriptine (2–10 mg q 8 hr po or NG tube), Sinemet, dantrolene sodium (2.5 mg/kg IV push q 5–10 min until sx subside or max 10 mg/kg/dose; follow with 4–8 mg/kg/d po divided tid–qid × 1–3 days to prevent recurrence)
• Serotonin syndrome	• Altered mental status, autonomic dysfunction, neuromuscular abnormalities, agitation, delirium, coma, mydriasis, hyperthermia, tachycardia	• SSRIs, SNRIs alone or in combination with other drugs (TCA, meperidine, MAOIs, cocaine)	• Cooling (**pack the pt in ice/** not only placing ice in neck, armpits, and groin) • Avoid succinylcholine • Serotonin-antagonist (cyproheptadine); benzodiazepines for sedation; oxygen, IV fluids; phenylephrine if hypotensive
• Malignant hyperthermia	• Hyperthermia, rhabdomyolysis, disseminated intravascular coagulation, darkened urine, arrhythmias, hypotension, muscle rigidity, risk of death	• Succinylcholine; seroflurane, halothane, desflurane, isoflurane, enflurane • Generally genetic defect in the ryanodine receptor present	• Dantrolene sodium IV; cessation of anesthesia; wrap pt in cooling blanket; administer lidocaine or beta-blocker for cardiac sx; IM or po fluid maintenance for renal function
• Sympathomimetic poisoning	• Hyperthermia, hypertension, intracranial hemorrhage, cardiac arrhythmias, tachycardia, diaphoresis	• Tricyclic antidepressants; MAOIs	• No clear antidote—general supportive tx; cooling measures; benzodiazepines for sedation
• Drug overdose (such as TCAs)	• Hyperthermia, confusion, agitation, hallucinations, hyperreflexia, anticholinergic signs (dry skin, dilated pupils), arrhythmias; mydriasis; seizures; prolonged QT interval; risk of death if untreated	• TCAs, cocaine	• Sodium bicarbonate if arrhythmias, physostigmine with cardiac monitoring; IV fluids if hypotensive; benzodiazepines for sedation
• Anticholinergic poisoning syndrome	• Hyperthermia, altered mental status, flushing, dry skin, mydriasis, tachycardia, hypertension	• Antihistamines (Diphenhydramine); anticholinergics; antipsychotics; cyclic antidepressants	• GI decontamination if recent ingestion; benzodiazepines for sedation; cardiovascular agents if TCA overdose; physostigmine
• Lethal catatonia	• Hyperthermia, anxiety, agitation, psychosis; rigidity, delirium, risk of death if untreated	• Lead poisoning	• Lorazepam, no antipsychotics; benzodiazepines;
• Autonomic hyperreflexia	• Hyperthermia, hyperreflexia, agitation	• Amphetamines	• Trimethaphan
• Simple hyperthermia	• Hyperthermia, diaphoresis • Febrile seizures in children	• Atropine, lidocaine, meperidine, thyrotoxicosis, NSAID toxicity	• Acetaminophen, diazepam for seizures

Adapted from Sadock, B. J., & Sadock, V. A. (2002). *Kaplan and Sadock's Synopsis of Psychiatry: Behavioral Sciences/Clinical Psychiatry* (9th ed.). Baltimore, MD: Lippincott Williams & Wilkins. p. 998.

OFF-LABEL USE OF PSYCHOTROPIC MEDICATIONS

Refers to prescribing a psychotropic medication outside of the scope of FDA-approved labeling: for a disorder other than its FDA-approved indication, unapproved dose, in an unapproved format (opening a capsule, crushing the tablet), for longer than the approved time, at a different dose schedule, for different populations not included in the labeling. In the past, off-label prescribing was generally permitted. However, under new legislation FDA may now limit prescribing to certain physicians, specialties, and the like, and may limit dispensing to certain pharmacies and/or require informed consent, special training of prescribers, and so on, under "Risk evaluation & mitigation strategies." The prescriber should be sure to read the package insert (labeling) of all drugs prescribed to be aware of any special conditions or limitations of prescribing.

TABLE 5.10.   Most Frequent Risks of Litigation

1. The drug is given at significantly **higher doses** than the label recommendation
2. The drug is given for **an indication not on the label**
3. The pt is **not a part of a population included in the clinical trials** listed on the label (children, geriatric pts)
4. **Bad outcome**

TABLE 5.11   Some Guidelines for Using Medications Off-Label

1. Check latest official prescribing information (www.fda.gov and http://www.accessdata.fda.gov/scripts/cder/drugsatfda/index.cfm FDA's Web site with drug labeling)
2. Be aware of **news and scientific evidence about specific drug** uses, effects, interactions, adverse effects
3. **Keep articles on off-label uses**, separate from pts' files
4. **Support your treatment choice** in explaining how the previous articles contributed to the choice of this particular drug for this particular pt at this particular time
5. **Explain to your pt** your reasoning and document this in the pt's chart
6. **Obtain informed consent and get a new one if change in treatment**
7. **Document** informed consent to describe the collaborative decision between you and your pt or pt's guardian, document in readable notes why this was decided, reflecting the conversation with the pt, the risks and benefits of the rx vs doing nothing, the effects of previous rx, and the understanding of the pt

FDA RESOURCES

- **FDA: Information sheets on hundreds of FDA-approved drugs, listed alphabetically.** www.fda.gov/cder/drug/DrugSafety/DrugIndex.htm. Check Drugs@fda.gov: great web site to look at the package labels

- Averse Event Reporting: **MedWatch. FDA.** 5,600 Fishers Lane, Rockville, MD 20852–9787. Fax: 1-800-FDA-0178, http://www.fda.gov/medwatch/safety.htm. **If side effects: Phone to the FDA: 1-800-FDA-1088. Online reporting: https://www.accessdata.fda.gov/scripts/medwatch/medwatch-online.htm. May also call the manufacturer to report the AE. FDA encourages the reporting of ALL adverse events, not just serious or severe ones.**

NOTE:
- As defined by the FDA, **a serious adverse event is a** reaction to a drug, a biologic, or a medical device at any dose that is associated with one of the following: "death," is "life-threatening," "requires hospitalization," "leads to disability," "causes congenital anomaly," and/or "requires an intervention" to prevent permanent impairment or damage whether or not it is felt to be due to the drug, biologic, device.

POLYPHARMACY

The use of multiple drugs in a patient at the same time

- Incidence ↑, ↑ risk of drug–drug interactions (DDIs).
- **Factors affecting polypharmacy**: comorbid medical and psychiatric conditions, ↑ number of approved psychoactive drugs, ↑ use of nonprescription drug (OTC medicines, herbal preparations, smoking), ↑ Internet availability (danger of getting fake, contaminated, substandard, and potentially dangerous medicines), syndromic nature of psychiatric disorders, ↑ prescription medicine coverage, rx of SEs (e.g., EPS, metabolic syndrome), lack of communication with multiple doctors each of whom is prescribing, ↓ use of behavioral and social techniques (e.g., sleep hygiene in insomnia), aging population, use of illicit drugs

- **Treatment considerations**
  - **Potential DDIs** (changes in magnitude, nature, or duration of the action of one drug as a result of the presence of another drug). This is influenced by pharmacodynamics (drug's affinity for the site of action in the body, or its biochemical and physiologic effect and mechanism of action), pharma-

cokinetics (conc. of the drug at the site of action and its action/including absorption, distribution, localization in tissues, biotransformation, excretion) and biologic variability among pts.

- **Intestinal motility and gastric pH** change absorption of drugs.
- **Liver disease**: may change the clearance of drugs by interfering with their metabolism or may alter plasma proteins affecting free drug concentration and distribution
- **Renal disease**: classic drugs cleared through the kidneys are lithium, gabapentin.
- **Medications used for physical conditions**: may also affect psychiatric medications
- **Older pts**: more susceptible to anticholinergic SE from psychiatric drugs or combinations, depression from antihypertensives, anxiety from SSRIs or prescriptions for other medical problems.
- **Noncompliance** ↑ with polypharmacy
- **Alcohol use**
- **Fatal outcomes** (e.g., MAOIs and meperidine, MAOIs and fluoxetine with development of serotonin syndrome).

GENERIC DRUGS

NOTE:

FDA requirements for generic drug approval: a generic drug must:
- contain the same active ingredients as the innovator drug (inactive ingredients may vary)
- be identical in strength, dosage form, and route of administration
- have the same use indications
- be bioequivalent: bioavailability must be 80–125% of innovator, defined as the area under the curve (AUC) and the max. plasma conc. (C_{max}) at 2 time points
- meet the same batch requirements for identity, strength, purity, and quality
- be manufactured under the same standards of FDA's Good Manufacturing Practice regulations required for innovator products.

Resources

- **National Alliance for the Mentally Ill (NAMI)**: http://www.nami.org/
- **www.schizophrenia.com**
- See practice guidelines for the treatment of patients with schizophrenia, 2nd ed. (2004). *American Journal of Psychiatry, 161*(Suppl 2), 1–56.

Scales for schizophrenia and psychosis: Brief Psychiatric Rating Scale, Schedule for Affective Disorders and Schizophrenia (SADS), Scale for the Assessment of Negative Symptoms (SANS), Thought Disorder Index (TDI), Quality of Life Scale (QLS), Scale for the Assessment of Positive Symptoms (SAPS).

History: see works of Emil Kraeplin (distinguished dementia precox from manic-depressive psychosis) and Eugen Bleuler (who gave the term schizophrenia, and stressed that it does not need to have a deteriorating course)

GENERALITIES

Psychosis: state of grossly impaired sense of reality, implies a degree of severity, may be coupled with emotional and cognitive disabilities leading to an inability to function, frequently producing confusion, disorientation, hallucinations, and delusions and often a lack of insight. In psychotic disorders, while there is severe impairment at times, a pt may not present as psychotic for long periods of time.

Etiologies: psychotic disorders may be of organic or nonorganic etiology (usually with a clear sensorium).

- **Think of organicity +++ if:**

- **Acute,** rapid onset (hours, days)
- **No family or personal hx of psychiatric illness**
- **Chronic, serious medical illness with periodic relapses**
- **A degree of delirium** (memory loss, confusion, disorientation, clouding of consciousness)
- **Drug abuse**

- **Always obtain a complete hx and physical** (identify any underlying medical, neurological causes or substance intoxication or withdrawal)

- **Many psychiatric conditions may have psychotic features when they reach a severe level**:

  Major depressive disorder or bipolar disorder: an affective component (depression or mania) often preceded the psychotic process.
  Brief psychotic disorders during stress in individuals with personality disorders.
  Panic attacks of psychotic proportion.
  Rage episodes of psychotic intensity in intermittent explosive disorders.
  Psychotic disorders in PDD and autism.
  "Psychotic states" can be seen in factitious disorders and malingering.

Clinical presentation of psychosis: may be acute or insidious, lasting brief episodes, months or years, with or without recurrence, leaving or not residual symptoms.

Early signs may be restlessness, nervousness, anhedonia (inability to experience pleasure), insomnia, problems in concentration.

Psychosis is a mixture of the following sx:

(1) **Formal thought disorder: (thinking may be illogical, difficult to understand)**:

- **Loosening of association**: lack of logical, inherent relationship between contiguous thoughts or ideas
- **Neologism**: inventing new words having a meaning to the pt but not to others
- **Thought blocking**: sudden cession in train of thought or mid-sentence
- **Clang associations**: rhyming combination of words or phrases because they share similar sounds
- **Autistic thinking**: subjective and highly individualized special meaning to thought
- **Circumstantiality**: proceeding to goal with many tedious details and overinclusive, irrelevant additions
- **Echolalia**: repetition of words or phrases without an apparent need to communicate
- **Alogia**: poverty of speech

- **Concreteness**: poor abstract thinking if normal intelligence
- **Tangentiality**: inability to have goal-directed thoughts
- **Flight of ideas**: continuous rapid skipping from one idea to another, related, not disjointed or bizarre
- **Perseveration**: persistence of a single response or idea

(2) **Content thought disorder**:

- **Poverty of content**: vagueness, obscure phrases
- **Delusions**: fixed false beliefs, based on incorrect inference about external reality, not corrected by reasoning. May be mood-congruent (associated to the mood) or mood-incongruent (not associated to the mood)

TABLE 6.1.   Types of Delusions

Persecutory delusions (paranoid delusions include persecutory delusions and delusions of reference)	Being followed, spied upon, monitored by the government, betrayed by one's mate, delusions of poverty
Delusions of guilt	Having committed a crime or a sin, deserving to be punished
Grandiose delusions	Having special powers, talents, ability to achieve great things, to control events, erotomania (belief that someone is deeply in love with them), unio mystica (oceanic feeling of mystic unity with an infinite power, if not congruent with cultural milieu), religious delusions
Somatic delusions	Believing one's body is changed, diseased
Delusions of reference	Thinking people in a room or on TV are talking about the patient, that events refer back to oneself or have a special meaning
Thought broadcasting	Hearing own thoughts out loud or feeling that they are broadcasted and heard by others
Thought insertion	Feeling thoughts are being put in one's head by an outside source
Thought withdrawal	Feeling thoughts are taken away by some outside source
Bizarre delusions	Absurd, strange false belief

- **Lack of insight**: unawareness of one's illness and need for rx

(3) **Disorder of perceptions**:

- **Hallucinations**: false sensory perception in the absence of an actual external stimulus. Most frequently auditory (1 or x voices, noises), may comment about the pt or events, may be derogatory, threatening, or giving orders (command hallucinations), perceived as real, coming from outside of the head. May be visual, olfactory, gustatory, or tactile (more when organicity); may be mood-congruent or mood-incongruent
- **Illusions**: misinterpretation of a real sensory experience
- **Depersonalizations**: loss of the sense of one's identity as related to surroundings
- **Derealizations**: the world seems unreal

(4) **Disturbance of emotions**: psychotic pts may switch from one emotion to another quickly.

- **Affect**: observed expression of emotion, may be **inappropriate** (disharmony between the feeling tone and the idea, thought, or speech accompanying it), **blunted** (severe ↓ in intensity of externalized feeling tone), **flat** (no affective emotion), **labile** (rapid changes in emotional tone unrelated to external stimuli)
- **Mood**: pervasive and sustained emotion experienced, reported by the pt and observed by others

(5) **Disturbance of behavior**:

- **Echopraxia**: pathological imitation of movements
- **Catatonia and postural abnormalities**: **catalepsy** (immobile position constantly maintained), **excitement**, **stupor** (marked slowed motor activity to the point of immobility; seeming unawareness of surroundings), **posturing**, **waxy flexibility** (when a position can be molded and then maintained), **rigidity** (rigid posture held against efforts to be moved), **akinesia** (↓ physical movements)
- **Mutism**
- **Aggressiveness, agitation**
- **Grimacing, excessive silliness**
- **Sexual inappropriateness, ritual behaviors**

CATEGORIES

- **Schizophrenia**: to be considered schizophrenia, as per *DSM-IV-TR*, *symptoms* **must be >6 months**

TABLE 6.2.   Diagnosing Schizophrenia

Symptoms (2 or more), present for >1 month	**Positive** (delusions, hallucinations, disorganized speech or behavior) or **negative** (alogia, flat affect, lack of motivation, asociality, inattention)
Duration (may include prodromal or residual symptoms)	**At least 6 months**
Exclusion of	Schizoaffective disorders (no mood disorder concurrently in active phase of schizophrenia) Mood disorder with psychotic features (in schizophrenia, mood episodes are brief during active sx) Organic condition (substance abuse, medical condition, medication)
In PDDs (autism or PDD-NOS)	Schizophrenia is diagnosed if active psychotic sx are >1 month
Subtypes	**Disorganized type**: has disorganized speech, behavior, and inappropriate affect **Catatonic type**: may have a combination of several forms of catatonia (stupor or mutism, negativism, rigidity, posturing, excitement excessive motor activity which may be life threatening due to exhaustion; repetition of others words/echolalia or actions/echopraxia) **Paranoid type**: develops usually later than other subtypes, most stable with consistent, often, paranoid delusions **Undifferentiated type**: does not fit the other subtypes **Residual type**: remission from active psychosis but presence of attenuated sx
Specifications given after 1 year	Episodic or continuous or single episode; with residual sx or none; with prominent negative sx or none; with partial or full remission; or unspecified pattern
Prognosis	**Chronic disorder** **Associated with good prognosis are**: Rapid onset of acute psychotic sx; precipitating stress to the acute psychosis Onset after 30 in women Good premorbid social and occupational functioning No CNS abnormalities No family hx of schizophrenia **Postpsychotic depression**: 25–50% during recovery of acute episode, often rx resistant, **suicide risk**, differentiate from medication-induced akinesia **Poor outcomes are** Demographic factors: male gender, early onset, poor premorbid functioning, low IQ, family hx of schizophrenia, no precipitating factor, hx of substance abuse, dysfunctional family Clinical factors: blunted affect, severity of negative sx, high incidence of soft neurological sx, TD, late rx initiation, neurocognitive deficit, disorganized type Noncompliance, medical factors, comorbidity
Biology	**Hypothesis**: **Dopamine** (neuroleptics block D2 postsynaptic dopamine receptors; amphetamines can cause psychosis by releasing central dopamine), **Serotonin** (↑ in CNS), **NE** (↑ in limbic forebrain), and **glutamate** (hypofunction in NMDA subtype of glutamate receptors; PCP acts on glutamate receptors) **On brain MRI**: more enlarged ventricles over time, ↓ volume of gray matter (parts of frontal lobe, parts of superior temporal lobes and corpus callosum) **Neurodevelopmental hypothesis**: nonstatic, abnormal reorganization of brain connections during adolescence?
Genetics	Neuronal growth defect prenatally, possibly genetically controlled. Familial risks (highest in monozygotic twins: 48%; nonidentical: 17%; normal population: 1%)

TABLE 6.3.   Cognitive Deficits in Schizophrenia

Verbal fluency	Muscarinic receptors M1 may be reduced in schizophrenia, contributing to the cognitive dysfunction Most antipsychotics have anticholinergic activity Anticholinergic medicines used for rx of the antipsychotic SEs impair learning and memory Acetylcholinesterase inhibitors and muscarinic agonists may improve cognition without affecting the psychosis (NDMC/N- desmethylclozapine, a metabolite of clozapine; donepezil)
Reasoning/problem solving	
Working memory	
Social learning	
Verbal learning memory	
Visual learning memory	
Attention/vigilance	

- **Schizophreniform disorder**: *symptoms are* **>1 month and <6 months,** begin and end more abruptly, are more acute than in schizophrenia, better premorbid adjustment, better recovery. Eliminate organic psychosis. The first 6 months of schizophrenia may need to be diagnosed as schizophreniform disorder.

- **Brief psychotic disorder**: *symptoms are* **>1 day and <1 month,** with or without a stressor, may be post-partum if onset is within 4 weeks, R/O medical conditions and substance abuse. Can be very dramatic mimicking other psychiatric disorders with psychosis. Possible recovery in a few days with good prognosis.

- **Schizoaffective disorder**: **mixed disorder with mood disorder sx** (depression, or mania, or mixed episode) **and sx of schizophrenia.** *Hallucinations or delusions must be >2 weeks in the absence of mood episode.* Mood sx are present during active and residual time (bipolar type or depressive type). Not due to substances or medical condition

- **Shared psychotic disorder or "folie a deux"**: a normal individual adopts the delusions of someone close and dominant. Separation of the two individuals is the rx

- **Delusional disorder**: nonbizarre delusions >1 month with little impairment in behavior or functioning. Types are: erotomanic, grandiose, jealous, persecutory, somatic, mixed, and unspecified

- **Psychotic disorder due to a general medical condition**: the psychosis does not occur only during a delirium, is not due to another mental disorder, is directly due to the medical condition

TABLE 6.4.   Medical Disorders Presenting with Psychotic Features

Space-occupying lesions	Primary or metastatic tumors Subdural hematoma Brain abscess
Central hypoxia	Severe anemia Pulmonary insufficiency Severe heart diseases Carbon monoxide intoxication
Metabolic and endocrine disorders	Endocrine disorders (thyroid, pituitary, adrenal, pancreas) Calcium metabolism disorders Electrolyte imbalance Uremia Hepatic failure Porphyria
Exogenous substances	*Substance abuse*: alcohol (intoxication, withdrawal), amphetamines, cannabis, cocaine, stimulants, hallucinogens *Medications*: antihistamines, anticholinergics, baclofen, barbiturates, cephalosporines, chloroquine, cimetidine, corticosteroids, cycloserine, digitalis, disopyramide, disulfiram, ephedrine, indomethacin, INH, Levodopa, methyldopa, propoxyphene, propanolol, reserpine, salicylates, theophylline, TCAs, vincristine
Nutritional deficiencies	Thiamine, niacin, cyanocobalamin, folic acid
Vascular abnormalities	Cerebral hemorrhage, collagen diseases, aneurysms, hypertensive encephalopathy
Infections	Meningitis, encephalitis, endocarditis, malaria, typhoid
Others	Normal pressure hydrocephalus, temporal epilepsy, dementias, Wilson's disease

- **Substance-induced psychotic disorder**: developing during or within 1 month of substance intoxication or withdrawal or due to a medication use, not occurring exclusively during a delirium

- **Psychotic disorder NOS**: psychotic sx do not fit criteria for any specific psychotic disorder

TREATMENT—BIOLOGICAL: ANTIPSYCHOTICS FOLLOW-UP

- **Suggested baseline assessments and frequency**:

Assess for physical conditions:

TABLE 6.5.   Medical Monitoring of Patients on Antipsychotic Medications

Vital signs	When
Body weight and height and body mass index (BMI), waist size	Each visit for 6 months then q 3 months
CBC	When indicated (regularly if on clozapine)
Electrolytes, renal, liver, thyroid function tests	Annually
Pregnancy test	If indicated
Toxicology (drug screen, heavy metal screen)	When indicated
Infectious diseases (syphilis, hepatitis C, and HIV)	If indicated
EEG, brain imaging	If clinically indicated

TABLE 6.6.   Body Mass Index*

BMI	Classification	4' 10"	5' 0"	5' 4"	5' 8"	6' 0"	6' 4"
<19	Underweight	<91	<97	<110	<125	<140	<156
19–24	Healthy weight	91–119	97–127	110–144	125–163	140–183	156–204
25–29	Overweight	120–143	128–152	145–173	164–196	184–220	205–245
30–40	Obese	144–191	153–204	174–233	197–262	221–293	246–328
>40	Very obese	>191	>204	>233	>262	>293	>328

Height in feet and inches; weight in pounds.

*BMI = kg/m^2 = (weight in pounds) (703)/(height in inches)^2. Anorectants appropriate if BMI ≥30 (with comorbidities ≥27); surgery an option if BMI > 40 (with comorbidities 35–40).

An increase in 1 BMI unit suggests need for intervention (closer monitoring, weight management program, possible adjunctive treatment to reduce weight, change of antipsychotic medication).

Source: National Institutes of Health's National Heart Lung and Blood Institute, www.nhlbi.nih.gov.

TABLE 6.7.   Assess for Side Effects of Treatment

Diabetes; fasting blood sugar and/ or Hb A1c	Rx onset, 4 months, then annually
Lipid panel	q yr
QTc prolongation (ECG, K+)	If cardiac risk factor; if change in dose of medications; if use of medications that can affect QTc
Hyperprolactinemia (amenorrhea, galactorrhea, menstrual irregularities, osteoporosis, may be associated with prolactin-secreting pituitary adenomas?)	Check levels if presence of sx and annually, if use of medication is known to increase the prolactin level. Consider other causes of hyperprolactinemia if very elevated (if > 200 ng/mL: MRI scan of sella turcica). Prolactin levels should be measured in the AM and hyperprolactinemia is defined as levels >25 ng/mL
Extrapyramidal signs, akathisia	Weekly until dose stable then q visit
Tardive dyskinesia (abnormal involuntary movements)	q 6 months if use of first-generation antipsychotics (3 if at risk patients), q 12 months for second-generation antipsychotics (6 if at risk); use AIMS
Vision	Ask if change, exam q 2 yr if pts <40, q yr in pts >40

TABLE 6.8.   Metabolic Syndrome: The New International Diabetes Federation (IDF) Definition

Central obesity: waist circumference ≥ 94 cm (>40 inches) for Europid men and ≥ 80 cm (>35 inches) for Europid women (specific values for other ethnic groups)

Plus any 2 of the following 4 factors:
- Raised TG level: ≥150 mg/dL or current specific rx for this
- Reduced HDL cholesterol: <40 mg/dL in males and <50 mg/dL in females, or current specific rx for this
- Raised blood pressure: systolic BP ≥ 130 or diastolic BP ≥ 85 mm Hg, or rx of previously diagnosed hypertension
- Raised fasting plasma glucose (FPG) ≥ 100 mg/dL or previously diagnosed type 2 diabetes

If above 100 mg/dL, OGTT is strongly recommended but is not necessary to define presence of the syndrome

TABLE 6.9.   Lipids Guidelines (National Cholesterol Education Program, NCEP)

Total cholesterol	Desirable if <200 mg/dL
Triglycerides	Normal if <150 mg/dL
LDL cholesterol	Normal if <100 mg/dL
HDL cholesterol	Low if <40 mg/ dL

Source: International Diabetes Federation, www.idf.org

TABLE 6.10.   ADA Criteria for Diagnosis of Diabetes

Fasting plasma glucose	Diagnosis	2-Hr OGTT
≥126 mg/ dL	Diabetes mellitus	≥200 mg/dL
100–125 mg/dL IFG	Prediabetes	140–199 mg/dL IGT
<100 mg/dL	Normal	<140 mg/dL

Source: American Diabetes Association. (2006). Standards of medical care in diabetes. *Diabetes Care, 29* (Suppl. 1), s4–s42. Retrieved October 28, 2010 from: http://care.diabetesjournals.org/content/29/suppl_1/s4.full

Fasting is defined as no caloric intake for 8 hours; for oral glucose tolerance test (OGTT): loading glucose should contain 75 g of anhydrous glucose dissolved in water and glucose is measured 2 hours after loading dose; random plasma glucose of ≥200 mg/dL indicated diabetes diagnosis.

HbA1c values reflect changes in glycemic control over a period of 120 days, thus will lag several months behind abnormalities in fasting and post-prandial glucose.

Many medications ↑ glucose levels (e.g., antipsychotics, diuretics, β-blockers, clonidine, protease inhibitors, corticosteroids, hormones, lithium, oral contraceptives, phenytoin).

Many medications ↑ lipid levels (e.g., antipsychotics, interferons, β-blockers, hormones, diuretics, protease inhibitors, oral contraceptives).

TABLE 6.11.   Recommendations for Weight Gain

Prior to treatment	Discuss life style, start nutrition (low fat, reduced calorie meals) and exercise education
Exercise	Walking, jogging, swimming at least 30 min each time, at least 3× wkly or "10,000 steps a day"
Diet	Eat smaller portions of 3 meals a day. ↓ Excess fats; eat lean meats, ↑ vegetables, salads, fruits; ↓ Carbohydrate like soft drinks, desserts, candy, gravies, potatoes, white bread. Avoid snacks
Monitoring from the onset of treatment	Monitor personal and family hx: q year **Monitor weight, height, BMI** at baseline, q wk in the first 2 months, at 3 months then q yr Monitor waist circumference at baseline and q yr **Monitor BP** at baseline, at 3 months then q yr **Monitor fasting glucose** at baseline, at 3 months and q yr **Monitor fasting lipids** at baseline, at 3 months then q yr
If weight gain >10 lbs in the first 4–6 wks	May add nizatidine (Axid) 300 mg bid or topiramate (Topamax) 100–200 mg/d or amantadine (Symmetrel) 100 mg bid to the antipsychotic. Continue adjunct until appetite ↓ then taper off. Continue to monitor weight, diet; at each visit; may need a nutritionist consultation (food intake diary, wellness clinic for exercise, diet program)

Other metabolic issues to consider with atypical antipsychotics:

- **Role of cytochrome P450 enzymes in antipsychotic metabolism**: significant; clozapine (metabolized by CYP1A2), risperidone (by 2D6), quetiapine and ziprasidone (by 3A4), aripiprazole (by 2D6 and 3A4). Hepatic metabolism → drug–drug interactions.
- **Effect of smoking**: ↑ metabolism of drugs via CYP 1A2 (clozapine and olanzapine). Caution pts who stop smoking in the hospital and restart after discharge.

Name: _____
Date: _____
Prescribing Practitioner: _____
INITIAL AIMS ASSESSMENT   **DATE OF LAST ASSESSMENT**
Complete AIMS examination procedure before rating.
CODES   0=None   1=Minimal, may be extreme normal   2=Mild   3=Moderate   4=Severe
Movement ratings:
Rate highest severity observed.
Rate movements that occur upon activation one less than those observed spontaneously
Either before or after completing the Examination Procedure: observe the pt unobtrusively at rest (eg, in waiting room).
  The chair to be used in this examination should be a hard, firm one without arms.

1: Ask pt whether there is anything in his/her mouth (e.g., gum, candy, etc) and if there so, to remove it.
2: Ask pt about the current condition of his/her teeth. Ask pt if he/she wears dentures. Do teeth or dentures bother pt now?
3: Ask pt whether he/she notices any movements in mouth, face, hands, or feet. If yes, ask to describe and to what extent
   they currently bother patient and/or interfere with his/her activities.
4: Have pt sit in chair with hands on knees, legs slightly apart, and feet flat on floor. (Look at entire body for movements
   while in this position).
5: Ask pt to sit with hands hanging unsupported. If male, between legs, if female, and wearing a dress, hanging over
   knees. (Observe hands and other body areas).
6: Ask pt to open mouth. (Observe tongue at rest within mouth). Do this twice.
7: Ask pt to protrude tongue. (Observe abnormalities of tongue movement).
8: Ask pt to tap thumb, with each finger, as rapidly as possible for 10–15 seconds: separately with right hand, then with
   left hand. (Observe facial and leg movements). [Activated]
9: Flex and extend pt's left and right arms, one at a time. (Note any rigidity and rate it).
10: Ask pt to stand up. (Observe in profile. Observe all body areas again, hip included).
11: Ask pt to extend both arms outstretched in front with palms down. (Observe trunk, legs, and mouth.) [Activated]
12: Have pt walk a few paces, turn, and walk back to chair. (Observe hands and gait.) Do this twice. [Activated]

Facial and Oral Movements	1. Muscles of facial expression (e.g., movements of forehead, eyebrows, periorbital area, cheeks) Include frowning, blinking, grimacing of upper face.	0 1 2 3 4
	2. Lips and perioral area (e.g., pouting, puckering, smacking)	0 1 2 3 4
	3. Jaw (e.g., biting, clenching, chewing, mouth opening, lateral movements)	0 1 2 3 4
	4. Tongue (rate only increases in movement both in/out of mouth, NOT inability to sustain movement	0 1 2 3 4
Extremity Movements	5. Upper (i.e., arms, wrists, hands, fingers) Include choreic movements (i.e., rapid, objectively purposeless, irregular, spontaneous), athetoid movements (i.e., slow, irregular, complex, serpentine). Do NOT include tremor (ie, repetitive, regular, rhythmic)	0 1 2 3 4
	6. Lower (i.e., legs, knees, ankles, toes) (e.g., lateral knee movement, foot tapping, heel dropping, foot squirming, inversion and eversion of foot	0 1 2 3 4
Trunk	7. Neck, shoulders, hip (i.e., rocking, twisting, squirming, pelvic gyrations) Include diaphragmatic movements	0 1 2 3 4
Global Judgments	8. Overall severity of abnormal movements	0 1 2 3 4
	9. Incapacitation due to abnormal movements	0 1 2 3 4
	10. Patient's awareness of abnormal movements (Pt report only) [Rating scale: 0 = no awareness; 1=aware, no distress; 2=aware, mild distress; 3=aware, moderate distress; 4=aware, severe distress]	0 1 2 3 4
Dental Status [Score 0 for No; 1 for Yes]	11. Any current problems with teeth and/or dentures?	No Yes
	12. Does pt wear dentures?	No Yes
	13. Edentia?	No Yes
	14. Do movements disappear in sleep?	No Yes
Score:		

FIGURE 6.1.   Abnormal Involuntary Movement Scale (AIMS).
Source: National Institute of Mental Health.

Commonly used antipsychotic medications:

TABLE 6.12. Overall Potency of the First Generation of Antipsychotics (FGA)

High-potency agents	Fluphenazine, haloperidol, pimozide, thiothixene, trifluoperazine
Mid-potency agents	Loxapine, molindone, perphenazine
Low-potency agents	Chlorpromazine, mesoridazine, thioridazine

TREATMENT GENERALITIES

(1) **Usual target dose is for FGA: 400–800 mg/d CPZ equivalents or 6–12 mg/d haloperidol equivalents** (doses lower for children and elderly) for control of positive symptoms without EPS. The objective is adequate rx of co-occurring syndromes, ↓ SE (specific issues with each antipsychotic), ↑ nonpharmacologic strategies

(2) **Minimum adequate duration: 4–6 weeks,** change antipsychotic if no response within 12 weeks

(3) **Depot antipsychotic if noncompliant**

(4) **Use clozapine within 6 months of nonresponse**

LIST OF ANTIPSYCHOTICS

TABLE 6.13. List of Antipsychotics

First-generation agents: FGA (dopamine receptor antagonists): Phenothiazines

Antipsychotic	Brand name	Half-life (h)	Dose range (mg/day) single usual dose: S.IM (mg)	EPS/TD	Prolactin	Weight	Glucose	Lipid	QTc Prol.	Sedation	Potency (mg of drug = 100 mg of chlorpromazine)	Anticholinergic	Hypotension	Particular risks
Chlorpromazine	Thorazine Only generic+	30 (tid)	300–1,000 start: 50–100 S.IM: 25–50	Low	+++	++			+	+++	Low 100	Moderate	High	Photosensitivity, rare cytopenia DDI: guanethidine, meperidine, paroxetine, pindolol, quinidones, β- blockers, ziprasidone
Fluphenazine	Prolixin Generic+	33 (tid)	5–20 start: 5 S.IM: 2–5	High	+++	+			+/-	++	High 1–3	Very low	Very low	GI upset, headaches, edema, leukopenia, akathisia DDI: guanethidine, paroxetine, quinidones
Mesoridazine	Serentil	24–48	150–400		+++	++			++	+++	Low 50	+++		Mesoridazine is the major metabolite of Melleril, may ↑ QTc
Perphenazine	Trilafon Generic+	10 (tid)	16–64 start: 4–8	High	+++	+	+ ?	+ ?	0	+	Medium 8–10	0	Low Low	Anorexia, rare cytopenias hepatotoxicity DDI: paroxetine, quinidones

Drug													Notes
Thioridazine Mellaril Only generic +	24	300–800	Low	++	+	+?	+?	+++	+++	Low 100	High	high	Retrograde ejaculation, ↓ libido, cardiotoxicity (T-wave inversions, dose-related ↑ QTC, torsade-de-pointe) (**Black box**); Check ECG, K+ DDI: fluoxetine, paroxetine, fluvoxamine, propanolol, pindolol
Trifluoperazine Stelazine Generic+	24 (bid)	5–20 start: 2–5 S.IM: 1–2	High	+++	+			+	++	High 3–5	Low	Low	DDI: alcohol, cisapride, guanethidine, metrizamide, paroxetine
First-generation agents: FGA (dopamine receptor antagonists): butyrophenone													
Haloperidol Haldol Generic+	20 (1–3× daily)	4–20 start: 2–5 S.IM: 2–6	+++	+++	+	0	0	0	++	High 2.5	0	0	Akathisia, anxiety, lethargy DDI: azole antifungals, carbamazepine, rifampin, rifabutin

Continued

TABLE 6.13. List of Antipsychotics Continued

Antipsychotic	Brand name	Half-life (h)	Dose range (mg/day) single usual dose. S.IM (mg)	EPS/TD	Prolactin	Weight	Glucose	Lipid	QTc Prol.	Sedation	Potency (mg of drug = 100mg of chlorpromazine)	Anticholinergic	Hypotension	Particular risks
Others (dopamine receptor antagonists)														
Loxapine	Loxitane Generic+	12–19 (1–2x daily)	50–150 start: 20 S.IM. 12.5–50	High	+++	+			+	++	Medium 10–20	Medium	Medium	DDI: barbiturates, general anesthetics, opiate agonists, radiopaque contrast agents, tricyclic antidepressants
Molindone	Moban	1.5 (3–4x daily)	50–150 start: 50–75	High	+++	+			+	++	Medium 6–10	Medium	Low	DDI: CNS depressants, anticonvulsants, tetracycline
Thiothixene	Navane Generic+	34 (2–3x daily)	15–50 start: 5–10 S.IM. 2–4	High	+++	+			+	+	High 2–5	Low	Low	Agitation, photosensitivity, hepatotoxicity DDI: guanethidine
Second-generation agents: SGA (novel or atypical or serotonin–dopamine antagonists)														
Aripiprazole	Ability	75 (once/day)	15–30 start: 10–15	0 akathisia	0	0	0	0	0	+	6–7.5	0	0	Nausea, anxiety vomiting headaches DDI: carbamazepine, fluoxetine, ketoconazole, paroxetine, quinidine, St John's wort

Drug	Brand		Dose													Comments
Clozapine	Clozaril Fazaclo Generic+	12 (bid)	150–600 start: 12.5 (half of a 25 mg tab)	0 akathisia	0	+++	+++	+++	+++	0	+++	50	+++	+++	Agranulocytosis, seizures, myocarditis, hypersalivation, weight gain DDI: barbiturates, caffeine, carbamazepine, cimetidine, erythromycin, phenytoin, rifampin, ritonavir, smoking, SSRIs, St John's wort
Olanzapine	Zyprexa	33 (once/day)	10–30 start: 5–10	0 akathisia	0	+++	+++	+++	+	0	+++	4–5	++	+	Headache, agitation, rhinitis, hepatitis. Avoid using in pts with diabetes, high triglycerides and / or low HDL DDI: carbamazepine, fluvoxamine, rifampin, smoking, St John's wort

Continued

TABLE 6.13. List of Antipsychotics   Continued

Antipsychotic	Brand name	Half-life (h)	Dose range (mg/day) single usual dose: S.IM (mg)	EPS/TD	Prolactin	Weight	Glucose	Lipid	QTc Prol.	Sedation	Potency (mg of drug = 100 mg of chlorpromazine)	Anticholinergic	Hypotension	Particular risks
Quetiapine	Seroquel	6 (bid)	300–800 start: 50	Akathisia	0	++	++	++	0	++	75–80	0	++	Cataracts? Agitation, headache DOI: erythromycin, fluconazole, ketoconazole, phenytoin, St John's wort, thioridazine, valproate
Risperidone	Risperdal Generic+	24 (once/ day)	4–6 start: 1–2	+	+++	++	++	++	+	+	1–2	0	+	Nausea, tremor, anxiety DOI: carbamazepine, cimetidine, fluoxetine, paroxetine, phenytoin, rifampin, tricyclic antidepressants. Valproic acid, topiramate, lamotrigine, mirtazapine, and venlafaxine Do not increase level of risperidone

Continued

Generic	Brand	Half-life (h)	Dose (mg/day)										Comments
Paliperidone	Invega	23 (once/day)	6–9 (max 12) start: 6mg in AM	+ / ++ if dose > 6 mg	+++ / ++++ if dose > 6 mg	++	++	++	+	+		+	Is the major active metabolite of risperidone. No adjustment needed if mild hepatic dysfunction. DDI: carbamazepine ↓ level of paliperidone
Iloperidone	Fanapt	18–31 (bid)	6–12 mg bid start: 1 mg bid, ↑ very slowly	+	+	++	?	?	+++	+	++	0	QTc prolongation, orthostatic hypotension. Not a first-line antipsychotic. Fanapt dose should be reduced by one-half when given with strong CYP2D6 inhibitors (fluoxetine, paroxetine) or strong CYP3A4 inhibitors (ketoconazole, clarithromycin)
Ziprasidone	Geodon	7 (1–2×/day, usually 1/3 in AM and 2/3 in PM)	120–200 start: 40–80	Oakathisia	+	0	0	0	++	0	5–20	0	Headache, weakness. DDI: Carbamazepine, diuretics, moxifloxacin, mefloquine, quinidine, sotalol, many antiarrhytmics, thioridazine, tricyclic antidepressants, chlorpromazine, mesoridazine, pimozide. Food increase absorption up to two-fold

TABLE 6.13.   List of Antipsychotics   Continued

Antipsychotic	Brand name	Half-life (h)	Dose range (mg/day); single usual dose: S.IM (mg)	EPS/TD	Prolactin	Weight	Glucose	Lipid	QTc Prol.	Sedation	Potency (mg of drug = 100 mg of chlorpromazine)	Anticholinergic	Hypotension	Particular risks
Asenapine	Saphris (sublingual only)	24 hr	Schizophrenia: 5 mg bid Bipolar disorders: 10 mg bid	+ Akathisia	+	++	?	?	++	++	?	0	+	In schizophrenia: akathisia, oral hypoesthesia, somnolence In bipolar disorder: somnolence, dizziness, EPS other than akathisia, and weight increased
First generation: FGA (dopamine receptor antagonist); diphenylbutylpiperidine														
Pimozide	Orap	50	1–10	High	+++	+			++	Low	High 1–2	Low	Low	Cardiotoxicity (↑ QT) DDI: clarithromycin (Biaxin), erythromycin, azithromycin (Zithromax), dirithromycin (Dynabac)

Abbreviations used: FGA: first-generation antipsychotics (typical); SGA: second-generation antipsychotics (atypical); DDI: drug–drug interactions.

TABLE 6.14. Management of Sedation Due to Antipsychotics

Can occur with first- and second-generation antipsychotics, **more severe with low potency FGA than SGA**

Distinguish **between sedation and negative sx** (avolition, withdrawal, anhedonia)

Is pt's **cognitive impairment** due to the sedative properties?

Give most of the dose **at bedtime**

R/O medical condition that produce sedation (hypothyroidism, obstructive sleep apnea, restless legs syndrome)

Review the pt's **medication list** to ↓ or eliminate sedating medications if possible; most sedating drugs are: TCAs and mirtazapine, mood stabilizers (VPA, but also carbamazepine, lithium, lamotrigine)

Reduce antipsychotic if possible

Consider **switching to a less sedating** one such as aripiprazole or ziprasidone

Caffeine in AM or off-label bupropion (75–100 mg 1–2 times/day)

Stimulants: **controversial** as risk is to ↑ psychosis

Modafinil: 200 mg in AM (risk of ↑ psychosis)

TABLE 6.15. Treatment-Resistant Psychosis and Schizophrenia

Is the diagnosis accurate?

R/O severe psychotic bipolar disorder

● Is it a schizoaffective disorder?

● Consider additional studies (metabolic profiles, vitamin and hormones levels, VDRL, neuroexam, neuroimaging) to R/O brain tumor or neurodegenerative disease

Review previous treatments and effects: medications used, adjunct medicines

Evaluation of efficacy and tolerability of the antipsychotic treatment:

● Clinical deterioration after ↓ dosages or skipping doses to reduce SEs

● Adherence to rx (41–50% nonadherence, effects of the disease on cognition, paranoia): supervised setting may be needed

Treatment goal to reevaluate and psychosocial planning

Safety (suicidal risks, aggressivity)

Social supports, risk of homelessness

Change in medications: ↑ meds, switch to a better tolerated one, add a mood stabilizer (lithium for antisuicide effects, clozapine)

TABLE 6.16.   Atypical Antipsychotics and FDA-Approved Indications

Drug	Trade name	Approved indications
Aripiprazole	Abilify	**Schizophrenia**: acute and maintenance rx in adults and adolescents 13–17 yo **Bipolar I disorder**: acute and maintenance rx of manic and mixed episodes with or without psychosis (monotherapy in adult and pediatric 10–17 yo); or adjunct rx for bipolar mania for adult and pediatric 10–17 yo (with lithium or valproate) **Major depressive disorder** (adjunct to antidepressants) Agitation in adults with schizophrenia or bipolar I (mania or mixed)
Olanzapine	Zyprexa	**Schizophrenia**: acute and maintenance in adults **Bipolar I disorder**: in adults acute and maintenance in monotherapy or combination rx with valproate or lithium in bipolar disorder (manic or mixed) Treatment-resistant depression in adults Depressive episodes associated with bipolar I disorder in adults Agitation in schizophrenia and bipolar I mania in adults
Quetiapine	Seroquel	Bipolar depression **Bipolar I disorder**: either monotherapy or adjunct rx to lithium or divalproex for mania or maintenance rx for bipolar I disorder (as an adjunct to lithium or divalproex) **Schizophrenia**: acute and maintenance rx of schizophrenia (Seroquel and Seroquel XR)
Risperidone	Risperdal	**Schizophrenia**: in adults and adolescents 13–17 yo **Bipolar I disorder**: in adults (acute manic or mixed episodes: alone or with lithium or valproate) and alone in children and adolescents (10–17 yo) Treatment of irritability associated with autistic disorder in children and adolescents 5–16 yo
Ziprasidone	Geodon	Schizophrenia: in adults **Bipolar I disorder**: mania or mixed with or without psychotic features in adults Acute agitation in schizophrenia in adults
Clozapine	Clozaril	**Schizophrenia**: refractory schizophrenia Bipolar I disorder: mania Acute agitation in schizophrenia Reducing the risk of recurrent suicidal behavior in patients with schizophrenia or schizoaffective disorder
Paliperidone	Invega	**Schizophrenia**: acute and maintenance in adults **Schizoaffective disorders**: acute treatment as monotherapy; acute treatment as an adjunct to mood stabilizers and/or antidepressants in adults
Iloperidone	Fanapt	**Schizophrenia**: acute treatment in adults
Asenapine	Saphris	**Schizophrenia**: acute treatment in adults Manic or mixed episodes associated with bipolar 1 disorder: acute treatment in adults

Source: Manufacturers' prescribing information.

TABLE 6.17. Neurological Adverse Effects of Antipsychotics

Type	Disorder	Symptoms	Treatment	Prevention
Extrapyramidal (mostly typical antipsychotics or higher doses of risperidone)	Acute dystonic reaction, dystonic reactions	Sustained muscular spasm can involve neck, jaw, tongue, or entire body Oculogyric crisis (eyes' upward lateral movement), blepharospasm, glossopharyngeal dystonia, can be painful **(laryngospasm is life threatening)** Rare after 1 wk of treatment	IM or IV anticholinergics (diphenhydramine 50 mg, or benztropine 1–2 mg IM) or lorazepam 1–2 mg IM. May be prevented by benztropine 1 mg bid or tid at beginning of tx or trihexyphenidyl (Artane) 2–5 mg tid	More in young men R/O: seizures, TD Rx: Anticholinergic drugs; sometimes need to change antipsychotic Prevention: anticholinergics or not? Yes: may help compliance, use if higher risk for dystonia (>45), treat 4–6 wk if dystonia, then taper to stop; restart if return of symptoms No: 30–50% do not need it, use may ↑ risk of TD and toxicity, abuse liability
	Parkinson-like syndrome	Muscle stiffness (cogwheel), parkinsonian tremor (coarse tremor of upper extremities, tongue, jaw, occurs with movement and rest, slow), akinesia (zombie-like with slowness, blunted or flat affect, fatigue), cognitive impairment Mimic negative sx of schizophrenia or motor retardation of depression	↓ Dose, divide dosing, bed time dosing Rx: benztropine 1–2 mg bid, or diphenhydramine 25–50 mg bid–tid, or propanolol 20–30 mg tid or trihexyphenidyl (Artane) 2–5 mg tid	Use lowest dose possible Think quickly of "**mental parkinsonism**" (emotional indifference, blunted affect, anhedonia), "**social parkinsonism**" (↓ initiative, apathia, ↓ energy and social drive), "**cognitive parkinsonism**" (slow thought process, poor concentration)
	Akathisia	Restlessness, constant moving, dysphoria (risk of suicide) Frequently mistaken for anxiety, agitation, psychotic behavior	Propanolol 20–30 mg tid, or clonidine 0.1 mg tid or lorazepam 1 mg bid or clonazepam 0.5–1 mg bid, rare use of anticholinergics, possibly use of mirtazapine; reduce antipsychotic if possible or switch to atypical or clozapine	Use lowest dose possible, more frequent in women, older age, high potency antipsychotics, negative sx, iron deficiency, cognitive dysfunction, an associated affective disorder
	Rabbit syndrome	Involuntary chewing movements	Symmetrel 100–200 mg/d (max 300)	
	Tardive dyskinesia (see following table for rx)	Slow choreiform or tic-like movements (mostly tongue and facial muscles or whole body). ↑ risks in aged, organic brain syndrome, ♀, high doses of medications, simultaneous multiple antipsychotics, long duration of tx. Develops over months or years. **May be irreversible**	No real rx Try to discontinue the antipsychotic if possible May change to another class of antipsychotic if medication still needed, possibly SGA See agents used in Fogel's cocktail	If typical antipsychotics: use lowest dose possible Use atypical antipsychotics (10× less TD than with typical) Clozapine has very low risk of TD Consider ECT Risk of vicious cycle as sx may disappear with ↑ dosage of antipsychotic Drug holidays may worsen it Use Abnormal Involuntary Movement Scale (**AIMS**)

Continued

TABLE 6.17.   Neurological Adverse Effects of Antipsychotics   Continued

Type	Disorder	Symptoms	Treatment	Prevention
Sedation		Mistaken for oppositional behavior	↓ Dose or use less sedative antipsychotic	Use a q hr schedule
Central anticholinergic effects		Mild anxiety up to toxic delirium or coma; restlessness, agitation up to confusion, incoherence disorientation, V/A hallucinations, memory problems, seizures, stupor, vasodilatation (warm dry skin, flushed face, dry mouth, fever), blurred vision, dilated pupils, absent bowel sounds	Stop antipsychotic Close supervision (cardiac monitor) Physostigmine 1–2 mg IM or slow IV (1 mg/ min) to be repeated q 30 min then q 12 hr as needed (not if bladder, bowel obstruction, asthma, glaucoma, heart Pbs). Risk cholinergic overdosage (salivation, sweating) needing to be treated with atropine (0.5 mg for each mg of physostigmine)	Monitor
Epileptogenic effects	Evaluate for organic cause (particularly if acute onset of psychosis)	Differentiate postictal psychosis, complex partial seizures, absence seizures The majority of pts with psychotic disorders and treated with antipsychotics have tonic-clonic seizures		Avoid rapid ↑ doses Risk ↑ if organic brain lesion or prior seizures, ↑ with low potency drugs Usually at the start of the antipsychotic or if unstable blood levels Molindone may have a higher seizure threshold, or use a drug effective at a lower dose Caution with drug interactions Adapt antiseizure medication to the types of seizures: **Grand mal**: carbamazepine, valproate, phenytoin Secondary absence seizures: valproate **Primary absence seizures**: first line = ethosuximide; second line: valproate, clonazepam **Partial seizures**: first line: carbamazepine, phenytoin; second line: phenobarbital, primidone, valproate
Neuroleptic malignant syndrome (see Table 6.19)		Muscular rigidity, cogwheeling, fever, confusion, tachycardia, sweating, hypertension developing in hours or 1–2 days. ↑↑↑ CPK. Look for rhabdomyolysis with myoglobinemia	Stop meds immediately Medical support Consider rx with dantrolene or bromocriptine	If hx of NMS, keep well hydrated particularly in hot weather. If happened on FGA, change to SGA May not reoccur until later reexposure to antipsychotics

TABLE 6.18. Neuroleptic Discontinuation Syndromes

Acute motor syndromes: acute dystonias, dyskinesias, akathisias, emergent parkinsonism **Chronic motor syndromes**: chronic tardive dyskinesia, chronic akathisia **Acute nonmotor syndromes**: nausea, vomiting, insomnia, diarrhea, myalgia, fatigue, anxiety, paresthesias, disturbance in temperature regulation, hyperalgesia **Chronic nonmotor syndromes**: dysthymias, concentration problems	Avoid abrupt discontinuation

Adapted from Tranter, R., & Healy, D. (1998). Neuroleptic discontinuation syndromes. *Journal of Psychopharmacology, 12,* 401–406.

Treatment of tardive dyskinesia (TD); Fogel's cocktail: the goal is to reduce glutamatergic neurotransmission with a temporary rx (6–18 months) to alleviate TD (utilizing agents that act as NMDA-type glutamate receptor antagonists and GABA-A receptor agonists). It is possible to use a single agent, for example, acamprosate (*Campral*) that has both activities.

Separate agents having these activities can be combined. An ion channel blocker can be used as an adjunct.

TABLE 6.19. Treatment of Tardive Dyskinesia

Possible agents to start with*	**Omega-3 fatty acids**: Start: 2–4 g of EPA (or EPA +DHA)/d; Max: 6–10 g total omega-3/d **Vitamin E**: Start: 400 IU bid, max dosage: 800 IU bid. May be used at higher doses if used alone (1,200–2,000 IU) **Taurine**: Start: 500 mg bid, max 2,000 mg bid **Magnesium salts**: start dose: 200–250 mg elemental Mg++ bid, max: 500 mg bid (caution if renal failure), works as an ion channel blocker; can be administered alone **May change the antipsychotic to Clozapine**: blood toxicity **Pyridixin (vitamin B6) may be given+++**: start 100 mg/d, increasing weekly in 100 mg increments to a total of 400 mg/d (some go up to 1,400 mg/day) **Melatonin**: 10 mg/d

Medications used:
Nimodipine *(Nimotop)*: Calcium channel blocker (officially approved only for subarachnoid hemorrhage): Start: 30 mg bid, max 30 mg qid. Could use verapamil instead
Dextrometorphan *(Robitussin)*: is a glutamate antagonist; dosage: 30 mg bid–qid
Acamprosate *(Campral)*, approved in the United States for prevention of ETOH relapse; interacts with glutamate and is also a GabaA agonist; dosage: 666 mg tid, SE: nausea
Namenda *(Memantine)*: approved in the United States for Alzheimer's type dementia; dopamine agonist, NMDA antagonist or partial agonist, dosage: 5 mg tid; SE: dizziness, lightheadedness

To prevent TD (as per Hawkins):
• Vitamin B3 (niacin or niacinamide): 3,000 mg
• Vitamin C: 3,000 mg
• Vitamin B6: 400 mg
• Vitamin E: 400 IU
Treatment of TD with manganese/B3 (as per Kunin): between 15 and 60 mg Mn-chelate (begin with low dose of 5 mg tid) and increase accordingly to symptoms; may aggravate dyskinesia at high doses; it is possible that about 20 mg/d can prevent TD; vitamin B3 is used in refractory cases (divided doses 500–1,500 mg/d)
Lecithin (phosphatidylcholine) treatment: 20 g or more for general cases; 50 g/d or more for difficult cases

See also Lemmo, *W. Nutritional Treatment of Tardive Dyskinesia.* Retrieved September 4, 2010 from: http://www.alternativementalhealth.com/articles/td.htm; Lerner, V., Miodownik, C., Kaptsan, A., Cohen, H., Matar, M., Loewenthal, U., & Kotler, M. (2001). Vitamin B(6) in the treatment of tardive dyskinesia: A double-blind, placebo-controlled, crossover study. *American Journal of Psychiatry, 158*(9), 1511–1514.

TABLE 6.20. Neuroleptic Malignant Syndrome (NMS)

Signs of NMS	Trunk or total body rigidity Diaphoresis, dysphagia, tremor, incontinence Delirium, confusion, coma Masseter spasm or trismus Tachycardia/tachypnea, labile BP Mixed respiratory and metabolic acidosis Increased temperature (may be a late sign) Leukocytosis Myoglobinuria Observe in PACU or ICU for at least 12 hr CPK levels > 10,000 IU/L is a presumptive sign of rhabdomyolysis and myoglobinuria
Risk factors	Dehydration, heat exhaustion, poor nutrition; prevalence 0.02–2.4% of pts exposed to neuroleptics
Treatment of NMS	Needs supportive measures, cooling, dantrolene (*Dantrium*) or bromocriptine (*Parlodel*): 7.5–45 mg/d tid; mortality is 10–20%

For more information, contact the Malignant Hyperthermia (MH) Hotline at (800) 644-9737 (for people outside the United States: (315) 464-7079). See also http://medical.mhaus.org/

TABLE 6.21.   Nonneurological Side Effects (SE) of Antipsychotics

Type	Mechanism/signs	Medications involved	Treatment
Sudden death	Premature to blame dopamine receptor antagonist action alone. Cases associated with other medical Pbs, treated also with other drugs Temperature dysregulation (heat stroke)	Pimozide prolongs QT Risk if concomitant use of drugs that inhibit the metabolism of the antipsychotic drug by the hepatic enzyme cytochrome P450 Antipsychotics may increase the risk of death in patients with dementia	
Orthostatic hypotension	Adrenergic blockade Syncopes, postural hypotension	More with low potency (chlorpromazine, thioridazine, clozapine) First few days of rx, more with IM injections	**Prevention**: monitor BP, rise gradually from bed, support hose, avoid caffeine, drink fluids, and add salt to food if no HTN Pure α-adrenergic pressor agents are the drugs of choice: metaraminol (Aramine) and NE (Levophed) **Do not give epinephrine** (paradoxical worsening of hypotension due to the β-adrenergic stimulating effect)
Hematological	Transient leucopenia (3,500 WBC), agranulocytosis (Mostly first 3 months, 1/10,000 pts, mortality: 30%) CBC if sore throat, fever. Rare thrombocytopenia, purpura, hemolytic anemia, pancytopenia	More with chlorpromazine, but seen with all Elderly females: rare Avoid combination of clozapine and carbamazepine or mirtazapine	Stop medication, transfer to medical facility
Peripheral anticholinergic effects	Dry mouth, dry nose, blurred vision, constipation, urinary retention, mydriasis, nausea, vomiting	Chlorpromazine (1%), mesoridazine, loxapine Particularly if multiple anticholinergic drugs are used together	Dry mouth: rinse mouth with water, use sugar-free candies or gum Constipation: laxatives Decrease dosage or switch to less anticholinergic drug Urinary retention: bethanechol (*Urecholine*) 20–40 mg/d
Endocrine	Blockade of dopamine receptor in tuberoinfundibular tract (increased prolactin) Galactorrhea, amenorrhea, gynecomastia, impotence	Clinical sx generally appear if prolactin levels $\geq$60–100 ng/mL Prolactin levels $\uparrow$ with haloperidol, risperidone, only high doses of olanzapine ($\geq$20 mg/d)	Change the antipsychotic drug: ziprazidone, quetiapine, clozapine are not associated with increased prolactine levels If hyperprolactinemia is not due to pregnancy, hypothyroidism, renal failure, pituitary, or parasellar tumor: consider adding a small dose of aripiprazole (will $\downarrow$ prolactin due to partial dopamine-agonist properties). Occasionally use bromocriptine (*Parlodel*) or cabergoline (risk of $\uparrow$ psychosis)

Continued

TABLE 6.21. Nonneurological Side Effects (SE) of Antipsychotics   Continued

Type	Mechanism/signs	Medications involved	Treatment
Sexual	Adrenergic blockade Impotence, ejaculatory disturbances, anorgasmia, painful orgasms Men and women Decreased libido	Thioridazine: ↓ libido, retrograde ejaculation	Selective phosphodiesterase (PDE) type 5 inhibitor: contraindicated with nitrates, caution with CYP3A4 inhibitors, little experience with women (Sildenafil 25–100 mg, 30 min to 1 hr prior to sex, Tadalafil 10–20 mg, 30 min to 1 hr prior to sex, Vardenafil 5 mg, 30 min to 1 hr prior to sex) Ciproheptadine 4–8 mg given shortly before intercourse (serotonin receptor antagonist, caution in mood disorders) Ejaculation problems: brompheniramine (*Dimetane*), ephedrine, phenylpropanolamine, imipramine (*Tofranil*)
Weight gain	Usually >5 kg within 2 months ↑ Type 2 diabetes mellitus (DM prevalence is increased even prior to rx in schizophrenia). DM may appear suddenly and with severe diabetic ketoacidosis even without weight gain	↑ Risk with clozapine, olanzapine (weight, diabetes) > risperidone > quetiapine	Monitor, diet, exercise. Risk of noncompliance. See Table 6.11 (strategies for managing weight) Less with molindone, loxapine, aripiprazole, ziprazidone
Dermatological	Allergic dermatitis, photosensitivity (sunburn) Skin eruptions (5%) in first few weeks (may remit spontaneously)	Chlorpromazine (also associated with blue–gray discoloration in areas exposed to sunlight)	Spend less than 30 min in the sun, use **sunscreens**
Ophthalmological	Retina pigmentation, blindness, benign pigmentation, lens deposits, cornea deposits Acute angle-closure glaucoma (due to anticholinergic SE)	Thioridazine if given 800 mg/d: risk of irreversible pigmentation of retina (starts with difficulty in night vision) Chlorpromazine: benign granular deposits (if ingestion of 1–3 kg of the drug during lifetime, no retinal damage, no impaired vision)	
Jaundice	Cholestatic jaundice in first 2 months of rx (abdominal pain, vomiting, flu-like sx, rash, eosinophilia, bilirubine in urine, ↑ bilirubinemia, ↑ hepatic transaminases). Sensitivity reaction?	Chlorpromazine; 1/1,000, also with promazine, thioridazine, prochlorperazine (Compazine) Rare with fluphenazine, trifluoperazine Haloperidol is the safest	Discontinue the medication

Continued

TABLE 6.21. Nonneurological Side Effects (SE) of Antipsychotics Continued

Type	Mechanism/signs	Medications involved	Treatment
Overdose	Suicide possible but with large doses	Thioridazine, mesoridazine can lead to heart block, ventricular fibrillation, death	Activated charcoal, if possible gastric lavage Supportive rx: seizures (diazepam, phenitoin), hypotension (norepinephrine, dopamine). **No epinephrine**
Cardiac	↑ QT and PR intervals, abnormal T wave, torsade de pointes QT > 0.44 ms: risk of sudden death (ventricular tachycardia or fibrillation)	Low potency drugs are more cardiotoxic: chlorpromazine, thioridazine Ziprazidone may prolong QTc interval	

TABLE 6.22. Neuroleptics and Pregnancy

Gradually stop during the first trimester if possible Gradually taper off before childbirth Resume medication postpartum by gradually increasing the dose Discourage breast-feeding **If used during pregnancy: minimize teratogenicity of typical antipsychotics** with low doses and high potency agents (risk of complicated childbirth, neonatal hepatic dysfunction, anticholinergic SE, EPS)	Close monitoring

TABLE 6.23. Antipsychotics in the Elderly

Antipsychotics are not FDA approved for treatment of dementia-related psychosis: **See black box warnings**
Risk of stroke and sudden cardiac death
Restrict antipsychotics to those with primary psychotic disorders or complex and dangerous behaviors that do not respond to nondrug treatments
Review and document risk factors for cardiovascular diseases (physical exam, lipid profile, fasting glucose, ECG, consultation with specialist)
Try nonpharmacological approaches first, document results
Review antipsychotics risks and benefits with pt and family
Use low dosages and increase gradually (risk is dose related)
Monitor effectiveness
Monitor CV symptoms: HR, BP, and BMI
Avoid using sedating antipsychotics for insomnia: if no psychiatric disorder

TREATMENT PRINCIPLES

- **Drug of choice**: the choice is on SE profile, prior response of the pt or family member, prior medical problems, affordability
- **Major principles**:
  - Define target sx.
  - **Use prior successful antipsychotic or base choice on adverse effect profile.**
  - **Minimal length of trial is 4–6 weeks**: if unsuccessful, use a different class. If negative experience at first dose, use a different drug (if not, may mean poor response, poor compliance); needs at least 4 weeks of rx with one antipsychotic (3 months for clozapine) to say that pt is not responding.
  - **Rare use of more than one antipsychotic at a time.**
  - If rx resistant, may add another drug.
  - **Use the lowest possible effective dosage.**
- **Acute psychosis**:
  1. **Select a neuroleptic**: start with one typical (FGA) or atypical (SGA). Usually atypical are better tolerated (risperidone, aripiprazole, quetiapine, olanzapine, or ziprasidone). Evaluate benefits and risks. If partial or nonresponse, switch to another of the typical or atypical that was not tried. If partial or nonresponse: Clozapine should be used alone. Do not switch if pt is unstable and do not switch multiple medications at once. Before switching, consider an adjuvant medication.

2. Switching strategies:

TABLE 6.24. Oral Antipsychotic Switching Strategies

Discontinue drug A completely and abruptly start drug B at full dosage: more convenient, risk of acute withdrawal
(as with clozapine: in this case extend cross-taping to ↓ rebound psychosis and cholinergic sx)
Slowly tapering drug A while starting drug B at full dosage (↓ risk of relapse but ↑ SE, more confusing if cognitive
impaired pts)
Slowly tapering drug A while slowly increasing drug B up to full dosage (↓ risk of relapse but ↑ SE, more confusing if
cognitive impaired pts)
NOTE (for 2 and 3): 3–7 days on an in-patient unit; 1–3 weeks in OPU

TABLE 6.25. Side Effects of Antipsychotics and Options for Switching to Other Neuroleptics

Akathisia: clozapine, olanzapine, quetiapine
Hyperprolactinemia: any atypical except risperidone
Insomnia: olanzapine, quetiapine at hs
Orthostatic hypotension: ziprasidone
Cardiac dysfunction: aripiprazole, olanzapine, quetiapine, risperidone
Diabetes: aripiprazole, quetiapine, ziprasidone
Sedation: aripiprazole, risperidone
Severe weight gain: aripiprazole, quetiapine, risperidone, ziprasidone

3. **First episode psychosis usually responds to lower dose of FGA or SGA.**

4. **Continue same treatment if adequate response and no intolerable SEs.**

- **Refractory illness**: 30% of pts with schizophrenia are considered "treatment refractory."

  - **If partial or nonresponse after clozapine alone**: add one atypical or a typical to the clozapine, or add ECT. If no response, consider combination rx: SGA + FGA or SGA + SGA or FGA + ECT or SGA + ECT or FGA + mood stabilizer or SGA + mood stabilizer such as lithium or anticonvulsants

  - **Failure to respond in the acute state**: possibility of an organic lesion, noncompliance, insufficient time; reexamine the stressors and the diagnosis.

  - **Looking at the main treatment-resistant syndrome**:

    - **If positive sx**: **use** clozapine, olanzapine, risperidone, high dose of quetiapine, augmentation with mood stabilizers, atypical + typical combination, ECT

    - **If hostility and aggression**: use clozapine, risperidone, quetiapine, olanzapine, augmentation with mood stabilizers (valproate), high dosages of β-blockers, benzodiazepines (but for short periods only), addition of SSRIs, ECT

    - **If negative sx**: use olanzapine, risperidone, clozapine, atypical + SSRI, clozapine + methylphenidate

    - **If obsessive-compulsive sx**: use atypical + SSRI; atypical + clomipramine; typical + SSRI

    - **If suicidal sx with or without depressive sx**: use clozapine; atypical + SSRI; atypical + TCA; atypical + mood stabilizer; ECT

  - **Use of megadose is rarely indicated**: A too "high" dose is when EPS side effects occur: usually for risperidone: 6 mg/d; olanzapine: mixed results on high doses 40–60 mg/d; quetiapine up to 1,800 mg/d; ziprasidone: 200 mg/d; aripiprazole: 30 mg/d; clozapine: 450 mg/d; haloperidol: 25 mg/d ; ↑↑ SE (EPS and hyperprolactinemia increases when D2 receptors occupancy >70–80%; fatal arrhythmias reported with high doses of olanzapine; dose-related EPS with ziprasidone) with rare advantages.

  - **Consider early use of clozapine if**: recurrent suicidality, violence, comorbid substance abuse, persistence of positive sx; More than 2 years, two failed trials with atypicals and one with typicals. Used in schizophrenic pts who cannot tolerate or are refractory to traditional antipsychotics; marked improvement in 30% of chronic pts and modest in 10–20%; may improve apathy, withdrawal, anhedonia, flat affect; risk reduction for suicidality.

TABLE 6.26.   Use of Clozapine: Clozaril National Registry at 1-800-448-5938

Indications	FDA approved for resistant schizophrenia, for ↓ in risk of recurrent suicidal behavior in pts with schizophrenia or schizoaffective disorder Non FDA approved: rx resistant bipolar disorder, violent pts with psychosis or other brain disorders not responsive to other rx, pts with tardive dyskinesia
Forms	Tablets: 12.5 mg scored, 25 mg, 50 mg, 100 mg scored, 200 mg (generic) Orally disintegrating tablets (Fazaclo ODT): 12.5, 25, 100 mg (scored)
Dosage	Start with 12.5 mg on day 1, then ↑ to 25 mg on day 2 then 25 mg bid on day 3. On day 6: ↑ to 25 mg in AM and 50 mg PM. On day 9: ↑ to 50 mg bid. On day 12: ↑ to 75 mg bid. On day 15: ↑ to 100 mg bid. On day 18: ↑ to 125 mg bid. On day 21: ↑ to 150 mg bid. On day 24: ↑ to 100 mg in AM and 200 mg PM. Then, might be ↑ wkly or biwkly by up to 100 mg **Target dose: 300–900 mg/d.** Do serum level for doses >600 mg/d. Steady-state clozapine levels > 350 ng/mL are usually therapeutic Doses > 300 mg/d should be divided; if need dose > 450 mg/d: increase only q wk up to max of 900 mg/d Max dose: 900 mg/d **Schedule:** 1/3 of the dose in AM and 2/3 in PM or tid. When dose reached is 400 mg, try to give bid **To discontinue:** gradually reduce dose over 1–2 wk It may take 6 months to see a full response. If no significant benefit after 6 wk, consider discontinuation to avoid risk of agranulocytosis Once a response has been achieved, the dose may often be gradually reduced, often to 300 mg without loss of effectiveness Retitrate if stopped for >3–4 days: +++
Monitoring +++	**Complete blood count**: before rx, q wk for 6 months, biweekly for months 6–12, then q 4 wk and 4 wk after discontinuation. Agranulocytosis risk: 1–2% Contraindicated if WBC < 3,500 or ANC < 2,000/mm³ **Patients rechallenged** after an episode of moderate leucopenia are at increased risk of agranulocytosis and must undergo wkly monitoring × 12 months Discontinue if ANC is < 1,000/mm³ or WBC < 2,000/mm³ or eosinophil count > 4,000/mm³ **Definitions**: **WBC**: White blood cell or leukocyte **ANC**: Absolute neutrophil count (total WBC count × %neutrophiles) **Neutrophils**: also known as: polymorphonuclear (poly), segmented cells or segs (mature polys), bands (immature polys). Add bands and segs to get total neutrophil percent **To calculate ANC**: total WBC count × percentage of neutrophils in the differential count Normal values: WBC ≥ 3,500/mm³ and ANC ≥ 2,000/mm³ WBC abnormalities: mild leukopenia: 3,000 to <3,500 moderate leukopenia: 2,000 to <3,000 severe leukopenia: <2,000 ANC abnormalities: mild granulocytopenia: 1,500 to <2,000 moderate granulocytopenia: 1,000 to <1,500 severe granulocytopenia: <1,000 Agranulocytosis: ANC < 500 (neutrophils/mm³) Start or continue Clozapine when: WBC ≥ 3,500 and ANC ≥ 2,000 Check WBC and ANC wkly for first 6 months, every 2 wk for the next 6 months and then every 4 wk If Clozapine is stopped, WBC count is to be continued for 4 wk Like all antipsychotics, monitor regularly: weight, BMI, waist circumference, BP, fasting blood glucose, liver function tests, ECG, general physical exam, baseline cardiac status, fasting lipid profile If to be discontinued: **rebound psychosis** may be seen unless slow tapering by 100 mg/wk or less over 6–8 wk especially if starting a new antipsychotic (cross-titration) Lack of consensus on optimal clozapine plasma level for therapeutic response: possibly > 350 ng/mL (is a high dosage with possible adverse effects; individualize dosing because levels may vary 50-fold among pts taking the same dosage)

Continued

TABLE 6.26.   Use of Clozapine: Clozaril National Registry at 1-800-448-5938   Continued

Side effects (SEs)	**Life-threatening SE**: (if need to abruptly stop clozapine: adding an anticholinergic drug such as benztropine may minimize the cholinergic rebound) **Agranulocytosis** (also if flu-like symptoms or infections) **Seizures** (are dose related): may require concomitant anticonvulsant use if doses > 550 mg/d **Hyperglycemia**: ↑ risk for diabetes Myocarditis or cardiomyopathy Pulmonary embolism **Cerebrovascular events** in elderly with dementia-related psychosis Neuroleptic malignant syndrome **Eosinophilia**: stop if >4,000/mm³ until count ↓ <3,000/mm³ **Hepatitis**: monitor LFTs **Others**: sedation (can wear off over time, frequent, if significant → give at q hr); weight gain (weight loss, exercise programs, and medical management as needed); sweating; increase salivation (may use hyoscine patches releasing 1 mg of hyoscine over a 72-hr period, or oral hyoscine or atropine drops but bitter taste; may use clonidine patch as well); hypotension If decision to stop clozapine and switch, 3 wk taper, starting after pt has reached full dosage on the new antipsychotic
Drug interactions	Cimetidine ↑ clozapine levels (use Ranitidine); Fluvoxamine ↑ clozapine levels by 2×; TCAs ↑ seizures risk, sedation, cardiac changes; risk of respiratory and cardiac arrest with other sedatives (benzo); smoking ↓ clozapine levels; caution with antihypertensive drugs; do not use with agents causing agranulocytosis
Special population	Caution in pts with glaucoma, enlarged prostate, uncontrolled epilepsy, hepatic, cardiac or renal impairment, elderly (lower doses), children and adolescents (↑ monitoring), Category B in pregnancy. Not to use when breast-feeding
Possible augmenting combinations (if partial response or rx-resistance)	Trial must be long enough (>3 months) with therapeutic plasma levels (250–350 ng/mL). Caution with valproic acid, lamotrigine, other anticonvulsants (carbamazepine, oxcarbazepine), other antipsychotics, lithium, benzodiazepines

- If poor compliance, consider long-acting medications: **Fluphenazine D (Prolixin decanoate), Haloperidol D (Haldol Decanoate), Risperdal Consta, Invega Sustena, Zyprexa Relprevv** (Zyprexa Relprevv Patient Care Program: requires prescriber, health care facility, pt, and pharmacy enrollment); see zyprexarelprevv.com to mitigate the risk of negative outcomes associated with postinjection delirium/sedation syndrome (PDSS).

TABLE 6.27.   Conversion Guide for Depot Antipsychotic Agents: Switching from Oral to Depot and from Depot to Oral

- Pt should be stabilized first on oral form of the medication
- Prophylactic antiparkinsonian medication should be considered. Use caution not to use excessive doses
- PO antipsychotic should be temporarily continued after pt received the depot form as follow:

Risperdal Consta: 3 wk of Risperdal PO

Haldol decanoate: ≤4–12 wk of Haldol PO

Prolixin decanoate: ≤2–4 wk of Prolixin PO

Invega Sustena: no need for oral supplementation

Risperdal Consta: 25–50 mg IM q 2 wk = 2–6 mg/d PO risperidone. Therapeutic levels sustained\<4–6 wk after Consta discontinuation

Invega Sustena: Day 1: 234 mg (deltoid); 1 wk later: 156 mg; then maintenance q 4 wk with 117 mg IM

Haldol decanoate: 100–200 mg q 4 wk IM = 10 mg/d PO Haldol (max initial dose of 100 mg IM due to risk of EPS); large range used from 50 mg IM q month (ineffective in 25% pts), to 100 mg IM q month (ineffective in 23% pts) to 200 mg IM q month (ineffective in 15%). This form requires 3–4 months to reach a steady-state plasma level

Prolixin decanoate: 12.5 mg q 2 wk IM = 8–10 mg/d of PO Prolixin

- Switching from depot to oral agents: start oral drug 1 month prior to discontinuing the depot medication

TABLE 6.28. Long-Acting Antipsychotics

Product	Brand name	Presentation	Starting dose	Maintenance dose	Frequency	Problems
Haloperidol	Haldol decanoate	50 mg of haldol (as 70.5 mg/ mL of haldol decanoate) 100 mg of haldol (as 141.04 mg/ mL of haldol decanoate)	Initial dose: 10–15 times the previous oral dose if on low doses (up to 10 mg/d) or up to 20 times the oral dose if pt on higher doses of the oral form Max initial dose is 100 mg. If higher dose needed, inject the remainder 7 days later	Only if pt has stabilized on oral form	q 4 wk with total dose. Half-life 3 wk	Deep IM gluteal injection
Fluphenazine	Prolixine decanoate	25 mg/mL	12.5 (0.5 mL)–25 mg (1 mL) IM or SC, usually given at 1/3–1/2 the oral dose. 12.5 mg (0.5 mL) is equivalent to 10 mg PO/d	12.5 mg (0.5 mL)–50 mg (2 mL)	q 2–4 wk Mean half-life: 6.8–9.6 days	Contraindicated in children <12
Risperidone	Risperdal-Consta	25 mg vial/kit, 37.5 mg vial/kit, 50 mg vial/kit	Only if pt tolerates well PO **Onset of action can be delayed for 2 wk,** continue or give oral antipsychotic for 3 wk after first injection	25—50 mg titration only q 4 wk Steady-state plasma conc. is reached after 4 injections of the Consta, and maintained for 4–6 wk after last injection	q 2 wk Max recommended dose is 50 mg q 2 wk Half-life: 3–6 days Elimination: 7–8 wk after last injection	If injection is missed for >28 days, cover with oral antipsychotic for 3 wk while reinitiating rx. If missed injection of <28 days, may not need oral coverage Must be kept refrigerated Drug is not in a solution and the whole syringe must be given **A new form** was marketed as a solution which may be given in the deltoid and is not painful In special populations: administer only if at least 2 mg/d/orally was tolerated (25 mg IM q 2 wk)
Paliperidone	Invega–Sustenna	234 mg, 156 mg, 117 mg, 78 mg. 39 mg	Initiation dosing: Day 1: 234 mg (deltoid) 1 wk later: 156 mg No need for oral supplementation	Maintenance: 117 mg (deltoid/ gluteal)	q 4 wk	R/O first any sensitivity to Risperdal or Invega; reduce dose if renal impairment If missed dose: • 4–6 wk late: resume monthly dosing • >6 wk–6 months late: dosing at previously stabilized dose with a first injection in deltoid and same dose 1 wk later, then one month later after the second dose (if pt was stabilized on 234 mg, the first 2 doses should be 156 mg each) • >6 months late: restart as an initiation dosing for the 2 first injections at 1-wk interval and then resume to previous stabilized dose
Olanzapine	Zyprexa Relprevv	Eq 210 mg base/ vial; eq 300 mg base/vial; eq 405 mg base/vial	See full prescribing information	See full prescribing information	q 2 or q 4 wk	Not studied in children <18 yr IM gluteal injection **Risk of postinjection delirium/sedation syndrome (PDSS):** pt must be observed in a registered facility for at least 3 hr after the injection (pt, health care provider, healthcare facility, and pharmacy must be enrolled in the Zyprexa Zyprevv Patient Care Program) 877-772-9390

- **Maintenance treatment in schizophrenia: is absolutely necessary to prevent relapses: +++**
  - 52% pts relapse on placebo vs 20% on maintenance tx. 10% may not relapse.
  - There is no measure to pinpoint who will or will not relapse.
  - The percentage of pts relapsing over time increases month after month.
  - Abrupt withdrawal of medication may produce a higher relapse rate than gradual withdrawal.
  - Untreated psychotic episodes may have deleterious effects on the natural course of schizophrenia.
  - Relapse rate after DC of medicine is 15% per month vs 1.5% when taking oral medication.
  - Depot medication prevents much rehospitalization.
  - Chronic rx with dosages titrated to the severity of remaining sx.
  - Dose adjustments are usually not more than q 3–4 months.
- **ECT**: *for catatonic pts or pts who cannot take antipsychotic drugs*

TREATMENT—NONBIOLOGICAL

All treatment should include psychoeducational interventions aimed at family functioning, problem solving, communication skills, relapse prevention, social skills training (to enhance socialization and vocational skills). Individual, supportive psychotherapy may be beneficial. Cognitive–behavioral therapy techniques may be helpful to manage suicidality, some residual symptoms such as hallucinations and delusions. Healthy lifestyle programs may be recommended (to prevent weight gain, encourage medical followups). Case management programs are also very useful in the community.

7 ■ ADJUSTMENT DISORDERS

Definition: Short-term maladaptive reactions to a psychosocial stressor; remit soon after the stressor ceases; sx appear within 3 months of the stressor's onset, resolve in 6 months or more if chronic stressor or one with lasting consequences.

Epidemiology: 2–8% of the population; more in single ♀; ♀ > ♂, stressors (school problems, parental rejection, divorce, substance abuse, moving, marital or financial problems), the most frequent psychiatric diagnosis in pts hospitalized for medical or surgical problems. 1 or x stressors; the severity of the stressor does not predict the severity of the disorder.

Etiology: psychodynamic factors (nature of the stressor, conscious and unconscious meaning of the stressor, pt's preexisting vulnerability/personality disorder, dysfunctional family, loss of a parent, relationship with parents, defense mechanisms, coping skills, life cycle time); family and genetic factors.

Diagnosis and clinical features: clinically significant sx (marked distress, impaired functioning), may start up to 3 months after the stressor and may last up to 6 months after the stressor ceases; acute or chronic. Sx vary with depressive, anxious, mixed features; possible physical sx (greater in children and elderly); others sx: assaultive behaviors, ↑ drinking, restless driving, withdrawal, insomnia, suicidal thoughts.

(1) **Adjustment disorder with depressed mood**: differential diagnosis is: MDD, uncomplicated bereavement

(2) **Adjustment disorder with anxiety**: differential diagnosis is anxiety disorders

(3) **Adjustment disorder with mixed anxiety and depressed mood**

(4) **Adjustment disorder with disturbance of conduct**: e.g., vandalism, fighting, truancy; differential diagnosis is: CD, antisocial personality disorder

(5) **Adjustment disorder with mixed disturbance of emotions and conduct**

(6) **Adjustment disorder unspecified**: other atypical reactions to stress.

Differential diagnosis: uncomplicated bereavement, MDD, brief psychotic disorder, GAD, somatization disorder, substance-related disorder, CD, identity problem, PTSD, acute stress disorder (trauma is outside of the range of normal human experience: rape, military combat, death camps, mass catastrophes)

Course and prognosis: usually good; adolescents may develop mood disorders or substance-related disorders and may need more time to recover.

Treatment: individual, group, family rx; be aware of secondary gains, make sure that the pt is held responsible for behaviors; crisis intervention, case management, rare hospitalizations. Pharmacotherapy: for specific sx, short periods of time (antianxiety or antidepressant/SSRIs agents, rarely antipsychotics).

Definition: sustained emotional states where the sense of control is lost and there is distress.

National organizations:

- **National Depressive and Manic Depressive Association**: http://www.ndma.org
- **Child and Adolescent Bipolar Foundation**: www.bpkids.org
- **Depressive Bipolar Support Alliance (DBSA)**: www.manicdepressive.org
- **National Institute of Mental Health**: http://www.nimh.gov/publicat/bipolar-menu.cfm

Resources:

- Practice parameters for the assessment and treatment of children and adolescents with bipolar disorder (*J Am Acad Child Adolesc Psychiatry*, 46(1), January 2007)
- National Collaborating Centre for Mental Health. Bipolar disorder: the management of bipolar disorder in adults, children, and adolescents, in primary and secondary care. Leicester (UK): British Psychological Society, Royal College of Psychiatrists; 2006.

Scales for mood disorders: Standard Assessment of Depressive Disorders (SADD), Mania Rating Scale, Manic State Rating Scale, Center for Epidemiologic Studies Depression Scale (CES-D), Geriatric Depression Rating Scale, Goldberg Depression Questionnaire, Quick Inventory of Depressive Symptomatology—Self-Report (QIDS-SR), Wakefield Self-Report Questionnaire, Beck Depression Inventory (21 questions, pt's self-rating), Hamilton Rating Scale for Depression (17–21 questions, therapist's rating); Mood Disorder Questionnaire (MDQ), the Goldberg Mania Questionnaire.

MAJOR DEPRESSION (MDD) AND BIPOLAR DISORDER (BPD)

Generalities

TABLE 8.1. Classification

Mood disorders	Type	Description
Depressive disorders	Major depressive disorder (MDD or unipolar disorder)	*Lasting >2 wk* may be superimposed on dysthymic disorder (double depression)
	Dysthymic disorder	>2 yr of depressed mood but not as severe as in a major depressive episode
Bipolar disorders	Bipolar I disorder	Either manic and depressive episodes or manic episodes alone (manic episode lasting >1 wk) A mixed episode is one (lasting >1 wk) in which a manic episode and a depressive episode occur almost daily
	Bipolar II disorder	*Episodes of major depression and hypomania* (episode of manic symptoms but not as severe and lasting >4 days)
	Cyclothymic disorder	>2 yr of hypomanic episodes and lower degree of depressive episodes

Specify the most recent episode: with psychotic features, with melancholic features (profound vegetative and cognitive sx including psychomotor retardation or agitation, sleep disturbances, anorexia or weight loss, and/or excessive guilt), with atypical features, with catatonic features, with postpartum onset.

Dysthymic and cyclothymic disorders may be at risk of developing bipolar I disorder.

TABLE 8.2. Etiology

Biologic factors	• **Biogenic amines**: 5-hydroxyindolacetic acid/5-HIAA (serotonin metabolite), homovanillic acid/HVA and 3-methoxy-4-hydroxyphenylglycol/MHPG (norepinephrine metabolite) ↓ in blood, urine, CSF of some pts. **Norepinephrine**: Antidepressant ↓ the sensitivity of 5-HT2 receptors; antidepressant action of noradrenergic drug like desipramine. **Serotonin**: Some pts with suicidal impulses have ↓ CSF conc. of serotonin metabolites and ↓ conc. of serotonin uptake sites on platelets; SSRIs block serotonin reuptake. **Dopamine**: DA activity may be ↓ in depression and ↑ in mania. Reserpine ↓ DA conc. → depression; Parkinson disease (has ↓ DA conc.) is associated with depression. Drugs that ↑ conc. of DA (tyrosine, amphetamine, bupropion) ↓ depression

Continued

TABLE 8.2.   Etiology   Continued

	• **Other factors**: GABA, vasopressin, endogenous opiates, second-messenger system (adenyl cyclase, phosphatidylinositol), calcium regulation • **Neuroendocrine regulation**: **adrenal axis**: ↑ secretion of cortisol in depression (stress → ↑ cortisol release). Dexamethasone-suppression test (DST): >50% of depressed pts fail to have a nl cortisol suppression response to a single dose of dexamethasone (limited validity). **Thyroid axis**: one-third pts with depression have a blunted release of TSH to an infusion of TRH (limited validity); possible association between a rapid cycle bipolar I disorder and hypothyroidism. **Growth hormone**: possible role. **Others**: ↓ nocturnal secretion of melatonin, ↓ FSH, ↓ LH, ↓ testosterone levels • **Sleep abnormalities**: delayed sleep onset, ↓ REM latency, ↑ length of first REM period, abnormal δ sleep • **Circadian rhythms**: transient ↓ depression with sleep deprivation; antidepressants change the internal biologic clocks • **Kindling suspected**: anticonvulsants are used in mood disorders (bipolar); Research on possible Biomarkers for Rapid Identification of Treatment Effectiveness in Major Depression, or BRITE-MD, measuring changes in brain-wave patterns using quantitative electroencephalography (QEEG) • **Brain imaging**: inconsistent ventricular enlargement: bipolar I disorder > MDD. Possible pathology of the limbic system (emotions), the basal ganglia, (posture, motion, cognition), the hypothalamus (sleep, appetite, sexual behavior, endocrine, immunologic, chronobiologic changes)
Genetic factors	• **Families studies**: In pts with bipolar I disorder: risk in first-degree relative is 8–18× for bipolar I and is 2–10× for MDD than in controls. 50% of all bipolar I disorder pts have at least one parent with a mood disorder. One parent with bipolar I disorder → 25% chance that any child will have a mood disorder; if both parents, the risk is 50–75% • **Twin studies**: concordance rates for bipolar I disorder is 33–90% in monozygotic twins, 5–25% in dizygotics; for MDD: concordance rate is 50% for monozygotic, 10–25% for dizygotic twins • **Linkage studies**: chromosomes 5, 11, and X may be involved
Psychologic factors	• **Stress** precedes the first episode of mood disorder in 25% of pts, 50% in elderly (loss of a spouse) • **Personality factors**: ↑ depression in oral dependent, obsessive-compulsive, hysteric personalities • **Psychodynamic factors in depression**: **Freud** (directing inward anger originally connected toward another person); **Melanie Klein** (inability to work successfully through the depressive position in childhood, the loved good object has been destroyed by the pt's own destructiveness; because of the lack of good object, the depressed person feels persecuted by the hated bad object); **Bibring** (tension is within the ego itself and not between the ego and superego); **Kohut** (when a parent does not validate a child's sense of self-esteem, the loss of self-esteem presents as depression). In mania: mania may be a defense against depression • **Cognitive theories**: negative distortions of life experiences, self-evaluation, pessimism, learned helplessness

Diagnosis and overview of treatment for each type

The goals are **safety** of the pt, complete diagnostic evaluation, and a treatment plan that addresses the acute and maintenance phases.

TABLE 8.3.   Hospitalization Necessary (Voluntary or Involuntary)

• Risk of suicide or homicide behaviors   • Hopelessness   • Out of control behaviors   • Need for special procedures   • Patient's inability to get food and shelter, and to take care of self   • Acute progressing symptoms   • Lack of support system

MAJOR DEPRESSIVE DISORDER (SINGLE OR RECURRENT)

Epidemiology: lifetime prevalence: 5–12%; M : F is 1 : 2; onset in the mid-20s; <40 yo in 50%, 10% after age 60. Depression may be missed (in ethnic minorities, pts with lower education).

Symptoms: episodes of depression lasting from **at least 2 wk** to 1 yr, during which the following sx appear:

TABLE 8.4.   Symptoms of Depression

Emotional	Cognitive	Physical	Other
• Depressed mood (sadness), irritability, helplessness, anxiety, hopelessness/despair, possible agitation, pervasive loss of interest (apathy), anhedonia (loss of pleasure in activities), interpersonal withdrawal, preoccupation with death/suicide	• Self-criticism, sense of worthlessness, guilt, pessimism, hopelessness, poor concentration, indecisiveness, obsessions, somatic complaints (elderly), ↓ memory, delusions, hallucinations (mood congruent such as guilt-ridden, self-condemning), rare catatonic stupor	• Anergia (lack of energy), insomnia (trouble falling asleep; awakening in the middle of the night, not going back to sleep; early awakening), or hypersomnia, anorexia or ↑ appetite, ↓ or ↑ weight (5% change in body weight), psychomotor retardation or agitation, ↓ libido, diurnal variation (most severe sx in AM), tachycardia, dry mouth and skin, constipation, dyspnea; if vague chronic pains (GI, cardiac, headaches, backaches unrelieved by analgesics) → think atypical depression	• Slow moving, tearful, sad facies

Adapted from Tomb, D. A. (1995). *Psychiatry* (5th ed.). Baltimore, MD: Williams & Wilkins. p. 44.

Differential diagnosis:

- **Mental disorders**: grief, bereavement (sadness, irritability, insomnia, ↓ concentration, ↓ functioning, preoccupation with the deceased; starts shortly after the loss of a loved one; is limited in time [<6 months]. R/O: MDD: vegetative sx exist >2 months after the loss, include guilt, worthlessness, psychomotor retardation, functional impairment, hallucinatory experiences); BPD (episodes of depression and episodes of mania; *a hx of a manic episode rules out the diagnosis of MDD*; bipolar disorder starts frequently with a depressive episode and the manic episode will start usually in less than 10 yr after the first depressive episode and not after five depressive episodes); dysthymia (chronic, low grade sx); PMS (in luteal phase); postpartum depression (only during postpartum); generalized anxiety disorder (no anhedonia or middle or terminal insomnia).

- **Medical disorders**: mood disorders due to a gl medical condition, or caused by a substance such as alcoholism (depression clears after 4 wk of abstinence), or due to stimulant withdrawal (clears in 1 wk of abstinence); any medication could be a factor; neurologic conditions (Parkinson, epilepsy, cerebrovascular diseases, tumors, dementias). Depression is more common in anterior brain lesions than posterior, if the epileptic focus is on the right side, if the tumors are in the diencephalic and temporal regions.

- **Pseudodementia**: depressed pts have cognitive deficits of an acute onset, with diurnal variation, guilt, and answer questions with "I don't know" instead of confabulating like in dementias.

- **Occupational problem**: includes job dissatisfaction, occupational distress, ↓ functioning at work and psychiatric sx (↓ self-esteem, anger, acting-up, sense of insecurity); problems with career choice, changes in career, adjustment to retirement, place of women in the work organizations, dual-career families; possible need for vocational rehabilitation.

Laboratory: DST (+ if failure to the nl suppression of plasma cortisol 6–24 hr after one po dose of dexamethasone; frequent false negative).

Course: one or more depressive episodes during lifetime. Intervals may be free of sx or with mild residual ones. Episodes' duration varies among pts but is rather stable within the same pt. Identify early to prevent the full development of depression. Untreated episode lasts 6–13 months, 3 months if treated; if treated <3 months, sx reappear; frequency and lengths of the episodes ↑ with disease progression. Less than 50% has only one episode, 50–60% have more than two episodes (recurrent), 10% are chronically, severely depressed. *Recurrent depressive episodes are frequently bipolar disorders before age 25 and unipolar disorders if onset after age 25.*

Note on dysthymia: more than 2 yr of depressive sx but not as severe as in MDD; pt is not free of sx for more than 2 months at a time. Episodes of major depression may appear but only after 2 yr (the combination of dysthymia and MDD is called "**double depression**," which has a worse prognosis than MDD alone).

Complications: ↓ occupational functioning, ↓ interpersonal relationships. Self-medication with alcohol, use of anxiolytics, suicidal attempts; completed suicide: 4%.

Prognosis: good if: mild episodes, no psychosis, good previous social functioning, lack of comorbid psychiatric illness, late onset, no personality disorder; poor if: presence of a dysthymic disorder, substance abuse, >1 depressive episodes, male.

Treatment: acute, continuation, and maintenance phases; CBT: effective in mild and moderate depressions; antidepressants: effective in all three phases.

ACUTE PHASE

- **Life-threatening depression**: ECT (also if pt unresponsive or not tolerating pharmacotherapy)
- **All antidepressants are equally effective**. SSRIs are the most widely used. Consider past response to the medication, potential SE, DDI (less for escitalopram, nortriptyline, bupropion, mirtazapine, venlafaxine, and more for MAOIs), risks in OD (MAOIs, heterocyclics). All have sexual SE (impotence, delayed ejaculation, ↓ vaginal lubrification, delayed orgasm, ↓ libido), with less for nefazodone, mirtazapine, bupropion. See Table 8.18 for FDA approved antidepressants
- **Use at an adequate dose**: start SSRI at the average therapeutic dose. Young, elderly, medically impaired: start lower and ↑ slowly to ↓ SE. Nortriptyline has a therapeutic window.
- **Assess SEs**: switch if not well tolerated.
- **Treat for adequate duration**: no response usually before 2 wk; if partial response, continue 4–6 wk more before switching; reassess the diagnosis if minimal response (look for hypothyroidism)
- **Treatment resistance**: ↑ dose (except for nortriptyline if max), or switch to a different class. If the situation is urgent, consider ECT or combination rx
- **Combination rx**:
  - Lithium + heterocyclic, or lithium + SSRI
  - Triodothyronine (T3): 25–50 mcg q day + heterocyclic, or T3 + SSRI (T3 more effective than T4). If augmentation with T3 successful, continue 2 months, then taper of 12.5 µg/d q 3–7 days. Liothyronine (Cytomel) is also used. Caution: frequent undiagnosed subclinical hypothyroidism, possible ↑ thyroid antibody levels, possible rapid antidepressant response to thyrotropin-releasing hormone, ↑ risk of antidepressant-induced rapid mood cycling
  - MAOI + tricyclic (potential dangers, tyramine-free diet): start with low dosages for each and ↑ slowly. Avoid imipramine + MAOI and avoid trimipramine + MAOI (↑ toxicity: convulsion, ↑ temp, twitching, sweating, risk of death).
  - Antidepressant + neuroleptic: fluoxetine + olanzapine (*Symbyax*) or SSRI + aripiprazole/*Abilify* 2 mg/d
  - Other combinations: with dextroamphetamine or methylphenidate; produce a rapid mood improvement (in <1 wk, closely monitor)
- **If failure** of combination treatment: **ECT,** transcranial magnetic stimulation (**TMS**)

CONTINUATION PHASE

Until depressive episode resolves. After 6 months of no sx, taper the dose of one third q 3 months until discontinued or sx reappear; if so, raise back the dose to the last effective dose; if *x* medications, ↓ the adjunct medication first. Maintain rx in pts with frequent or severe episodes.

MAINTENANCE TREATMENT

Same as the effective rx.

BIPOLAR I DISORDER (SINGLE OR RECURRENT)

Epidemiology: lifetime prevalence is 1.3–1.6%; M : F is 1 : 1. Incidence in children and adolescents: 1%; onset: late teens, early 20s (onset as early as 8 yo, poor prognosis).

Symptomatology: usually during lifetime there are >1 manic and >1 depressive episodes; **more than 50% pts start with depression** (often with hypersomnia, psychomotor retardation, psychosis, hx of postpartum depression), and the manic episode starting 6–10 yr later; family hx of bipolar I disorder, hx of antidepressant-induced mania are frequent.

- **Manic episodes**: gradual or acute; last from weeks **(at least 1 wk)** to months; 3 stages: **stage I** (hypomania, heightened mood, grandiosity, pressured speech, flight of ideas, distractibility, hyperactivity, ↑ energy, ↓ need for sleep); **stage II** (acute mania, same intensified sx, and delusions of grandeur or persecution); **stage III** (intense sx with often auditory hallucinations, incoherence, bizarre behaviors like catatonia). The episode reaches its peak and resolves backward. May be precipitated by: drugs (antidepressants, stimulants, sympathomimetics, theophylline, levodopa-carbidopa, bromocriptine, and corticosteroids), drug withdrawal (alcohol, benzodiazepine, clonidine), light therapy, sleep deprivation. Many pts do not complain as they feel too good or irritable but "full of life."

TABLE 8.5.   Symptoms of Mania

Emotional features	Cognitive features	Vegetative features	Other signs
● Excited, elevated mood, euphoria, emotional lability, irritability, low frustration tolerance, demanding behavior, egocentricity	● Elevated self-esteem, grandiosity, speech disturbances (loud, clanging, pressured speech, flight of ideas, incoherence), poor judgment, disorganization, paranoia, delusions, hallucinations	● Boundless energy, insomnia, little need for sleep, ↓ appetite	● Psychomotor agitation

- **Depressive episodes**: appear gradually (weeks or months), with depressed or irritable mood, ↓ concentration or memory, anhedonia, fatigue, ↓ or ↑ appetite, psychomotor changes (agitation or retardation), insomnia or hypersomnia. Delusions of guilt and auditory hallucinations (condemning type) are frequent. The episode lasts about 6 months and ↓ gradually. *The depression of bipolar disorder usually is "atypical" or agitated.*

- **Mixed manic episodes**: in a minority of pts; sx **must last nearly every day for at least 1 wk. Risk of suicide** ↑

Course: the sequence of the episodes varies; most pts have a preponderance of one type over the other. The intervals between episodes vary (few weeks to a decade or more; sx free or with mild residual sx). 1–2 episodes per lifetime to ≥4 per year (rapid cycling in 5–15% of cases). An untreated manic episode lasts 3 months. 90% of pts have more than one manic episode. 7% will not have a recurrence of sx, 40% have a chronic disease; time between episodes ↓ as disease progresses.

Note on cyclothymia: *more than 2 yr of hypomanic episodes and lower degree of depressive episodes* (chronic cyclic episodes of mild depression and sx of mild mania), during which the pt is not free of sx for more than 2 months at a time. **Differentiate with bipolar II disorder (hypomania and episodes of major depression).** Thirty percent of pts have a family hx of BPD; prevalence 1%; onset 15–25 yo; F : M is 3 : 2.

Complications: in mania: spending sprees, promiscuity, aggressive behaviors, suicide (10–20%). In depression: occupational and relationship problems, self-medication with anxiolytics or alcohol, suicide (4–10% completed). **Bipolar disorder is a lethal disease+++.**

Prognosis: poor: premorbid social functioning, psychotic features, alcohol abuse, males, poor adherence with medications (more relapses and future lower treatment response). Good: short manic episodes, late age of onset, few suicidal thoughts, lack of coexisting medical or psychiatric problems, compliance with effective treatment…

DIFFERENTIAL DIAGNOSIS

- **Mental illnesses**: MDD (no manic episode), cyclothymia (mild sx), *schizoaffective disorder of bipolar type (manic episodes and depressive episodes, but during the euthymic intervals, the pt remains psychotic)*; in bipolar disorder, even if the pt is psychotic during the episodes, the euthymic intervals do not present any psychotic sx, postpartum psychosis (only during postpartum period), schizophrenia (in mania: more elation, manic mood, rapid and pressured speech, hyperactivity, onset is more acute, frequent family hx of mood disorder, catatonic sx are frequent in BPD; BPD is underdiagnosed in blacks and Hispanics).

- **Medical conditions**: secondary depression, secondary mania (due to medical illness). *Antidepressants may precipitate mania.*

TREATMENT

■ **Acute episode**

1- MANIA AND MIXED MANIA

Mood stabilizers (gabapentine, lamotrigine, topiramate are not effective). Stage I is treated with a mood stabilizer alone, stages II and III will need adjunctive rx.

MOOD STABILIZERS

- **Divalproex**: start at 20 mg/kg, divided in bid, blood therapeutic range is 50–100 mcg/mL, ↓ doses if elderly or debilitated; SEs (nausea, vomiting, hair loss, sedation, weight gain, hepatitis, hyperammonemia, ↓ platelets); response in 2–4 days; metabolized in the liver

- **Lithium**: start with 900–1,800 mg/d (divided into tid–qid), can be switched later on to time-release preparations (q hr); therapeutic blood level is 0.6–1.2 meq/L; ↓ doses if renal failure, pts on other medications (DDI), elderly, debilitated. SEs: nausea, vomiting, diarrhea, weight gain, hair loss, tremor, hypothyroidism/check TSH q 6 months particularly if depression appears, nephrogenic diabetes insipidus, ↑ acne, ↑ psoriasis. Diuretics, NSAIDs, ACE inhibitors, metronidazole: ↑ lithium levels (risk of toxicity); Theophylline ↓ lithium level. Risk of seizures with lithium + fluvoxamine. Response seen in 7–10 days; is excreted in the urine; to stop lithium: taper over 2–3 wk to ↓ risk of relapses. Types of *mania less responsive to lithium are*: *mixed mania, rapid-cycling mania, secondary mania, mania with other psychiatric or medical disorders*

- **Carbamazepine**: start at 300–800 mg/d divided tid–qid; can be switched later to a time-released preparation (given bid), blood therapeutic level is 4–12 mcg/mL; ↓ doses if elderly, debilitated, liver failure. SEs: sedation, ataxia, dizziness, constipation, dry mouth, blurred vision, rash, hyponatremia due to SIADH, agranulocytosis, aplastic anemia; response seen in 7–10 days; not routinely used for treating acute mania

ATYPICAL ANTIPSYCHOTICS

- **Olanzapine (Zyprexa)**: monotherapy for acute manic or mixed episode: start 10–15 mg po daily; ↑ by 5 mg/d at intervals ≥24 hr. Effective doses: 5–20 mg/d, max 20 mg/d (also for maintenance tx); adjunctive tx for acute mixed or manic episodes: start 10 mg po daily; effective dose: 5–20 mg/d, max 20 mg/d; agitation in acute bipolar mania: start 10 mg IM (2.5–5 mg in elderly or debilitated pt; may repeat in ≥2 hr to max 30 mg/d; use for short-term (3–4 wk) acute manic episodes associated with BPD. May cause significant ↑ weight, dyslipidemia, hyperglycemia or new onset of diabetes; monitor weight, fasting blood glucose, and triglycerides before initiation + regular intervals during tx. Monitor for orthostatic hypotension when given IM. IM injection can also be associated with bradycardia, hypoventilation especially if used with other drugs that have these effects (caution with benzodiazepines).

- **Quetiapine (Seroquel)**: acute bipolar mania, as monotherapy or adjunctive; start 50 mg PO bid on day 1, then↑ to 100 mg bid on day 2, 150 mg bid on day 3, and 200 mg bid on day 4; may ↑ as needed to 300 mg bid on day 5 and 400 mg bid thereafter; effective dose: 400–800 mg/d; max is 800 mg/d; also used for bipolar depression; for maintenance, continue dose required to maintain sx remission. May cause ↑ weight, dyslipidemia, hyperglycemia or new onset of diabetes; monitor metabolic panel before initiation and at regular intervals; use lower doses and slower titration in the elderly or pts with hepatic dysfunction; eye exam for cataracts q 6 months; low risk for EPS and TD; extended-release tabs to be taken without food or after light meal.

- **Risperidone (Risperdal)**: bipolar mania: start 2–3 mg po daily; ↑ by 1 mg/d q 24 hr to max 6 mg/d; FDA approved for pediatric bipolar mania (age 10–17 yo): start 0.5 mg po daily and ↑ by 0.5–1.0 mg/d at intervals ≥24 hr to 2.5 mg/d, max 6 mg/d. More EPS than other atypicals (also in neonates following use in third trimester of pregnancy; may cause ↑ weight, dyslipidemia, hyperglycemia or new onset of diabetes; monitor metabolic panel before initiation and at regular intervals; pts with Parkinson disease and dementia have ↑ sensibility to SE such as EPS, confusion, falls, neuroleptic malignant syndrome

- **Aripiprazole (Abilify)**: acute tx for manic or mixed episodes, monotherapy or adjunctive to lithium or valproate: start 15 mg po daily; may ↑ to 30 mg/d (also for maintenance). For agitation associated with BPD: 9.75 mg IM; may consider 5.25–15 mg if indicated, may repeat in >2 hr up to max 30 mg/d. Approved for pediatric BPD (acute + maintenance for manic or mixed episodes, monotherapy or adjunctive to lithium or valproate for 10–17 yo): start 2 mg po daily; may ↑ to 5 mg/d at ≥2 days and to target dose of 10 mg/d after 2 more days; ↑ by 5 mg/d to max 30 mg/d; has low EPS and TD risk; ↑ dose by one-half if used with CYP3A4 inducers (carbamazepine); ↓ dose by at least half if used with CYP3A4 or CYP 2D6 inhibitors (ketoconazole, fluoxetine, or paroxetine); ↓ dose when inducer is stopped.

- **Ziprasidone (Geodon)**: in bipolar mania: start 40 mg po bid with food; may ↑ to 60–80 mg bid on day 2; effective dose is 40–80 mg bid; DDI with carbamazepine and ketoconazole

- **Asenapine (Saphris)**: acute treatment of manic or mixed episodes associated with bipolar I disorder in adults (start 10 mg sublingually bid; the dose can be ↓ to 5 mg twice daily if AEs; the tablet cannot be swallowed; no food or drink for 10 min after administration). Caution with fluvoxamine and paroxetine; SE: somnolence, dizziness, EPS other than akathisia, and ↑ weight.

- **Texas Medication Algorithm Project (TMAP)** may be followed (http://www.dshs.state.tx.us/mhprograms/TMAPover.shtm), BPD I, manic or mixed acute with no psychosis: start with a mood stabilizer or an atypical antipsychotic BPD I, manic or mixed acute with psychosis: start with a mood stabilizer + an atypical antipsychotic.

ADJUNCTIVE TREATMENTS

- **For agitation**: lorazepam (2 mg q 1–2 hr IM, max 12 mg/d), haloperidol (5 mg q 1–2 hr IM/caution with EPS reactions, max 60 mg/d), chlorpromazine (50–100 mg q 1–2 hr/caution with hypotension, max 1,000 mg/d), or ziprasidone (10–20 mg IM; may repeat 10 mg dose q 2 hr or q 4 hr, to max 40 mg/d)

- **For control of manic symptoms**: olanzapine (15 mg/d), ziprasidone (120–160 mg/d), risperidone (2–6 mg/d)

PREVENTIVE TREATMENT RECOMMENDED IF

Episodes (mania or depression) have occurred q 2 yr or more frequently, have been very severe or if very acute onset.

2- DEPRESSION

Antidepressants in the absence of mood stabilizers usually make bipolar pts worse: treat first with a mood stabilizer (do not use lamotrigine as a single, first-line agent in bipolar I disorder); if no response, add antidepressant (SSRIs, or bupropion or venlafaxine). Caution: when depression has cleared, taper and DC the antidepressant alone to ↓ risks of switching to mania and of rapid cycling (different from rx of unipolar depression). Caution with paroxetine and venlafaxine (greater risk of withdrawal sx).

An alternative to antidepressants is lamotrigine (ineffective for mania), quetiapine (FDA approved for bipolar depression): start with 50 mg PO hs on day 1, 100 mg hs on day 2, 200 mg hs on day 3 and 300 mg hs on day 4; may increase prn to 400 mg hs on day 5 and 600 mg hs on day 8).

Avoid antidepressants in depressed pts who have: rapid-cycling BPD, a recent hypomanic episode, and recent impairing rapid mood fluctuations. Instead, consider ↑ dose of the antimanic agent or adding a second antimanic agent (including lamotrigine).

Incomplete response: reassess for substance misuse, stressors, physical health problems, comorbid disorders (anxiety, severe obsessional sx) and poor adherence to medication. Consider: ↑ antidepressant dose, individual tx focused on depressive sx, switching to another antidepressant (mirtazapine, venlafaxine), adding quetiapine or olanzapine, or adding lithium.

TABLE 8.6. The Use of ECT in Severe Manic and Depressive Episodes

● Indications	● For rapid and short-term improvement of severe sx, after adequate trial of other rx options has been ineffective and/or the condition is potentially life threatening, such as severe depression, catatonia, or a prolonged severe manic episode
● Assess	● Risks associated with the anesthetic ● Current comorbidities ● Anticipated adverse events, particularly cognitive impairment ● The risks of not having treatment
● Precautions	● Stop or ↓ lithium or benzodiazepines before giving ECT ● Monitor the length of fits if the patient is taking anticonvulsants ● Monitor mental state for evidence of switching to the opposite pole

■ Long-term drug treatment

For at least 2 yr after an episode of BPD, and up to 5 yr if risk factors for relapse (hx of x relapses or severe psychotic episodes, comorbid substance misuse, ongoing stressful life events, poor social support).

BIPOLAR II DISORDER

Major depressive disorder combined with hypomanic episode: earlier onset than bipolar I disorder; **more suicidal risks** (more than in bipolar I and MDD). R/O: other mood disorders, psychotic disorders, borderline personality disorder; it is a chronic disease.

SOME CONSIDERATIONS

TABLE 8.7. Distinguishing Bipolar from Unipolar Depression

Features	Bipolar I or II depression	Unipolar depression
● Substance abuse	● Very high	● Moderate
● Gender parity	● Equal	● More likely female
● Family history	● Very frequent	● Sometimes
● Suicidal ideation	● Frequent	● Sometimes
● Seasonality	● Common	● Occasional
● Age at first episode	● Likely <25 yr	● Likely >25 yr
● Rapid cycling	● Typical	● Unusual
● Psychotic features <35 yr	● Highly predictive	● Uncommon
● >3 recurrent major depressive episodes	● Common	● Unusual
● Antidepressant monotherapy	● Insufficient	● Common
● Antidepressant-induced mania/hypomania	● Frequent	● Uncommon
● Mixed depressions (presence of hypomanic features within the depressive episode)	● Frequent	● Rare

Adapted from Kaye, N. S. (2005). Is your depressed patient bipolar? *Journal of American Board of Family Practitioners*, *18*, 271–281.

TABLE 8.8. FDA-Approved Treatments for BPD

Acute depression	Acute mania	Longer term treatment
● Olanzapine/fluoxetine combination	● Lithium	● Lithium
● Quetiapine (Seroquel or Seroquel XR) ● Depressive episode associated with BPD: Day 1: 50 mg; Day 2: 100 mg; Day 3: 200 mg; Day 4: 300 mg	● Chlorpromazine	● Lamotrigine
	● Divalproex ER	● Olanzapine

Continued

TABLE 8.8. FDA-Approved Treatments for BPD   Continued

Acute depression	Acute mania	Longer term treatment
	• Olanzapine	• Aripiprazole
	• Risperidone	• Quetiapine (adjunct to lithium or valproate) • (Seroquel or Seroquel XR) 400 mg/d to 800 mg/d
	• Quetiapine	• Risperidone *LAI* (monotherapy and adjunct to lithium or valproate)
	• Ziprasidone	• Ziprasidone (adjunct to lithium or valproate)
	• Aripiprazole	
	• Carbamazepine	
	• Asenapine	

LAI = long-acting injectable.

PARTICULAR FORMS OF MOOD DISORDERS

(1) Postpartum onset:

Postpartum depression:

Epidemiology: 10–15%, usually after the second or third child; *may be a manifestation of a bipolar disorder.*

Symptomatology: gradual onset, 3 wk–5 months postpartum; same sx as in MDD, possible disturbing obsession of an urge to kill the infant.

Course and complications: gradual spontaneous remission in <1 yr or chronic depression. High risk of recurrence after subsequent pregnancies (50%), ability to care for the infant may be compromised, *possible suicide, rarely infanticide.*

Etiology: sensitivity to falling sexual hormones?

Scale: The depression component of the Structured Clinical Interview (SCID) Edinburgh Postnatal Depression Scale.

Differential diagnosis: postpartum blues (earlier onset, a few days after delivery), postpartum psychosis (only psychotic process present), major depression (occurs outside of the puerperium), Sheehan syndrome (↓ lactation, no menses, loss of hair).

Treatment: same as in MDD. Most medications are excreted in the breast milk, consider bottle feeding. Possible effectiveness of estradiol patches (0.2 mg/d). The infant might need to be cared for by others until the mother recovers; have supervised visits if mother has infanticide urges. Preventive rx in the next puerperium.

Postpartum blues:

Epidemiology: 50% of postpartum women.

Symptomatology: acute onset, a few days after giving birth, lability of mood and affect, fatigue, poor concentration, insomnia.

Course and complications: remits fully and spontaneously in 2 wk.

Differential diagnosis: postpartum depression (>3 wk postpartum), postpartum psychosis (within 3 days postpartum, lability, psychosis).

Etiology: severe ↓ progesterone.

Treatment: reassurance, extra help, medications (caution with breastfeeding).

Postpartum psychosis (PPP):

Risk factors: sleep deprivation, hormonal shifts after birth, stressors (marital problems, older age, single mother, low socioeconomic status), hx of bipolar or schizoaffective disorder with or without prior hospitalization, hx of postpartum psychosis, cessation of lactation, obstetric factors (first pregnancy, delivery complications, preterm birth, acute C section, long labor). **Postpartum psychosis may be a manifestation of bipolar disorder** (mixed with depression and mania).

Clinical signs: depression with rapid mood changes suggests postpartum psychosis rather than postpartum depression alone.

Medical work-up: R/O delirium and organic causes (metabolic, neurologic, cardiovascular, infectious, substance- or medication-induced, thyroiditis, tumor, CNS infection, head injury, embolism, eclampsia, substance withdrawal, electrolyte anomalies, anoxia, and vitamin B_{12} deficiency).

Treatment: PPP usually requires hospitalization and is a psychiatric emergency (risks of suicide, infanticide, and child maltreatment). Mood stabilizers, including antipsychotics such as conventional ones/ haloperidol (lower risk of weight gain or of sedation that could impair a mother's ability to respond to her infant) are mainstays of rx. ECT yields rapid improvement for mothers with postpartum mood or psychotic sx. Discharge plans are necessary (notify child protective services if child is at risk): meet with the pt + family to discuss rx, engage visiting nurses, schedule frequent outpatient appointments, family rx.

Prevention: manage proactively BPD during pregnancy. Anticipate that depressive or psychotic sx could develop within days after delivery; seek rx immediately if this occurs (mood stabilizers or atypical antipsychotics in the postpartum). Prophylactic lithium may be given late in the third trimester or immediately after delivery or prophylactic mood stabilizers immediately in the postpartum. Use atypical antipsychotics in pregnancy and lactation if necessary. The antipsychotics in women at risk for PPP may help prevent or treat both manic and psychotic sx.

TABLE 8.9.   Women with Bipolar Disorder Who Are Planning a Pregnancy, Are Pregnant, or Breastfeeding

• General principles of management	• Discuss problems associated with both treating and not treating the bipolar disorder during pregnancy • ↑ contact by mental health specialist because of ↑ risk of relapse during pregnancy and the postnatal period • A written plan for managing a woman's bipolar disorder during the pregnancy, delivery, and postnatal period should be developed as soon as possible with the pt and significant others, shared with all providers of care • If a pregnant ♀ is stable on an antipsychotic and likely to relapse without medication: maintain on the antipsychotic, and monitor for ↑ weight and diabetes • Avoid the following drugs: *Valproate*: risk to the fetus and child development; Carbamazepine: limited efficacy, risk of harm to the fetus; *Lithium*: risk of harm to the fetus (cardiac problems); *Lamotrigine*: risk of harm to the fetus; *Paroxetine*: risk of cardiovascular malformations in the fetus; Long-term rx with *benzodiazepines*: risks during pregnancy and after birth (cleft palate and floppy baby syndrome)

• Women planning a pregnancy	• Pt will be advised to stop taking valproate, carbamazepine, lithium, and lamotrigine, and consider alternative prophylactic drugs (such as an antipsychotic)
	• Some antipsychotics ↑ prolactin levels and ↓ chances of conception (may need to switch antipsychotic)
	• If a pt needing antimanic medication plans a pregnancy, use a low-dose typical or atypical antipsychotic (least known risks)
	• If a woman taking lithium plans to become pregnant, consider:
	   ° If the pt is well with low risk of relapse: gradually stop lithium
	   ° If the patient is not well with high risk of relapse: switch to an antipsychotic; stop lithium and restart it in the second trimester (if sx have responded better to lithium than to other drugs in the past); continue with lithium (after full discussion of the risk), while trying to conceive and throughout the pregnancy, if manic episodes have complicated the woman's previous pregnancies, and sx have responded well to lithium
	   ° If pt remains on lithium during pregnancy, check lithium levels q 4 wk, then q wk from the 36th wk, and less than 24 hr after childbirth. Adjust serum levels. Maintain adequate fluid intake
	• If a ♀ plans a pregnancy and becomes depressed after stopping prophylactic medication: CBT therapy to be preferred to an antidepressant (risk of switching to mania). If an antidepressant is used, choose SSRI (not paroxetine: risk of cardiovascular malformations in the fetus). Monitor closely

• Women with an unplanned pregnancy	• Confirm the pregnancy quickly; advise to stop taking valproate, carbamazepine, and lamotrigine • The pregnancy is confirmed in the first trimester and the ♀ is stable, stop the lithium over 4 wk, and inform that this may not remove the risk of cardiac defects in the fetus • If the woman remains on lithium during pregnancy: check lithium q 4 wk, then q wk from the 36th wk, and less than 24 hr after childbirth; adjust the dose; maintain adequate fluid intake • An antipsychotic should be offered as prophylactic medication • Offer counseling about the continuation of the pregnancy, the need for ↑ monitoring and the risks to the fetus if the ♀ stays on medication • The newborn baby needs a full pediatric assessment; social + medical help to be provided for mother and child

Continued

TABLE 8.9. Women with Bipolar Disorder Who Are Planning a Pregnancy, Are Pregnant, or Breastfeeding   Continued

• **Pregnant women with acute mania or depression**	• Acute mania:
	  ○ Pregnant woman, not taking medication, develops acute mania: consider an atypical or a typical antipsychotic. Keep the dose as low as possible; monitor carefully
	  ○ Pregnant woman develops acute mania while taking prophylactic medication: Check the dose of the prophylactic agent and adherence
	  ○ ↑ the dose if the woman is taking an antipsychotic, or change to an antipsychotic if she is not
	  ○ If no response to changes in dose or drug and the pt has severe mania: consider the use of ECT, lithium, and, rarely, valproate (if no alternative to valproate: inform of the ↑ risk to the fetus and the child's intellectual development). Use the lowest dose possible and ↑ it with additional antimanic medication (not carbamazepine). The maximum dosage should be 1 g/d, in divided doses and in the slow-release form, with 5 mg/d of folic acid
	• Depressive sx:
	  ○ Mild depressive sx: self-help approaches, brief psychologic interventions, antidepressants
	  ○ Moderate to severe depressive sx: Psychologic rx (CBT) for moderate depression; medication + psychologic rx for severe depression; quetiapine alone or SSRIs (not paroxetine) in combination with prophylactic medication (less switching with SSRIs than the TCA). Monitor closely, stop the SSRI if development of manic or hypomanic sx.
	  ○ Inform of the potential but short-lived adverse effects of antidepressants on the neonate

• **Care in the perinatal period**	• Women taking lithium: deliver in hospital with the obstetric medical team. Monitor fluid balance (risk of dehydration and lithium toxicity) • After delivery, and ♀ on no medication with high risk of developing an acute episode, reinstate medication as soon as possible once the fluid balance is established • If a woman maintained on lithium is at high risk of a manic relapse in the immediate postnatal period, augment rx with an antipsychotic • If a woman with bipolar disorder develops severe manic or psychotic symptoms and behavioral disturbance in the intrapartum period: rapid tranquillization with an antipsychotic in preference to a benzodiazepine (risk of floppy baby syndrome). Collaborate with an anesthetist
• **Breastfeeding**	• If taking psychotropic medication and wish to breastfeed: advise on risks/benefits of breastfeeding; advise not to breastfeed if taking lithium, benzodiazepines, or lamotrigine. Offer prophylaxy that can be used when breastfeeding: an antipsychotic should be the first choice (but not clozapine) • Use an SSRI if an antidepressant is used (but not fluoxetine or citalopram)
• **Care of the infant**	• Monitor in the first few weeks for adverse drug effects, toxicity, or withdrawal (floppy baby syndrome, irritability, constant crying, shivering, tremor, restlessness, ↑ tone, feeding and sleeping difficulties, seizures). If mother on antidepressants in third trimester: R/O serotonergic toxicity syndrome rather than withdrawal, and monitor carefully the neonate

(2) **Rapid cycling**: mostly females; R/O stress, drug rx, thyroid disorder, substance abuse; can be applied to bipolar I or II disorders; **must have >4 episodes in 1 yr** (episodes separated by full or partial remission for >2 months or a switch to an episode of opposite polarity); difficult to treat: may be less responsive to lithium, avoid antidepressant, may need a combination of antimanic agents (including valproate). Treat manic and depressive episodes. Optimize long-term rx; trials of medication should be >6 months; psychoeducation (mood diary to monitor changes in severity and frequency of sx + impact of interventions).

TABLE 8.10.   Long-Term Management of Rapid-Cycling Bipolar Disorder

• Consider as first-line rx a combination of lithium and valproate • Consider lithium monotherapy as second-line rx • For patients already taking lithium: ↑ dose • Avoid the use of an antidepressant • Consider combinations of lithium or valproate with lamotrigine, especially in bipolar II disorder • Check thyroid function q 6 months, with levels of thyroid antibodies if indicated by the thyroid function tests

(3) **Acute mixed**: avoid antidepressant; treat like an acute manic episode and monitor closely (at least wkly) for *suicide risk.*

(4) **Atypical depression** (hypersomnia, weight gain, hyperphagia, $\uparrow$ sensitivity to every stressor, not just to interpersonal rejection), may respond better to MAOIs than to TCAs.

(5) **Seasonal pattern**: F : M is 2–4 : 1; depression usually the fall or winter (seasonal affective disorder), with normality or hypomania during spring or summer; frequent atypical depression. Phototherapy (2–6 hr/d, response in 2–3 days) alone or in combination with pharmacotherapy

(6) **Depression in children and adolescents**: may present as school problems, truancy, promiscuity, antisocial behavior, substance abuse, oppositional behaviors, somatic complaints

(7) **Depression in older people**: underdiagnosed and undertreated; $\uparrow$ somatic complaints

(8) **Mania in adolescents**: may present with psychosis, substance abuse, antisocial behaviors (promiscuity, aggressivity), suicide attempts, irritability.

(9) **Depressive disorders NOS**

　　Minor depressive disorder (5% of population), F > M, less severe sx; rx: SSRIs, bupropion, psychotherapies

　　Recurrent brief depressive disorder: multiple brief episodes (<2 wk) of depression, common, higher in young adults, more chaotic lives, differentiate from major depression with seasonal pattern and BPD, same rx as in MDD. Lithium may be useful.

　　Premenstrual dysphoric disorder/PMS: 2–1% of $\female$; high estrogen-to-progesterone ratio? Is it a chronobiological phase disorder? One week free of sx during each menstrual cycle; rx: progesterone, fluoxetine.

　　Postpsychotic depressive disorder of schizophrenia: a major depressive episode that occurs during the residual phase of schizophrenia.

(10) **Bipolar disorder NOS**: very rapid alternation between manic and depressive sx, or recurrent hypomanic episodes without depressive episodes, or manic or mixed episode superimposed on a psychotic disorder.

(11) **Secondary mood disorders**

TABLE 8.11.　Mood Disorders Due to a Medical Condition

Depression	Mania
• **Focal CNS lesions**: strokes; traumatic brain injury, subdural hematoma;	• **Focal CNS lesions**: caudate nucleus lesion/infarct, frontal or temporal lobe cortex lesion, brain tumor
• **Tumors** (brain, lung, pancreatic cancer 50% may develop depression before cancer is detected)	• **Infectious diseases**: AIDS, syphilis, influenza, encephalitis, cryptococcosis
• **Infectious diseases**: AIDS, neurosyphilis, influenza, mononucleosis, Lyme, hepatitis, encephalitis	• **Metabolic disorders**: hemodialysis, postoperative state, vitamin B_{12} deficiency
• **Endocrine disorders**: Cushing syndrome, adrenocortical dysfunction, steroid abuse, hypothyroidism, hyperthyroidism, hypoparathyroidism, hyperparathyroidism, Turner syndrome, menopause	• **Epilepsy**: right temporal; ictal, postictal
	• **Surgery**: right hemispherectomy
	• **Cerebrovascular accident**: thalamic stroke
• **Vitamin deficiency**: B_{12}, pellagra	• **Dementing diseases**: Huntington, adrenoleukodystrophy, metachromatic leukodystrophy
• **Dementing diseases**: Alzheimer, Parkinson, Huntington, Wilson	• **Miscellaneous**: multiple sclerosis, Wilson disease, head trauma, hyperthyroidism, cerebellar atrophy, SLE, chorea gravidarum
• **Miscellaneous**: MS, electrolyte disorders, post-MI, epilepsy, SLE, PMS	

Adapted from Tomb, D. A. (1994). *Psychiatry* (5th ed). Baltimore: Williams & Willkins. p. 51–52.

TABLE 8.12.　Substance-Induced Mood Disorders

• Depression	• **Drugs of abuse**: alcohol, sedative-hypnotics, opioids, PCP • **Medications**: oral contraceptives, corticosteroids, reserpine, alpha-methyldopa, guanethididne, levodopa, indomethacin, benzodiazepines, opiates, cimetidine, propanolol, anticholinesterases, amphetamine withdrawal • **Miscellaneous**: heavy metal poisoning
• Mania	• **Drugs of abuse**: cocaine, amphetamines, hallucinogens, PCP, alcohol intoxication • **Medications**: steroids, L-dopa., INH, procarbazine, cyproheptadine, thyroxin, L-glutamine, alprazolam, metrizamide, captopril, yohimbine, clonidine withdrawal • **Miscellaneous**: organophosphates, petroleum distillates

(12) Bipolar mania with psychosis

TABLE 8.13. Particular Treatment Issues in Bipolar Disorder with Psychotic Features

- **Misdiagnosis in bipolar disorder with psychosis**: 70% misdiagnosis rate, one third of these pts wait >10 yr for the right diagnosis (caution if a family hx of bipolar disorder and suicide in a first-degree relative), risk of antidepressant-induced mania. Bipolar disorder (particularly hypomania in young pts) is frequently misdiagnosed as ADHD; R/O schizophrenia and schizoaffective disorder
- **Stimulant use in bipolar disorder**: may precipitate mania; may delay remission of a bipolar disorder or contribute to rx resistance
- **Selection of antipsychotic medication in bipolar disorder**: eliminate any medication that could ↑ mania or psychotic sx; use mood stabilizer at adequate doses; if adding an antipsychotic, balance efficacy and SE, consider doses and adequate time trial for the antipsychotic, rx compliance; *bipolar pts may be more susceptible to tardive dyskinesia than pts with schizophrenia* (with equivalent doses of neuroleptics)
- **Monitor appearance of depression**: *postmanic depression is frequent* (consider fluoxetine-olanzapine combination, lamotrigine, quetiapine which is effective in treating psychosis, mania, and bipolar depression). *Lithium may be useful as a suicide preventing agent*; Aripiprazole works well as an adjunct to unipolar depression but not for the treatment of bipolar depression or the prevention of the same

COEXISTING DISORDERS

- **Anxiety**: frequent. Are there two comorbid disorders or is it a bipolar mixed disorder (if irritability, overstimulation, family hx of bipolar disorder: consider BPD)? In mixed episodes: SSRIs worsen mania, do not help with the depression, and an antipsychotic such as quetiapine is to be used. If presence of OCD: add an SSRI only when the pt is protected with a mood stabilizer and/or an antipsychotic. Quetiapine has strong antianxiety effects. **In "agitated depression": R/O mixed BPD, bipolar II disorder.**
- **Alcohol dependence**: in depressed women more than in depressed men.
- **Other substance abuse**: precedes the mood disorder or may represent a way for the pt to ↓ the sx of the mood disorder (e.g., use of cocaine or amphetamines in depressed pts). Think about energy drinks, anabolic, and herbal preparations.
- **Medical conditions**: rx of the MDD may improve the course of the medical condition.

TABLE 8.14. Late Life Depression Associated with Some Common Medical Conditions

Disease	Depression	Treatment
• Stroke	• Poststroke depression **common 3–6 months post stroke**, 20–50% within 1 yr • Predisposing factors: older age, females, past depression, size of infarct, severity of sequelae, speech impairment, stroke in left front cerebral hemisphere • Depression may predispose to stroke	• If pt stays depressed after 6 wk following a stroke: treat with antidepressants • Methylphenidate (5–10 mg/d): useful on apathy (Ritalin LA) • Integrated care: liaison with a stroke specialist, primary care physician, telephone tracking system, management of vascular risks factors, screening for depression
• Coronary heart disease	• Link between the two; association with: heart rate variability, atherosclerosis, vascular inflammation (↑ levels of interleukin-6 and C-reactive protein), smoking, social isolation, ↑ cholesterol, poor compliance with rx	• Treat with SSRIs (also ↓ platelet activity) • TCAs are type 1A antiarrhythmics that ↓ heart rate variability • Avoid venlafaxine (↑ BP, risk of ventricular arrhythmia)
• Diabetes mellitus	• ↑ Risk for depression. Depression ↑ risk for diabetic complications, poor glycemic control, subcortical encephalopathy (small vessel pathology)	• TCAs may impair diabetic control, but may be useful for painful neuropathy • Fluoxetine can cause hypoglycemia • Mirtazapine ↑ weight • Lithium toxicity ↑ if nephropathy • Valproic acid may give false-positive result for glucose urine test

Continued

TABLE 8.14. Late Life Depression Associated with Some Common Medical Conditions Continued

• **Parkinson disease**	• Depression: 50–80% of pts with Parkinson disease. Causes are neurodegeneration, ↓ multiple neurotransmitters, social isolation, duration of illness, cognitive impairment • Sx of depression may be masked by the almost identical motor sx of Parkinson disease	• Antidepressants, ECT, exercise, CBT, support groups, self-help programs • SSRIs: do not combine with selegiline (serotonine syndrome) • TCAs: not recommended (anticholinergic effects) • Moclobemide (selective and reversible MAOI) (Aurox, Manerix) • Dopamine receptor agonist: pramipexole (Mirapex), combined with L-dopa may be useful • Modafinil (provigil) • Deep brain stimulation is a rx for both disorders
• **Chronic obstructive pulmonary disease**	• 40% depression; factors: anoxia, smoking, lack of exercise, social isolation	• Avoid benzodiazepines (respiratory distress) • Paroxetine and mirtazapine; useful if ↑ anxiety • CBT
• **Vascular depression** (depression in the context of a vascular disease)	• Abnormalities in basal ganglia and white matter, 50% of late life depressions, evidence of microvascular disease	• Standard antidepressants are less effective • Fluoxetine (augmentation with nimodipine, a Ca-channel drug used in delayed ischemic deficits [DIDs]/Nimotop: risk of hypotension, bradycardia) • Target apathy (problem solving, behavioral activation) • SNRIs?

- **Personality disorder**: withhold a diagnosis of personality disorder until secure in the assessment.

REFRACTORY BIPOLAR DISORDERS: DRUG AUGMENTATION STRATEGIES

- **Mood stabilizer combinations in refractory bipolar disorders**: frequent

TABLE 8.15. Mood Stabilizer Combinations

• Patient on lithium	• May add: divalproex or gabapentin or tiagabine
• Patient is on divalproex	• May add: carbamazepine or gabapentin or topiramate
• Patient is on carbamazepine	• May add: gabapentin

For gabapentin or tiagabine, the data suggesting efficacy are sparse.

- **Other combinations**:
  - Mood stabilizer + antipsychotic is the most frequent combination+++
  - Mood stabilizer + clonazepam
  - **Lamotrigine**: usually used alone or as an adjunct in bipolar disorders. **Caution**: rashes ↑ early in treatment, if ↑ conc., if given with valproic acid. Valproic acid ↑ lamotrigine conc. (→ decrease dosage of Depakote)
- **Refractory mania: clozapine** (in rare cases)

REFRACTORY DEPRESSIONS: DRUG AUGMENTATION STRATEGIES

- **Antidepressant combinations**:

TABLE 8.16. Augmentation of an Antidepressant with Another Antidepressant

• **Patient is on TCA**	• **May add**: SSRI	• Noradrenergic TCAs (desipramine, nortriptyline) ↑ action of SSRI but risk is ↑ TCA levels (less with sertraline, citalopram). Monitor TCA levels
• **Patient is on SSRI**	• **May add**: bupropion or venlafaxine	• Venlafaxine: less CV risks than with TCA (which may be lethal in OD; many SE: including sedation, antimuscarinic effects) • Bupropion (Wellbutrin): may be added to fluoxetine, or paroxetine; May reverse SSRI-associated sexual dysfunction, no weight gain, antismoking effects; do not use if seizure or bulimia history
• **Patient is on Venlafaxine**	• **May add**: bupropion	
• **Patient is on Nefazodone**	• **May add**: bupropion or SSRI	
• **Patient is on Mirtazapine**	• **May add**: bupropion or SSRI	• Bupropion may ↓ sedation associated with mirtazapine

- **Other drugs to augment antidepressant drugs action**:

TABLE 8.17.   Augmentation of an Antidepressant Action with a Nonantidepressant Drug

• **Lithium**	• Works well; 600–1,200 mg/d. May enhance action of antidepressants including MAOIs as well as TCAs	• Lesser dosages than in bipolar disorders; blood levels: 0.4–0.8 mEq/L. Monitor Li levels, thyroid, and renal functions
• **Thyroid hormones**	• Works with TCA, may work with other antidepressants	• Liothyronine (Cytomel: 25–75 µg) works better than levothyroxine (Levoxyl, Synthroid). Monitor thyroid function, bone loss, and cardiac rate if high doses
• **Sympathomimetics**	• In pts who do not tolerate antidepressants, or as an adjunct to ↓ fatigue, apathy in medically ill or if comorbid ADHD	• Monitor BP. Risk of abuse? Initial weight loss, ↓ sleep, rare paranoia, and/or agitation. Prescription regulations
• **Benzodiazepines**	• Help with associated anxiety	• Risks of sedation, withdrawal, long-term dependence (alprazolam if >2 months) • Xanax: 0.25–0.5 mg tid and Xanax XR: 1–2 mg tid; high abuse and withdrawal seizure risk
• **Buspirone**	• Helps with bruxism and sexual dysfunction due to SSRI	• Buspar: 20–50 mg/d. Start low if added to fluvoxamine or nefazodone as they ↑ buspirone levels. May reverse SSRI-associated sexual dysfunction; if nausea: may add ginger root
• **Antipsychotics**	• If associated psychotic sx; useful in nonpsychotic depressed refractory pts	• Risperidone (↑ prolactin), olanzapine, quetiapine, clozapine are anxiolytic and sedative. Quetiapine is approved for bipolar depression. Little weight gain risk with aripiprazole (is approved as an adjunct) or ziprasidone. Caution with MAOIs: risk of hypotension with low potency antipsychotics
• **Anticonvulsants**	• Fair response	• Monitor drug interactions
• **Concentrated fish oil**	• EPA supplements are more effective than DHA supplements	• OmegaBrite: Start with 1 g EPA, increase to 1.5–3 g/d, max 6 g/d. No fishy aftertaste; many brands (check content and EPA: DHA ratios); may be added to SSRIs

MEDICATIONS USED IN MOOD DISORDERS

ANTIDEPRESSANTS

TABLE 8.18.   FDA-Approved Indications for Antidepressants

(1) SSRIs
- **Fluoxetine (Prozac)**: MDD (acute and maintenance rx in adults and pediatric pts aged 8–18 yr); OCD (acute and maintenance in adult and pediatric pts aged 7–17 yr); bulimia nervosa (acute and maintenance in adults), panic disorder with or without agoraphobia (acute rx in adults), premenstrual dysphoric disorder
- **Prozac and olanzapine in combination (Symbyax)**: Bipolar I disorder (depressive episodes in adults associated with bipolar I disorder); in rx-resistant depression in adults (acute rx for adults who have not responded to 2 separate trials of different antidepressants of adequate dose and duration in the current episode)
- **Paroxetine (Paxil, Paxil CR)**: MDD (adults; Paxil and Paxil CR), OCD (adults), panic disorder with or without agoraphobia (adults; Paxil and Paxil CR), PTSD (adults), social phobia (adults; Paxil and Paxil CR), GAD (adults), premenstrual dysphoric disorder (Paxil CR)
- **Sertraline (Zoloft)**: MDD (adults), OCD (adults and children), panic disorder with or without agoraphobia (adults), PTSD (adults), PMDD/premenstrual dysphoric disorder (adults), social phobia (adults)
- **Fluvoxamine (Luvox)**: OCD (adults and children aged 8–17)
- **Citalopram (Celexa)**: MDD (adults)
- **Escitalopram (Lexapro)**: acute rx of GAD (adults), MDD (acute and maintenance rx of adults and children aged 12–17)

(2) Tricyclics and tetracyclics:
- Tertiary amines
   - **Imipramine (Tofranil)**: MDD
   - **Amitriptiline (Elavil)**: depression, endogenous depression
   - **Trimipramine (Surmontil)**: depression, endogenous depression
   - **Clomipramine (Anafranil)**: OCD (adults and children >10)

Continued

TABLE 8.18.　FDA-Approved Indications for Antidepressants　Continued

　　Doxepine (Sinequan): pt with depression and/or anxiety (psychoneurotic or associated with alcoholism, or associated with organic disease), psychotic depressive disorders with associated anxiety, involutional depression, and manic-depressive disorder
- Secondary amines
　　Desipramine (Norpramin): MDD
　　Nortriptyline (Pamelor): MDD
　　Protriptyline (Vivactil): depression

(3) Tetracyclic drugs
- **Maprotiline (Ludiomil):** depression
- **Amoxapine (Asendin):** neurotic or reactive depression, endogenous and psychotic depressions, depression with anxiety or agitation

(4) MAOIs:
- **Isocarboxazid (Marplan):** depression
- **Phenelzine (Nardil):** depressed pts characterized as "atypical," "nonendogenous," or "neurotic"
- **Selegiline (EMSAM/transdermal system, Eldepryl/oral):** MDD (transdermal), Parkinson disease or symptomatic Parkinsonism (adjunctive, oral form)
- **Tranycypromine (Parnate):** major depressive episode without melancholia

(5) Atypical antidepressants:
SNRIS
- **Venlafaxine (Effexor, Effexor XR):** MDD, GAD, social anxiety disorder, panic disorder in adults
- **Desvenlafaxine (Pristiq):** MDD in adults
- **Duloxetine (Cymbalta):** MDD, GAD, fibromyalgia, diabetic peripheral neuropathic pain (all adults)
- **Duloxetine (Cymbalta):** MDD, GAD, fibromyalgia, diabetic peripheral neuropathic pain (all adults)

Others
- **Mirtazapine (Remeron):** MDD in adults
- **Nefazodone:** depression, relapse prevention in MDD in adults (Serzone was discontinued due to hepatotoxicity
- **Trazodone (Desyrel, Oleptro):** MDD in adults
- **Bupropion (Wellbutrin):** MDD, Seasonal affective disorder in adults

(1) **SSRIs: first-line agents** for rx of depression, inhibit the reuptake of serotonin by presynaptic neurons with little effect on the reuptake of NE and almost no effect on the reuptake of dopamine.

TABLE 8.19.　SSRIs

Drug	Half-life	Start dose (mg)	Dosage (mg/d)	Interactions of clinical importance
• Fluoxetine (Prozac)	• 4–6 days, 4–16 days for metabolites	• 20 q AM	• 10–80	• Desipramine, carbamazepine, ↑ phenytoin, ↑ haloperidol, lithium, benzodiazepines (↑ alprazolam), antineoplasic agents, ↑ clozapine, ↑ TCAs, MAOIs (serotonin syndrome), ↑ warfarin
• Fluvoxamine (Luvox)	• 15 hr	• 50–100 q AM	• 100–300	• ↑ Warfarin, ketoconazole, ↑ level of benzodiazepines (not lorazepam), theophylline, clozapine, carbamazepine, methadone, ↑ propanolol level, diltiazem • Haloperidol ↑ fluvoxamine • Fluvoxamine: ↑ olanzapine, ↑ clozapine (↑↑ seizures, do not use together) • MAOIs (serotonin syndrome) • ↑ risk of seizures with lithium
• Paroxetine (Paxil)	• 21 hr	• 20 q AM	• 10–50	• ↑ Phenytoin, procyclidine, tranylcypromine, tramadol (serotonin syndrome) • Cimetidine ↑ conc. of Paxil • Phenytoin, phenobarbital: ↓ conc. of Paxil • ↑ clozapine, ↑ TCAs, MAOIs (serotonin syndrome), ↑ warfarin, ↑ level of phenytoin

Continued

TABLE 8.19.   SSRIs   Continued

Drug	Half-life	Start dose (mg)	Dosage (mg/d)	Interactions of clinical importance
• Sertraline (Zoloft)	• 26 hr	• 50 q AM	• 50–200	• Lithium, Cimetidine: ↑ conc. of Zoloft • ↑ clozapine, ↑ TCAs, MAOIs (serotonin syndrome), ↑ warfarin, ↑ level of phenytoin
• Citalopram (Celexa)	• 35 hr	• 10–20 q AM	• 20–80	• Cimetidine ↑ conc. of Celexa • ↑clozapine, ↑ TCAs, MAOIs (serotonin syndrome), ↑ warfarin, ↑ level of phenytoin
• Escitalopram (Lexapro)	30 hr	10 q AM	10–20	↑ clozapine, ↑TCAs, MAOIs (serotonin syndrome), ↑ warfarin, ↑ level of phenytoin

Adapted from Sadock, B. J., & Sadock, V. A. (2002). *Kaplan and Sadock's Synopsis of Psychiatry: Behavioral Sciences/Clinical Psychiatry* (9th ed.). Baltimore, MD: Lippincott Williams & Wilkins. p. 1094, 1101.

TABLE 8.20.   Side Effects of SSRIs: Minimum due to Lack of Antihistaminergic and Anti-α-Adrenergic Receptor Activities, but Mild Anticholinergic Activity; Very Low Cardiac Conduction Effects, no Orthostatic Hypotension (Very Low for Fluoxetine)

Types	Treatment
• ↓ Sexual functioning	• ↓ Dosage, switch to bupropion or nefazodone, or addition of bupropion, or of yohimbine, or of cyproheptadine, or of dopamine receptor agonists, use of sildenafil, use of amphetamine • More with paroxetine?
• Gastrointestinal	• Nausea, loose stools (more diarrhea with sertraline); are dose related, transient. Weight loss due to fluoxetine is usually transient
• Weight gain	• Mostly with paroxetine: switch
• Serotonin syndrome (diarrhea, diaphoresis, changes in VS, tremor, ataxia, myoclonus, confusion, rigidity, fever, delirium, coma, seizures, shock, death)	• Remove the SSRI, provide supportive care, transfer to ICU
• Headaches	• Mostly with fluoxetine: switch
• Central nervous system	• Anxiety: mostly with fluoxetine • Insomnia: mostly with fluoxetine → give AM, may be treated with benzodiazepines, trazodone • Somnolence: (sertraline, fluvoxamine, citalopram, paroxetine); switch to another SSRI (fluoxetine) or bupropion • Nightmares: transient or use another SSRI • Seizures: when high doses of SSRIs • Extrapyramidal sx: mostly with fluoxetine >100 mg/d. Rare cases of TD or ↑ motor sx of Parkinson disease • Bruxism: give small doses of buspirone • Amotivational or apathy syndrome: to differentiate from depression; ↓ SSRI, or augment with a stimulant or an antidepressant with noradrenergic (secondary amine TCA) or dopaminergic activity (bupropion), or switch to a different class of antidepressant, or add olanzapine • "Poop-out" syndrome (loss of potency while on the SSRI): ↑ dose or switch the SSRI or adding an adjunct
• Anticholinergic: blurred vision, constipation, ↓ salivation, ↓ sweating, retrograde ejaculation, delirium, memory problems, narrow-angle glaucoma, photophobia, tachycardia, urinary retention	• Dry mouth, mostly with paroxetine (sedation, constipation/ dose dependent)
• Hematologic	• ↑ Bruises. Rare neutropenia with paroxetine and fluoxetine
• Electrolytes and glucose	• ↓ Blood glucose (caution in diabetes) • Hyponatremia, SIADH
• SSRI withdrawal (dizziness, ataxia, paresthesis, numbness, lethargy, headache, tremor, sweating, anorexia, insomnia, nightmares, nausea, vomiting, diarrhea, irritability, agitation	• Mostly with paroxetine, fluvoxamine. If rx <6 wk, resolves spontaneously in 3 wk. May use fluoxetine to treat it
• Allergies	• Rashes, rare pulmonary fibrotic lesions: discontinue

(2) **SNRIs**:

    Venlafaxine (Effexor): fast acting, good for depression with melancholic features. Start dose: 75 mg/d in 2–3 divided doses or ER form at hs (max 200 mg). ↑ Dose by 75 mg/d q 4 days. Dosages are 225–375 mg/d. If to be stopped, taper over 2–4 wk to **avoid discontinuation syndrome.** May give more nausea and vomiting than SSRI. Cimetidine ↑ levels of venlafaxine. Venlafaxine ↑ levels of haloperidol, ↑ TCAs, risk of NMS-like syndrome with MAOIs. SE: nausea (less with ER form), somnolence, dry mouth, anxiety, constipation, blurred vision, sexual dysfunction, ↑ **in BP (if >300 mg/d)**. Has an anti-OCD effect. Not to give in bipolar depression or mixed BPD (↑ agitation and risk of suicide). Difficulty in withdrawing venlafaxine.

    Duloxetine (Cymbalta): doses are 60 mg/d to 60 mg bid. SE: nausea, dry mouth, fatigue, constipation, sweating, dizziness. Avoid discontinuation syndrome (sleep disruption, anxiety, agitation, headaches, N/V, flu-like sx).

    Desvenlafaxine (Pristiq): doses are 50 mg/d. SE; nausea, dizziness, hyperhidrosis, constipation, ↓ appetite, hyponatremia, mydriasis, ↑ BP. Caution with aspirin, NSAIDs, warfarin (↑ bleeding events), serotonergic drugs (serotonin syndrome). Do not use with MAOIs; if to be discontinued: gradual reduction (giving 50 mg less frequently).

(3) **Tricyclics and tetracyclics (TCAs)**

TABLE 8.21. Tricyclic and Tetracyclic Antidepressants

Drug name	Starting dose/day (mg); divide doses, increase q wk in OPU setting	Usual adult dose (mg/day)	Therapeutic plasma concentration (ng/mL)	Side effects				
				Anti-cholin.	Sed.	Hypotension	Seizures	Cardiac conduction
Tertiary amines								
Imipramine (Tofranil)	75	150–300	150–300 The level should include the active metabolite desipramine: toxicity risk	+++	+++	++++	+++	++++ quinidine-like antiarrhythmic effects
Amitriptyline (Elavil)	75 (give q hs due to sedative effects)	150–300	100–250 The level should include the active metabolite nortriptyline: toxicity risk	++++	++++	+++	+++	++++
Clomipramine (Anafranil)	75	150–250	?	++++	++++	+++	+++	++++
Trimipramine (Surmontil)	75	150–200	?	++++	++++	+++	+++	++++
Doxepine (Adapin, Sinequan)	75	150–300	100–250	+++	++++	++	+++	++
Secondary amines								
Desipramine (Norpramin)	75	150–300	150–300	++	++	+++	++	+++
Nortriptyline (Pamelor, Aventyl)	50	50–150	50–150	+++	+++	+	++	+++
Protriptyline (Vivactil)	15	15–60	75–250	+++	+	++	++	++++
Tetracyclics								
Amoxapine (Asendin)	150	150–400	?	+++	++	+	+++	++
Maprotiline (Ludiomil)	75, increase slowly due to possible seizures	150–225 (usually 175–200)	150–300	+++	+++	++	++++	+++

Adapted from Sadock, B. J., & Sadock, V. A. (2002). *Kaplan and Sadock's Synopsis of Psychiatry: Behavioral Sciences/Clinical Psychiatry* (9th ed). Baltimore, MD: Lippincott Williams & Wilkins. p. 1127, 1130.

TABLE 8.22. Precautions in Using TCAs

• **Inducing a manic episode** (pts with a hx of bipolar disorder): use low dosages or use fluoxetine or bupropion
• **Exacerbate a psychotic disorder**
• **Anticholinergic effect**: dry mouth (use sugarless gum or candies, fluoride lozenges), constipation, blurred vision, pupillary dilatation, precipitation of glaucoma (narrow-angle glaucoma) (use miotic eye drops), urinary retention and impotence (bethanechol such as Urecholine 25–50 mg 3–4×/d, may be given 30 min before sex), delirium (IM or IV physostigmine/Antilirium is a diagnostic tool)
• **Sedation**: the most sedating are amitriptyline, trimipramine, and doxepin
• **Orthostatic hypotension**: fludrocortisone (0.05 mg bid)
• **Cardiac effects**: tachycardia, flattened T waves, ↑ QT intervals, depressed ST (contraindicated in pts with preexisting conduction defects); **in OD: risk is arrhythmias**. Discontinue the drug a few days prior to surgery (risk of hypertensive episodes). **Stop during ECT**
• **Neurologic**: myoclonic twitches, tongue tremor, upper extremities tremor, ataxia. Amoxapine can cause parkinsonism, neuroleptic malignant syndrome. All ↓ the seizure threshold (caution in pts with epilepsy or brain lesions)
• **Allergy and blood**: skin rashes, rare jaundice, agranulocytosis, leukocytosis, leucopenia, eosinophilia (stop the drug)
• **Weight gain**: change to a different class
• **Sexual**: more with amoxapine (impotence, hyperprolactinemia), amenorrhea, inappropriate secretion of antidiuretic hormone
• **During pregnancy and breastfeeding**: to avoid (clomipramine may be safer)
• **Drug interactions**: blocks effects of guanethidine, propanolol, clonidin. TCAs with methyldopa may cause agitation. Birth control pills, vitamin C, barbiturates, nicotin, primidone, and lithium: ↓ TCA plasma conc. Acetazolamide, aspirin, cimetidine, thiazide diuretics, SSRIs (fluoxetine >>> paroxetine > sertraline > citalopram): ↑ TCA plasma conc. If + antipsychotics: ↑ anticholinergic and sedative SE. If + sympathomimetics: ↑ serious CV effects by ↑ TCA. With MAOIs: risk of hypertension crisis. TCAs ↑ Phenytoin level. TCAs with class I antiarrhythmic (quinidine, disopyramide, procainamide) may lead to quinidine toxicity with arrhythmias
• **Overdoses are serious** (see OD management in psychiatric emergencies chapter)+++   **Symptoms**: agitation, delirium, convulsions, mydriasis, abnormal BP and temperature, coma, respiratory depression, cardiac arrhythmias (risk for 4 days after the OD → monitor in ICU)   **Prescriptions should be given for <1 wk and nonrefillable for pts at risk for suicide**

Adapted from Sadock, B. J., & Sadock, V. A. (2002). *Kaplan and Sadock's Synopsis of Psychiatry: Behavioral Sciences/Clinical Psychiatry* (9th ed). Baltimore, MD: Lippincott Williams & Wilkins. p. 1127, 1130.

(4) Trazodone and Nefazodone

Trazodone (Desyrel, Oleptro): antidepressant with no anticholinergic SE, very sedative (used for insomnia, fluoxetine-induced insomnia/dose is 50–100 mg at hs, half-life 6–12 hr), does not worsen psychotic sx, rather safe in OD. SE: orthostatic hypotension, headache, nausea, priapism (if untreated → risk of impotence/stop the drug; rx of priapism may be intracavernosal injection of a 1 µg/mL solution of epinephrine), neutropenia. DDI: with buspirone (↑ SGPT), ↑ phenytoin, ↑ digoxin; serotonergic syndrome reported. Oleptro is the extended-release form (forms: 150, 300 mg tabs; given once/day in PM)

Nefazodone (Serzone): Rarely used (hepatotoxicity); similar structure to trazodone. Starting dose: 50 mg bid, ↑ with 100–200 mg/d q wk. Average dose is 300–600 mg/d in bid doses (max 400 mg in elderly); may be taken 1×/d at hs. SE: orthostatic hypotension, sinus bradycardia (caution if cardiac condition, past stroke, dehydration, pts on antihypertensive drugs). It rarely induces mania in pts with hx of BPD. May ↑ levels of triazolam, alprazolam, digoxin, haloperidol, and may ↑ the SE of lithium. No priapism.

(5) **Mirtazapine (Remeron)**: very sedating (50% of pts) but ↓ in 1 wk. Starting dose: 15 mg q hr may be ↑ by 15 mg q 5 days up to 45 mg q hr (max 72 mg). SE: somnolence, dizziness, orthostatic hypotension, ↑ appetite and weight, may ↑ lipids, ALT levels, ↓ neutropenia (0.3% of pts; if pt develops fever, chills, sore throat, or signs of infection, discontinue drug and treat), ↑ sedation with benzodiazepines and alcohol. Risks: hypertensive crisis with TCAs, serotonin syndrome with MAOIs.

(6) **Bupropion (Wellbutrin, Zyban, Aplenzin)**: for depression, smoking cessation; starting dose: 100 mg bid (or 150 mg 1×/d of the SR form); ↑ to 100 mg tid or 150 mg bid (or 300 mg in AM of SR form). Max/d is 450 mg of regular form (400 mg of the SR form). Do not exceed 150 mg per dose of the regular form (300 mg/dose of SR form). Combination with a dopaminergic agent (levodopa-carbidopa or bromocriptine) may induce dyskinesia and delirium. May ↑ seizures. Not useful for anxiety. Rare psychosis (avoid in pt with MDD and need for detoxification: seizure risk ↑).

(7) MAOIs

> • **Caution with MAOIs**: (not to combine with other antidepressants. In rare cases, these have been used with TCAs/see precautions. Do not use with SSRIs and SNRIs/risk of HTN and serotonin syndrome). The original MAOIs require a strict tyramine-free diet. Peripheral MAO-A is required for the breakdown of tyramine in the diet. MAOI given po inhibits gut MAO-A, creating the risk of food-related hypertensive crises (transdermal selegine enters the circulation directly; high brain levels are obtained with little inhibition of MAO-A in the gut → no diet restriction if used at low dosage: 6 mg/d). However, all MAOIs have DDIs at any dosage with high risk of serotonin syndrome (may be fatal). Do not give large prescriptions to impulsive or suicidal pts.

TABLE 8.23.   MAOI Diet: Eliminate the Following Foods

• Cheese	• English Stilton, blue cheeses, old cheddar, mozzarella, cheese spreads, feta, parmesan; avoid soft cheeses (Brie, cream cheese, sour cream, Boursin, Ricotta), soy milk, yogurt (one should not eat more than 2 oz of sour cream, yogurt, cottage cheese, American cheese, or mild Swiss cheese per day). All other cheese products or food involving fermentation should be avoided
• Fish, meats	• Cured meats, sausages, pâtés, organs, salami, mortadella, bologna, pepperoni, dried meats, chicken liver, fish, smoked fish or meat, shrimp paste, pickled herring, liverwurst, dried salted fish, spoiled meat, fermented meats
• Alcoholic beverages	• Liqueurs, beer and ale, concentrated alcoholic drinks, red or Chianti wines, sherry, scotch (one may occasionally have a single cocktail or 2–3 oz of white wine; gin and vodka have no tyramine content)
• Others	• Yeast extracts (e.g., Marmite; bread is safe), fermented food, fermented soy products, monosodium glutamate/MSG, sauerkraut, banana, avocado, old yogurt, chocolate (not more than 2 oz of chocolate candy per day; chocolate-flavored cookies, cake, and ice-cream may be consumed), broad beans, canned figs, coffee (should drink decaffeinated coffee or decaffeinated cola drinks, or limit the intake to a total of 2 cups or glasses of caffeine-containing beverage per day)

A high tyramine-containing meal contains approximately 40 mg tyramine; a high-tyramine content food contains ≥2 mg of tyramine per serving.

TABLE 8.24.   MAOI Contraindications

• Never use +++	• Antiasthma drugs • Buspirone (risk of hypertensive crisis) • Levodopa, methyldopa, L-tryptophan • Opioids (meperidine, dextromethorphan, propoxyphene, tramadol, morphine, codeine, fentanyl, methadone, buprenorphine, oxycodone) • Antihypertensives (reserpine, methyldopa, guanethidine) • Cold medications containing sympathomimetics, dextromethorphan. Avoid nasal decongestants and inhalers (can take chlorpheniramine, brompheniramine, guaifenesin, aspirin) • SSRIs (risk of serotonin syndrome), SNRIs, nefazodone, mirtazapine, St. John's wort, clomipramine, venlafaxine, sibutramine • Sympathomimetics (amphetamines, cocaine, methylphenidate, dopamine, epinephrine, NE, ephedrine, pseudoephedrine, isoproterenol, phenylpropanolamine, diet pills): risk of hypertensive crisis • Other MAOIs • Over-the-counter pain medications (can take acetaminophen and ibuprofen, aspirin) • Certain triptans: sumatriptan, zolmitriptan, rizatriptan • Carbamazepine • Meperidine
• Avoid	• Antihistamines • Bromocriptine • Disulfiram • Hydralazine • Sedative-hypnotics (phenobarbital, secobarbital, pentobarbital) and alcohol • Anticholinergics • Tricyclics and tetracyclics (imipramine, chlomipramine, trimipramine, desipramine, nortriptyline), SSRIs • Propranolol • Closely monitor stimulants

Adapted from Sadock, B. J., & Sadock, V. A. (2002). *Kaplan and Sadock's Synopsis of Psychiatry: Behavioral Sciences/Clinical Psychiatry* (9th ed). Baltimore, MD: Lippincott Williams & Wilkins. p. 1079.

TABLE 8.25. Switching Medications from or to an MAOI

• Switching from an MAOI to another type of antidepressant	• **Wait 14 days** after last dose of MAOI prior to starting the new drug
• Switching from an antidepressant to MAOI	• Wait 10–14 days (5 wk for fluoxetine) after the last dose prior to starting the MAOI
• Switching from a RIMA to another type of antidepressant	• Wait 3 days after the last dose of RIMA
• Treatment gap to and from MAOIs in unstable patients (controversial)	• Caution (discuss risks with pts, be prepared for possible hypertensive crisis) with: • Bupropion, atypical antipsychotics, tricyclics (predominant NE action), stimulants, trazodone, lamotrigine, some opiates (oxycodone, hydrocodone), T3, lithium, benzodiazepines (alprazolam) • Dietary supplements: EPA (omega-3 fatty acids), SAMe, chromium, magnesium, selenium, inositol, DHEA, L-tyrosine, L-Tryptophan

TABLE 8.26. Available MAOIs in the United States: Monitor Liver Enzymes, MAOIs ↓ the Blood Sugar (Caution in Diabetes), May Cause False-Positive Test Results for Pheochromocytoma or Neuroblastoma (↑ Urinary Metanephrine Conc.); Usually a 1–4 Wk Delay in the Clinical Response

- **Phenelzine (*Nardil*)**: start with 15 mg on first day, increase to 15 mg tid during 1st wk then ↑ 15 mg/d/wk up to 4 wk and up to 30–90 mg/d. Has a greater sedating and antianxiety effect than parnate
- **Isocarboxazid (*Marplan*)**: start with 10 mg/d, increase to 10 mg tid during 1st wk up to 10–50 mg/d
- **Tranylcypromine *(Parnate)***: start with 10 mg/d, increase to 10 mg tid during 1st wk up to 20–40 mg/d. Is more activating and has less hepatotoxic risks. Divide the doses to prevent hypotension. May have a more rapid onset of action than the 2 other MAOIs
- **Selegiline, an oral selective inhibitor of MAO-B** (↑ dopaminergic neurotransmission) at recommended doses, but if greater doses, blocks both MAO-A and MAO-B from breaking down NE, serotonin, and dopamine (↑ noradrenergic, serotonergic, and dopaminergic neurotransmission) and blocks metabolism of tyramine in the gut: Selegiline: metabolized to L-amphetamine and L-methamphetamine (lesser risk of abuse than D isomers), may be detected on urine toxic screens:
    - *Eldepryl*: not approved for depression (may need high doses; 20–60 mg/d) but used for Parkinson disease (10 mg/d)
    - *Emsam* (transdermal selegiline): is MAO-A and MAO-B inhibitor in brain and relatively selective MAO-B inhibitor in the gut; no dietary restriction at low dose/6 mg/d but restricted diet if 9–12 mg/d; same drug interactions as original MAOIs

TABLE 8.27. Side Effects of MAOIs

- **Orthostatic hypotension**: rx is avoidance of caffeine, intake of >2 L of fluids/d, ↑ salt intake (unless CHF), fludrocortisone (0.1–0.2 mg/d, use with caution) or licorice extracts, dividing the daily dose. Use lowest dose possible; R/O drug interaction etiology
- **Hypertensive crisis tyramine-induced or spontaneous nontyramine-induced with tranylcypromine** (Parnate >30–40 mg all at once): Educate pt: sx (severe, occipital headache, may be accompanied by photophobia, palpitations, stiff neck, N/V, sweating)
- **Intervene early**: α-adrenergic antagonists like phentolamine (slow administration of Regitine/5 mg IV) or chlorpromazine (Thorazine: 25–50 mg po, may be used at home) to lower BP; ↓ fluids with a diuretic, and control tachycardia with β-adrenergic receptor antagonist. Nifedipine (Procardia): 10-mg capsule-squirt under the tongue or swallowed, used if sx were intolerable but caution due to sudden low BP (not recommended anymore). Have pt sit or lie down
- **RIMAs**: ↓ risk of tyramine-induced hypertensive crisis if taking RIMAs/reversible inhibitors of MAOI such as moclobemide or befloxatone, not available in the United States and the recommendations then were not to eat tyramine-containing foods for 2 hr after taking the drug; Cimetididne and fluoxetine ↓ the elimination of moclobemide
- **Weight gain, edema**: switch to another agent
- **Insomnia**: MAOIs may ↓ REM sleep; divide the dose, do not give after dinner, use lowest dosage in AM; use trazodone (Desyrel) or estazolam (ProSom) or quazepam (Doral) to ↑ slow-wave and REM sleep
- **Sexual dysfunction**: switch to another drug
- **Muscle pains**: due to pyridoxine deficiency (pyridoxine 100–400 mg/d) administration of vitamin B_6 may minimize the jumping movements and muscular irritability
- **Possible hepatotoxic effects**: discontinue
- **Less risks of epilepsy and of cardiotoxicity than tricyclics and tetracyclics**
- **May trigger mania in pts with bipolar disorder, psychosis in pts with schizophrenia**
- **In overdose**: 1–6 hr after ingestion, agitation progressing to hypertension, coma, tachypnea, dilated pupils, involuntary movements. Rx: acidification of urine, dialysis, treatment of hypertension

MOOD STABILIZERS

(1) LITHIUM (Eskalith, Eskalith CR, Lithobid, Lithium carbonate tablets, Lithium citrate syrup)

FDA-approved manic episodes of manic depressive illness, maintenance rx for manic depressive pts with a hx of mania for manic episodes of manic depressive illness, maintenance rx for manic depressive pts with a hx of mania but also used for bipolar depression, antidepressant augmentation, schizoaffective disorder, mixed manic states, recurrent unipolar depression.

Lithium may have **neurotrophic properties** (↑ the density of gray matter in the brains of pts with bipolar disorder). **Is a suicidality-reducing agent with a nine-fold reduction (works on depression and mania). Lithium can be used on low-dosage therapy for suicidal depression,** like starting on 300 mg, increasing to 450 mg/d.

TABLE 8.28.   Available Forms: Converting from One Form to Another: Substitute on an Equal Milligram Equivalency

• **Immediate-release lithium carbonate:** Eskalith, Lithium carbonate (usually 150-, 300-, 450-, and 600-mg pills)	• More variability in plasma lithium levels in 24 hr → more side effects
• **Slow-release forms:** (Eskalith CR, Lithobid): 450 mg pills may be given once/d	• No advantage with regard to renal toxicity
• **Lithium citrate** (8 mEq/5 mL or 300 mg/5 mL syrup)	• 4 mEq of the citrate = 150 mg of lithium

Pharmacokinetics: absorbed in 8 hr, peak plasma level in 1–3 hr (4 hr for controlled-release lithium, 0.5 hr for citrate), is not protein bound, is excreted by the kidney. Monitor blood conc. (draw blood 12 hr after the last dose/usually before breakfast). Lithium half-life is 18–36 hr (fastest in youth, slowest in elderly). A constant oral dosage needs 5–8 days to reach a steady state.

TABLE 8.29.   Monitoring Lithium Treatment

• Prior to treatment	• Physical evaluation • CBC • Kidney function tests (serum creatinine, urine specific gravity, electrolytes) • Thyroid function tests • ECG • Pregnancy test • Weight: Pt is overweight if BMI is 25–30, obese if BMI > 30 • Check for prediabetes (fasting plasma glucose: 100–125 mg/dL), or diabetes (fasting plasma glucose >126 mg/dL) • Check for dyslipidemia

• During treatment	• Kidney function 1–2×/yr (q 2–3 months for the first 6 months)
	• Plasma lithium levels:
	   acute treatment (1.0 mEq/L–1.5 mEq/L)
	   chronic treatment (0.6–1.2 mEq/L)
	• Monitor weight and BMI
	• Possible effects on tests: ↑ WBCs, ↑ glucose, ↑ Mg, ↓ K, ↓ uric acid, ↓ thyroxin

InstaRead Lithium System from ReliaLab available and used to use finger-sticks/point of care test, office-based/www. relialab.com. Kit includes the machine, 12 pts test packs, instruction manual. Call (866) INSTAREAD (FDA CLIA-waived test) or (866) 467–8273 for more information.

TABLE 8.30.   Clinical Guidelines for Lithium Treatment

• **Starting doses**	• 300 mg tid for adults unless previous effective dose is known, possibly up to 1,800 mg/day. Response in acute mania may take 7–14 days	• Usually:
		   900–1,200 mg/d → level of 0.6–1 mEq/L
		   1,200–1,800 mg/d → level of 0.8–1.2 mEq/L

• **Maintenance doses**	• Usually divided in 2–3 doses for the regular form or in a single dose for the sustained-released (= to the total daily dose of the regular form)	• Divided doses better for GI side effects • Check levels every 2–6 months once stable • Blood sample must be drawn 12 hr after a given dose • Usually effective for mania at levels 1.0–1.5 mEq/L and maintenance at 0.4–0.8 mEq/L
• **Discontinuation**	• If ineffective or not well tolerated	• Risk of recurrence • Risk of failure when rx is reinstituted • Rapid discontinuation ↑ risk of relapse and possibly suicide (taper slowly over 3 months)

Continued

TABLE 8.30.   Clinical Guidelines for Lithium Treatment   Continued

• Patient education	• ↑ Na intake→ ↓ in lithium conc. • ↓ Na intake→ ↑ in lithium conc. (↑ toxicity) • Dehydration, sweating → ↑ toxicity	• Caution with salt-restricted diets and diuretics
• Special precautions	• Toxic levels are near therapeutic levels → monitor toxicity (tremor, ataxia, vomiting, sedation) • Monitor for dehydration → lower dose • Monitor pts with thyroid disorders • Do not use: if allergy to lithium, severe kidney disease, severe CV disease, severe dehydration, sodium depletion	• Elderly: lower doses needed, more SE. Steady state usually reached within 5 days but can take up to 10 days in elderly or renally impaired pts (draw levels later on to avoid any toxicity). Serum levels as low as 0.4–0.6 mEq/L may be needed (↑ neurotoxicity if >) • Children, adolescents: caution, efficacy and safety not established if <12 yo • Pregnancy: category D: ↑ major birth defects; ↑ cardiac anomalies (Ebstein's); premature birth, nephrogenic diabetes insipidus, hypoglycemia, euthyroid goiter, neonatal hypothyroidism in infants; if used during delivery: ↑ hypotonia in infant; discontinue slowly prior to pregnancy and restart after delivery; no breastfeeding while on lithium; atypical antipsychotics are preferable to lithium or anticonvulsants during pregnancy for bipolar disorders. Lithium clearance ↑ 50–100% early in pregnancy and returns to normal at delivery (risk of toxicity). If given during pregnancy: fetal echocardiogram, ultrasound exam at 16–18 weeks of gestation

TABLE 8.31.   Variations in Lithium Levels

• Serum level of lithium is too low	• Serum level of lithium is too high: Avoid lithium level >1.2 mEq/L (toxicity occurs >1.5 mEq/L)
• Incorrect blood sample timing: (forgotten dose, sample taken more than 12 hr after dose): recheck • Dosage decrease: if dose forgotten, recheck 4–5 days later after correction: if pt has decreased the doses due to SEs, reassess the dosage with the pt • Change in dosage schedule: switching from a single daily dose to a divided dose schedule may ↓ the level. Do not correct if well tolerated • Dietary changes: if dietary salt intake ↑, serum lithium ↓; adjust by ↑ lithium dosage if a low-salt diet is stopped • Drug interactions: see Table 8.32 • Sweating and exercising: Lithium is excreted in sweat • Polyuria: most pts with polyuria secondary to lithium usually do not need higher doses of lithium. Treat the polyuria rather than ↑ the lithium dose (if diuretic used to treat polyuria, lithium dose reduction may be needed), Caution as polyuria may result in dehydration and ↑ serum lithium level • Blood sample storage: in clotted whole blood, lithium levels ↓; in frozen plasma, lithium conc. is stable • Poor compliance: very frequent	• Incorrect blood sample timing: repeat the level on blood drawn 12 hr after last dose • Dosage increased or double dose taken: if sx of toxicity, hold lithium until sx resolve and then restart at a lower dose. If no toxic sx, repeat the level 4 days after correction of the dosage • Change in dosage schedule: when switching from divided to single daily dose, there is a 10–26% increase in the 12-hr value. Do not change the dosage if no toxicity • Kidney disease: adjust. Consider an anticonvulsant alternative • Dehydration: correct it • Dietary changes: ↓ in salt intake (serum Li ↑: ↓ dose or ↑ salt) • Drug interactions: see Table 8.32 • Pharmacy error: pt must know size, shape, name, and dose • Collection error: if collected in a tube containing a lithium-heparin anticoagulant (green top) instead of a standard red-top tube • Mood state: ↑ levels during depression? (controversial), adjust the dose • Postpartum: in pregnancy, GFR↑ (need for greater doses of lithium); after delivery: risk of toxicity → stop lithium shortly before delivery and restart at lower dosage shortly after delivery • Posture: higher levels after ambulatory activity than after being in bed (caution in shift workers) • Laboratory variability: check

TABLE 8.32. Lithium Treatment: Side Effects and Their Remediation

Gastrointestinal	Anorexia, nausea, vomiting, diarrhea	Divide the dosage, give with food, switch to another lithium preparation (less diarrhea, loose stools, abdominal cramping with lithium citrate, and regular release forms; if nausea, switch to a slow-release or lithium citrate), move the entire dose to bedtime; sustained-release form may ↓ gastric irritation; antidiarrhea drugs (Imodium, Pepto-Bismol, Lomotil)
Neurological	Rapid, fine, intention tremor EEG: ↑ amplitude and generalized slowing Headaches, anxiety Memory problems Muscular weakness, myoclonus Dulling	↓ dosage; switch to sustained-release form ↓ caffeine intake, check other medicines pt is on, treat anxiety, propanolol (30–120 mg/d in divided doses), primidone (50–250 mg/d), adding a benzodiazepine If low K+: supplement Suspect lithium toxicity Memory problems: low dose cholinesterase inhibitors?
	Cognition changes (within 6–8 months of rx): lack of spontaneity, dulling, dysphoria, loss of memory, fatigue, sedation	May decrease over time
	Mild parkinsonism, ataxia, dysarthria, peripheral neuropathy, **pseudotumor cerebri**, ↑ risk of seizures, organic brain syndrome (confusion, lethargy with normal or low Li levels) may be seen	Rarely
Renal	Polyuria (urine vol. >3–4 L/24 hr, nocturia), ↑ thirst, dry mouth, and polydipsia (reversible)	Evaluate renal function, fluid replacement, lowest possible dose of lithium, single daily dosing. Possible addition of a diuretic (chlorothiazide 50 mg/d or amiloride 5–10 mg/d) while ↓ the dose of lithium by 50% and monitoring lithium levels
	Interstitial fibrosis, renal failure (rare, serious, if administration >10 yr, 20% develop renal insufficiency on long-term lithium), nephrotic syndrome (may be chronic, irreversible)	Check renal function regularly
Thyroid	Hypothyroidism: clinical or subclinical, 7–10%, F > M, > in rapid-cycling BPD, > in first 2 yr of rx (by impaired release of thyroxine), goiter (↑ with smoking) Hyperparathyroidism (↑ serum Ca → bradycardia, and ↑ parathyroid hormone), loss of bone mineral density (↑ osteoporosis)	Frequent ↑ TSH (check q 6–12 months), check if depression appears during lithium rx Treat with levothyroxine (Synthroid) 0.05 mg/d, ↑ q 6 wk as needed following the TSH level. Check antithyroid antibodies (pt may need ongoing rx) Lithium-induced hypothyroidism may be transient: try to ↓ the daily T4 dose after several years of rx and check TSH regularly (T4 can precipitate mania in bipolar pts not treated with a mood stabilizer)
Cardiac	T wave flattening or inversion (reversible), sinus arrhythmia, heart block, syncope (obtain Holter monitor in elderly) No QTc changes, no BP changes	Caution in pts on a low-salt diet, on diuretics, on ACE-inhibitors, with renal failure, with electrolyte imbalances. Discontinue Lithium if dysrhythmias (↑ death risk in older males with cardiac pathology). Risk↑ if used with phenothiazines
Skin	Acne, rash, alopecia, ↑ psoriasis Lithium does not affect visual acuity but ↓ the retinal sensitivity to light (role of melatonin?)	Tetracycline ↑ lithium level Benzoyl peroxide (5–10%) sol., erythromycin (1.5–2%) sol. for acne
Metabolism	Weight gain (dose related) Leukocytosis (benign: 10,000–14,000 WBCs/ neutrophilia) Mild hypercalcemia (usually not progressive, range 10.5–11.5 mg/dL with normal levels of parathyroid hormone: check Ca 1, 6, 12 months after starting lithium and q yr)	If edema, spironolactone (50 mg/d)

Note: Most SE will disappear by waiting ↓ the dose, taking the entire dose at night, changing to a different lithium preparation, reducing from tid to bid.

TABLE 8.33. Drug Interactions with Lithium

• **Antipsychotics**	• Haloperidol: reports of encephalopathy similar to NMS • Quetiapine: somnolence • Ziprazidone: ↑ tremor • Chlorpromazine: possible ↑ of lithium excretion • Risk of NMS • Clozapine: may improve leucopenia, but questionable due to risks of neurotoxicity, seizures, agranulocytosis, psychosis, NMS
• **Antidepressants**	• TCAs: risk of switch to mania, ↑ tremors, acts synergistic with lithium • ECT: discontinue lithium 2 days prior to rx • Fluvoxamine: risk of seizures • SSRI: risk of serotonin syndrome
• **Diuretics**	• Most diuretics ↑ lithium levels: distal tubule diuretics (thiazide), potassium sparing (spironolactone, amiloride, trimterene), loop (furosemide, ethacrynic acid) • Osmotic diuretics, xanthines (caffeine, theophylline), carbonic anhydrase inhibitors: ↓ lithium levels
• **Angiotensin-converting enzyme inhibitors**	• ↑ Lithium conc.
• **Nonsteroidal anti-inflammatory**	• ↓ Lithium conc. Aspirin and sulindac do not change lithium conc.
• **Anticonvulsants**	• Start combination at a lower dosage of each medication. Lithium + valproate: better tolerated than lithium + carbamazepine • May be safely and effectively combined with lamotrigine, and perhaps with topiramate
• **Calcium channel inhibitors**	• ↑ Neurotoxicity (may appear with lower lithium levels)
• **Succinylcholine**	• Lithium prolongs the neuromuscular blocking effect
• **Marijuana**	• Unclear if there are interactions
• **Antibiotics**	• ↑ Lithium levels with spectinomycin, metronidazole, tetracyclines, levofloxacin

TABLE 8.34. Lithium Toxicity

- Real toxicity is about 2× the therapeutic levels of lithium
- 0.8–1.2 mEq/L: tremor, polyphagia, polydipsia, nausea, weakness
- 1.2–1.5 mEq/L: same as above + memory and concentration problems, fine hand tremor, GI upset, fatigue
- 1.5–2.5 mEq/L: diarrhea, vomiting, slurred speech, tinnitus, blurred vision, poor motor coordination, sedation, abdominal pain
- >2.5 mEq/L: nystagmus, coarse tremor, hallucinations, dyskinesia, seizures, coma, death

Best response to lithium: classical BPD (bipolar I disorder without mood-incongruent delusions and without comorbidities, pts who get completely well during episodes). Lithium works better for "highs" (euphoric mania, better in manic episodes than depressive episodes, preventing manic relapses) than depressive relapses. Divalproex is better for mixed bipolar episodes and in comorbid substance abusers.

(2) ANTICONVULSANTS

- **Note 1**: Basic actions of anticonvulsants:
  - Inhibitory (GABAergic) drug: such as gabapentin (Neurontin), vigabatrin (Sabril), tiagabine (Gabitril), which enhance GABA activity, possibly also valprotate
  - Antiexcitatory effects by action on glutamate/by decreasing the excitatory neurotransmitter glutamate and blockage of sodium channels (carbamazepine, oxcarbamazepine, valproate, lamotrigine, topiramate). Topiramate also blocks the AMPA/ampa/kainite type of glutamate receptor
  - Combining an antiexcitatory drug with an inhibitory drug may be better in BPD
- **Note 2**: Black box warning: monitor for suicidality and other unusual changes in behavior

TABLE 8.35.   Psychiatric Adverse Effects of Anticonvulsant Drugs

• Types	• Behavioral disorders (agitation, aggression); depression; mania, hypomania; delirium; psychosis; pseudodementia; encephalopathies
• Drugs involved	• Vigabatrine, phenobarbital > phenytoin > carbamazepine, valproic acid, benzodiazepines > lamotrigine, gabapentin
• Guidelines	• Use monotherapy if possible, minimal effective dosage, escalate doses slowly, awareness of toxicity or withdrawal, folic acid deficiency • Preexisting psychiatric/behavioral disorders and organic brain damage predispose to these reactions • Discontinuation of the offensive drug may be needed • If psychiatric disorders are associated with epilepsy: is it coincidental? Related to epileptic seizures or underlying brain damage? Associated with psychosocial handicaps of epilepsy? Adverse reaction to the AED drug?

Valproate (Depakene, Depakote, Depakote ER)

- **Forms**
  - **Valproate or valproic acid** (Depakene syrup: 250 mg/5 mL; Depakene capsules: 250 mg)
  - **Divalproex** (Depakote: 125 mg, 250 mg, 500 mg; Depakote-ER: 250 mg, 500 mg; Depakote sprinkle capsules: 125 mg): better tolerated than valproic acid
  - **Valproate sodium injection** (Depacon injection: 100 mg valproic acid/mL; IV use only)
- **Pharmacokinetics**: half-life is 8–17 hr, protein binding; peak: 3–8 hr; may be given 1–4×/d, hepatic metabolic pathway, renal elimination, interacts with many drugs that are metabolized by the liver: enzyme inducers ↓ conc. of valproic acid.
- **Used**: acute episodes and prophylaxis of bipolar I disorder, schizoaffective disorder, other mental disorders (intermittent explosive disorder, aggression, adjunct of other medications), seizure disorders.
- **FDA approval**: bipolar I disorder: acute mania (divalproex) and mixed mania (divalproex, divalproexER) (in adults, not in children <10), epilepsy: complex partial seizures that occur in isolation or in association with other types of seizures (monotherapy and adjunctive), simple and complex absence seizures in adults and children >10 (monotherapy or adjunctive), multiple seizure types which include absence seizures (adjunctive), migraine prophylaxis (divalproex, divalproex ER).

TABLE 8.36.   Valproate Treatment: Side Effects and Their Remediation

• Prior to treatment	• R/O hepatic and pancreatic disease (do not give if such exists)
• Starting dose	• 250 mg with a meal, ↑ to 3×/d (over the next 3–6 days, may go faster in hospital)
• Assess plasma levels	• In AM before the first daily dose (better: 12 hr after the most recent dose); therapeutic doses: 50–100 μg/mL (for maintenance) if well tolerated (sometimes up to 150 μg/mL for acute mania), usually on a daily dose of 1,200–1,500 mg divided. Higher doses have been used (up to 4,200 mg). Effects appear between 5 and 15 days. Note: levels > 125 mcg/mL ↑ SE risks. Adjust on rx response and tolerance. Therapeutic levels for acute bipolar depression are not yet established

TABLE 8.37.   Side Effects, Adverse Reactions, Remediation

• GI	• Nausea, vomiting, and diarrhea	• Use the sprinkle or delayed-release forms; histamine H2 receptor antagonists (*Pepcid*); give after meals; give 4–6 glasses of water with a dose • Diarrhea may ↑ with slow or controlled-release lithium
• Nervous system	• Sedation, ataxia, dysarthria, tremor • Risk of encephalopathy, coma, death in OD • Dulling	• Tremor: β-adrenergic receptor antagonists or gabapentin • ↓ Dosage
• Weight gain	• Frequent; edema	• Low calorie diet, ↓ dosage
• Hair loss	• Chelation of selenium or zinc?	• Vitamin supplements with zinc and selenium such as *Centrum Silver*: ingest divalproex and the vitamin separately in time

Continued

TABLE 8.37. Side Effects, Adverse Reactions, Remediation   Continued

• Blood	• **Thrombocytopenia** with high dosages • Coagulation disturbances • Agranulocytosis • Hyponatremia (SIADH) • ↑ **Liver transaminases** (up to 3 times the upper normal limit) is asymptomatic	• ↓ Dosage
• Liver	• Potential **fatal hepatotoxicity in pts <3 yo**, taking phenobarbital (lethargy, anorexia, vomiting, and abdominal pain). Possible hyperammonemic encephalopathy (do not use if urea cycle disorder)	• Discontinue drug • If hyperammonemia: ↓ dose or discontinue dietary supplementation with carnitine (1–2 g/d) and monitoring
• Pancreas	• **Rare pancreatitis** (usually in first 6 months of rx, risk of death, in pts <20 yo with chronic encephalopathy)	• Discontinue the drug
• Miscellaneous	• **Polycystic ovary disease** (hirsutism, acne, alopecia, menstrual abnormalities, obesity, ↑ serum testosterone, ↑ LH, ↑ prolactin, ↓ FSH, insulin resistance) • False-positive results in urinary ketone, false abnormal thyroid function tests	• Assess benefit–risk for the use of valproate in women with reproductive capacity
• Pregnancy	• **Neural tube defects** (spina bifida) if taken during first trimester; cognitive problems in children exposed in utero, also heart defects, multicystic dysplastic kidney, postaxial polydactyly type B, inguinal hernia, penile hypospadias • Pregnancy registry for women on antiepileptic medication	• **Should not be used during pregnancy or lactation:** ↓ risk with folic acid (1–4 mg/d, started 3 months prior to conception and taken during pregnancy) • Note: lamotrigine and carbamazepine may be safer on the fetus (but not risk-free)

TABLE 8.38. Drug–Drug Interactions with Valproate

Drug	Adverse effects	Action/remediation
• Lithium	• ↑ Tremors • (Divalproex + lithium is better tolerated than divalproex + carbamazepine)	• If tremors: use β-receptor antagonists (50 mg/d atenolol), or switch to a slow-release lithium
• Antipsychotics	• ↑ Sedation, ↑ EPS, delirium, stupor	• Antiparkinsonian drugs if EPS
• Anticonvulsants	• Ataxia, nausea, lethargy, acute psychosis	• Valproic acid: • **May ↑ serum levels** of carbamazepine, lamotrigine, phenobarbital • **May ↓ serum level** of phenytoin • Carbamazepine may ↓ level of valproate

• Antidepressants		• Valproic acid:
		  ↑ **Levels** of amitriptyline, nortriptyline
		  ↓ **Levels** of desipramine
		  Amitriptyline and fluoxetine↑ level of valproate

• Benzodiazepines		• Valproate ↑ conc. of diazepam
• Anticoagulants	• Bleeding risk	• Valproate ↑ effect of aspirin and warfarin
• Guanfacine		• ↑ Level of valproate

TABLE 8.39. Conversion from Depakote to Depakote ER

• Extended-release valproate is about 80% as bioavailable as immediate-release valproate
• When switching from regular to ER valproate: increase 8–20% the immediate-release dose
• Divalproex ER improves GI side effects and alopecia

Carbamazepine (Tegretol, Tegretol XR, Carbatrol, Equetro) and oxcarbazepine (Trileptal)

- **Forms**
  - **Carbamazepine**: 100 and 200 mg tablets, suspension (100 mg/5 mL). Extended-release form/*Equetro and Carbatrol* (100, 200, and 300 mg tablets); *Tegretol XR* (100, 200, 400 mg). Store in a cool, dry place.
  - **Oxcarbazepine**: 150, 300, and 600 mg tablets, oral suspension 300 mg/5 mL.

- **Indications**: BPD (acute mania, prophylaxis of both manic and depressive episodes), rapid cycling. Tolerance for the antimanic effects may appear. Also used for MDD, schizophrenia, schizoaffective disorders, and impulse-control disorders.

- **FDA approved**
  - **Carbamazepine**: epilepsy (partial seizures with complex symptomatology, grand mal seizures, and mixed seizure patterns), bipolar disorder/mania (acute mania/mixed mania), neuropathic pain (pain associated with true trigeminal neuralgia), approved in children for epilepsy.
  - **Oxcarbazepine**: partial seizures in adults with epilepsy (monotherapy or adjunctive), partial seizures in children aged 4–16 with epilepsy (monotherapy or adjunctive).

- **Pharmacology**: better absorbed if taken with meals, peak plasma levels in 2–8 hr, half-life varies over time (after 1 month of rx, there is an induction of hepatic enzymes and half-life ↓ to 12–17 hr), is metabolized in the liver.

TABLE 8.40.   Clinical Guidelines for the Use of Carbamazepine and Oxcarbazepine

● **Pretreatment evaluations**	● Hematological, hepatic, cardiac diseases are relative contraindications ● CBC with platelet count, liver function tests, serum electrolytes, ECG
● **Starting doses**	● Carbamazepine: Start 200 mg bid (may be divided in 3×/d. Increase slowly ● (<200 mg/day or q 2–7 days in OPU) up to 600–1,800 mg/d ● Oxcarbazepine: Start 150 mg bid, ↑ to optimal doses of 900–2,400 mg/d
● **Plasma levels monitoring**	● Therapeutic levels: 4–12 μg/mL, after a steady dosage for at least 5 days. Draw level in AM prior to giving the first AM dose ● **Carbamazepine autoinduces its own metabolism**: doses given 5–10 days after initiation of tx may need to be increased 4–6 weeks later (decreased blood levels as a result of the autoinduction, which may be misinterpreted as noncompliance) ● Usual therapeutic doses/day: 400–1,600 mg/d ● **Follow-up levels regularly** when stable q 2–3 months
● **Laboratory monitoring**	● **Risks: agranulocytosis and aplastic anemia** ● Check q month for 6 months then q 3–6 months CBC, liver, and renal functions ● Discontinue rx and consult hematologist if: WBC <3,000/mm³ with neutrophil count <1,500/mm³, hematocrit <32%, Hb <11 g/100 mL, platelet count <100,000/mm³, reticulocyte count <0.3%, iron <150 mg/100 mL ● Transient ↓ in T4 and T3 (with normal TSH), and ↑ total cholesterol ● May give false-positive pregnancy test results ● Serum electrolytes to be checked occasionally to r/o hyponatremia

- **Side effects, adverse reactions, remediation**

Most are dose related if plasma levels >9 μg/mL.

TABLE 8.41.   Side Effects, Adverse Reactions, Remediation in Carbamazepine Treatment

● **Blood**	Aplastic anemia, thrombocytopenia, **agranulocytosis (life threatening**: fever, sore throat), petechiae, bleeding	Emergency → hospitalization **Discontinue drug**
● **Hepatitis**	● In a few weeks of rx: ↑ transaminases, cholestasis (↑ alkaline phosphatase, ↑ bilirubin)	● Discontinue drug if hepatic enzymes ↑ above 3× the upper normal limit
● **Exfoliative dermatitis**	● Rash, exfoliative dermatitis, **Stevens-Johnson syndrome**, erythema multiform, toxic epidermal necrolysis	● **Discontinue drug**; life threatening; higher risk than for valproic acid
● **GI**	● N/V, constipation, diarrhea, abdominal pain	● Will improve if dosage is slowly increased and kept as low as possible

Continued

TABLE 8.41. Side Effects, Adverse Reactions, Remediation in Carbamazepine Treatment   Continued

• **Neurologic**	• Confusion (mostly if + lithium or + antipsychotics), particularly in elderly, pts with cognitive disorders • Dizziness, ataxia, sedation, clonus, tremor, diplopia	• Increasing dosages very slowly will prevent it. Similar cognitive disturbances among carbamazepine, lithium, valproic acid • Check electrolytes
• **Others**	• ↓ Cardiac conduction • Caution in pts with glaucoma, prostate diseases, diabetes, alcohol abuse • **Risk of hyponatremia** (by ↑ vasopressin-receptor function, not like the renal effects of lithium) • Rare immune disorder (myocarditis) • Hypothyroidism (may have additive effect with lithium) • Overdose risk similar to TCAs • Multiorgan hypersensitivity reactions	• Hyponatremia may be reversed by demeclocycline or lithium
• **Pregnancy**	• Cranial facial malformations, fingernail hypoplasia, spina bifida in infants, neural tube defects	• Do not use unless absolutely necessary • Folic acid during pregnancy: 1–4 mg/d • Is secreted in breast milk • **See special registry: the North American Antiepileptic Drug Pregnancy Registry (888-233-2334)**

TABLE 8.42. Drug–Drug Interactions with Carbamazepine: +++

• **Carbamazepine ↓ levels of**	• Acetaminophen, • Benzodiazepines (alprazolam, clonazepam) • Antidepressants (bupropion, clomipramine, desipramine, doxepine, imipramine, amitriptyline) • Antipsychotics (clozapine, fluphenazine, haloperidol) • Anticonvulsants (ethosuximide, lamotrigine, methsuximide, phenytoin, primidone, valproate, felbamate, phensuximide) • Antibiotics (doxycycline) • Hormonal contraception • CNS drugs (methadone, fentanyl) • Immunosuppressants (cyclosporine) • Anticoagulants (dicumarol, warfarin) • Calcium channel blockers (nimodipine) • Anesthesia drugs (pancuronium) • Theophylline
• **Drugs that ↑ the levels of carbamazepine**	• Antibiotics (clarithromycin, erythromycin, isoniazid ↑ metabolites, ketoconazole, itraconazole, macrolides) • Anticonvulsants (valproate ↑ active metabolites, lamotrigine) • Xanthine oxidase inhibitor (allopurinol) • Histamine receptor antagonists (cimetidine) • Steroids (danazol) • Diuretics (diltiazem) • Lipid regulating agent (gemfibrozil) • Antihistaminics (loratadine) • Antidepressants (nefazodone, fluoxetine, fluvoxamine) • Calcium channel blockers (verapamil)
• **Drugs that ↓ the levels of carbamazepine**	• Anticonvulsants (carbamazepine by autoinduction, phenitoin, primidone, felbamate, valproate, phenobarbital) • Theophylline • Rifampin • Antineoplastic drug (cisplatin, doxorubicin)

Adapted from Sadock, B. J., & Sadock, V. A. (2002). *Kaplan and Sadock's Synopsis of Psychiatry: Behavioral Sciences/Clinical Psychiatry* (9th ed.). Baltimore, MD: Lippincott Williams & Wilkins. p. 1039.

Other anticonvulsants: gabapentin (Neurontin), lamotrigine (Lamictal), topiramate (Topamax), tiagabine (Gabitril), pregabalin (Lyrica)

- **Indications: as alternative or adjuncts in BPD**, anxiety disorders, pain, substance abuse, agitation. Have mood stabilizing and antidepressant effects, usually added to first-line mood stabilizers (lithium, valproic acid, or carbamazepine); sometimes used in monotherapy. Lamictal is used for acute and prophylactic rx of pts with depressive episodes of bipolar I disorders and pts with rapid cycling. All are used for rx of seizures. Gabapentin is used to treat polyneuropathy. Pregabalin is used for fibromyalgia.

- **Pharmacokinetics**
  - **Gabapentin**: poor gut absorption, not protein bound, half-life 5–9 hr, peak reached in 2 days, given bid, not metabolized, excreted unchanged in the urine. No real evidence of effectiveness in BPD
  - **Lamotrigine**: well absorbed, half-life 25 hr, **increase dosage slowly**, given bid, protein bound, excreted in urine
  - **Topiramate**: well absorbed, half-life 21 hr, 15% bound to protein, excreted in urine

TABLE 8.43. Clinical Guidelines for the Use of Gabapentin, Lomotrigine, and Topiramate

• Gabapentin	• Capsules of 100, 300, 400 mg • Tablets of 600 and 800 mg • Oral sol: 250 mg/5 mL	• Start: 300 mg 3 tid, ↑ up to 1,800 mg tid in a few days • Usual dosage is 600–900 mg/d	• Mild sedation • To discontinue, taper slowly • False-positive reading for urine protein	• FDA approved: postherpetic neuralgia (in adults); in partial seizures with or without secondary generalization (in pts > age 12); as an adjunctive therapy in rx of partial seizures in children 3–12 • Not FDA approved: anxiolytic effect (may be more useful in depression than mania)
• Lamotrigine*	• Tablets of 25, 100, 150, 200 mg	• Start: 25 mg/d during wk 1–2 • Increase slowly to 50 mg/d during wk 3–4 then to 100–200 mg/d during wk 4–5 • Max: 500 mg/d • If used with valproic acid: give half of the dose to begin up to a max of 200 mg/d • Risk for rash rare with low starting dose and very slow increases Caution if used with other drugs	• Caution: • If <16 yo (risk of rash) • Valproic acid slows the elimination of lamotrigine • ↓ Dosage • If renal insufficiency • Rash: stop immediately the drug • Taper down to discontinue over 2 wk (unless rash)	• FDA approved: maintenance treatment of bipolar I disorder; partial seizures (adjunctive; adults and children >2); generalized seizures of Lennox-Gastaut syndrome (adjunctive; adults and children >2); conversion to monotherapy in adults with partial seizures who are receiving treatment with carbamazepine, phenytoin, phenobarbital, primidone, or valproate • Efficacy in depression and rapid cycling
• Topiramate	• Tablets of 25, 100, 200 mg	• ↑ Slowly up to 200 mg bid over 8 wk	• Mild sedation, glaucoma, hyperthermia, cognitive deficits?	• FDA approved: partial onset seizures (adjunctive; adults and children 2–16); primary generalized tonic-clonic seizures (adjunctive; adult and children 2–16); seizures associated with Lennox-Gastaut syndrome (2 yr of age or greater than); migraine prophylaxis • Not FDA approved: adjunct in mania

*When offering lamotrigine to women taking oral contraceptives, prescribers should explain that the drug may decrease the effectiveness of the contraceptive and discuss alternative methods of contraception. If a woman taking lamotrigine stops taking an oral contraceptive, the dose of lamotrigine may need to be reduced by up to 50%.

TABLE 8.44. Gabapentin, Lomotrigine, and Topiramate: Side Effects and Their Remediation

• Gabapentin	• Somnolence, dizziness, ataxia, transient nystagmus (not dose related)
• Lamotrigine	• Neurologic: dizziness, ataxia, somnolence, headache, diplopia, blurred vision • Vision: lamotrigine accumulates in the pigmented retina • **Skin: Stevens-Johnson syndrome and toxic epidermal necrolysis** (if starting dose is too high, ↑ is too rapid, if concomitant use of valproic acid, after 2–8 wk of rx → **discontinue immediately**)
• Topiramate	• Psychomotor slowing, dizziness, ataxia, nystagmus, paresthesias, visual problems, weight loss, tremor, renal calculi

TABLE 8.45. Drug Interactions with Gabapentin, Lomotrigine, and Topiramate

• Gabapentin	• Antiacids ↓ absorption of gabapentin
• Lamotrigine	• Lamotrigine's action on anticonvulsants: • ↓ Valproic acid level by 25% • ↑ Side effects of carbamazepine (dizziness, blurred vision, diplopia, ataxia) by ↑ conc. of its metabolites • Anticonvulsants' action on lamotrigine: • Carbamazepine, phenytoin, and phenobarbital: ↓ lamotrigine levels by 40–50% • Valproic acid ↑ level of lamotrigine (doubled or greater than) • **Sertraline**: ↑ lamotrigine levels • **Oral contraceptives**: lamotrigine ↓ effectiveness of oral contraceptives
• Topiramate	• Topiramate's action on anticonvulsants: • ↑ levels of phenytoin and ↑ levels of valproic acid • No change in levels of carbamazepine, phenobarbital, primidone • Anticonvulsants' action on topiramate: • Carbamazepine ↓ levels of topiramate • Valproic acid ↓ levels of topiramate • Phenytoin ↓ levels of topiramate • **Digoxin**: topiramate ↓ levels of digoxin • **Oral contraceptives**: topiramate ↓ efficacy of contraceptives • **Carbonic anhydrase inhibitors** (acetazolamide, dichlorphenamide): adding topiramate ↑ risk of renal calculi

ECT AND OTHER TREATMENTS

CONDITIONS TO BE MET

• Imminent risk of death
• Inanition or malnutrition severe enough that will not allow other rx to be taken and be successful
• Resistance to other treatments
• Inability to tolerate other treatments
• Pts' preference

ELECTROCONVULSIVE THERAPY (ECT)

It is a procedure in which electric currents are passed through the brain, deliberately triggering a brief seizure, induced in anesthetized patients.

TRANSCRANIAL MAGNETIC STIMULATION (TMS)

See Web site as there are limited number of rx centers: (www.NeuroStarTMS.com), phone (877–6000-7555). (Neuronetics, Inc.).

FDA approved on October 7, 2008: for pts with MDD, after failure of four adequate antidepressant trials (in dose and duration).

Mechanism of action: noninvasive rx, TMS delivers intense intermittent magnetic pulses produced by an electrical charge into a ferromagnetic coil (placed on the scalp over the left dorsolateral prefrontal cortex/DLPFC).

Standard outpatient treatment: Five daily sessions of 40 min each/wk, for up to 6 wk. Determine the motor threshold (level of stimulation required to produce contractions in the contralateral target muscle/contraction of the thumb), frequency of stimulation (10 cycles/s/Hz), stimulation train (= duration of the stimulation: 4 s), intertrain interval (ITI; time between stimulation train: 26 s), total stimulations given in a session (3,000 stimulations per session).

TMS vs ECT: five studies reported equivalency, three studies reported some superiority for ECT.

Safety: headache, pain at the site of stimulation, rare seizures. No development of mania, no change in cognitive functioning. TMS is contraindicated in pts with implanted metallic devices in or around the head (except for dental hardware or braces).

VAGUS NERVE STIMULATION

http://www.vnstherapy.eu/depression/cyberonics.php

First developed for refractory seizure disorders; seems to be effective for moderate rx-resistant MDD (approved by the FDA in 2005); is still a controversial rx.

A pacemaker-like pulse generator is implanted under the skin in the upper left chest, and a stimulation electrode, connected to the generator, goes from the chest to the neck where it is attached to the left vagus nerve.

SE: hoarseness, sleep-disordered breathing.

ACUPUNCTURE

Chinese healing technique; use of sterilized needles inserted at specific points into the skin to correct any imbalance of energy flow; may be beneficial in pain conditions and detoxification programs.

SLEEP DEPRIVATION

May precipitate mania in bipolar I pts; may relieve depression in unipolar pts (transient benefit). The most effective strategy combines sleep deprivation with pharmacologic rx of depression (delaying the time when pt goes to sleep each night: pt may stay awake from 2 AM to 10 PM daily + use of antidepressant or lithium); may accelerate the response to antidepressants (fluoxetine, nortriptyline); may also improve premenstrual dysphoria.

PHOTOTHERAPY (LIGHT THERAPY)

Used for sleep disorders and seasonal affective disorder (F > M); using bright light in the range of 1,500–10,000 lux (light box sitting on the table, pt being in front of it for 1–2 hr before dawn each day, not looking directly at the light); is well tolerated (possible switch into mania); jet lag may respond to light therapy. http://www.litebook.com; http://www.bio-light.com/; http://www.fullspectrumsolutions.com.

PSYCHOSURGERY

rare, improving techniques; major indications in the presence of a debilitating, chronic mental disorder that has not responded to any other rx (>5 yr and debilitating); mostly intractable MDD and OCD; controversial for extreme aggression; is not indicated for schizophrenia or mania; deep brain stimulation (DBS): potential treatment for disorders of mood, behavior, and thought (problems with the location of the surgical implantation of the device, the efficacity vs safety); the need for a multidisciplinary team; is still an investigational procedure not approved by the FDA.

9 ■ DELIRIUM, DEMENTIA, AMNESTIC DISORDERS, COGNITIVE DISORDERS NOS

Common, particularly in the elderly. First, identify the syndrome, then the likely organic cause.

TABLE 9.1.   Classification of Delirium, Dementia, Amnestic Disorders, and Cognitive Disorders NOS

● **Delirium**	● Usually brief, reversible
	● Marked by short-term confusion + changes in cognition
	● Four categories:
	  ○ Due to a general medical condition
	  ○ Substance induced
	  ○ Due to multiple causes
	  ○ Delirium NOS

● **Dementia**	● Longer-lasting, more often irreversible
	● Marked by severe impairment in memory, judgment, orientation, and cognition
	● Six categories:
	  ○ Dementia of the Alzheimer's type (>65 yo, progressive intellectual decline, delusions, depression)
	  ○ Vascular dementia
	  ○ Due to other medical conditions
	  ○ Substance induced
	  ○ Multiple etiologies
	  ○ NOS

● **Amnestic disorder**	● Marked by memory impairment and forgetfulness
	● Three categories:
	  ○ Due to medical conditions
	  ○ Due to toxin or medication
	  ○ NOS

● **Cognitive disorder NOS**	● Cognitive disorder that does not meet the criteria for the above 3 disorders

Includes:

- **Full psychiatric hx**
- **Comprehensive neuropsychiatric mental status examination**
  - General description (appearance, level of consciousness, arousal, level of attention, posture, gait, movements, demeanor, response to the examiner)
  - Language and speech (comprehension, output, repetition, object naming, color naming, body part identification, response to commands)
  - Thought (form and content)
  - Mood and affect (internal and demonstrated emotional status)
  - Suicidal and homicidal thoughts
  - Insight and judgment
  - Cognition:
    - Premorbid intellectual functioning
    - Intellectual functioning
    - Attention/concentration
    - Memory: spontaneous and tested (immediate repetitions, delayed recall, cued recall, visual recognition, verbal). To test verbal memory: use prose passages; to test rote verbal learning tasks: use word list learning tasks. Visual memory is assessed by memory of geometric designs, memory of faces, and spatial memory.
    - Visuospatial skills
    - Constructional ability

- Mathematics
- Reading
- Writing
- Fine sensory functions
- Finger gnosis
- Right–left orientation
- Executive functions: planning, organizing, sequencing
- Abstraction

TABLE 9.2.   Mini-Mental State Examination (MMSE) Questionnaire

- A score of ≤23 indicates cognitive impairment suggesting dementia
  - Orientation: (score 1 each if correct: max 10): name this building or hospital; what city are you in? What year is it? What month is it? What is the date today? What state are you in? What county are you in? What floor of the building are you on? What day of the week is it? What season of the year is it?
  - Registration: (score 1 for each object correctly repeated: max 3):
    - Name 3 objects that the pt will repeat (score). Name the 3 objects many times for the pt to be able to repeat (record trials)
  - Attention and calculation
    - Subtract 7 from 100 to 65 (max score is 5)
  - Recall: do you recall the 3 objects named previously? (score 1 for each: max 3)
  - Language tests:
    - Ask pt to name shown objects: watch, pen = 2
    - Repetition: "No ifs, ands, or buts" = 1
    - Comprehension: pick up the paper in your right hand, fold in half, and set it on the floor = 3
    - Read and perform the command: "close your eyes" = 1
    - Write any full sentence = 1
  - Construction: copy the design below

Adapted from Crum, R. M., Anthony, J. C., Bassett, S. S., & Folstein, M. F. (1993). Population-based norms for the Mini-Mental State Examination by age and educational levels. *Journal of the American Medical Association, 18,* 2386–2391.

The Clock Drawing Test

Examines planning, abstract reasoning, constructive abilities with assessment of the four criteria that best discriminates between AD pts and healthy individuals (12 numbers present, number 12 at the top, 2 distinguishable hands, correct reading of the time)

     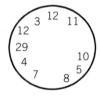

FIGURE 9.1.   The clock drawing test.

1 point for the clock circle
1 point for all the numbers being in the correct order
1 point for the numbers being in the proper special order
1 point for the two hands of the clock
1 point for the correct time.

A normal score is four or five points.

Adapted from Agrell, B., & Dehljin, O. (1998). The clock-drawing test. *Age and Ageing, 27,* 399–403.

● **Full physical examination with screening tests**:

TABLE 9.3. Laboratory Screen and Other Tests for Delirium, Dementia, Amnestic Disorders, and Cognitive Disorders NOS

● **CBC (Hb, WBC, RBC)**: R/O anemia, infection
● **Chemical panel (Na, K, glucose, BUN, Ca, Mg, bilirubin, liver enzymes, creatinine)**
● **Selective testing**: HIV antibodies, RPR
● **Serum ammonia, PT, aPTT**
● **Cortisol, TSH, phosphorus, and parathyroid levels if suspected endocrine cause**
● **Toxicology (serum and urine), U/A**
● **Head CT scan without IV contrast**: if CNS infection, trauma, or a CVA is suspected. A CT scan is excellent for detecting acute hematomas and most subarachnoid hemorrhages (SAH); follow-up lumbar puncture may be needed to rule out SAH ● **MRI**: MRI helps distinguish between AD and vascular causes of dementia
● **ECG**
● **EEG (if paroxysmal onset)**
● **LP (if encephalitis suspected)** for CSF studies, including cryptococcal antigen or India ink prep, and VDRL
● **Oxygen saturation and, in some cases, arterial blood gases (ABGs) with a carbon monoxide level**
● **B_{12} and folate levels**

DELIRIUM

Epidemiology: seen in 10–30% of all pts on a medical-surgical ward (40% > age 65), directly due to a medical condition. Onset: acute (hours to days), sudden (stroke), or paroxysmal (complex partial seizure). Most likely in children and the elderly; Whites greater than other races; F > M.

Pathophysiology:

● **Risks factors**: predisposing factors: age (>75), male, living alone, sensory impairment, medical comorbidity (renal insufficiency, cardiopulmonary alterations, anemia, history of alcohol abuse, fever, malnutrition, hip fracture), altered brain function (dementia). Precipitating factors: acute cardiac event, anemia, bed rest, drug withdrawal, fecal impaction, electrolyte disturbance, indwelling devices, acute infections, medications, restraints, pain, and urinary retention.

● **Three molecular mechanisms** may play a role: cholinergic transmission disruption (anticholinergic substances ↑ delirium), monoaminergic dysfunction (dopamine and serotonin agonists can cause psychosis), stress-released glutamate may produce psychosis), cytokine release (interleukins and interferon-alpha from tissue injuries cross the blood–brain barrier interfering with neurotransmitter synthesis + transmission).

Symptoms: fluctuating symptoms (waxing and waning), characterized by **sudden confusion** (clouding of sensorium, ↓ degree of arousal) and **short-term memory loss** (disorientation to time, place; inability to recall objects after 5 min), **alteration in attention** (inability to focus). Frequency but nonessential presence of formal thought disorder (circumstantiality, tangentiality, incoherence), and content thought disorder (hallucinations: visual > auditory; delusions: often persecutory; misinterpretations). Pt may be agitated or underactive.

Laboratory and other tests: see Table 9.3.

Differential diagnosis

● *In dementia: no confusion +++*

● *Differentiate a formal thought disorder from the cognitive disorder of a delirium*: a formal thought disorder gives the impression of a code linking the loose associated thoughts and there is consistency of the arousal and attention level in the formal thought disorder.

Causes

TABLE 9.4. Causes of Delirium "I WATCH DEATH"

Infectious	Encephalitis (herpes simplex, mononucleosis, mumps, zoster, arbovirus) Meningitis Syphilis **AIDS**, other immunocompromised states (TB, mycoses, toxoplasmosis, cytomegalovirus) **Sepsis** (fever, tachycardia, tachypnea, leucocytosis) Febrile delirium (temp > 105–106°F)
Withdrawal	**Alcohol (delirium tremens) or sedative-hypnotic**
Acute metabolic	Hyperglycemia (thirst, polyuria, glucose 300–600 mg/dL in diabetic ketoacidosis, 600–2,000 in nonketotic hyperglycemia), hypoglycemia (tremor, glucose < 45 mg/dL) Hypernatremia (Na > 160mEq/L if acute; >170 if gradual), hyponatremia (asterixis and myoclonus, Na < 120 mEq/L if acute; <110 if chronic) Hypokalemia (hyporeflexia, K < 2.5 mEq/L) Hypermagnesemia (hyporeflexia, Mg > 5 mEq/L), hypomagnesemia (myoclonus, Mg < 1 mEq/L) Hypercalcemia (vomiting, abdominal pain, constipation, Ca > 14 mg/dL), hypocalcemia (muscle cramping, paresthesia, tetany, seizures, Ca < 7 mg/dL) Uremia (asterixis, myoclonus, BUN > 100 mg/dL if acute; >200 if chronic) Hepatic encephalopathy (asterixis, NH_3 > 55 mcg/dL, caution as NH_3 may be normal) Respiratory failure (PaO_2 < 50 mmHg; PCO_2 > 70 mmHg if acute; PCO_2 > 90 mmHg if chronic) Hepatic porphyria ($\uparrow$ serum delta-aminolevulinic acid, abdominal pain, polyneuropathy) Pancreatitis (abdominal pain, $\uparrow$ lipase, $\uparrow$amylase) Dialysis disequilibrium syndrome
Trauma	Delayed radiation encephalopathy, subdural hematoma, subarachnoid hemorrhage
CNS pathology	**Febrile delirium**, postictal confusion, status epilepticus, **complex partial seizure** (40% of these pts will have no diagnostic available on EEG), MS, paraneoplastic limbic encephalitis (PLE), acute hydrocephalus, stroke, systemic lupus erythematosus (pleurisy, arthritis, rash, ANA+), chorea (Sydenham, chorea gravidarum), brain abscess, neoplasms
Hypoxia	Postanoxic delirium, respiratory insufficiency, carbon monoxide poisoning (arterial blood gases), fat emboli syndrome (after fractures of long bones)
Vitamin deficiencies	**Thiamine** (Wernicke's encephalopathy: acute syndrome, "confusion, ataxia, ophthalmoplegia" with nystagmus, abducens and conjugate gaze palsies, confabulation, lethargy, indifference, mild delirium, peripheral neuropathy; 84% will develop Korsakoff syndrome; treat with thiamine until ophthalmoplegia resolves, may also need magnesium). Niacin (encephalopathic pellagra), folate deficiency
Endocrinopathies	Cushing syndrome, adrenocortical insufficiency, hyperthyroidism, Hashimoto's encephalopathy
Acute vascular etiology	Hypertensive encephalopathy, confusional migraine, thrombotic thrombocytopenic purpura
Toxins and drugs	**Medications:** ● **Anticholinergics**: atropine, benztropine mesylate, diphenhydramine, eyes and nose drops, scopolamine, thioridazine, trihexyphenidyl hydrochloride ● **Neuroleptics** (neuroleptic malignant syndrome): ● **Serotoninergic** (serotonine syndrome): ● **Dopaminergic drugs**: amantadine, bromocriptine, levodopa ● **Others**: digoxin, quinidine, prednisone, theophylline, bismuth, podophyllin, meperidine, disulfiram, codeine, warfarin, furosemide, nifetidine, ergotamine tartrate, thyroid hormones ● **Histamine H2 antagonists**: ranitidine, cimetidine ● **Anticonvulsants**: phenytoin, barbiturates, valproate ● **Beta adrenergic blockers**: propanolol, timolol ● **Gamma aminobutyric acid agonists**; baclofen, benzodiazepines ● **Antiarrhythmics**: diisopropamide, lidocaine hydrochloride, quinidine ● **Antibacterials**: aminoglycosides, amodioquine hydrochloride, amphetoricine B, cephalosporines, chloramphenicol, chloroquine, ethambutol, gentamicine sulfate, INH, metronidazole, rifampin, sulfonamides, tetracyclines, vancomycin hydrochloride ● **Antihypertensives**: captopril, clonidine, methyldopa, reserpine ● **Anti-inflammatory drugs**: ibuprofen, indomethacin, naprosyn, sulindac ● **Antiviral agents**: acyclovir, interferon ● **Immunosuppressives**: L-Asparaginase, 5-Azacytadine, Cytarabine, 5-Fluorouracil, Methotrexate at high dose, procarbazine, tamoxifen, vinblastine, vincristine ● **Steroids, ACTH** ● **Tricyclic antidepressants, MAOIs** ● **Lithium** ● **Amphetamines** **Pesticides** **Solvents** **Intoxications**: methanol, cannabis, inhalant, PCP, amphetamine, cocaine, ephedrine, phenylephrine
Heavy metals	Lead, thallium, arsenic (vomiting, abdominal pain, blood levels), manganese, mercury

Sources: Moore, D. P. (2006). *The Little Black Book of Psychiatry* (3rd ed). Sudbury, MA: Jones & Bartlett Learning; Wise, M. G. and Brandt, G. T. (1992). Delirium. In: S. C. Yudofsky & R. E. Hales (Eds.), *The American Psychiatric Press Textbook of Neuropsychiatry* (2nd ed.). Washington, DC: American Psychiatric Press. p. 291–310

Course: fluctuates, ↑ at night (sundowning), ↓ in AM. Reversible.

Complications: delirium worsens the prognosis of the underlying condition: nursing home placement × 3, risk of death × 2 (more if previous dementia, or elderly).

Treatment:

- **Treat underlying cause**
- **Nonpharmacologic approaches**:
  - **Modify environment**: ↑ light (day + PM, ↓ light at night), ↓ noise and clutter, check room temperature, put environmental clues (signs, labels, large calendar, and large digital clock), call button in easy reach, a view from a window, good supervision
  - **Use consistent daily routines**
  - **Optimize stimulation**: maintain routines, validation, special interests, familiar objects (family pictures, clothes), ↑ contacts with family + friends, religious support, music, recreation, food, exercise
- **Medications for agitation** (doses to be decreased for an elderly, debilitated pt or pt in hepatic failure)
  - **Haloperidol**: regularly dose with prn doses; increase until pt is calm, max dose is reached, or side effects occur. Start: 0.25–2 mg po/IV/IM bid or tid; prn dose 2 mg q 4 hr. Average: 5–10 mg/d, max: 20 mg/d. SE: akathisia, acute EPS reactions, ↑ QTc interval with IV haloperidol (>100 mg), risk of torsades de pointe, dysrhythmia, ventricular tachycardia, fibrillation. Note: IV administration may be preferable to IM in some cases (poor absorption in distal muscles if delirium associated with circulatory compromise; if paranoid pt and repeated painful IM injections; IM can complicate interpretations of muscle enzyme studies and need for enzyme fractionation; IV haloperidol is less likely to produce EPS). **10 mg of haloperidol po corresponds to 5 mg IV or IM. CAUTION: if haloperidol is going to be used via IV: strictly follow hospital protocol +++ as it would be used off label; warning by FDA (**QT-interval prolongation, torsades de pointes, other ventricular arrhythmias, and sudden death)
  - **Risperidone**: start: 0.25–1 mg bid; prn: 0.5–1 mg q 4 hr. Average: 3–4 mg/d. Max: 6 mg/d. SE: EPS, sleepiness, parkinsonism, hypotension, mild akathisia
  - **Quetiapine**: start: 12.5–25 mg bid; prn: 12.5–25 mg q 4 hr. Average: 100–200 mg/d. Max: 500 mg/d. Some pts continue to improve cognitively 3 months after stabilization of delirium.
  - **Olanzapine**: start: 2.5 mg/d po/IM. Average: 10 mg/d. Max: 15 mg/d.
  - **Lorazepam**: 0.5–2 mg po or IV q 4–8 hr; only as an adjunct except in delirium induced by alcohol or benzodiazepine withdrawal

DEMENTIA

National organizations

- **Alzheimer's Association**: www.alz.org or http://www.alz.org; 800-272-3900
- **Alzheimer's Association Safe Return Program**: www.alz.org/services/SafeReturn.asp; 800-272-3900
- **Alzheimer's Disease Education and Referral (ADEAR) Center**: PO Box 8250, Silver Spring, MD 20907-8250; 1-800-438-4380, 301-587-4352 (fax); http://www.alzheimers.org
- **Family Caregiver Alliance**: www.caregiver.org; 800–445-8106
- **National Institute on Aging**: www.nia.nih.gov; 800–222-2225
- **American Geriatric Society**: www.americangeriatrics.org; 212–308-1414
- **Alzheimer's Caregiver Support Online**: www.alzonline.net; 866–260-2466

Scales: Clinical Dementia Rating Scale (CDR), Standardized Alzheimer's Disease Assessment Scale (SADAS), the Functional Assessment Staging Tool (FAST), Cornell Scale for Depression in Dementia (CSDD), Mini-Mental State Examination (MMSE), the Cornell-Brown Scale for Quality of Life in Dementia (CBS), Global Deterioration Scale (GDS), Alzheimer's Disease Caregiver Questionnaire (ADCQ)

Epidemiology: 5–10% if >65 yo; 30% if >80 yo; atypical dementias (4–6 millions of Americans) in 20–30% of cases (care plan must be individualized); younger patients: mostly AIDS-related dementia, certain familial forms of AD, and some cases of variant Creutzfeldt–Jakob disease (i.e., bovine spongiform encephalopathy or mad cow disease)

Symptoms: insidious onset (Alzheimer's) or acute (stroke); severe **global ↓ in intellectual functioning** (memory, abstract thinking, calculations) with a **clear sensorium (without confusion)**: dementia means intellectual decline with or without memory loss (involves memory when advanced)

- **Memory defect**: **more anterograde** (inability to recall words after 5 min, losing things, forgetfulness of things just said or done/wallets, keys/food cooking on the stove/difficulty navigating around the house or the neighborhood) **than retrograde** (↑ with progression of the disease, inability to recall past events like schooling, jobs, children, etc.). Memory loss is often not an early or cardinal sx in certain dementias such as vascular dementia, frontotemporal dementia, and Parkinson-related dementias among others. Nearly all dementias do eventually involve memory when advanced.

- **Abstracting defect** (poor proverb interpretation, concreteness)
- **Calculating ability defect** (serial 7s)
- **Clear sensorium** (exceptions seen in late Alzheimer disease, diffuse Lewy body disease, multi-infarct dementia)
- **Possible personality, mood changes** (disinhibited behaviors, depression, apathy), psychosis, agitation, anxiety (catastrophic reactions), sleep disturbances, motor disturbances, speech changes, poor judgment
- **Findings such as** parkinsonism, chorea, neurologic focal sx point out to some etiologies. Various physical sx may be associated with dementia: the grasp, glabellar, blink, palmomental, Babinski, and sucking reflexes
- **Variations due to**: premorbid personality, culture, lifelong preferences, regions of the brain affected, size of the damage, histopathology, external demands

Tests

- **See Table 9.3.**
- **Others**:
  - **CAT scan or MRI is the routine initial evaluation** (SPECT not superior and not recommended). In normal aging, the volume of the brain shrinks about 0.4% per year but in AD it is about 4% per year (tests need to be repeated)
  - Genetic testing not recommended for dementia with Lewy bodies and Creutzfeldt–Jakob disease
  - Routine Apo-E genotyping or other genetic markers not recommended in pt suspected of AD
  - Testing for tau mutations in pt with frontotemporal dementia or AD gene mutations is not routine
  - No cerebrospinal fluid or other biomarkers for routine use in diagnosis of AD
  - CSF 14-3-3 protein is recommended for confirming or rejecting the diagnosis of Creutzfeldt–Jakob disease

In mild cognitive impairment (MCI) cases: transition stage between the cognitive decline of normal aging and the more serious problems caused by Alzheimer disease; *slowing of memory/word-finding are a normal feature of brain aging, 50%* of patients with MCI and normal day-to-day functioning will develop the onset of dementia within 3 yr. *No accurate way exists to predict which pts will develop progressive dementia.*

TABLE 9.5.   MCI Criteria

- Memory complaint, corroborated by an informant
- Objective memory impairment
- Normal general cognitive function
- Intact activities of daily living
- Not demented

- Monitor for cognitive and functional decline (for subsequent dementia): MMSE, Kokmen Short Test of Mental Status, 7-Minute Screen, and Memory Impairment Screen
- Screen with brief cognitive assessment instruments like the clock drawing test (see Fig. 9.1).
- Neuropsychologic batteries in at risk populations (i.e., Neuropsychologic Battery, Mattis Rating Scale, Halifax Mental Status Scale, and Fuld Object Memory Test)
- Interview-based techniques (i.e., Blessed Roth Scale, Clinical Dementia Rating, Informant Questionnaire on Cognitive Decline in the Elderly): to identify pts with dementia
- **Check for the presence of amnesia or not**:
  - **If the disturbance is in multiple domains and nonamnestic**: it is primarily an executive dysfunction or difficulty with problem solving and abstraction (use preventive measures to limit progression toward dementia/aerobic exercise, Mediterranean diet, moderate wine consumption, ↑ mental activities and social + leisure activities, stop smoking, treat hypertension, legal decisions/buy long-term care insurance, plan with advanced directives, financial planning, hook up with the Alzheimer's Association)
  - **If it is a true memory-related amnesty disturbance with MCI**: *80% → dementia within 5 yr* (pts lose about 4 points on the MMSE test per year); 25% of MCI pts present as depressed.

Distinguishing subcortical and cortical dementias (not always accurate)

TABLE 9.6. Subcortical Dementia vs Cortical Dementia

Characteristics	Subcortical	Cortical
● Types	● Huntington disease ● Parkinson disease ● AIDS dementia complex	● Alzheimer ● Creutzfeldt–Jakob
● Language	● No aphasia ● Anomia in severe cases	● Early aphasia +++
● Memory impairment	● Impaired recall (retrieval greater than encoding) but less than in cortical dementia	● Recall (retrieval) and recognition (encoding) impaired +++
● Visuospatial skills	● Impaired	● Impaired
● Calculation	● Preserved until late	● Involved early
● Frontal systems (executive functions)	● Impaired	● Impaired
● Speed of cognitive processing	● Slowed early +++	● Normal until late in the disease
● Personality	● Apathetic +++, frequent depression (often treatment resistant)	● Unconcerned
● Mood	● Depressed	● Euthymic
● Speech	● Dysarthric	● Articulate until late
● Posture	● Bowed, gait dysfunction	● Upright
● Coordination	● Impaired	● Normal until late
● Motor speed	● Slowed	● Normal
● Abnormal movements	● Chorea, tremor, tics, dystonia	● Absent, possible myoclonus

Adapted from Pajeau, A. K., & Roman, G. C. (1992). HIV encephalopathy and dementia. *Psychiatric Clinics of North America, 15,* 457; Sadock, B. J., & Sadock, V. A. (2002). *Kaplan and Sadock's Synopsis of Psychiatry: Behavioral Sciences/Clinical Psychiatry* (9th ed). Baltimore, MD: Lippincott Williams & Wilkins. p. 334.

Differential diagnosis:

- **Amnestic syndromes**: no global intellectual decrease
- **Delirium**: clouding of sensorium and confusion (↓ ability to maintain and shift attention, fluctuation of the cognitive deficits). Some dementia may present with some confusion, chronic (late Alzheimer's) or episodic (new stroke in multi-infarct dementia, or early diffuse Lewy body disease)
- **MR**: Onset <18 yr, cognitive development goes up to a certain point (usually normal memory), then stabilizes. In dementia, the intellectual functions ↓
- **Depression**: with problems in concentration and memory **is called pseudo-dementia**: must be treated as depression

TABLE 9.7. Organic Dementia vs Pseudo-Dementia +++

Features	Organic dementia	Pseudo-dementia
● Age	● Usually elderly	● Nonspecific
● Onset	● Vague	● Days–weeks
● Course	● Slow, ↑ at night	● Rapid
● History	● Systemic illness or substances	● Affective disorder
● Awareness	● Unaware, unconcerned	● Aware and distressed
● Organic signs	● Often present	● Absent
● Cognition	● Prominent impairment	● Variable deficits
● MSE	● Consistent, spotty deficits, confabulates, approximates, perseverates ● Shallow, labile mood ● Emphasizes trivial accomplishments	● Apathetic ● Depressed mood ● Emphasizes failures
● Behavior	● Appropriate to degree of impairment	● Incongruent with the degree of impairment
● Cooperation	● Cooperative, frustrated	● Uncooperative, little effort
● CT/EEG	● Abnormal	● Normal

- **Schizophrenia**: less severe cognitive deficits, and + specific psychotic sx
- **Malingering and factitious disorders**: more inconsistencies over time
- **Age-related cognitive decline**: nonprogressive, no functional impairment

TABLE 9.8.   Fundamental Questions in Making the Diagnosis of Dementia

- *Is it dementia or MCI?* Where does aging stop and dementia begin?
- Acute vs rapid or slow progressive onset?
- R/O delirium, depression (pseudo-dementia)?
- Are the sx only cortical or also subcortical (localization)?
- Any focal neurologic sx (localization, typical vs atypical dementias)?
- Physical sx leading toward some possible specific etiology?
  - **Primary neurodegenerative disorders**: AD (Alzheimer disease), FTD (frontotemporal degeneration), DLB (diffuse Lewy body disease), PDD (Parkinson disease dementia), PSP (progressive supranuclear palsy), HD (Huntington disease), WD (Wilson disease), CJD (Creutzfeldt–Jakob disease)
  - **Vascular**: multi-infarct, Binswanger's, CADASIL (cerebral autosomal dominant arteriopathy with subcortical infarcts and leukoencephalopathy)
  - **Inflammatory**: multiple sclerosis, vasculitis
  - **Infectious**: syphilis, Lyme, HIV, other viral, fungal
  - **Cancers**: primary, metastatic, paraneoplastic
  - **Other/physical**: hydrocephalus, trauma
- *Most frequent dementias*: (1) Alzheimer disease, (2) vascular, (3) diffuse Lewy body disease and dementia of Parkinson disease, (4) multiple others (think AIDS-related dementias)

TABLE 9.9.   Suggestive Features of Some Dementing Disorders

Types	Suggestive features
● Alzheimer disease	● Amnesia, agnosia, aphasia, apraxia (the 4 As)
● Vascular dementia	● **Fluctuating, stepwise deterioration; focal neurologic signs**, brain imaging evidence of cerebrovascular disease (see NINDS—AIREN criteria for the diagnosis of vascular dementia: dementia + cerebrovascular disease + a relationship between the two disorders such as (a) onset of dementia within 3 months following a recognized stroke; (b) abrupt deterioration in cognitive functions; or fluctuating, stepwise progression of cognitive deficits) http://strokecenter.org/trials/scales/ninds-airen.html
● Dementia with Lewy bodies	● **Fluctuation in** performance; visual hallucinations, delusions; **bilateral symmetric parkinsonism**; hypersensibility to neuroleptics
● Frontotemporal dementia	● **Early personality changes**; frontal dysexecution syndrome; early language dysfunction; relatively preserved memory and visuospatial functions
● Parkinson disease dementia	● **Asymmetric parkinsonism** features; later onset of the dementia; subcortical dementia with impairment of executive functions

Course

- Depends on underlying cause: progressive (Alzheimer's), static (head trauma), reversible sometimes: ¼ of demented pts have some treatable illness (B_{12} deficiency, depression)
- **Stages**: (mild, moderate, severe, profound, terminal). **Dementia symptom continuum (functional assessment staging: FAST)**:
  - stage 1: no deficit
  - stage 2: subjective functional deficit
  - stage 3: objective functional deficit and interference with complex social tasks
  - stage 4: deficient performance of complex ADL
  - stage 5: deficient performance of basic ADL
  - stage 6: decreased ability to dress, bathe, and toilet
  - stage 7: loss of speech, locomotion, and consciousness

Complications: behavioral problems. In advanced cases: falls, decubiti, dehydration, weight loss, aspiration pneumonia, sepsis, death

Treatment: multimodal, guided by the stages, focused on the specific sx, psychotherapy, psychosocial rx, safety, psychoeducation of the pt, the family and care givers, support groups for care givers (use of computer networks, telephone support groups), long-term education to delay nursing home placement, advise on levels of care, educate staff of long-term facilities to ↓ use of unnecessary psychotropics, financial and legal issues, somatic rx, development of a treatment plan, rx of comorbid conditions + underlying cause

- **Environmental measures**: risk of falls, injuries, behavior modification, scheduled toileting and voiding, ↑ functional independence with graded assistance, practice, positive reinforcement, low lighting levels at night, ↑ light during the day, ↓ clutter, put signs and labels and other environmental cues (familiar objects), light exercise (allow some wandering), music, multimodality group training, use of family videotapes, contact with family and friends, massage, pet therapy, cognitive remediation

- **Level of care decisions**: special care units within long-term care facilities; home-like physical setting, traditional nursing homes; short-term hospitalizations; out-patient care, adult day care, respite services think quickly about home health care with disease management

- **Somatic treatments: general principles treating an elderly population**: lower starting doses, smaller ↑ in doses, go slow, be alert to gl medical conditions, DDI, medication SE (sedation, EPS, orthostasis), avoid polypharmacy

- **Depression**:
  - SSRIs: (fewer anticholinergic SE, cardiovascular SE, N/V, agitation, akathisia, Parkinsonism, sexual dysfunction, ↓ weight, hyponatremia, falls, drug interactions (cytochrome P450 system). Citalopram (start 5–10 mg/d, ↑ q few weeks to max of 40 mg/d). Sertraline (start 12.5–25 mg/d, ↑ at 1–2 wk intervals up to a max of 150–200 mg/d)
  - SNRIs: Venlafaxine: start 25 mg/d (for ER form: start 37.5 mg/d), ↑ q wk to max of 375 mg/d in divided doses (for ER, 225 mg/d), less medication interactions, risk of ↑ BP; Duloxetine (start 20–40 mg/d), ↑ slowly to max of 60–80 mg/d, in divided doses; Mirtazapine (risk of sedation, weight gain, liver toxicity, neutropenia. Start 7.5 mg at hs, ↑ by 7.5 mg up to 45–60 mg at hs)
  - Bupropion: start at 37.5 mg once or twice/d (SR: 100 mg/d), ↑ slowly to max 300 mg/d in divided doses (SR: 300 mg/d). Less than 150 mg of immediate release bupropion should be given within any 4-hr period due to risk of seizures
  - Trazodone: sedative SE can be used when insomnia or severe agitation; risk of postural hypotension and priapism. Trazodone: start 25–50 mg/d, ↑ up to max 150–250 mg/d (ER form exists now/*Oleptro*, to be given once a day in PM)
  - Dopaminergic agents: psychostimulants (*d*-amphetamine, methylphenidate), amantadine, bromocriptine, and bupropion if severe apathy in demented pts. Start dextroamphetamine and methylphenidate: 2.5–5 mg in AM, ↑ by 2.5 mg q 2 or 3 d to a max of 30–40 mg/d (do not give in PM)
  - ECT in life-threatening cases

- **Psychosis and agitation**:
  - Antipsychotics:
    - **Atypical antipsychotics are not approved by the FDA for the rx of pts with dementia-related psychosis; FDA black box: antipsychotics may increase the risk of death in dementia pts.** If used off-label: check levels of K+, Mg++, check LFTs, QTc (risk of torsade de pointe is greater in F), avoid using if pt + recent heart attack or stroke; check drug interactions (quinidine, procainamide, disopyramide, amiodarone, sotalol, bepridil, prenylamine, astemizole, metochlopramide), reassess need regularly, use lowest effective dose, stop when pt is stable and use prn to avoid decompensation
    - Standing doses rather than as prn: start low (e.g., 0.25–0.5 mg/d of haloperidol; 0.25–1 mg/d of risperidone; 12.5 mg/d of clozapine; 1.25–5 mg/d of olanzapine; 12.5–50 mg/d of quetiapine; 5 mg/d of aripiprazole). Usual max dosages for pts with dementia: 2 mg/d of haloperidol; 1.5–2 mg/d of risperidone (less EPS if <1 mg/d); 75–100 mg/d of clozapine; 200–300 mg/d of quetiapine; 10 mg/d of olanzapine; and 15 mg/d of aripiprazole. These medications take time to work, if ↑ doses too rapidly: → SE but no more rapid efficacy. Atypical may be better tolerated than traditional
  - Benzodiazepines: occasionally useful for agitation if anxiety is ↑. Avoid long-term use (disinhibition, sedation, falls, ↑ delirium, dependence). Oral lorazepam (or IM in emergency): 0.5–1 mg every 4–6 hr prn, standing oral doses of 0.5–1 mg may be given 1–4 ×/d. Oxazepam; slower absorption, less useful as a prn, standing doses of 7.5–15 mg.

- **Insomnia**: establish regular sleep and waking times, calming bedtime rituals, daytime physical + mental activities. Limit daytime sleeping, fluid intake in the PM. Treat underlying medical and psychiatric conditions. Adjust medications interfering with sleep. Trazodone 25–100 mg q hs or nonbenzodiazepine hypnotics (zolpidem 10 mg at hr, zaleplon 5–10 mg at hs)

- **Treatments for cognitive losses**:
  - No FDA-approved rx for MCI

The only FDA-approved medications for dementia or cognitive impairment (mild to moderate AD) are **the cholinesterase inhibitors** (tacrine, donepezil, rivastigmine, and galantamine) and are the standard rx. Note: increased rates of syncope, bradycardia, pacemaker insertion, and hip fracture with cholinesterase inhibitors These medications should be used early in the disease: the gains may be better maintained if tx started early

Tacrine (Cognex): has reversible hepatic toxicity. Must be given 4×/d. Start: 10 mg po qid × 4 wk, incr. 10 mg qid q 4 wk prn; Max: 40 mg po qid. Very poor efficacy and poorly tolerated; rarely prescribed

Donepezil (Aricept, Aricept ODT) is given once/d, usually starting at 2.5–5 mg hs. ↑ Dose in 2.5 mg increments. May be ↑ to 10 mg hs if tolerated. The minimal effective dose is 5 mg/d. Does not slow the disease progression

Galantamine (Razadyne, Razadyne ER): start at 8 mg/d in divided doses, ↑ gradually up to 16–24 mg/d in divided doses, max up to 32 mg/d; minimal effective dose: 16 mg/d. A once-daily formulation (Razadyne ER: start: 8 mg po q AM, incr. 8 mg/d q 4 wk to 24 mg q AM as tolerated; max: 24 mg/d; info: give w/food).

Rivastigmine (Exelon, Exelon patch): start at 3 mg/d in divided doses, ↑ gradually up to 6–12 mg/d in divided doses. The minimal effective dose is 6 mg/d. Doses may be ↑ q 4 wk.

TO NOTE

AChE inhibition (acetylcholine esterase): → but GI side effects (N/V, weight loss, and diarrhea). Rivastigmine is more selective for the form of AChE present in hippocampus neurons (+++ for cognition)

BuChE inhibition (butyrylcholine esterase): in Alzheimer disease, neuronal dropout is replaced by glia which contains BuChE. Rivastigmine is the only one which inhibits it, may be more useful in advanced cases of AD (?)

Nicotinic receptors: may cause ↑ release of ACh, DA, serotonin, GABA, glutamate, NE. Galantamine helps modulating nicotinic receptors and may cause more ACh and other neurotransmitters release (improving attention, cognition, depression, anxiety)

Memantine (Namenda): *NMDA antagonist.* Combination rx with donepezil is more effective (usually donepezil is started first). Begin at 5 mg/d, increase by 5 mg/d q wk up to 10 mg bid

Ergoloid mesylates (Hydergine: approved for nonspecific cognitive decline)

- **Vitamin E** (<400 IU, avoid if vitamin K deficiency, has been used up to 1,000 IU po bid to slow the disease but not recommended), **ginkgo biloba** (ginkgotoxin found in seeds may provoke seizures), **and selegiline** (approved by the FDA for Parkinson disorder and in the patch form for depression) have shown a lack of efficacy and safety. **NSAIDs, statin medications, antioxidants, and estrogen supplementation** (with conjugated equine estrogens) are occasionally used (uncertain efficacy and safety; estrogen only should not be prescribed to treat AD) no evidence to support their use.

- **Avoid medications with anticholinergic activity** (caution if CV disease, prostate, bladder diseases, ↑ cognitive impairment, confusion, delirium)

Etiology

TABLE 9.10. Etiologies of Dementias

Specific dementias	Etiologies and frequency
• Dementia of the Alzheimer type (plaques + tangles)	• Alzheimer disease (most frequent dementia: 50–60%)
• Mild cognitive impairment (MCI)	• Nonprogressive deficits or prodromal of Alzheimer disease, or of other dementias
• Vascular dementia (also known as multi-infarct or poststroke dementia or vascular cognitive impairment)	• Multi-infarct dementia (2nd in dementia frequency: 10–20%) • Lacunar dementia • Cerebral amyloid angiopathy • Binswanger's disease • Cortical microinfarctions
• Dementia of Parkinson disease (nigral LB + nigral cells loss) and dementia with Lewy bodies (neocortical + nigral LB + nigral cell loss)	• Parkinson disease: 1% • Diffuse Lewy body disease (3rd in dementia frequency) • Arteriosclerotic parkinsonism (focal deficits) • Progressive supranuclear palsy (PSP; vertical gaze palsy, falls, axial extension): 1% • Striatonigral degeneration is a variant of multiple system atrophy (MSA): neurodegenerative disease (dementia with mild ataxia, impotence, orthostatic dizziness, incontinence) • Dementia pugilistica (distant h/o repeated head trauma, ataxia) • Corticobasal ganglionic degeneration (CBGD): neurodegenerative dementia (asymmetric parkinsonism, ideomotor apraxia, myoclonus, dystonia, and the alien hand syndrome)
• Dementia due to frontotemporal dementia spectrum disorders	• Pick disease (1%) • Frontotemporal degeneration (2–5%)
• Other progressive dementing disorders	• Huntington disease (1%) • Creutzfeldt–Jakob disease
• Dementia due to other diseases	• Structural lesions: Brain tumors: 1–5% (glioma, metastasis); Subdural hematoma; Slowly progressive or normal-pressure hydrocephalus (NPH): (1–5%) with triad: ataxia + dementia + urinary incontinence (can present with sx of depression): is treatable • Head trauma: 1–5% (e.g., dementia pugilistica, anoxia, chronic subdural hematoma) • Endocrine conditions (e.g., hypo or hyperthyroidism, hypercalcemia, hypoglycemia, pituitary disease) • Nutritional conditions (e.g., deficiency of vitamin B_{12}, of thiamine or vitamin B_1: 1%, of niacin or vitamin B_3, of folate acid, of B_6 or nicotinic acid with "dementia, dermatitis, and diarrhea") • Infectious conditions (e.g., AIDS: 1%, neurosyphilis, Cryptococcus, progressive multifocal leukoencephalopathy, Behcet syndrome, end stages of some meningitis and encephalitis) • Renal (dialysis dementia), hepatic insufficiencies • Neurologic conditions (e.g., multiple sclerosis, Wilson disease) • Medications (e.g., benzodiazepines, beta-blockers, anticholinergics) • Autoimmune diseases (e.g., lupus erythematosus, vasculitis, Hashimoto's encephalopathy, neurosarcoidosis) • Lipid storage diseases • Toxins (e.g., heavy metals, organic hydrocarbons), long-standing substance abuse, especially alcohol abuse: 1–5%, absinthe

ALZHEIMER DISEASE

Epidemiology: most frequent cause of dementia: (50–60%); 5% if >56 yr; 20% if >80 yr; early onset <65, late onset >65; less common and older age of onset in Japan, China, and Scandinavia.

Pathophysiology: **in AD, the hippocampus** (located inside the medial temporal lobe, beneath the cortical surface) is one of the first regions of the brain to suffer damage; memory problems and disorientation appear among the first sx. **Senile or neuritic plaques** (made of β amyloid deposits/neurotoxic and other components such as cytokines, complement factors, activated glia/autoimmune pathophysiology, role of nonsteroidal anti-inflammatory?; amyloid plaques start 20 yr before the dementia) and **intraneuronal neurofibrillary tangles in the cortex**, in some subcortical structures (nucleus basalis of Meynert/loss of cholinergic cell bodies → ↓ activity of cerebral cortical choline acetyltransferase). Five percentage of cases are familial (mutations on chromosomes 1, 14, 21). Chromosome 14 locus is associated with very early onset (age <50, autosomal dominant inheritance). Early-onset pts may have β-amyloid precursor protein (BAPP) mutations linked to a gene on chromosome 21 (*relationship between AD and Down syndrome?*). Some cases present with ApoE epsilon 4 allele (Apo-E gene on chromosome 19). The presence of Apo E epsilon 2 allele may reduce the risk for late onset AD. Research is done concerning the ratio: tau/Aβ 42 in CSF (tau ↑ and Aβ 42 ↓ → ratio ↑) in AD.

Symptoms: insidious onset, gradual progression, usually >50 yr, **with multiple cognitive deficits manifested by amnesia** (first anterograde and only later on retrograde) **and one or more cognitive disturbances** (**aphasia**: language disturbance; **apraxia**: inability to carry out motor activities despite intact motor function; **agnosia**: failure to recognize objects despite intact sensory function; **disturbance in executive functioning**: such as planning, organizing, sequencing, abstracting) or personality changes (apathy, irritability, or disinhibition), progressing to global deficits. Possible associated depression (25%), hallucinations (visual > auditory), delusions (persecutory). **The 4 As of Alzheimer disease: Amnesia, Agnosia, Apraxia,** and **Aphasia.**

TABLE 9.11.   Symptoms Rarely Seen in Alzheimer Disease

Symptoms generally inconsistent with Alzheimer disease	Signs atypical for Alzheimer disease
• Sudden onset • Presenting focal neurologic findings (hemiparesis, hemianesthesia, hemianopia) • Seizures early in the course of the illness • Abnormal gait or coordination • Preservation of memory function	• Dominant nonmemory symptoms (language, praxis, visuospatial function) • Behavioral, personality, psychotic symptoms • Early parkinsonism (resting tremor, bradykinesia, cogwheeling) • Bulbar/brainstem signs • Motor or reflex asymmetries • Unexplained UMN signs (e.g., Babinski) • Unexplained LMN signs (e.g., fasciculations)

Tests: MRI (widespread cortical atrophy particularly in temporal and parietal lobes). Apolipoprotein E (ApoE), genotyping is not specific.

Differential diagnosis: Binswanger's disease (focal deficits, widespread leukoencephalopathy on MRI), normal pressure hydrocephalus (NPH; early ataxi-apraxic gait and urinary incontinence), Pick's disease, and frontotemporal dementia (personality changes ++, mild cognitive deficits). **Vascular dementia (vs Alzheimer's type)**: more deterioration accompanying cerebrovascular disease over time; common focal neurologic sx; presence of risk factors for CV disease.

Note: Half of pts with AD have concomitant vascular disease or cortical Lewy bodies.

Course: progressive, depression, death from intercurrent illness in 8–10 yr.

Stages

- **Stage I: duration of disease 1–3 yr** (new learning defective, ↓ remote recall; topographic disorientation, poor constructions, anomia, apathy, occasional sadness, normal motor function, normal brain scan)
- **Stage II: duration of disease 2–10 yr** (severe ↓ recent and remote recall, spatial disorientation, poor construction, fluent aphasia, ↓ comprehension, acalculia, ideomotor apraxia, apathy, restlessness, slowing background rhythm on EEG, normal or ventricular dilatation, sulcal enlargement)
- **Stage III: duration of disease 8–12 yr** (severe intellectual deficits, echolalia, dysarthria, mutism, limb rigidity, flexion posture, urinary + fecal incontinence, diffuse slowing on EEG, ventricular dilatation, sulcal enlargement)

Treatment: see general rx of dementia.

ATYPICAL DEMENTIAS

Unlike Alzheimer disease, these atypical dementias are often associated with neurologic symptoms (reflecting the localization of the degenerative process rather than the nature of the underlying histopathology):

■ Pathology

TABLE 9.12. Pathology in Atypical Dementias

● **Frontotemporal dementia**: cerebral atrophy in the frontal and anterior temporal lobes
● **AD**: affects the hippocampal, posterior temporal, and parietal regions

■ Signs

TABLE 9.13. Signs in Atypical Dementias

● Sudden onset of symptoms
● Focal neurologic signs (hemiparesis, hemianesthesia, hemianopia)
● Seizures early in the course
● Abnormal gait or coordination
● Preservation of memory function
● Dominant nonmemory signs:
Language, praxis, visuospatial dysfunction
Prominent behavioral, personality, or psychotic signs
Early parkinsonism (resting tremor, bradykinesia, cogwheeling)
Early prominence of bulbar/brainstem signs, unexplained motor or reflex asymmetries

■ Types of atypical dementias

● *Cortical degenerative syndromes*

(1) **Frontotemporal lobe degeneration (FTLD)**: is a heterogeneous disorder; highly familial in 50% cases, **younger age than AD**; associated with **profound personality changes**, social incompetence, language, and stereotypic behaviors, yet with preserved visuospatial skills; lesions destroy areas of the brain that govern behaviors; M : F is 1 : 1; 25% of presenile dementias.

TABLE 9.14. Clinical Criteria for Frontotemporal Dementia

● **Presence of all core diagnostic features: (personality and behavior changes prior to cognitive changes)**
● Insidious onset and gradual progression
● Early decline in social interpersonal conduct
● Early impairment in regulation of personal conduct (apathy and emotional bluntness or overactivity and disinhibition)
● Early affective symptoms: depression, anxiety, somatization, aspontaneity, indifference
● Early loss of insight
● Supportive diagnostic features:
Behavioral disorders: decline in ADLs; mental rigidity; distractibility; hyperorality; perseveration and stereotyped behaviors (verbal, ritual, motoric), social withdrawal, social impropriety (partial clothing, urinating, defecating in front of others, loss of empathy), disinhibition, impulsivity
Early speech and language impairment: lack of spontaneity and poverty of speech, echolalia, stereotypy, perseveration, mutism
Relative preservation of praxis and visuospatial skills (manual dexterity remains good and the pt doesn't get lost or wander off)
Physical signs: primitive reflexes, incontinence, akinesia, rigidity, tremor
● Tests:
Neuropsychology: impaired frontal lobe tests (deficits in abstraction, planning, insight, problem solving), **no amnesia** or perceptual deficits
EEG: normal
Brain imaging: predominant frontal and/or anterior temporal abnormality

TABLE 9.15.   Frontotemporal Lobe Degeneration Spectrum

- Frontotemporal dementia (FTD)
- Pick disease (FTLD-Pick)
- FDT lacking distinctive pathology
- **Progressive aphasias**: difficulty in verbal expression, anomia, shortened phrase length with relative preservation of comprehension (mainly asymmetric atrophy in left frontotemporal lobe); memory of daily events, visual and spatial skills, and behavior remain intact; may be nonfluent, fluent, anomic, mixed, or associated with motor neuron disease
- **Semantic dementia** (fluent): difficulties in finding words, naming objects, circumlocutions, impaired comprehension of single words
- Some of the "tauopathies": **corticobasal degeneration (CBD), familial tauopathies linked to chromosome 17 (FTDP-17: frontotemporal dementia and parkinsonism)**

Note:
- **ALS amyotrophic lateral sclerosis-dementia**: is recognized as a frontal dementia in which there is motor-neuron disease (frontal dementia with lower motor neuron signs/fasciculations, muscle atrophy, weakness, gait disorder, dysarthria, dysphagia, EMG/NCV confirm motor neuropathy)
- **Progressive supranuclear palsy (PSP) or Steele-Richardson-Olszewski syndrome**: is a parkinsonian disorder and a frontotemporal type of dementia (supranuclear gaze deficits: vertical > horizontal, parkinsonism, axial rigidity and multiple falls, pseudobulbar palsy, subcortical dementia, language impairment
- **Corticobasal degeneration (CBGD)**: not strictly a frontotemporal dementia; may still be considered one of the frontal dementias: subcortical dementia, aphasia, obsessiveness, apraxias (ideomotor and ideational), asymmetric sensory and motor findings, parkinsonism, cortical sensory loss, alien limb phenomenon
- **Huntington disease**: not strictly a frontotemporal dementia; may still be considered one of the frontal dementias: personality change (disinhibition, substance/ETOH use, promiscuity), psychosis (delusions, rarely hallucinations), subcortical dementia (↓ drives, ↓ executive functions, ↓ spontaneous speech), chorea (UE > LE), gait change

TABLE 9.16.   Frontotemporal Dementia vs Alzheimer Disease

Frontotemporal dementia	Alzheimer disease
• Early: interpersonal or personality changes with loss of executive abilities and relative preservation of memory • New learning is spared • Disturbed behaviors (compulsive, obstinate acts, verbal stereotypes, changes in eating behaviors) are more common • Bifrontal and anterior temporal atrophy with enlargement of sylvian fissures and volume loss of hippocampus and entorhinal cortex on MRI	• Early: amnesia with preserved social skills and personal propriety • New learning is impaired • On MRI: more severe degree of hippocampal atrophy

(2) **Parietal and parietotemporal symptoms** (see neurologic examination): two functional regions in the parietal lobes: one integrates sensory information to form a single perception (cognition) and the other integrates sensory input, primarily with the visual system, constructing a spatial system that represents the world around us; damages to the parietal lobes → striking deficits such as abnormalities in body image and spatial relations.

● *Other specific dementias:*

Different disorders may occur in an overlapping fashion

(1) **Diffuse Lewy body disease** (Lewy body dementia, senile dementia of the Lewy body type, cortical Lewy body disease)

Epidemiology: *common, third cause* of dementia after AD.

Symptoms: gradual onset in the 60s or 70s; **starts with dementia or dementia with mild parkinsonism** (parkinsonism does not appear for the first time at a stage of severe dementia, *rule of 1 yr* between appearance of dementia and parkinsonism to differentiate with Parkinson disease dementia where parkinsonism is already well established).

TABLE 9.17.   Criteria for Lewy Body Dementia

- **Essential features**: **dementia**; persistent ↓ memory evident with progression; deficits of attention, executive function and visuospatial ability
- **Core features**: fluctuating cognition; recurrent, bizarre, fixed **detailed visual hallucinations**; spontaneous features of **parkinsonism**
- **Suggestive features**: severe neuroleptic hypersensitivity; REM sleep behavior disorder
- **Supportive features**: common falls, syncopes; transient loss of consciousness; severe autonomic dysfunction (orthostatic hypotension, urinary incontinence; depression, other hallucinations, delusions)

Tests: MRI shows mild cortical atrophy and ventricular dilatation, relative preservation of the hippocampal and medial temporal lobe (vs AD).

Differential diagnosis: arteriosclerotic parkinsonism, progressive supranuclear palsy, striatonigral variant of multiple system atrophy (MSA), dementia pugilistica.

Etiology: **Lewy bodies** (aggregates of protein: alpha-synuclein + others in the cytoplasm of nerve cells) **throughout the cortex and in the nucleus basalis of Meynert and substantia nigra**. LBs are also often found in AD, PD, Down syndrome, and other disorders.

Course: progression with death in 1–20 yr.

Treatment: general rx of dementia. Usually there is no need to treat mild motor parkinsonian sx with levodopa-carbidopa.

(2) **Vascular dementias**: Heterogeneous group; three most common mechanisms (simple stroke, multiple infarcts due to thrombosis or emboli of the large or medium size arteries, and subcortical small-vessel disease).

TABLE 9.18.   Probable Vascular Dementia

- **Dementia**
- **Cerebrovascular disease**:
  - Focal signs on neurologic exam (hemiparesis, lower facial weakness, Babinski sign, sensory deficit, hemianopia, dysarthria)
  - Evidence of vascular disease on brain imaging
- **Presence of one or more**: onset of dementia within 3 months of a stroke, abrupt decrease in cognitive functions, stepwise deterioration of cognitive functions
- **Clinical features**: such as early gait disturbance, multiple falls, urinary incontinence, pseudobulbar palsy, personality and mood changes
- **Vascular dementia vs Alzheimer disease**: difficult differentiation, strong association (mixed dementia), existing vascular factors for dementia, including AD

Multi-infarct dementia

Epidemiology: *second most common* after Alzheimer disease; M > F. Preexistence of hypertension, heart disease, or other cardiovascular risk factors; many pts have mixed forms (AD + MID).

Symptoms: **starts with a stroke in** the 50s or 60s, and **then multiple strokes**, sx of **global cognitive deficit, multiple focal sx** due to multiple infarctions (hemiplegia, aphasia, apraxia, aprosodia, pseudobulbar palsy), depression, lability. Multi-infarct dementias have *mixed characteristics (cortical and subcortical)*. Pseudo-bulbar palsy is the bilateral impairment of the function of the lower cranial nerves 9, 10, 11, and 12, which control eating, swallowing, talking (result of an upper motor neuron lesion).

Tests: **multiple cortical or subcortical lesions secondary to infarction or intracerebral hemorrhages on MRI**; Hachinski Ischemic Index.

Differential diagnosis: amnestic syndromes, delirium, MR, depression. **Vascular dementia vs transient ischemic attacks**: in TIA, briefs episodes of focal neurologic dysfunction <24 hr (usually 5–15 min), resulting from microembolization → transient brain ischemia resolving without tissue alteration; one third will have a brain infarction later. Differentiate sx coming from the vertebrobasilar system (disturbance in the brainstem or the occipital lobe) and those coming from the carotid arterial system (unilateral retinal or hemispheric abnormality).

Etiology: arteriosclerosis, cerebral amyloid angiopathy, polyarteritis nodosa, vasculitis secondary to cocaine or amphetamines, cranial arteritis, systemic lupus erythematosus, meningovascular syphilis.

Course: deterioration with each new stroke, which brings short-term delirium and ↑ of the dementia. Complications: same as in all dementias

Treatment: No FDA approval for cholinesterase inhibitors in this indication although individual pts may benefit from them.

Lacunar dementia

Epidemiology: uncommon.

Symptoms: onset in the 50s or 60s; sx depend on size and locations of the lacunar infarctions. Dementia appears only with accumulation of lacunae. Evidence of **global deficit**, elements of a **frontal lobe syndrome, pseudo-bulbar palsy**, one or more **lacunar syndromes** (motor hemiplegia, sensory hemiplegia, ataxic hemiperesis).

Tests: MRI shows **multiple lacunae, bilaterally in subcortical structures** (thalamus, internal capsule, basal ganglia).

Differential diagnosis: Alzheimer disease (no lacunar syndromes, only late appearance of pseudo-bulbar palsy), multi-infarct dementia (hx of major cortical infarct).

Etiology: multiple small cystic infarctions, or lacunae. Pts usually have HTN.

Course: progressive. Complications: same as in all dementias.

Treatment: Treat HTN but avoid hypotension, which may lead to another lacunar infarction. Use prophylactic Aspirin (65 mg/d), general rx of dementias.

- **Binswanger disease (subcortical arteriosclerotic encephalopathy)**

Epidemiology: rare.

Symptoms: gradual onset in the 50s or 60s. It starts with forgetfulness, concreteness, depression, evolving toward a global intellectual deficit, sometimes + minor focal sx (aphasia, apraxia); possible pseudo-bulbar palsy, psychotic sx, and agitation.

Tests: MRI shows **widespread patchy leukoencephalopathy**.

Differential diagnosis: Alzheimer disease (late appearance of focal signs, no leukoencephalopathy on MRI)

Etiology: widespread arteriolar lipohyalinosis and demyelinization; may be seen in pts with or without HTN.

Course: progressive over years.

Treatment: general rx of dementias; aspirin for prevention.

(3) AIDS dementia (see Chapter 15)

Epidemiology: >50% of AIDS pts will develop dementia. The **AIDS dementia complex (ADC)** is one of the most common and clinically important CNS complications of late HIV-1 infection.

Symptoms: *complex* emphasizes that this disease not only impairs the intellect, but also concomitantly alters motor performance and, at times, behavior; onset is insidious, 10 yr after HIV infection usually, in rare cases the dementia presents as the first sx of AIDS; frequent sx of apathy and psychomotor retardation, then cognitive deficits ↑ with appearance of ataxia (myelopathy), tremor, possible psychosis.

TABLE 9.19.   Clinical Manifestations of ADC

• Cognition	• **Early**: inattention, low concentration, slow thinking • **Late**: global dementia
• Motor performances	• **Early**: slow movements, ataxia • **Late**: paraplegia, urinary incontinence
• Behavior	• **Early**: apathy, change in personality, possible agitation and mania • **Late**: mutism

Tests: HIV serology is positive. MRI shows cortical atrophy, ventricular dilatation, and widespread patchy leukoencephalopathy. In CSF: mononuclear pleocytosis, ↑ protein, ↑ IgG index and oligoclonal bands.

Differential diagnosis: opportunistic infections: TB, CMV encephalitis, toxoplasmosis, mycoses; primary CNS lymphoma; hydrocephalus.

Etiology: HIV crosses the blood–brain barrier. ADC is thought to be caused by HIV-1 itself, rather than an opportunistic infection; evidence of: multinucleated giant cells and microglial pallor and vacuolization.

Course: 5-step ADC Staging System (limited survival if > stage 2); rapid, progressive death in months to 1 yr.

Treatment: general rx of dementia, highly active antiretroviral therapy (**HAART**). Avoid neuroleptics which produce parkinsonism. Selegiline (<10 mg/d) may produce mild cognitive improvement.

(4) Dementia due to head trauma

Epidemiology: more in young males.

Symptoms: three types:

- **Diffuse axonal injury (DAI)**: due to severe acceleration-deceleration: coma is immediate with serious damage, vegetative state or dementia, personality changes, irritability, violent outbursts
- **Cerebral contusions**: usually in the temporal lobes and the inferior portions of the frontal lobes (cognitive deficits or personality changes)
- **Subdural hematoma**:
  (1) **Acute**: arterial bleeding is a neurosurgical emergency
  (2) **Subacute**: slow venous bleeding happens in days or weeks, appears as a delirium or a dementia
  (3) **Chronic**: slow venous bleeding, appears in months to years, and shows a progressive dementia. May be caused by minor trauma particularly in the elderly

Tests: MRI shows contusions and subdural hematomas. In DAI: cortical atrophy and ventricular dilatation. Petechial hemorrhages are possible.

Differential diagnosis: if apparent stabilization and secondary worsening, consider hydrocephalus.

Etiology: shearing, strain, and rupture of axons and arterioles

Course: some recovery in DAI then becomes static. Complications: gl complications of dementias.

Treatment: general rx of dementias, evacuation or not of a subdural hematoma. Violent outbursts may respond to propanolol (240–480 mg/d). Irritability: antidepressant (nortriptyline, citalopram).

(5) Parkinson disease (PD)

Epidemiology: 0.25% of the population, **one third will develop dementia**. PD is the most common neurologic disorder seen clinically.

Pathophysiology: Degeneration of dopamine-producing cells in the substantia negra. Loss of DA leads to ↑ excitatory drive from the subthalamic nucleus and the resulting excessive (inhibitory) output from the pallidum (pallidotomy used for rx of refractory cases). Excessive inhibition of activity in the thalamus, cortex, and brain stem is critical. Environmental toxins (MPTP: byproduct of meperidine, drinking well water, heavy metals: iron, zinc, copper, mercury, manganese, magnesium), free radical production (↑ concentration in oxidative products due to DA metabolism → neurotoxicity), mitochondrial abnormalities and genetic factors (45% concordance rate for monozygotic twins and 29% for dizygotic twins). Lewy bodies and cell loss are found in the substantia negra, throughout the cortex in dementia, and in the dorsal raphe nucleus of the midbrain in depression; **imbalance between dopamine (deficiency) and acetylcholine (relative predominance of acetylcholine or insufficient dopamine to maintain the balance with acetylcholine) in the striatum of parkinsonian pts**.

Types of dementia in Parkinson disease: varied and inconsistent pathologic findings; possible relationship between AD and Parkinson disease dementia (which may have heterogeneous causes):

- DA deficiency alone
- DA and ACh deficiency (DA system and atrophy of the nucleus basalis of Meynert, the source nucleus of choline acetyltransferase that synthesizes cortical Ach)
- Cortical Lewy bodies (cortical + brainstem Lewy bodies): *third* in dementia frequency
- Alzheimer-type changes in 40% of PD pts with dementia
- Alzheimer-type changes and cortical Lewy bodies: Lewy body dementia or Lewy body variant of Alzheimer disease

TO NOTE

- Typically a "subcortical dementia" with psychomotor retardation, memory abnormalities, cognitive impairment, and mood disturbances; but cognitive deficits are mostly in the frontal-executive functions
- **More cortical pathology → more severe dementia**
- **More dementia in older PD pts**
- Pts with **dementia have more adverse effects from drugs** (psychosis), **more sensitivity to anticholinergic drugs** (risk of delirium)

Symptoms: motor sx of Parkinson disease start first: tremor (rhythmic, frequency of 3 cycles/s, at rest, pill-rolling movements), rigidity (generalized and cogwheel type), bradykinesia (generalized slowness of movements and thoughts), postural instability, then mild dementia. No focal sx; delusions, hallucinations, depression (30–40%), anxiety, possible apathy.

Differential diagnosis of the dementia associated with parkinsonism (frequent atypical signs): diffuse Lewy body disease (the dementia precedes the motor parkinsonian sx, which are usually mild), arteriosclerotic parkinsonism (focal deficits and hx of strokes), progressive supranuclear palsy (vertical gaze palsy, falls, axial extension), striatonegral variant of multiple system atrophy or MSA (mild ataxia, mild autonomic failure with impotence, orthostatic hypotension, incontinence), dementia pugilistica (past head trauma, ataxia).

TABLE 9.20. Etiology of Parkinsonism

• **Primary parkinsonism**	• Parkinson disease • Juvenile Parkinson disease
• **Secondary parkinsonism**	• **Drugs**: DA-receptor-blocking agents (neuroleptics, metoclopramide, prochlorperazine), DA-depleting agents (reserpine), lithium, fluoxetine and paroxetine, Divalproex, calcium-channel blockers, disulfiram • **Vascular**: multi-infarct, Binswanger encephalopathy • **Toxins**: MPTP, CO, manganese, methanol, ethanol, posthypoxic • **Infections**: postencephalitis, prion disease, AIDS • **Others**: pellagra, focal lesions of the basal ganglia
• **Parkinson plus another disease**	• Progressive supranuclear palsy • **Multiple system atrophy** (striatonegral degeneration, Shy-Drager syndrome, Olivopontocerebellar degeneration) • **Parkinsonism-amyotrophy-dementia complex, cortical-basal degeneration, Lewy body dementia, dementia pugilistica**
• **Parkinsonism associated with heterodegenerative diseases**	• Wilson disease • Huntington disease • Hallervorden-Spatz disease • Autosomal dominant Lewy body disease • Familial basal ganglia calcification (Fahr disease) • Neuroacanthocytosis

TREATMENT

- **For Parkinson disease: symptomatic**
  - **Increase dopaminergic transmission:**
    - **Dopamine precursors: levodopa or L-DOPA is the most effective** (levodopa with action of dopa-decarboxylase → DA): only 1% administered enters the brain. Mostly effective for bradykinesia and rigidity

TABLE 9.21. Motor Complications Associated with Levodopa (LD): (28–84% of Patients Treated with LD, after 5–7 yr of Use)

Type	Management
• **Wearing off**: episodic reemergence of parkinsonian sx, ≥3 hr after each dose of levodopa (temporary insufficiency of DA)	• ↓ LD dose interval, use sustained-release LD, use DA agonist, use MAOI or COMTI
• **Diphasic dyskinesia**	• Increase LD, use sustained-release LD, or use DA agonist as primary therapy and levodopa as ancillary therapy
• **Off-period dystonia**, painful cramps, early morning dystonia	• Use nighttime LD, use baclofen, use DA agonist as primary rx and levodopa as ancillary rx
• **Freezing**: severe temporary deficiency in NE in progressively depleted and damaged NE pathways, manifests as irregular episodes of sudden freezing, usually of short duration, with the pt unable to move, also accompanied by hypotonia and postural instability	• ↑ LD, use DA agonist
• **Peak-dose dyskinesia** (involuntary movements occurring at the time of peak plasma level/too much DA)	• Reduce LD, or use DA agonist
• **On-off**: temporary insufficiency of dopamine, described as a rapid alteration between a state of satisfactory motility, usually with oral-facial dyskinesias, and a rigid akinetic state without dyskinesias	• Use DA agonist, or selegiline, or switch to a slow-release levodopa
• **Myoclonus**	• ↓ LD, use clonazepam, use methylsergide

- **Peripheral dissipation of levodopa → DA**: SE: (nausea, vomiting, cardiac arrhythmia, orthostatic hypotension) and need for high doses: this is controlled by adding peripheral inhibitors of dopa-decarboxylase to LD (**carbidopa/Lodosyn**: start 25 mg po/d with first daily dose of carbidopa + levodopa; may give additional 15.5–25 mg with each dose as needed, max 200 mg/d). Food delays absorption and reduces peak plasma conc. **Levodopa + benserazide (*Prolopa*)** may be used as well. Vitamin B_6 (pyridoxine) is a cofactor of decarboxylase, will increase the peripheral conversion of levodopa to DA, resulting in ↑ SEs and ↓ therapeutic effects (if use of carbidopa, no need to avoid vitamin B_6)

- **Limitations of Levodopa due to**: loss of efficacy, fluctuations in motor performance (due to intermittent stimulation of the striatal dopaminergic receptor by exogenous LD, possibly becoming toxic to dopaminergic neurons/long-acting formulations of levodopa may prevent the fluctuations), mental disturbances/levodopa-induced psychosis

- **Carbidopa + L-DOPA** combination or ***Sinemet*** (10/100, 25/100, 25/250 mg): start 1 tab 25/100 mg po tid, increase by 1 tab/d q 1–2 days prn. Use 1 tab 25/250 mg po tid–qid when higher levodopa doses needed; ***Parcopa*** (**disintegrating tabs**: Start: 10 mg/100 mg po tid–qid or 25 mg/100 mg po tid, incr. 1 tab/d q 1–2 days; max 200 mg/2,000 mg/d)

Info: 70–100 mg/d carbidopa needed to saturate peripheral Dopa decarboxylase and minimize adverse effects

- **Sustained-release carbidopa + levodopa**: ***Sinemet-CR, carbidopa + levodopa ER***: 25/100, 50/200 mg: start 1 tab 50/200 mg po bid, separate doses by ≥4 hr. Increase as needed at intervals ≥3 days. Typical max dose is 1,600–2,000 mg/d of levodopa, but sometimes more

- **Carbidopa + levodopa + entacapone (*Stalevo* 50** = 12.5/50/200 mg; ***Stalevo* 100** = 25/100/200 mg; ***Stalevo* 150** = 37.5/150/200 mg): To substitute for IR carbidopa/levodopa and entacapone previously administered as individual products or to replace IR carbidopa/levodopa therapy (without entacapone) when pts experience the sx of end-of-dose "wearing-off" (only for pts taking a total daily dose of levodopa of 600 mg or less and not experiencing dyskinesias (max 6 tabs/d).

- **Enzymatic degradation blockers**:

  - **Selegiline (*Eldepryl, Zelapar ODT*): usually as adjunct to levodopa** (MAO-B inhibitor, metabolized to amphetamine and methamphetamine → release of DA, neuroprotective role is controversial, may prevent parkinsonism associated with toxin MPTP; Selegine: given 5–10 mg/d; if given at higher dose, it loses its selectivity for MAO-B and may produce a hypertensive crisis with tyramine found in some foods; cannot be administered with meperidine/Demerol). May retard the progression of the disease (controversial). Zelapar ODT: start 1.25 mg SL q AM for >6 wk, then ↑ prn to max 2.5 mg q AM

  - **Rasagiline (*Azilect*)** (MAO-B inhibitor); sometimes used with levodopa; 1 mg po qd. Info: start 0.5 mg po qd if levodopa adjunct. *Requires MAOI diet*

- **Dopamine reuptake blockers**: amantadine (*Symmetrel*) (NMDA antagonist): 100–300 mg/d divided in 2–3 doses, may lose its action after 6–12 months. SE: anticholinergic, livedo reticularis, edema. Useful as monotherapy for bradykinesia or tremors

- **Dopamine agonists**: effective for all features but not as effective as L-DOPA, more expensive

  - ↓ Dopamine turnover → less oxidative stress/neuroprotective effects? They may be used as monotherapy early on.

  - **Bromocriptine (*Parlodel*:** dose: 2.5–10 mg); **apomorphine (*Apokyn*)** is given subcutaneously, short therapeutic effect; longer half-life than levodopa, but less effective (used as adjuncts)

  - More SE: hypotension, abdominal bloating, fatigue, sedation, dry mouth, nausea, constipation, hallucinations, delusions, vivid dreams. Ergoline DA agonists (bromocriptine) can produce pulmonary, retroperitoneal fibrosis, and erythromelalgia (erythema, swelling, and a painful burning sensation primarily in the extremities)

  - New nonergoline agents:

    - **Ropinirole (Requip, Requip XL)**: Requip. Start 0.25 mg po tid for 1 wk. The second week: 0.5 mg po tid. In the third week: 0.75 mg po tid. In the fourth week: 1 mg po tid. Max of 24 mg/d. For XL form: start 2 mg once daily for 1 to 2 wk, ↑ of 2 mg/d at 1 wk or longer intervals, up to 24 mg/d

    - **Rotigotine (Neupro)**: transdermal patch delivering rotigotine, an agonist to treat Parkinson's and restless leg syndrome, was approved in the United States in 2007, and then in April 2008 it was withdrawn from the market (worldwide) due to crystallization (and potential ↓ in potency)

    - **Pramipexole (Mirapex)**: DA agonist; starting dose of 0.125 mg po tid for 1 wk, then ↑ to 0.25 mg po × 1 wk then ↑ by 0.75 mg/wk divided tid. Usual effective dose: 0.5–1.5 mg po tid

  - Addition of DA agonist to levodopa helps to ↓ dose of levodopa (↓ 20%) to a minimum and to provide more continuous dopaminergic stimulation.

  - Treatment of SE:

    - **Hypotension**: ↓ dose of DA agonist, add salt to the diet, fludrocortisone, midodrine (Orvaten:10 mg po tid)

- **Vomiting**: titrate slowly; give DA agonist with food, trimethobenzamide (Tigan: 250–300 mg po tid–qid)
- **Psychosis: common in late stage of PD; reduce levodopa (if psychosis does not clear and still need an agonist: add quetiapine)**

- **Reducing cholinergic transmission**: anticholinergics such as **benztropine (*Cogentin*:** start 0.5–2 mg/d; max 6 mg/d) or **trihexyphenidyl (*Artane*:** therapeutic dose: 8–12 mg, risk of delirium) and **biperiden (*Akineton*:** 2–20 mg/d). Peripheral SEs (dry mouth, constipation, mydriasis, poor visual accommodation, and urinary retention) + central SEs: confusion, delirium, visual hallucinations (6–38%). Best response: on tremor, then rigidity

- **COMT inhibitors: Entacapone (*Comtan*) and tolcapone (*Tasmar*)**: adjunctive; Entacapone: start 200 mg po with each dose of Carbidopa-levodopa. Max: 8 tabs (1,600 mg/d). Tolcapone: start 100 mg po, max 200 mg po tid. Tolcapone is more centrally active and entacapone is more peripherally active: both are COMT inhibitors/catechol-O-methyltransferase inhibitors → metabolite of COMT pathway, 3-O-methyldopa competes with levodopa for transport at the blood–brain barrier → selective inhibition of COMT may ↑ levels of levodopa in the brain. COMT inhibitors also prolong the effect of levodopa

- **When to initiate combination therapy?** With a dopamine agonist and levodopa; early combination is frequent

- **Conclusions**: For ameliorating motor and ADL disability: L-DOPA; Ropinirole, pramipexole are effective for PD pts who need dopaminergic rx. L-DOPA is more effective, but has more motor complications after 2.5 yr of follow-up. Ropinirole and pramipexole: more hallucinations, somnolence, and edema than L-DOPA; same rate of motor complications with immediate-release or sustained-release levodopa

- **Neural transplantation (fetal cells) and surgery (posteroventral pallidotomy), deep brain stimulation**, when other therapies fail

- **Glutamate antagonists** may have a role in preventing MPTP-induced parkinsonism. Lamotrigin inhibits the release of glutamate.

- **Treatment of behavioral changes**:
  - **Depression**: tricyclics with few anticholinergic SE (nortriptyline), SSRI (risk to↑ motor disability), ECT (useful on the depression and on the motor sx). Avoid Bupropion (risk of confusion and dyskinesia). Selegiline is a selective MAO-B inhibitor at ≤10 mg; if used >10 mg, it also inhibits MAO-A → risk of hypertensive crisis if a TCA is added or risk of serotonin syndrome if SSRIs are added.
  - **Sleep disorders**: ↓ dopaminergic agents. Give selegiline in AM.
  - **Anxiety treatment**: benzo. (Lorazepam, clonazepam), or buspirone. Dopamine agents may → OCD sx. Treat panic attacks with antidepressants or benzodiazepines.
  - **General treatment of the dementia**: donepezil (5–10 mg/d) may improve cognition.
  - **Psychosis**:
    - First, ↓ the dose of the dopamine agonist, or discontinue adjunctive medications (anticholinergics, amantadine, selegiline, and DA agonists).
    - If sx persist, use antipsychotic such as quetiapine.
    - Differentiate hallucinations due to dopaminergic drugs (intact sensorium) vs those due to anticholinergic agents (fluctuating arousal, ↓ attention, incoherence, threatening hallucinations)
    - Antipsychotics ↑ motor sx of PD. Use the ones with less EPS risks: such as quetiapine (less D2 blocking effect, less likely to complicate PD); rarely thioridazine (10–75 mg) but check ECG because of ↑ QTc risk; clozapine (12.5–100 mg) may be used if other atypical failed: follow protocol and monitor for agranulocytosis, may also ↓ severity of the motor sx).
  - **Mania/hypomania in 10% pts treated with dopaminergic agents**: ↓ dosage of dopaminergic agents; if ineffective use mood stabilizers (carbamazepine: 200–1,200 mg/d; valproate: 250–300 mg/d)
  - **Hypersexuality, other compulsive behaviors (gambling…)**: ↓ dosage of dopaminergic agents.

- **For the treatment of the dementia: as in general rx of dementias**
Course: progressive, severe disability in 15 yr. **Depression** is frequent (4–70%, due to the neurobiologic changes).

(6) Huntington disease (Huntington chorea)

Epidemiology: lifetime prevalence: 0.004–0.008%; greater in blacks and Japanese.

Symptoms: *insidious onset in the late 30s*; **may be with chorea or dementia** (personality changes, followed by a global intellectual deficit, with common psychotic sx, depression); chorea sx such as jumping, lightning-like, unpredictable movements, presents with clumsiness and restlessness, first in the face (forehead) or upper extremities, spreading later to lower extremities with dancing, prancing gait.

Tests: **MRI** later on shows atrophy of the heads of the caudate nuclei. **Genetic testing**: abnormal chromosome 4.

Differential diagnosis: neuroacanthocytosis (lip biting, increased acanthocytes on 3 wet preps), Wilson disease (copper studies), dentatorubropallidoluysian atrophy (genetic testing), acquired hepatocerebral degeneration (repeated episodes of hepatic encephalopathy in chronic alcoholics), tardive dyskinesia.

Etiology: *autosomal dominant*; cell loss throughout cortex but mostly in caudate nucleus.

Course: progressive, death in 10–30 yr.

Treatment: general rx of dementia; neuroleptics to ↓ chorea and psychosis (risperidone 3–6 mg/d; haloperidol 2.5–10 mg/d; olanzapine 5–10 mg/d); treat depression with SSRI or TCA (nortriptyline). Do not use bupropion (may ↑ the chorea). For mania: neuroleptic and/or mood stabilizer.

(7) Pick disease

Epidemiology: M > F; insidious onset, 50–70 yo.

Symptoms: **personality changes of the frontal lobe type (disinhibition), with possible elements of the Kluver-Bucy syndrome** (hypersexuality, placidity, hyperorality), with **evolution to a global cognitive deficit**; possible expressive aphasia or seizures.

Tests: MRI shows **cortical atrophy, mostly in frontal and temporal lobes**. Characteristically, the posterior portion of the superior temporal gyrus is spared.

Differential diagnosis:

- Alzheimer disease may present with frontal lobe syndrome but not with a Kluver-Bucy syndrome and usually no lobar atrophy.
- Frontotemporal dementia is a mixed entity: may include Pick disease, cases of amyotrophic lateral sclerosis (revealed by upper and lower motor neuron signs), other disorders described as: frontotemporal dementias and parkinsonism linked to chromosome 17 (FTDP-17) and dementia lacking distinctive histology features (DLDH). For some, frontotemporal dementia includes only FTDP-17 and DLDH.

Etiology: autosomal dominant transmission. Presence of **lobar, knife-like atrophy, with neuronal loss, gliosis, and characteristic Pick bodies,** which are made of straight or twisted tau neurofilaments.

Course: progressive with death from intercurrent disease in 3–10 yr.

Treatment: general rx of dementia.

(8) Creutzfeldt–Jakob disease

Epidemiology: very rare.

Symptoms: gradual or subacute onset. May present with nonspecific dementia or other sx (parkinsonism, **early appearance of myoclonus** in 90% of cases, ataxia, cortical blindness, hemianopia, pyramidal tracts sx), evolving toward both **dementia and other neurologic sx** (pyramidal sx, extrapyramidal sx, cerebellar sx, aphasia, visual impairment).

Tests: MRI shows progressive **cortical atrophy**; EEG with spike-slow wave complexes. CSF contains the 14–3–3 protein (in Creutzfeldt–Jakob disease and in acute neuronal disease).

Differential diagnosis: new-variant Creutzfeldt–Jakob disease (nvCJD) which is acquired by eating meat from cows that had bovine spongiform encephalopathy. Sx are: depression or psychosis with later dementia, ataxia and myoclonus, abnormal MRI, normal EEG.

Etiology: **prion disease** (the prion protein exists in the cell membrane). These prions are widespread with **neuronal loss, vacualization → spongiform aspect of the cortex**. Three forms: inherited (15%, onset in the 50s), transmitted (after a latency of 10–25 yr after iatrogenic infection/after transplants, grafts, human growth hormone), sporadic (any age but mostly in the 60s).

Course: **rapid progression** with akinetic and mute state in the terminal stage, rapid death in 1 yr.

Treatment: general rx of dementia. Prions are resistant to autoclaving and formalin but not to hypochloride bleach.

(9) Alcoholic dementia (alcohol-induced persisting dementia)

Epidemiology: 10% of all chronic alcoholics, 20% of all cases of dementia.

Symptoms: insidious onset; global intellectual deficit, personality changes, disinhibition, apathy, poor judgment, and possible focal sx (aphasia, apraxia).

Tests: MRI shows generalized cortical atrophy and ventricular dilatation.

Differential diagnosis: subdural hematoma (prominent focal sx like hemiplegia), acquired hepatocerebral degeneration (presence of chorea), Korsakoff syndrome (amnesia alone, no cognitive deficits).

Etiology: alcohol is a neurotoxin.

Course: progressive if continued drinking; if abstinence, possible improvement up to 1 yr then static.

Treatment: general rx of dementia, abstinence, adequate nutrition, thiamine supplementation.

(10) Inhalant-induced dementia

Epidemiology: not rare.

Symptoms: insidious onset; after years of chronic inhalant use appear dullness, apathy, concrete thinking, evolving into dementia, with possibility of cerebellar ataxia, and generalized hyperreflexia.

Differential diagnosis: alcoholic dementia if accompanied by cerebellar degeneration (hx of alcoholism), hypothyroidism may show dementia and ataxia (presence of myxedematous changes, constipation, hair loss), spinocerebellar ataxia (autosomal dominant), the olivopontocerebellar variant of multiple system atrophy (mild autonomic failure and mild parkinsonism).

Etiology: toluene is the most toxic; widespread demyelinization.

Course: progressive if continued use, static if discontinuation.

Treatment: general rx of dementia, abstinence.

AMNESTIC DISORDERS

Epidemiology: blackouts are very common, transient global amnesia (TGA) is very rare.

Scale: Wechsler Memory Scale-Revised (WMS-R)

Symptoms:

- Two components: **anterograde amnesia** (unable to lay down new memories), **retrograde amnesia** (unable to recall events previously remembered)
- Check short-term, intermediate, long-term memory.
- Episodic or chronic
  - **Chronic amnesia**: anterograde amnesia always present + variable retrograde amnesia (period of amnesia covering months or years of time before the amnesia began)
  - **Episodic amnesia**:
    - Pt tested during the amnesia period: anterograde amnesia + some retrograde amnesia (covering events that occurred before the start of the episode)
    - Pt tested after the episode has ended: can recall the events that preceded that episode but no recall of events experienced during that episode.

Tests: as per etiology

Differential diagnosis:

- **Delirium**: presence of confusion
- **Dementia**: presence of global intellectual deficit, amnesia, deficits in abstracting and calculating abilities; may present as pure amnesia
- **Dissociative amnesia**: (dissociative disorder), trigger is an emotional event; during rx, young adults may recall events that occurred while the amnesia was present.

Etiology:

- **Chronic amnesia**: **Korsakoff syndrome**, **paraneoplastic limbic encephalitis** (amnesia, followed by personality changes, seizures or dementia, MRI, antineuronal antibodies**), prodrome to dementia** (like Alzheimer disease)
- **Episodic amnesia**: **TGA (transient global amnesia), epileptic amnesia** (paroxysmal onset, no cloudiness of consciousness, no automatism, lasts minutes to hours, associated with other types of seizures, EEG, MRI), **blackouts, concussion, TIAs** (rare, may present as amnesia if they involve temporal lobes or anterior thalamus)

Course: as per etiology.

Complications: chronic: institutionalization? Episodic: frequently unrecognized; agitated episodes.

Treatment: supervision, treat the underlying cause.

Korsakoff syndrome (alcohol-induced persisting amnestic disorder)

Epidemiology: uncommon.

Symptoms: anterograde and retrograde amnesia, confabulation, no confusion.

Differential diagnosis: delirium, dementia, dissociative amnesia.

Etiology: sequela to Wernicke's encephalopathy due to alcoholism (after the delirium of Wenicke's encephalopathy clears, the pt is left with amnesia), protracted vomiting, lack of thiamine; focal bilateral lesions in the circuit of Papez (hippocampus, fornix, mammillary bodies, anterior nuclei of the thalamus). Lesions may be due to infections, infarctions, hypoxia, temporal lobectomy, tumors.

Course: supervision, institutionalization.

Treatment: treat etiology if possible.

Transient global amnesia (TGA)

Epidemiology: rare.

Symptoms: abrupt onset in the 60s, often preceded by high emotion, sex, or argument. During the episode, the pt may be able to engage in complex activities, but unable to keep track of ongoing events, or unable to recall events that had occurred a few hours before the onset. Lasts 4–18 hr with a gradual spontaneous resolution. After the episode resolves, the pt cannot recall events that occurred during the episode.

Differential diagnosis: epileptic amnesia (earlier onset, episodes <1 hr, recurring more often, with frequent more typical seizures); blackouts (usually after intoxication); concussion (head trauma), TIA (lasts a few minutes); dissociative amnesia (younger onset, dissociative disorder)

Etiology: unknown. Epileptic? Vascular?

Course: usually 1 episode, infrequent, rare complications if the pt is supervised.

Treatment: supervision, prophylaxis? (aspirin, divalproex).

COGNITIVE DISORDERS NOS

The sx do not meet the criteria for delirium, dementia, or amnestic disorders; the disorders may involve a specific general medical condition, a pharmacologically active substance, or both.

TABLE 10.1. Consider an Organic Condition of Psychiatric Symptoms

● Specific symptoms	● **Acute onset**
	● **First episode in an older pt**
	● **Hx of substance abuse with possible intoxication or withdrawal** (alcohol, amphetamine, cocaine, opioid, sedative-hypnotic, cannabis, hallucinogens)
	● **Current medical illness** (SLE, temporal arteritis, polyarteritis nodosa, migraines, MS, epilepsy, brain tumors)
	● **Physical trauma**: head injury
	● **Specific neurologic symptoms**:
	○ Loss of consciousness
	○ Seizures
	○ Focal sx:
	○ Aphasias
	○ Frontal lobe syndromes: changes in concentration, thinking, impulse control, reasoning ability
	○ Temporal lobe syndromes: psychosis, seizures, bizarre behaviors, personality changes
	○ Bilateral injuries: with hypersexuality, hyperorality, placidity, inability to recognize the emotional significance of visual stimuli, frequent shifts of attention like in Kluver-Bucy syndrome
	○ Right TLE personality: excessive emotionality
	○ Left TLE personality: humorless approach to life, interest in philosophic issues
	○ Parietal lobe syndromes: abnormal tactile sensations, visuospatial functions (if right side lesion), with reading or calculation (if left side lesion), hypomania
	○ Occipital lobe syndromes: cortical blindness with denial (Anton syndrome)
	○ Changes in movements and gait
	● **Specific mental status changes**: ↓ alertness, disorientation, ↓ memory, ↓ concentration, changes in speech, nonauditory hallucinations
	● **Poor ability to control fine and gross motor movements**: poor communication skills, abnormalities in drawing clock, Bender test
	● **Catatonia**: combativeness, rigidity, posturing, muteness, echopraxia, echolalia, grimacing
	● **Nonspecific clinical signs of chronic organicity**: intellectual, memory, and cognitive impairment (shallow thoughts, lack of intellectual flexibility, perseveration, poor judgment); change in personality; disinhibition (inappropriateness or exacerbation of underlying personality traits); poverty of speech with decreased vocabulary and use of clichés; prominent visual hallucinations, affect initially may be depressed, anxious and labile but may progress to be shallow, apathetic, empty
● CNS disorders requiring immediate treatment	● **Hypoglycemia**: fruit juice orally, dextrose 50% IV
	● **Wernicke's encephalopathy**: Thiamine 100 mg IV
	● **Opioid intoxication**: naloxone (Narcan) 4 mg IV
● Think organicity in particular syndromes	● **Delirium and dementia**: global impairment (see Chapter 9): **think about offending medications in delirium and dementia**
	● **Amnestic syndrome and organic hallucinosis**: selective areas of impaired cognition
	● **Amnestic syndrome**: Korsakoff psychosis (thiamine deficiency, bilateral lesions of mammillary bodies), head trauma (hippocampal region), tumors (bilateral temporal lobes, frontal lobe damage), herpes simplex encephalitis (attacks temporal lobes), ECT, seizures, cerebral anoxia, transient global amnesia
	● **Organic hallucinosis**: most common causes are alcohol (auditory), hallucinogens/LSD, mescaline, psilocybin, PCP (visual), also sensory deprivation, seizures (olfactory and gustatory hallucinations in TLE), cerebral tumors
	● **Organic delusional, mood, and anxiety syndromes**: similar to functional disorders but imply a probable organic origin
	● **Organic delusional syndrome**: amphetamine intoxication, Huntington chorea, temporal lobe epilepsy, endocrinopathies, deficiency states, connective tissue diseases, CNS disorders (MS), toxic/ medications, others
	● **Organic mood syndrome**: endocrine disorders, secondary mania associated with infectious diseases (influenza, Q fever) or tumors (meningiomas and gliomas) or TLE, medications, and illicit drugs
	● **Organic anxiety syndromes**: endocrine disorders, psychoactive substances (stimulants use, sedative withdrawal), brain tumors, epilepsy, COPD, vitamin B$_{12}$ deficiency, connective tissue disease (SLE), many others
	● **Organic personality syndrome** (usually involve structural brain damage): TLE, damage to the frontal lobes, metabolic factors, SLE
	● **Intoxication and withdrawal**: defined by etiology

TABLE 10.2.   Glasgow Coma Scale

Eye opening	Verbal activity	Motor activity
		● 6. Obeys commands
	● 5. Oriented	● 5. Localizes pain
● 4. Spontaneous	● 4. Confused	● 4. Withdraws to pain
● 3. To command	● 3. Inappropriate	● 3. Flexion to pain
● 2. To pain	● 2. Incomprehensible	● 2. Extension to pain
● 1. None	● 1. None	● 1. None

TABLE 10.3.   Evaluation to R/O Organic Mental Disorder

● Initial assessment	● Present episode: Pt's report of onset, hx of previous similar altered behavior, family's report of recent changes in behavior or personality ● Psychiatric history: previous psychiatric illness and psychiatric rx, family hx of psychiatric illness ● Medical history: recent illnesses and sx, specific hx of previous medical illness or injury, review of systems with emphasis on neurologic hx, exposure to toxic substances, social and family and work hx ● Drug history: prescribed medications, over-the-counter, illicit drugs, alcohol abuse ● Mental status examination: behavior, orientation, attention, concentration, language abilities, memory, higher cognitive functions, affect, thought process and content, perceptual abnormalities, judgment, focal cortical deficits ● Vital signs
● Physical examination and laboratory tests	● Physical examination, chest X-ray, skull X-ray, EKG, laboratory tests (SMA 12, electrolytes, CBC, U/A, drug screen, blood alcohol level)
● Guided selective tests	● EEG, blood glucocorticosteroid, thyroid panel, vitamin B_{12}, RBC folate, serum ceruloplasmin, antinuclear antibodies, red cell sedimentation rate, cerebrospinal fluid, arterial blood gases, serum heavy metal levels, blood carbon monoxide, VDRL, FTA (blood and CSF), other specific laboratory tests
● CAT scan and/or MRI	● As needed

TABLE 10.4.   Treatment of Agitation (Chemical Restraints)

● Benzodiazepine	● Lorazepam (Ativan: 2 or 4 mg/mL vials): 1–3 mg IM q hr up to 3 doses
● Benzodiazepine ± antihistamine	● Lorazepam (Ativan: 2 and 4 mg/mL vials): 1–3 mg IM ● ± Diphenhydramine (Benadryl: 50 mg/mL vials; generic: 10 mg and 50 mg/mL): 50–75 mg IM ● Lorazepam (Ativan: 2 and 4 mg/mL vials): 1–3 mg IM ● ± Hydroxyzine (Vistaril: 25 or 50 mg/mL vials): 25–50 mg IM
● Atypical antipsychotic	● Ziprasidone (Geodon: 20 mg/mL vials): Start with 10–20 mg IM. May repeat q 2 hr if 10 mg or q 4 hr with 20 mg IM (more effective). Max dose 40 mg/d. Warnings if used in pts at risk of ↑ QTc. Continue IM for up to 3 days before switching to po 80 mg bid ● Olanzapine (Zyprexa: 10 mg/mL vials): Start with 10 mg IM; may repeat q 2–4 hr with 10 mg IM. Max dose 30 mg/d. Risk of hypotension. Rapid onset; no ↑ of QTc ● Apiprazole (Abilify: 7.5 mg/mL; vials containing 9.75 mg/1.3 mL): Start with 9.75 mg IM; may repeat q 2–4 hr. Max dose is 30 mg/d. Adult pt may receive up to 15 mg (2 mL) in a single dose. In the elderly, start with 0.7 mL/5.25 mg
● Typical antipsychotic	● Chlorpromazine (Thorazine: 25 mg/mL vials): 50–75 mg IM ● Haloperidol (Haldol: 5 mg/mL vials): 5 mg IM. Give with Benztropine (Cogentin: 1 mg/mL vials): 1–2 mg IM to prevent EPS
● Possible combinations	● Haloperidol (Haldol: 5 mg/mL vials): 5 mg IM) + benztropine (Cogentin: 1 mg/mL vials: 1–2 mg IM) + Lorazepam (Ativan: 2 and 4 mg/mL vials: 2–3 mg IM). May repeat 30–60 min later (up to 3 doses). For elderly pts or children: use 1–2 mg IM of haloperidol + benztropine 1 mg IM + 0.5–1 mg of lorazepam IM

CAUTION WITH CHEMICAL RESTRAINTS

- Risk **of neuroleptic malignant syndrome (NMS)** with mechanical restraints, high potency neuroleptics (haloperidol), dehydration
- ↑ **CPK blood levels** with IM injections and agitation (differential diagnosis with NMS)
- Risk **of respiratory depression** with sedative-hypnotics (benzodiazepines), neuroleptics
- **Chlorpromazine IM**; painful, risk of hypotension
- **Haloperidol injection**: avoid in pts with "basal ganglia disease"
- **Droperidol**: mostly used in anesthesia; rarely used 5 mg IM or 2.5–5 mg IV (duration greater than halo-peridol, ↓ BP when given IM, may be superior to lorazepam for agitated pts with cocaine toxicity)
- **Benzodiazepines**: risk of aggressive dyscontrol, of dependency. Do not give valium IM (erratic absorption)
- **If pt can take po medication**: may use risperidone 2 mg po in combination with lorazepam 2 mg po.

Risperdal M tab. and Zyprexa Zydis are bioequivalent in speed of onset of efficacy to standard risperidone and olanzapine tabs, respectively.

Oral risperidone liquid + oral lorazepam was as effective as haloperidol IM + lorazepam IM to ↓ agitation in 30–60 min.

Monitor for cardiorespiratory depression in pts treated with olanzapine IM, especially if receiving concomitant benzodiazepine.

PHYSICAL RESTRAINTS

TABLE 10.5.   Indications and Contraindications of Restraints and Seclusion

	Indications	Contraindications	Regulations
• Seclusion	• To prevent any imminent harm to self or others • To prevent any serious disruption in the milieu • As part of the behavioral treatment plan • To decrease stimuli	• Unstable medical or psychiatric conditions • Seriously suicidal pt • Delirious or demented pt • Pt with an overdose or in drug withdrawal • For only the convenience of the staff	• Must be implemented only if the pt creates a risk to harm self or others and no less restrictive alternative is available • Must be implemented by a written order from a medical staff after evaluation of the pt • Order of confinement must be time limited for a specific episode. The physician must state the type of restraints, reason for use, and the times to be used. The maximum length of time must be written; it varies with the age of the pt • Pt's condition must be regularly reviewed (to give the patient an opportunity for hydration, eating, toileting, exercise, and other activities of daily living) and documented, following the **hospital, APA, JCAHO, state guidelines** • If the original order must be extended, it must be reviewed and reordered
• Restraints	• To prevent any imminent harm to self or others		

Adapted from Park, M., Tang J. H., & Ledford, L. (2005). Changing the practice of physical restraint use in acute care. Iowa City, IA: University of Iowa Gerontolofgal Nursing Interventions Research Center, Research Translation and Dissemination Core. Retrieved September 3, 2010 from: http://www.guidelines.gov/content.aspx?id=8626

TABLE 10.6.   Sample of an Order for Restraints

- Type of restraint:
  - Seclusion in the quiet room (door locked or open), or in pt's bedroom
  - 4-point leather restraint or soft restraints
- Reason for restraint:
  - Threat to self
  - Threat to others
  - Severe agitation, combativeness
- Time: start at … maximum of … hours
- Monitor the patient as per hospital policy (1:1 or q 15 min …)
- Staff may release gradually the restraints and completely if pt is calm and contracts for safety

The note accompanying the restraint must describe:

- The specific behaviors of the pt preceding the restraint
- What other less restrictive measures were considered or offered, and why were they found not useful at the time?
- What seclusion/restraints were given?
- What supervision was offered regularly as per protocol?
- Any prn medication po or IM given?
- Time started and time of release from the restraints
- A documentation of a debriefing session with the pt after being released from the restraints
- The note must be dated with the time written and signed

TABLE 10.7.   Treatment of Neuroleptic Adverse Reactions

• **Acute dystonia**: opisthotonos, oculogyric crises (rolling of the eyes, involves mostly neck, face (trismus), back, tongue (feeling of having a thick tongue, difficulty swallowing, or fixed protrusion of the tongue); is painful, frightening; usually sudden onset; risk of laryngeal dystonia and suffocation; usually a few days or weeks after drug initiation or dosage increase; R/O: malingering, seizures	• **Acute treatment**:
	   Benztropine (Cogentin): 1–2 mg IM
	   Or diphenydramine (Benadryl): 50–75 mg IM
	   May be given IV if respiratory problems
	   or lorazepam 1–2 mg IM
	 • **Prophylaxis**: ↓ antipsychotic dosage, or switch to a serotonin-dopamine antagonist, may give anticholinergics for a few weeks and try to discontinue

• **Akathisia** (= psychomotor restlessness, differentiate from ↑ agitation or ↑ psychosis): subjective (irritability, inner feelings of restlessness, urge to move, no circadian pattern, may ↓ with sleep) and objective features (rocking, pacing, fidgeting) present; absence of other causes of akathisia (restless legs syndrome, Parkinson disease, subthalamic lesions) and absence of peripheral neuropathy, myelopathy, myopathy; acute (sx begin within 6 wk of drug initiation or increase) or chronic (if more than 3 months). R/O: tardive akathisia has a delayed onset unrelated to drug initiation or ↑ dosage, may be unmasked by drug withdrawal (may be associated with choreoathetoid limb dyskinesias and orofacial dyskinesias)	• Propanolol (Inderal: 10–20 mg tid; long-acting propanolol (Inderal LA: 60–80 mg q d) • Or Clonazepam (Klonopin: 0.5–1 mg po bid) • Rarely: clonidine
• **EPS: Extrapyramidal sx** = dystonia, tremor (low-frequency, resting, "pill-rolling"), rigidity, cogwheeling, mask-like facies, bradykinesia with difficulty to initiate or arrest movement; R/O Parkinson disease, TD, dystonia	• Benztropine (Cogentin): 1–2 mg po bid • Or Diphenhydramine (Benadryl): 50–100 mg po tid • Or trihexyphenidyl (Artane): 2–5 mg tid • Or Amantadine (Symmetrel): 100 mg po bid, max 300 mg/d (risk of toxicity if elderly, renal failure) • Or Clonazepam (Klonopin): 0.5–1 mg po bid
• **NMS (neuroleptic malignant syndrome** = confusion, delirium, rigidity, autonomic instability with changes in pulse, BP, temp ↑, sweating, ↑ in CPK and WBC. Risk of death)	• Discontinue neuroleptic; transfer to MICU for supportive medical treatment; rehydrate; consider dopamine agonists or dantrolene • **NOTE: Malignant hyperthermia (MH) Hotline**: **1-800-644-9737** (outside the US: 1-315-464-7079) http://medical.mhaus.org/

Continued

TABLE 10.7.   Treatment of Neuroleptic Adverse Reactions   Continued

• **TD (tardive dyskinesia** = involuntary movements of the tongue, mouth, fingers, toes, and other body parts such as chewing, smacking, licking the lips, sucking, tongue protrusion, blinking, grimaces, facial distortions, choreic movements); delayed onset (not earlier than 3 months after initiation or ↑ dosage); R/O: EPS, akathisia, dystonia, idiopathic or hereditary or metabolic dyskinesias	• Discontinue antipsychotic. May switch later on to an antipsychotic from a different class (mostly atypical) or clozapine. There is no treatment for TD. Prevention is the best treatment • Vitamin C (500–100 mg/d) and vitamin E (1,200–1,600 IU/d). See Fogel's cocktail; *vitamin B6+++* • Accepted drug rx for TD sx: reserpine up to 2–4 mg/d (risk of severe depression). Stimulation of GABA-ergic system: baclofen (40–80 mg/d), clonazepam (1–8 mg/d), valproic acid (1–3 g/d) • Adjuncts: none appears to be definitively effective. Ondansetron (Zofran), used off-label at 12 mg/d. Melatonin has also been studied without conclusive results; tetrabenazine/Xenazine (used in chorea in Huntington disease; risk of depression, suicide)

See also: Worldwide Education and Awareness for Movement Disorders (WE MOVE), http://www.wemove.org/
Many medications might cause akathisia: first and second generation of antipsychotics, SSRIs, lithium, buspirone, amoxapine, calcium-channel blockers.

TABLE 10.8.   Treatment of Anticholinergic (Antimuscarinic) Side Effects and Toxicity

• **Anticholinergic drugs involved**	• Neurologic drugs: Amantadine (Symmetrel), Benztropine mesylate (Cogentin), Biperiden (Akineton), Procyclidine hydrochloride (Kemadrin), Trihexyphenidyl hydrochloride (Artane), Orphenadrine citrate (Norflex, Dispal) • Psychiatric drugs: most antipsychotics, TCAs, MAOIs, benzodiazepines, narcotic analgesics • Over-the-counter cold preparations: codeine (eliminated in most US states) • Multiple medications have anticholinergic SE: antihistamines, antiulcer drugs (cimetidine > ranitidine), bronchodilators (theophylline), cardiovascular drugs (angiotensin-converting enzyme inhibitors, anticoagulants/warfarin, digoxin, diuretics/furosemide, dyazide, and calcium channel blockers/nifedipine), muscle relaxants, prednisolone
• **Symptoms**	• Mnemonic used: **dry as a bone** (dry mucosae); **blind as a bat** (blurred vision, exacerbation of narrow-angle glaucoma, photophobia); **plugged as a pig** (constipation, urinary retention, delayed or retrograde ejaculation); **hot as a hare** and **red as a beet** (↓ sweat, ↓ salivation, ↑ temperature); **quick as a tick** (tachycardia); **mad as a hatter** (anticholinergic delirium) • **Anticholinergic intoxication**: delirium, coma, seizures, agitation, hallucinations, severe hypotension, supraventricular tachycardia, flushing, mydriasis, dry skin, hyperthermia, decreased bowel sounds

• **Treatment with cholinergic agonists**	• **Medications**:
	  Bethanechol (Urecholine): approved only for nonobstructive urinary retention (start: 10–20 mg po bid; max 200 mg/d in divided doses)
	  Cevimeline (Evoxac): approved only for Sjogren syndrome (start 30 mg po bid–tid; max 30 mg tid)
	  Pilocarpine (Salagen): approved for Sjogren syndrome, dry mouth from radiotherapy for head and neck cancer (start 5 mg po bid–tid; max 5 mg qid)
	  Physostigmine (generic IM, IV): is an inhibitor of anticholinesterase, 0.5–1 mg IV (img diluted in 10 mL of NS) given q 2 min or IM, may repeat q 30 min if severe sx persist or recur and no cholinergic sx; absorption of IM is erratic; have atropine available, use only with cardiac monitoring and life-support services available; only to treat the most serious sx of anticholinergic intoxication (seizures, severe hypotension, delirium)
	• **Contraindicated if**: hepatic dysfunction, CAD, uncontrolled asthma, narrow angle glaucoma, iritis, cardiac abnormalities
	• **Side effects**: sweating, diarrhea, drooling, nausea, changes in BP and pulse
	• **Drug interactions**: beta blockers (cardiac conduction problems)

TABLE 10.9. Serotonin Syndrome

Symptoms	Mild	Moderate	Severe
● CNS	● Confused, restless	● Agitated, somnolent, delirium	● Coma, seizures, death
● Autonomic	● Temp <38°C, mydriasis, diarrhea, ↑ HR	● Temp <39.5°C, BP low or high, mydriasis	● Temp >39.5°C, dyspnea, diaphoresis, ↑ HR, shock
● Neuromuscular	● Clonus, tremor, ataxia, akathisia, ↑ DTR	● Myoclonus, clonus, ataxia	● Muscle rigidity (rhabdomyolysis)

● Select causes; drug interactions with monoamine oxidase inhibitors (MAOIs), TCAs, SSRIs SNRIs, bupropion, nefazodone, trazodone, opioids (tramadol, fentanyl, pentazocine, buprenorphine, oxycodone, hydrocodone), CNS stimulants (amphetamine, sibutramine, methylphenidate, cocaine), 5-HT₁ agonists triptans, psychedelics (MDMA, MDA, 5-methoxy-diisopropyltryptamine, LSD), herbs St John's wort, Panax ginseng, Others (tryptophan, L-Dopa, valproate, buspirone lithium, risperidone, olanzapine, ritonavir). Compared to neuroleptic malignant syndrome, pts with serotonin syndrome have more rapid onset, more GI features (diarrhea, nausea), more hyperkinesis (myoclonus, ↑ DTR), and less muscle rigidity

● Treatment: Stop drug, transfer to MICU for medical support, manage complications (hyperthermia, rhabdomyolysis), and administer benzodiazepines. Some experts recommend cyproheptadine (Periactin: serotonin antagonist) 4–8 mg po q 8 hr (one author states that 30 mg is needed for efficacy). *Emergency Medicine Clinics of North America* (2007), *25*, 477.

Source: Reilly, T. H., & Kirk, M. A. (2007). Atypical antipsychotics and newer antidepressants. *Emergency Medicine Clinics of North America, 25,* 477–497.

TABLE 10.10. Cardiotoxicity of Selected Psychiatric Drugs

Agents	Effects

● Antidepressants	● TCAs: not to be given in cardiac pts
	  Slowing of conduction: ↑ QTc, QRS enlargement > 108 m, AV block
	  Arrhythmias
	  Orthostatic hypotension (α1-adrenergic blocking property)
	  ↑ heart rate (anticholinergic effect)
	● SSRIs: none (safer in cardiac patients)
	● Desyrel: rare ventricular ectopy and heart block
	● MAOIs: orthostatic hypotension

● Antipsychotics	● Orthostatic hypotension (α1-adrenergic blocking property) ● QTc prolongation: particularly with thioridazine, pimozide, ziprasidone to a lesser degree ● Chlorpromazine (Thorazine) has similar cardiac toxicity as TCAs ● Clozapine: cases of myocarditis (majority developing in first 2 months of rx, with 25% mortality, rate: 1/500–1/10,000) and cardiomyopathy (dilated cardiomyopathy mostly, usually pts <50 yo, 15% mortality)

Normal PR interval = 0.12–0.2 s; QRS duration = 0.04–0.1 s; **normal QTc = 350–440 ms.** (Caution if QTc 450–500; If > 500: high risk of torsade de pointes; risk ↑ if low K+, low Mg ++, polypharmacy with agents that prolong QTc, if long QT syndrome, CHF, recent MI.)

TOXICOLOGY

Contact local poison center for details concerning latest indications:

CONTACTS

● **Poison Help Number for nearest poison control center**: 1-800 (222-1222)
● **Phone numbers to identify HAZMAT (Hazardous Chemical Agents/Spills and Their Management)**: CDC? (ATSDR). 404-488-7100 & (CHEMTREC) 800-424-9300

TABLE 10.11. Heavy Metal Poisoning

● **Lead** (solder, ceramic glazes)	● Abdominal colic, lead neuropathy, lead encephalopathy (delirium, seizures, elevated BP, impaired memory and concentration, headache, tremors, deafness, transient aphasia, and hemianopia); possible vertigo, chronic headache, hyperesthesia for visual and auditory stimuli
● **Mercury**	● **Mad Hatter disease**: gastritis, bleeding gums, excessive salivation, coarse tremor, jerky movements, irritability, timid and shy, nervous, losing temper easily
● **Manganese** (in welding, dry batteries, workers involved in bleaching)	● Headache, asthenia, torpor, hypersomnia, impotence, uncontrollable laughter and crying, poor impulse control, late parkinsonism
● **Arsenic** (in fur, glass, insecticides industries)	● Chronic dermatitis, conjunctivitis, lacrimation, anorexia, headache, vertigo, apathy, intellectual impairment, peripheral neuropathy, amnesia, psychosis
● **Thallium** (in pesticides)	● Tingling, abdominal pain, vomiting, headache, tachycardia, offensive breath, alopecia, ataxia, paraesthesias, peripheral neuropathy, tremor, chorea, athetosis, myoclonic jerking, impaired consciousness, depression, seizures, delirium

TABLE 10.12.   General Approach to Poisoning

• Treat airway, breathing, and BP • Insert IV and apply cardiac monitor • Apply pulse oximeter, administer O$_2$	• Consider dextrose: 50 ml of D50, naloxone 2 mg IV, and thiamine 100 mg IV

TABLE 10.13.   Charcoal Administration

• Single-dose activated charcoal should not be administered routinely to poisoned patients (greatest benefit within the first hour of ingestion of a potentially toxic amount of a poison known to be absorbed by charcoal). Pt must have an intact or protected airway to administer charcoal
• Dose: initial dose: 25–100 g po or per NG mixed with cathartic such as sorbitol (70%): 1–2 g/kg po or NG
• Administer repeat charcoal doses q 3–4 hr (use cathartic only for 1st dose)

• Contraindications for charcoal (below)	• Drugs cleared by multidose charcoal (below)
• Unprotected airway • Corrosives, caustics (acids, alkalis) • Ileus, bowel obstruction • Drugs bound poorly by charcoal (arsenic, bromide, K+, toxic alcohols, heavy metals, iron, iodide, lithium)	• Chlorpropamide, dextropropoxyphene, diazepam, digoxin, nadolol, nonsteroidals, phenytoin, phenobarbital, salicylates, theophylline, tricyclic antidepressants

ACETAMINOPHEN TOXICITY

TABLE 10.14.   Acetaminophen Toxicity

Phase	Time after ingestion	Signs
1	30 min to 24 hr	Asymptomatic, or minor GI irritation
2	24–72 hr	Relatively asymptomatic, GI sx resolve, possible mild ↑ of LFTs or renal failure
3	72–96 hr	Hepatic necrosis (potential jaundice), hepatic encephalopathy, coagulopathy, and renal failure
4	4 days–2 wk	Resolution of sx or death

Acetaminophen overdose management: *ingestion of ≥140 mg/kg is potentially toxic*. Obtain acetaminophen level ≥4 hr after acute ingestion and plot on the Rumack-Matthews nomogram. A 4-hr level ≥140 µg/mL indicates need for *N*-acetylcysteine. On the nomogram, levels above the dotted line (…) indicate probable risk, whereas levels above the bottom solid line (–) indicate possible risk of toxicity. If time of ingestion is unknown, obtain level at time 0 and 4 hr later to calculate half-life. If half-life is >4 hr, administer antidote. NOTE +++: risk of hepatotoxicity when acetaminophen is used daily (max allowed 4 gm/d); risk ↑ if used as a supplement to other medicines containing it (such as Vicodin, Lortabs, Norco, and others).

TABLE 10.15.   Management of Acetaminophen Overdose

• Decontamination	• Charcoal is indicated only if toxic coingestants are present • Increase oral Mucomyst dose by 20% if charcoal given

• *N*-acetylcysteine (NAC)
  (Mucomyst)
  (Acetadote-IV formulation)
	• Assess toxicity based on nomogram
	• If drug level will return in <8 hr postingestion, treatment can be delayed until level known. NAC prevents 100% of toxicity if administered <8 hr from ingestion. If level will return >8 hr and ≥140 mg/kg ingested, administer first dose of Mucomyst. NAC is definitely useful ≤24 hr after ingestion and possibly up to 72 hr
	• Po dose: 140 mg/kg po, then 70 mg/kg q 4 hr × 17 doses. Shorter course (36 hr) may be effective if no liver toxicity at 36 hr. May dilute in cola to 5% solution. Contact poison center for short protocol specifics
	• IV dose: 150 mg/kg IV (in 200 mL D5W) over 4 hr, then 100 mg/kg (in 1,000 mL D5W) over 16 hr. Up to 18% develop anaphylactoid reaction (esp. if asthmatic or if prior NAC reaction). If this happens, discontinue and manage sx (e.g., antihistamines, epinephrine, inhaled β agonists, IV fluids). If sx stop and were mild, consider restarting NAC. Otherwise, do not restart. **Consult poison center for assistance with management (1-800-222-1222)**

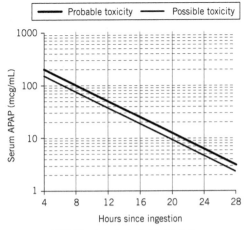

FIGURE 10.1.   Acetaminophen toxicity nomogram.

CLONIDINE TOXICITY

A CNS Clonidine: α-adrenergic agonist that $\downarrow$ BP and ameliorates opiate withdrawal; rapidly absorbed; $\downarrow$ BP within 30–60 min, peaking at 2–4 hr; half-life is 12 hr (6–24 hr): it $\downarrow$ BP at the presynaptic α2-agonist receptors $\rightarrow$ in $\downarrow$ sympathetic outflow. At high doses, it is a peripheral α-agonist + causes $\uparrow$ BP. It is also a depressant. When needs to be discontinued: taper off (if not: risk of rebound)

TABLE 10.16.   Clinical Features of Clonidine Toxicity

• CNS	• Lethargy, coma, recurrent apnea, miosis, hypotonia
• Cardiac	• Sinus bradycardia, hypertension (transient), later hypotension
• Other	• Hypothermia and palor

TABLE 10.17.   Treatment of Clonidine Overdose

• Monitor	• Apply cardiac monitor + pulse oximeter and observe closely for apnea. Apnea often responds to tactile stimulation
• Decontamination	• Charcoal ± gastric lavage. Avoid ipecac
• Atropine	• Indication: bradycardia. Dose: 0.5 mg IV
• Antihypertensives	• Hypertension is transient and usually no rx is required. If needed, use short-acting titratable agent (e.g., Nipride)
• Fluids/pressors	• Treat hypotension with fluids and dopamine prn
• Naloxone	• 2 mg IV may reverse CNS but not cardiac BP effects

COCAINE TOXICITY

See Chapter 20 for the effects of cocaine toxicity

Cocaine is the HCl salt of the alkaloi d extract of the Erythroxylon coca plant and is absorbed across all mucous membranes. It is a local anesthetic that blocks the reuptake of NE, DA, and serotonin.

TABLE 10.18.   Cocaine Absorption and Duration of Effects

Route	Peak effect	Duration
• Nasal	• 30 min	• 1–3 hr
• GI	• 90 min	• 3 hr
• IV/inhaled	• 1–2 min	• <30 min

TABLE 10.19.   Management of Cocaine Toxicity

● **General**	● Apply cardiac monitor, oxygen, and pulse oximeter; observe for arrhythmia, seizures, and hyperthermia ● Benzodiazepines: drugs of choice for agitation; Haldol is also effective (without ↑ cocaine seizure threshold)
● **Hyperthermia and rhabdomyolysis**	● Benzodiazepines to ↓ agitation and muscle activity. Cool with mist and fan. Continue rectal probe temperature. Check serum CK/CO_2. Administer IV fluids and bicarbonate to prevent renal failure
● **GI decontaminate**	● Body stuffers (rapid ingestion to hide drugs): charcoal and monitor for perforation/ischemia ● Body packers (hidden packets for transportation): X-ray and whole bowel irrigation. If rupture: laparotomy to remove cocaine
● **Cardiovascular** (arrhythmias and hypertension)	● Benzodiazepines for ↑ BP, ↑HR; follow standard ACLS protocols. Use sodium nitroprusside (Nipride) or phentolamine for severe HTN. In the past, experts have recommended avoiding β blockade (due to unopposed alpha effects) ● Limited studies suggest there may be a beneficial protective effect of β blockade. No current clear-cut recommendations (Dattilo et al., 2008)
● **Cardiovascular** (chest pain)	● Give benzodiazepines, aspirin, and IV NTG. Alternatively, phentolamine IV may reverse coronary vasoconstriction. PCI/PTCA is preferred over thrombolytics as CNS bleed/vasculitis/HTN ↑ risk of CNS bleed
● **Neurologic**	● Benzo for status epilepticus. Barbiturates are second line (phenytoin is not useful). Rx comorbidity (CT, glucose, electrolytes, R/O infection)

FLUNITRAZEPAM: ROHYPNOL "ROOFIES"

Benzodiazepine marketed outside of the United States for insomnia, sedation, and preanesthesia that is 10 times as potent as diazepam. It ↑ and prolongs the effects of heroin, methadone, alcohol, and ↓ the withdrawal of cocaine. It produces disinhibitions; used as a "date rape" drug.

TABLE 10.20.   Flunitrazepam (Rohypnol) Intoxication

● **Onset/duration**	● Maximal absorption is 0.5–1.5 hr with $T_{\frac{1}{2}}$ of nearly 12 hr
● **Major clinical effects**	● CNS: sedation, incoordination, hallucinations. Paradoxical excitement esp. with alcohol use. ↓ DTRs, mid to small pupils ● CV-Pulm: respiratory depression, hypotension. Aspiration
● **Management**	● Not routinely detected in urine benzodiazepine screen ● Lavage if <1 hr from ingestion, otherwise administer charcoal ● Protect airway and apply cardiac monitor, pulse oximeter ● Admit if lethargic or unstable after 2–4 hr of observation ● Routine use of flumazenil to reverse this drug's effects not recommended (possibility of seizures if current use of cyclic antidepressants, chronic benzodiazepine or flunitrazepam use, or underlying seizure disorder)

HALLUCINOGENS

see Chapter 20 for the sx of hallucinogens intoxication.

Include LSD (lysergic acid diethylamide), mescaline (peyote plant), psilocybin (mushrooms, esp. from cow pastures), morning glory seeds (similar to LSD), nutmeg, and toads (skin contains hallucinogenic bufotoxins).

NEUROLEPTICS

TABLE 10.21.   Neuroleptics OD Signs

● **Antiadrenergic**: ↓ BP, ↑ HR
● **Anticholinergic**: ↑ temp, dry, urine retention, ↑ pupils (phenothiazines may cause ↓ pupils), CNS and respiratory depression
● **Antidopaminergic**: dystonia, akathisia, motor disorders
● **Quinidine effect on heart** (↑ QT, ↑ PR, torsades). Low potency drugs (Thorazine, Serentil) have more anticholinergic/antiadrenergic effect, while high potency (butyrophenones, thioxanthenes) have more antidopamine effects. Thioridazine and mesoridazine have more quinidine-like cardiac effect

TABLE 10.22. Treatment of Neuroleptics Overdose

• Monitor	• Apply cardiac monitor + pulse oximeter and obtain ECG
• GI decontaminate	• Charcoal 1 g/kg po, consider lavage first if <1 hr since ingestion and potentially lethal overdose
• Hypotension	• NS IV, if unresponsive: use α-agonist (e.g., norepinephrine)
• Ventricular arrhythmias	• If wide QRS (SALT syndrome): IV NaHCO$_3$ 1–2 mEq/kg • Lidocaine or amiodarone • Magnesium 2–4 g IV over 15 min (if no renal insufficiency) • Avoid Class IA antiarrhythmics (e.g., procainamide)
• Medically admit	• If becomes symptomatic over 6 hr (e.g., ↓ BP, altered mental status, arrhythmia, ECG changes) • All Thioridazine or mesoridazine ingestions (delayed VF/VT)

PHENCYCLIDINE (PCP)

See Chapter 20 for the symptoms of PCP intoxication or withdrawal or treatment

Three stages of intoxication: (1) acute organic brain syndrome with violent behavior, (2) progressive stupor with intact pain response, and (3) deep coma.

SALICYLATES

Methylsalicylate (oil of wintergreen) is the most toxic form of salicylates. Absorption is within 1 hr of ingestion (absorption delayed ≥6 hr with enteric-coated and viscous preparations). At toxic levels, salicylates are renally metabolized. *Alkaline urine promotes excretion.* At different acidosis/alkalosis states, measurable salicylate levels change: need to measure arterial pH at the same time as drug level.

TABLE 10.23. Degree of Severity in Salicylates Overdose

Ingestion	Severity	Symptoms
• <150 mg/kg	• Mild	• Vomiting, tinnitus, and hyperpnea
• 150–300 mg/kg	• Moderate	• Vomiting, hyperpnea, diaphoresis, and tinnitus
• >300 mg/kg	• Severe	• Acidosis, altered mental status, seizures, shock

TABLE 10.24. Clinical Features of Salicylate Toxicity

• Direct	• GI irritation (reports of perforation)
• Metabolic	• Early: respiratory alkalosis from respiratory center stimulation • Later: metabolic acidosis (uncoupled oxidative phosphorylation) • Hypokalemia, ↑ or ↓ glucose, ketonuria, and either ↑ or ↓ Na+
• CNS	• Early: tinnitus, deafness, agitation, hyperactivity • Later: confusion, lethargy, coma, seizure, CNS edema
• GI	• Vomiting, gastritis, pylorospasm, ↑ liver enzymes, perforation
• Pulmonary	• Noncardiac pulmonary edema (esp. with chronic toxicity)

TABLE 10.25. Indicators of Salicylate Toxicity

• Clinical	• Features listed above are associated with toxicity
• Ingestion	• Ingestion of >150 mg/kg may be associated with toxicity
• Ferric chloride	• Mix 2 drops FeCl$_3$ + 1 mL of urine. Purple = salicylate ingestion but not salicylate toxicity
• Phenstix	• Dipstick test for urine. Brown indicates salicylate or phenothiazine ingestion (not toxicity). Adding 1 drop 20 NH$_3$SO$_4$ bleaches out color for phenothiazines but not salicylates
• Salicylate levels	• A level >30 mg/dL drawn ≥6 hr after ingestion is toxic. Clinical findings are more important than serum levels • Follow serial levels (q 2–3 hr) until downward trend established • Arterial pH must be measured at the same time as acidemia ↑ CNS penetration and toxicity at lower levels • Done nomogram has been proven unreliable
• Nontoxic ingestion	• If none of the following are present, acute toxicity is unlikely: (1) <150 mg/kg ingested, (2) absent clinical features, (3) level <30 mg/dL obtained ≥6 hr after ingestion (unless enteric-coated preparation, viscous preparation, or chronic ingestion)

TABLE 10.26.   Treatment of Acute Salicylate Toxicity

• General	• Rx dehydration, electrolyte abnormalities; CSF hypoglycemia occurs with normal serum glucose; add D5 or D10 to all fluids
• Decontaminate	• Multidose charcoal; whole bowel irrigation (if enteric-coated)
• Alkalinization	• Add 100–150 mEq NaHCO₃ to 1 L D5W (20–40 mEq/L K+ if no renal failure, since urine alkalinization often not possible until low K+ corrected). Infuse at 200 mL/hr. Goal: urine pH > 7.5
• Hemodialysis	• Indications: renal failure, noncardiogenic pulmonary edema, CHF, persistent CNS disturbances, ↓ BP, unable to correct acid–base or electrolyte imbalance, salicylate level >100 mg/dL

TABLE 10.27.   Treatment of Chronic Salicylate Toxicity

• Presentation	• Older, chronic users; altered CNS, noncardiogenic pulmonary edema, frequently misdiagnosed as infectious/neurodisease
• Drug levels	• Salicylate levels are often normal to therapeutic
• Treatment	• Supportive measures and urinary alkalinization. Dialyze if acidosis, confusion, or pulmonary edema even if nl level

SSRIs

TABLE 10.28.   SSRIs Overdose

• Signs	• OD relatively benign (morbidity due to coingestants). Common sx: ↑ HR, tremor, vomiting, drowsiness. ECG: ↑ HR, nonspecific ST-T changes. Seizures and cardiotoxicity (wide QRS/QTc) can occur at high levels (esp. fluoxetine); ↓ HR is seen with fluvoxamine at high or low doses
• Treatment	• Exclude coingestants • Observe for 6 hr; Nipride or phentolamine for HBP • Charcoal 1 g/kg • Sodium bicarbonate IV is useful if wide QRS, tachycardia • Observe for potentially lethal Serotonin syndrome (hyperthermia, myoclonus)

MAOIs

TABLE 10.29.   MAOI Overdose

• Signs	• OD: onset up to 12 hr later. Excess α + β adrenergic sx: headache, tremor, ↑ BP, ↑ DTR, rigidity, chest pain, ↑ Temp. • Later ↓ BP, ↓ HR, seizures
• Treatment	• Nipride or phentolamine for ↑ BP (no β blockers) • NS + Norepinephrine for ↓ BP • Charcoal • Benzodiazepines • Treat hyperthermia with aggressive cooling (see malignant hyperthermia management) • Treat rhabdomyolysis • Admit all intentional OD and all ingestions >2 mg/kg

OTHER ANTIDEPRESSANTS OVERDOSE

TABLE 10.30. Other Nontricyclic Antidepressants Overdose

● **SNRIs** (Effexor, Cymbalta)	● OD causes ↑ HR and ↓ level of consciousness, brief and limited seizures, and mild hypotension. Rx: supportive care, benzo. if seizures, saline and vasopressors for hypotension
● **NE and dopamine reuptake inhibitors** (Wellbutrin)	● OD causes lethargy (41%), tremors (24%), and seizures (21%). Mean onset of seizures is 3.7 hr: responds to benzodiazepines, phenytoin. One case report of prolonged QRS/QRc. Supportive rx
● **Noradrenergic and serotoninergic antidepressants** (Remeron)	● Mirtazapine inhibits presynaptic α2 receptors: ↑ serotonin and NE transmission. OD: rare sedation and drowsiness → rare intubation. No cardiac conduction effects or seizures noted to date
● **Serotonin-2-receptor antagonists** (Serzone, Desyrel)	● They block serotonin reuptake and inhibit serotonin 2 receptors. Nefazodone (Serzone) also blocks NE reuptake with minimal α1 receptor antagonism. Both (esp. Desyrel) cause sedation, GI upset, headaches. Desyrel: associated with nonsustained VT and other dysrhythmias. Rx for OD of either agent is supportive

SYMPATHOMIMETICS

TABLE 10.31. Sympathomimetics (Amphetamines and Derivatives)

● **Effects of amphetamines** are:
  1. Sympathomimetic: α & β adrenergic (mydriasis, ↑ HR, ↑ BP, ↑ temp, arrhythmia, MI, rhabdomyolysis, psychosis, CNS bleed, ↑ sweat, seizures)
  2. Dopaminergic: restlessness, anorexia, hyperactivity, movement disorders, paranoia
  3. Serotonergic: mood, impulse control, serotonin syndrome
● **Ice/crank (crystal methamphetamine):** one of the most commonly synthesized illicit drugs. Onset is in minutes, lasts 2–4 hr
● **MDMA-Ecstasy:** popular at "raves" and consumed orally. Low dose: euphoria, mild sympathomimetic sx last 4–6 hr. Potent serotonin releaser (no impulse control). High dose: effects (1–3) above in addition to hyponatremia
● **Treatment:**
  supportive care, cardiopulmonary, and neuro monitoring
  anticipate complications
  benzodiazepines for agitation
  Labetalol or Nipride: first line for ↑ BP. Some recommend phentolamine as first-line antihypertensive agent
  If ↓ BP: dopamine or norepinephrine
  Charcoal if oral ingestion
  Treat MI, dysrhythmias, hyperthermia, rhabdomyolysis

ETHANOL

See also Chapter 20 (Tables: 20.4 up to 20.14).

Ethanol (EtOH) ↑ serum osmolarity of 22 mOsm/L for every 100 mg/dL; mean elimination of ethanol is 20 mg/dL/hr (range 16–25). (Brennan et al., 1995).

Alcohol ketoacidosis: Ethanol binge in pt with ↓ caloric intake; ketoacids, β-hydroxybutyric acid (β-HB) and acetoacetate (AcA) ↑ in blood.

TRICYCLIC ANTIDEPRESSANTS (TCA)

TABLE 10.32.   Tricyclic Antidepressants (TCAs) Overdose

Clinical features in overdose of TCAs
• Are due: to α adrenergic block (↓ BP), anticholinergic effects (altered mentation, seizures, ↑ HR, mydriasis), inhabitation of NE uptake (↑ catecholamines), Na + channel blockade (quinidine like cardiac depression) • ECG findings in TCA overdose: ◦ Sinus tachycardia ◦ ↑ QRS > 100 ms*, ↑ PR interval, ↑ QT interval, BBB** (esp. right BBB) ◦ Right axis deviation of the terminal 40 ms of the QRS > 120° (prominent terminal R in AVR); ◦ AV conduction blocks (all degrees) ◦ Ventricular fibrillation or tachycardia 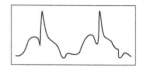 *ms= milliseconds; **BBB= bundle branch block

Treatment of TCA toxicity	
• General	• Cardiac monitor, baseline ECG with QRS width, QT interval
• Decontamination	• Administer charcoal 50 g po or NG q 2–4 hr. Consider lavage if <1 hr from ingestion (TCAs slow GI absorption) • Ensure pt airway and gag reflex prior to decontamination • Avoid ipecac as pts may have rapid mental status decline or seizures (do not use flumazenil)
• NaHCO₃	• Indications: ◦ acidosis ◦ QRS width >100 ms ◦ ventricular arrhythmias or ◦ hypotension ◦ Alkalinization enhances TCA protein binding and reverses Na+ channel blockade and toxic cardiac manifestations ◦ Dose: 1–2 mEq/kg IV. May repeat ◦ Goal: arterial pH of 7.50–7.55 ◦ NaHCO₃ is ineffective for CNS side effects (e.g., seizures)
• Fluids/pressors	• Administer 1–2 L NS for hypotension. Repeat 1–2× • If fluids ineffective, administer phenylephrine or NE (not dopamine) due to α-agonist effects
• Antiseizure medications	• Use lorazepam followed by phenobarbital if seizure • Phenytoin is ineffective in TCA-induced seizures
• MgSO₄	• 25 mg/kg IV (over 15 min) may be useful for cardiac toxicity
• Disposition	• Transfer to a psychiatric facility if all of the following are present: ◦ No major evidence of toxicity during 6 hr ED observation ◦ Active bowel sounds and ≥2 charcoal doses are given ◦ There is no evidence of toxic coingestant

THE VIOLENT PATIENT

- **Demography**: peaks in late teens + early 20s, M > F, lower social class, street violence, lower IQ
- **Epidemiology**: ↑ rate if: ↑ number of psych. diagnosis, substance abuse
- **Etiology**
  - Biologic (prefrontal cortex lesions, stimulation of amygdale + limbic system, ↑ androgens and CSF NE, or ↓ CSF serotonin and GABA)
  - Psychologic (impulsivity, ↓ frustration tolerance, inability to tolerate criticism, *x* antisocial acts, ego-centricity, entitlement, tends to dehumanize others, no introspection, first psychiatric hosp. <18)
  - Psychosocial (past phys. abuse, delinquency, prior arrests for assault, triad of enuresis + fire setting + cruelty to animals)
  - Cultural (living setting, access to weapons, probation, substance abuse)

- **Patterns**
  - Chronic (antisocial personality disorders, associated with drugs + alcohol abuse, onset in youth, delinquency, adult crime) or episodic (explosive rages with little provocation, daily to *x* times/yr, brief, sometimes amnesia and remorse)
  - Two types: **affective** (due to internal or external threat, intense activation of the autonomic system) and **predatory** (planned, purposeful, goal directed, not reactive, emotional detachment is the hallmark of a psychopathic character; very dangerous).
- **Mental disorders associated with violence**: (serious medical illness may also present with violent behavior)

TABLE 10.33. Mental Disorders Associated with Violence

● **Organic brain syndromes**: if confusion (delirium) or ↓ impulse control (dementia, drugs in the elderly, CNS infections, anoxia, metabolic disorders, ↓ glucose, brain damage, temporal lobe epilepsy, MS, poststroke, tumor)
● **Alcohol, drug abuse**: amphetamines, cocaine, PCP, inhalants, downers, anabolic steroids
● **Schizophrenia**, paranoid (more serious, more planned, access to weapons, more directed toward the "persecutor") and catatonic types. More if associated with command hallucinations, alcohol. Delusional disorders pose a danger to people incorporated in the delusional system (erotomanic, persecutory, jealous types)
● **Acute psychotic state** (if disorganized: less planned, less dangerous)
● **Mental retardation**: possibly Klinefelter syndrome or others
● **Severe ADHD**
● **Depression**: if despair (homicide prior to suicide)
● **Mania**: when limits are set, more assaults or threats than serious violence
● **PTSD**: ↑ with threatening hallucinations in flashbacks, irritability, substance abuse
● **Personality disorders**: paranoid, antisocial, borderline, histrionic
● **Intermittent explosive disorder**: paroxysmal explosive anger

- **Assessment of risk of future violence**:

TABLE 10.34. Assessment of Risk of Future Violence

● **Past violence**: assess pt's most violent act, frequency, reason, degree of injury, substance abuse, information (family, victim, and pt's legal + psychiatric records)
● **Patterns**: during psychosis, during interpersonal conflict, ego-dystonic vs ego-syntonic, remorse? Affective vs predatory, drugs or alcohol, weapons?
● **Prior history of**: x psychiatric admissions, escape from institution, problematic military hx or work hx, sexual aggression hx
● **Pt's characteristics** increasing the risks for violence:
○ Hx of past violence
○ Male gender
○ Adolescent or young adult
○ Intoxication
○ Low socioeconomic background
○ Low intelligence and limited education
○ Acute situation such as loss of job, loss of significant other
○ Labile mood and abusive language

- **Current assessment of dangerousness**: believe your subjective feelings of dangerousness +++

TABLE 10.35. Current Dangerousness

● **Ideas or threats of violence** have to be taken seriously
● **Assess risk factors**: mental disorders associated with violence
● **Assess mental state**: irritability, hostility? Agitation? Lack of empathy. Violent pts are often frightened pts. Is there any paranoia?
● **Detect discreet delusions** with nonbizarre content (difficult because of the plausible nature of the delusion and the reticence of the pt if paranoid) or appearing to be an overvalued idea in the context of anxiety or depression (assess reasoning process)
● **Assess any fixity of belief**, a tendency to jump to conclusions and misinterpret reality
● **Control of impulses and rage?** Any fear of losing control? Tension?
● **Is there an intended victim?** Any plan? Sadistic fantasies?
● **Weapon available?**
● **Lack of family support?**

- **Treatment**: hospitalization is appropriate when there is an imminent danger (involuntarily if necessary)
    - **Deescalation of violence**:

TABLE 10.36.   Tips and Verbal Interventions to Working with Violent Patients

Tips	Verbal interventions
• Be alert • Use intuition • Maintain optimal distance • Have available exits and a way to call for help • Keep environment free of objects that could be used as weapons • Make security staff available • Keep close light-weight objects that can be used as shields (cushion) • Think that a pt may carry a weapon • Establish a therapeutic alliance without expecting trust • Let the pt recount his theory and listen • Address any of the pt's fears • Separate thoughts and speech from actions: remind the pt of this • Understand the pt's sense of helplessness • Emphasize consequences of violence • Attend to all clinical concerns by finding solutions • Maintain a position of ethical integrity: be fair, consistent, and straightforward; honestly acknowledge one's mistakes; maintain a nonjudgmental attitude and respect • Consider prosecution if necessary	• Not if pt has lost control, is going off, or if altered mental status makes it impossible to cooperate: 　Keep calm voice, manner, and posture. Set clear limits 　No potential weapon available 　Easy access to the door for pt and therapist 　With or without a security present 　Offer food and drink. Be direct and reassuring 　Do not challenge, provoke, or openly disagree

- **Prn medications**: use lower doses and longer dosing intervals for the debilitated, elderly, youth, pts with liver problems. Be aware of SE.
    - **Neuroleptics**:
        - Haloperidol: 5–10 mg q 1–2 hr until calm, max 50 mg (↑ EPS). Can be given po/IM
        - Risperidone: 2 mg q 1–2 hr until calm, max 12 mg
        - Olanzapine: 10 mg q 1–2 hr until calm, max 40 mg
        - Chlorpromazine: 50–100 mg q 1–2 hr until calm, max 1,000 mg (↑ sedation, ↑ hypotension). Can be given po/IM
    - **Benzodiazepines**: Lorazepam: 2 mg IM q 1–2 hr until calm, max 12 mg (can be used if nonsevere liver impairment)
    - **Combination of a neuroleptic and lorazepam**: ↑ dosing interval to q 2–4 hr
        - **Seclusion, restraints**: if loss of control + pt not responding yet to prn medication. Seclusion might be sufficient in some cases to calm down. Restraints may ↑ agitation and cause hyperthermia. **Follow state laws and hospital regulations**. (See section Physical restraints above in this chapter.)
    - **Treat the underlying condition.**
        - **Symptomatic rx**: To ↓ violence: lithium, carbamazepine, divalproex, propanolol (160–600 mg/d; may take 4–6 wk for effect), SSRIs. Recognize early signs of internal tension; develop a support system (team work).
- **Duty to warn**: Tarasoff vs UC (1976): A legal duty to warn exists in every state of the United States, if there is a known intended victim; need to notify the possible victim and the police (jurisdictions of the pt and of the intended victim)
- **Develop a plan for the prevention of other episodes.**

THE SUICIDAL PATIENT

- **Organizations**:

Suicide Prevention Lifeline: 1-800-273-TALK; 1-800-273-8255, 24 hr a day, 7 days a week
Para obtener asistencia en espanol: 1-888-628-9454
TTY: 1-800-799–4TTY (1-800-799-4889)

- **Epidemiology**:
    - 30,000 reported suicides in the United States/yr; many are underreported (accidents?). Ninth leading cause of death.
    - 20 attempted suicides (3F : 1M), mostly overdoses, for one successful (3M : 1F), mostly shooting
    - One fifth is unanticipated. Most pts are not psychotic or incompetent.
    - US lifetime prevalence: suicidal ideations: 10%; suicidal attempts: 0.3%; completed suicide: 0.012%.
    - Two thirds of all suicide completers saw an MD, 1 month prior to killing themselves. 70% had a treatable psychiatric illness.
- **Evaluation**:

(1) **Identification of the potentially suicidal pts**:
    - Suicidal attempt: pts tend to minimize the attempt.
    - Talk or threat of suicide
    - Severe depression or anxiety
    - Recent loss (spouse, job, self-esteem)
    - Recent change in behavior (making a will, giving away possessions)
    - Recent change in demeanor (angry, cheerful, withdrawn)
    - Command hallucinations to kill self

(2) **Assess risk factors for completing suicide**:

TABLE 10.37.   Risk Factors for Completing Suicide

- >45 yr (↑ if >60 yr), M > F
- White > blacks, ↑ in Native Americans, Protestant > Catholic or Jewish
- Depression, alcoholism, poor, recent losses, no social ties, hopelessness
- Lethality of intended method, low probability of rescue
- Prior attempts within 2 yr

(3) **Assess in all suicidal pts**: intention (**why**), plan (**how**), method (**with what** weapon, lethality, access), **psychiatric or organic factors** (psychotic depression, thought disorder, organicity, self-medication), **losses** (loneliness, no support system), **level of intent** to commit suicide (hopelessness, unbearable psychologic pain), **frequency of suicidal thoughts** (how often), what prevents the pt from killing self (**why not**), ask if they tried before but didn't succeed, why not, and how many times, ask what the pt thinks will happen after his or her death. Assess the pt's judgment, level of impulse control, motivation for help, coping skills, resilience to stress.

TABLE 10.38.   Individual Risks Factors of Suicide

Individual risk factors	Comments
• **Internal negative feelings**	• Hopelessness, helplessness, extreme fatigue, delusions of sin, nihilistic delusions, anhedonia, insomnia
• **Psychiatric illness**	• **Major mood disorder** (50% of all suicides). Risk ↑ when pt starts to recover from depression due to ↑ energy • **Schizophrenia** (when chronic, lonely, with persecutory delusions, command hallucinations,↑ in younger pts and in pts in partial remission due to realization of inability to attain life goals) • **Psychoses** due to organic conditions, mixed bipolar disorders. Assess reality testing • **Personality disorders** (borderline, antisocial): 7× more suicide than in nl population • **Anorexia nervosa** • **Akathisia** due to psychotropic medications
• **Failing health**	• If previously independent (5% of all suicides), pts on dialysis, cancer, AIDS, MS, chronic complex partial seizures, chronic pain, Huntington disease, peptic ulcer disease, chronic obstructive pulmonary disease
• **Substance abuse**	• Intoxication, active use: • Alcoholism (25% of all suicides): ↑ if chronic, men, depression, poor social support • Drug addiction (10% die by suicide), ↑ with PCP, LSD
• **Prior hx of suicidal attempts**	• Particularly serious attempts, access to lethal weapon
• **Family hx of suicide**	• Genetics? Personal exposure to suicide
• **Lack of support**	• Single, widowed, separated, divorced, unemployed, retired
• **Family stress**	• Financial, conflicts, separations, losses, rejections, holidays, anniversaries, death of a loved one

TABLE 10.39.   Protective Factors Against Suicide

- Social ties (spouse, children, friends), religious affiliation
- Hope for the future
- Low lethality of the intended method (OD on vitamins vs shooting), probability of rescue (attempt in front of people)
- Positive coping or problem-solving skills
- Good pt–therapist relationship

- **Treatment**:
  - (1) **High risk**: **hospitalize pt (if necessary involuntarily)** in a locked ward. **"Better safe than sorry."** Communicate the decision to hospitalize decisively. Remove any dangerous items; put on close observation or 1 : 1 observation. Check on proper administration and swallowing of medications.
  - (2) **Low risk**: outpatient rx may be done but ↑ frequency of visits and ensure supervision at home. Make sure of no access to fire arms, potentially lethal medication. Limit the number of dispensed pills. Give instructions to pt and family if an emergency arises. Families must be an integral part of rx planning. Be careful about the no-suicide contracts and use your best judgment. Treat the underlying illness (depression, substance abuse, individual, family rx).
  - (3) **Make a crisis plan**

TABLE 10.40.   Crisis Plan to Prevent Suicide

• **Address risk factors**	• Relapse of mental illness, discontinuation of medications, noncompliance with rx, loss, alcohol or substance abuse relapse
• **Prepare for a crisis**	• Involve pt, family, treating team; build a therapeutic alliance; manage any countertransference issue
• **Help with access to emergency services**	• Give addresses, phone numbers
• **Communicate with rx systems and families**	• Assess the patient's ability to collaborate with care givers; educate involved member; do not rely on safety or suicide contracts only; get professional second opinions
• **Identify rx needs**	• Plan for follow-up appointments; reassess suicidal risks regularly, in particular at high-risk points (admission, discontinuation of 1:1 observation, any psychologic change, weekend passes, discharge, termination of rx)
• **Address medication safety**	• Provide only a limited and safe amount
• **Address safety of the environment**	• Removal of all firearms and ammunitions

Adapted from Jayaram, G., & Herzog, A. (2008). SAFE MD: Practical applications and approaches to safe psychiatric practice committee on patient safety. American Psychiatric Association. Approved by the Council on Quality Care and The Joint Reference Committee. Retrieved October 27, 2010 from: http://psych.org/Departments/QIPS/Downloads/SAFEMD.aspx

- **Medicolegal concerns**:
  - (1) No standards for the prediction of suicide
  - (2) Standard of care for suicidal patients is based on the concept of **"foreseeability"** (ability to take a thorough hx, to recognize relevant risk factors, to implement a rx plan that provides precautions against suicide, consideration of the benefits of exerting greater control over the pt (e.g., hospitalization, calling the family).
  - (3) If suicide occurs: seek support from colleagues. Consult with an attorney or a risk manager. Pt's confidentiality extends beyond the pt's death and this applies to medical records. If something needs to be added to the medical record, date it properly. Do not change anything in the medical record. Conversations with family members may be appropriate.

- **Nonsuicidal self-injury**:
  - (1) Are very common, ⅓–½ of the adolescent population in the United States
  - (2) Includes cutting or burning oneself without suicidal intent, hitting, pinching, banging, or punching walls or other objects to induce pain, breaking bones, ingesting toxic substances, interfering with healing wounds; report of feeling minimal or no pain; behavior may acquire addictive characteristics
  - (3) Frequently occurring in pts who at other times had suicidal thoughts or attempts (risk of suicide or suicide attempt)
  - (4) Association with developmental disabilities, eating disorders, borderline personality disorders, other psychiatric conditions (MDD, PTSD, GAD, CD, ODD, substance abuse disorders, past abuse); also associated with high emotional reactivity, hyperarousal, Goth subculture, self-harm in peers/contagion effect

    (5) Under standing the functions of the behavior: affect regulation (anxiety, anger, frustration, depression), change of cognitions (distraction from problems, stopping suicidal thoughts), self-punishment, stop dissociation, interpersonal situation (attention seeking, peer group)

    (6) Assessment: complete a full medical and psychiatric evaluation (comorbid psychiatric illness, suicide risk, hx of sexual and physical abuse, substance abuse, risk factors, family and social supports), functional behavioral analysis (antecedents/situations, stressors leading to self-harm, frequency, duration, intensity of the behaviors, consequences/emotional relief, attention from others).

    (7) Treatment: develop a therapeutic alliance, treat primary psychiatric disorders, target behavioral interventions for the behavior (affective language skills, self-soothing skills, communication skills), provide psychoeducation for the pt and the family, initiate cognitive problem-solving skills rx and monitor response of the behavioral rx, consider family rx and DBT.

- **Suggested readings**:
  - APA practice guidelines : Assessment and treatment of patients with suicidal behaviors, http://www.psychiatryonline.com/pracGuide/pracGuideTopic_14.aspx

RAPE

National Organizations::

    RAINN or Rape, Abuse and Incest National Network: http://www.rainn.org/

    National Sexual Assault Hotline: 1-800-656-HOPE (4673). Or 202-544-3064 (RAINN business office)

    Violence Against Women: http://womenshealth.gov/violence/

    National Domestic Violence Hotline: 1-800-799-SAFE (7233) or TTY 1-800-787-3224

    The National Center for Victims of Crime: http://www.ncvc.org/ncvc/Main.aspx: (1-800-394-2255); TTY: 1-800-211-7996. Has information about stalking

    National Sexual Violence Resource Center: http://www.nsvrc.org/contact/nsvrc

    The National Teen Dating Abuse Hotline number: 1-866-331-9474

Epidemiology: affects adults, children, $\female$ + $\male$; associated with depression, generalized phobic anxiety, and PTSD. False allegations of rape and sexual assault are rare. W : M is 1/6 : 1/33; frequent underreporting and secondary or sanctuary victimization of the survivor.

Risks: Most victims do not develop mental illness following rape, but may experience difficulties. Some will develop PTSD. The persistence of rape-related PTSD >3 months postassault predicts a long-term disorder. Risk for chronic PTSD for: those who were injured during the attack or were threatened by the perpetrator (of being hurt or killed), have hx of prior assault, or have experienced negative interactions with family, peers, or law enforcement systems.

Acute intervention: Need for specially trained forensic nurses providing 24 hr/d, first-response medical care and crisis intervention to rape survivors in hospitals or clinic settings; will provide:

- Sensitive crisis intervention; referral for ongoing counseling and support must be made available. Rx is client-centered, time-limited rx: providing psychoeducation; give time to consolidate memories of the assault and to ventilate the survivor's distress (**Rape is never the victim's fault. It's the perp's fault.**)

- Comprehensive, consistent **postrape medical care** (e.g., emergency contraception, sexually transmitted disease [STD], prophylaxis)

- Documenting the **forensic evidence** of the crime completely and accurately

- Improving the prosecution of sexual assault cases by providing better forensics and expert testimony

- Creating community change by bringing multiple service providers together to provide **comprehensive care** to rape survivors.

Multimodal approach to treat rape survivors: includes: psychoeducation, psychotherapy (supportive, behavioral, group, family), support groups. Rx considerations: sociocultural influences on a person's response to rape, the hx of victimization, the specific nature of the assault, and the experiences with victim-blame.

Possible psychiatric findings in child victims of rape:

- **In children who are preverbal**: sexualized behaviors, screaming attacks, clinging to a carer, acute stranger anxiety, nightmares, bed wetting, soiling, and possible eating disturbances

- **Age 5–12 yr**: may be able to describe the event verbally or through play with toys or dolls, or by drawing the incident; frequent psychosomatic problems (recurrent abdominal pain, ↑ asthma, enuresis, soiling, dysphagia (if forced oral rape), constipation and anal retention (if anal rape), dysuria.

ABUSE (SEE CHAPTER 27)

Child abuse hotlines: Where to call to get help or report abuse

- If you suspect a child is in immediate danger, contact law enforcement as soon as possible: 911
- **To get help in the U**nited States, **call**:
- Child Help National Child Abuse Hotline **1-800-4-A-CHILD (1-800-422-4453)**
- To get help for child sexual abuse, call: 1-888-PREVENT (1-888-773-8368)—Stop It Now
- Rape, Abuse & Incest National Network (RAINN), 1-800-656-HOPE

Department of Social Services: NYS: 1-800-342-3720

National Coalition Against Domestic Violence: http://www.ncadv.org/resources/StateCoalitionList_73.ht

Domestic Violence Hotline number: in English: 1-800-942-6906; in Spanish: 1-800-942-6908

The National Domestic Violence Hotline number: 1-800-799-7233

The National sexual Assault Hotline number: 1-800-656-4673

The National Teen Dating Abuse Hotline number: 1-866-331-9474

11 ■ ANXIETY DISORDERS

National organization: Anxiety Disorders Association of America: www.adaa.org

Scales for anxiety disorders: Anxiety States Inventory, Fear Questionnaire, Social Avoidance and Distress Scale, Leyton Obsessional Inventory, Hamilton Anxiety Rating Scale, Yale-Brown Obsessive-Compulsive Scale.

GENERALITIES

- **Anxiety**: unpleasant, unjustified sense of apprehension with or without physiologic sx. It **is an alerting signal**.
- **Anxiety disorder**: possibly only anxiety may be present, or with other sx like phobia + obsessions (anxiety may be seen only when the other sx are opposed). The sx are ego-alien or ego-dystonic (feeling unnatural or alien); significant distress and dysfunction are due to the anxiety.
- **Fear** is universal and a response to an obvious cause.
- **Biology**:
  - Neurotransmitters:
    - **NE** (poor regulation, bursts of activity)/**locus ceruleus**, cerebral cortex, limbic system, brainstem, and spinal cord are involved; α_2-adrenergic receptor antagonists (yohimbine) and β-adrenergic receptor agonists (isoproterenol) produce anxiety; α_2-receptor agonist (clonidine) relieves anxiety.
    - **Serotonin**/raphe nuclei in the brainstem, cerebral cortex, limbic system (amygdale, hippocampus), and hypothalamus; SSRI ↓ anxiety; serotonin 5-HT1A receptor agonist (buspirone) ↓ anxiety
    - **GABA** (γ-aminobutyric acid): benzodiazepines ↑ activity of GABA and ↓ anxiety
    - Genetic: partially (variation in the gene for the serotonin transporter?)
- **Neuroanatomy**:
  - Brain imaging: ↑ size of cerebral cortex? Cerebral asymmetries, abnormal frontal, occipital, and temporal areas; **caudate nucleus in OCD**; asymmetric metabolism in the **parahippocampal gyri**
  - **Limbic system** receives noradrenergic and serotonergic innervation and has a high conc. of GABA A receptors
  - The **frontal cerebral cortex and the temporal cortex** are implicated (some clinical similarities between temporal lobe epilepsy and OCD)
- **Peripheral manifestations of anxiety**: *GI* (upset stomach, diarrhea), *cardiologic* (palpitations, tachycardia, hypertension, syncope, dizziness), *neurologic* (hyperreflexia, tremors, restlessness), *sweating, urinary frequency, pupillary mydriasis, respiratory* (tachypnea)

PANIC DISORDERS AND AGORAPHOBIA

- **Definitions**:
  - **Panic disorder**: dramatic, acute sx that define panic attacks (peak in less than 10 min), lasting minutes to hours, self-limited. The **first panic attack is spontaneous**. May be multiple in 1 day or a few per year; may occur on pts with or without chronic anxiety. The mixture of sx lasts >1 month. Sx are similar to an intense autonomic discharge (chest pain, heart pounding, tremor, abdominal pain, dizziness, confusion, depersonalization, sense of impending doom and death, and an urge to escape). Sx may disappear quickly or gradually, leaving the pt drained. Can become chronic. One third of cases have also agoraphobia. In few pts, panic attacks may happen at night during NREM sleep.
  - **Agoraphobia**: fears of open and/or closed spaces (trains, airplanes, elevators, tunnels), unfamiliar or crowded places, of being alone; avoidance of being in such spaces without a companion; refusal to leave the house. Often complicates a panic disorder. May exist without panic attacks.
- **Epidemiology**: lifetime prevalence: 1–5%; F : M is 2–4 : 1, mean age of onset: 20 yr, recent hx of divorce, separation; exists in children, adolescents
- **Etiology**: familial, agents provoking panic attacks: lactate infusion, inhalation of 5% CO_2, cholecystokinin, isoproterenol, flumazenil (benzodiazepine antagonist)
- **Comorbidity**: most have ≥1 other psychologic disorders (depression with ↑ risk of suicide, specific phobias, PTSD, separation anxiety disorder, OCD, hypochondriasis, substance abuse, personality disorders).

No evidence cause and effect with mitral valve prolapse. Panic disorders may be with or without agora-phobia. Agoraphobia may exist without panic disorder.

- **Differential diagnosis**:
  - (1) **Medical disorders**:
    - Need for complete medical hx and physical exam, CBC, electrolytes, fasting glucose, Ca, liver function, urea, creatinine and thyroid, U/A, drug screen, ECG. If normal, suspect a panic disorder. If atypical sx (loss of bladder control, loss of consciousness) or late onset (>45 yo), reconsider a medical condition. If cardiac sx exist in a pt with cardiac risk factors: pursue tests (24-hr ECG, stress test, chest X-ray, cardiac enzymes)
    - Panic disorders **can mimic multiple medical diagnosis**:

TABLE 11.1.   Medical Diagnosis Mimicking Panic Disorders

Types of medical disorders	Examples
● **Cardiovascular diseases**	● Anemia, angina, congestive heart failure, hypertension, mitral valve prolapse, arrhythmias
● **Pulmonary diseases**	● Asthma, pulmonary embolus, hyperventilation
● **Neurologic diseases**	● Epilepsy, tumors, cerebrovascular diseases, infections, MS, migraines, Meniere disease, Parkinson disease
● **Endocrine diseases**	● Diabetes, hypoglycemia, pheochromocytoma, hyper- or hypothyroidism, Cushing syndrome, menopause, carcinoid syndrome, Addison disease
● **Drug intoxications**	● Amphetamine, cocaine, hallucinogens, marijuana, caffeine, nicotine, theophylline, anticholinergics, PCP
● **Drug withdrawal**	● Alcohol, opiates, sedatives, antihypertensives
● **Others**	● Electrolytes disturbances, anaphylaxis, infections, temporal arteritis, uremia, acute intermittent porphyria

  - (2) **Mental illnesses**:
    - **Unexpected panic attacks and nonfocused anxiety are the hallmark of panic disorders**. Situational panic attacks may indicate a social phobia, a specific phobia, OCD, major depression.
    - Eliminate: malingering, factitious disorders, hypochondriasis, depersonalization disorders, PTSD, depressive disorders, specific phobias, and schizophrenia.
- **Course**:
  - **Panic disorder**: onset in late adolescence, early adulthood. Can be chronic. 30–40% become sx free, 50% have mild sx, and 10–20% have severe sx later on. Frequency, severity of the attacks may vary. Caffeine and nicotine ↑ sx. Depression exists in 40–80% of the pts (↑ risk of suicide). Substance abuse, alcohol abuse in 20–40% of cases
  - **Agoraphobia**: if + panic disorder: rx of the panic disorder will improve agoraphobia. If alone: often becomes chronic
- **Treatment**: chronic (>8–12 months); 30–90% of pts relapse at discontinuation. CBT can prevent attacks, may be used with medications. Relaxation techniques, in vivo exposure, respiratory training, family rx, insight-oriented therapy, alone or in combination may be useful
  - **Antidepressants**: start at a low dose to avoid ↑ in attacks, ↑ slowly. It may require a full antidepres-sant dose. Wait 6 wk for full result: (starting dose in mg [S], maintenance dose in mg/d [M]).
    - SSRI like fluoxetine (S: 2–5, M: 20–60) may be activating; paroxetine (S: 5–10, M: 20–60) has sedative effects; sertraline (S: 12.5–25, M: 50–200); fluvoxamine (S: 12.5, M: 100–150); citalo-pram (S: 10, M: 20–40); escitalopram (S: 5, M: 10–20)
    - Tricyclics like nortriptyline (S: 5–25, M: 150–200); desipramine (S: 5–25, M: 150–200); imipramine (S: 5–25, M: 150–200); clomipramine (S: 12.5, M: 50–200)
    - MAOIs like phenelzine (S: 15, M: 30–90), with need for dietary restrictions +++
  - **Benzodiazepines**: alprazolam (S: 0.25 tid, M: 0.5–2 tid); clonazepam (S: 0.25 bid, M: 0.5–2 bid). May be titrated up in 1 wk. If rx is >6 wk: risk for withdrawal; will need to be tapered down very slowly (>10 wk). Can be used as a first agent (rapidity of action), or while the antidepressant becomes effective. *Alprazolam dependence is difficult to overcome +++.*
  - **Anticonvulsants**: Divalproex (S: 125 bid, M: 500–750 bid). May help in resistant cases for anxiety and mood instability
- **Treatment resistance**:
  - Check comorbid disorders
  - Switch from one class of drugs to another

- Use a combination like: SSRI + Benzo or Tricyclic + Benzo or SSRI + Lithium or SSRI + Tricyclic
- Nefazodone and venlafaxine have been used
- Other anticonvulsants: carbamazepine
- Augment with buspirone

SPECIFIC PHOBIA (SIMPLE PHOBIA)

- **Definition**: excessive, irrational fear of a specific object, situation; strong, persistent, with conscious avoidance of it, distress in its presence or in thinking of it, with anticipation of being harmed (being bitten by a dog, losing control, being stuck in an elevator, fear of blood, spiders, storms, heights)
- **Epidemiology**: 5–10% of population. Lifetime prevalence: 11%. F : M is 2 : 1. Peak age is 5–9 yr for the fear of injury type vs mid-20s for the situational type.
- **Comorbidity**: other anxiety disorders, mood disorders, substance abuse
- **Etiology**: Association between a specific object or situation with the emotions of fear and panic, modeling (learning theories), psychoanalytic factors (phobia or "anxiety hysteria" from unresolved childhood oedipal situation → fear of castration → defense mechanisms like displacement, projection onto an object or situation → signal anxiety → object to avoid). Runs in families.
- **Diagnostic**: The fear is excessive, irrational. The exposure to the phobic stimulus provokes an immediate anxiety response that could become a panic attack. The stimulus needs to be avoided. If pts <18 yr, the duration is >6 months.
- **Types**: animals (fear of animals: zoophobia; of dogs: cynophobia; of cats: ailurophobia), natural environment (fear of heights: acrophobia; of water: hydrophobia), situational types (fear of open places: agoraphobia; of closed spaces: claustrophobia; of strangers: xenophobia), blood, injection, injury, other types (fear of dirt and germs: mysophobia; of fire: pyrophobia)
- **Differential diagnosis**: hypochondriasis (fear of having a disease vs fear of contracting one in phobia), OCD, paranoid personality disorder (more generalized fears)
- **Course and prognosis**: most specific phobias start in childhood and persist for many years. Early onset phobias tend to remit in adulthood, in opposite to adult-onset ones. Severity seems constant.
- **Complications**: minimal if phobic object can be avoided. If not, may be disabling.
- **Treatment**: Behavior rx (mostly systematic desensitization) is done in a gradual way, with intensive exposure (flooding) through imagery or in vivo. Exposure therapy is the most used. Insight-oriented psychotherapy is rarely used now. Hypnosis, supportive rx, family rx may be useful. Pharmacotherapy (benzodiazepines) may be needed.

SOCIAL PHOBIA/SOCIAL ANXIETY DISORDER

- **Definition**: A marked and persistent fear of a social or performance situation that will be avoided (fear of humiliation), even though it is recognized as being an excessive fear. Exposure to the situation provokes intense anxiety interfering with the pt's normal life. If <18 yr, the duration is >6 months.
- **Epidemiology**: Lifetime prevalence: 3–13%. F : M is 3 : 2. Peak age: teens
- **Comorbidity**: other anxiety disorders, mood disorders, substance abuse, bulimia nervosa
- **Etiology**:
    - Familial: biologic trait (pattern of behavioral inhibition)?
    - Psychologic situation: some parents being more rejecting, overprotective, less caring?
    - Neurochemical hypotheses: adrenergic theory (performance phobias with ↑ release of epinephrine and NE) and dopamine theory (↓ homovanillic acid concentration, ↓ striatal dopamine reuptake site density)
- **Types**: Circumscribed social phobia: one or more social or performance situation involved (public or private) or generalized social phobia (includes most social situations)
- **Differential diagnosis**:
    - Major depression: other signs of depression
    - Schizoid, schizotypal personality disorder: isolation with little interest in social contacts
    - Avoidant personality disorder: may be a form of generalized social phobia
    - Body dysmorphic disorder: the source of embarrassment is the imaginary disfigurement
    - Agoraphobia: fear of leaving home vs fear of encountering a social situation

Treatment:

- Circumscribed social phobia:
  - Psychotherapy: desensitization
  - Pharmacotherapy:
    - See pharmacologic rx of simple phobias.
    - Phobia associated with performance situation (speaking, writing, eating, performing in public): β-adrenergic receptor antagonists (atenolol: 50–100 mg q AM or 1 hr before the performance; propanolol: 20–60 mg taken 2 hr before)
- Generalized social phobia:
  - CBT: less effective than medications
  - See pharmacologic rx of simple phobias. SSRIs (escitalopram, paroxetine, sertraline), as both the first-line and longer term tx; SNRIs (venlafaxine); β-adrenergic receptor antagonists (propanolol, atenolol); Benzodiazepines as short-term adjuncts; Gabapentin is also effective (daily doses of ≤2,400 mg; efficacy varies among the anxiety disorders: social anxiety disorders respond better to gabapentin than panic disorders)

OBSESSIVE-COMPULSIVE DISORDER

- **National organization**: **Obsessive-Compulsive Foundation**: www.ocfoundation.org
- **Epidemiology**: Lifetime prevalence: 2–3%. M : F is 1 : 1. Fourth most common after phobias, substance abuse, and depression. Onset ~20 yr up to late 30s; onset is earlier in boys. Two thirds of pts have onset at age <25; singles > married; whites > blacks
- **Etiology**:
  - *Genetic*: high concordance rate for monozygotic twins; a high percentage of first-degree relatives of OCD pts are afflicted; Tourette disorder and OCD may have some communality of genes involved.
  - *Anatomy*: **head of the caudate and the orbito-frontal cortex**
  - *Biology*: serotonergic system (serotonergic drugs are effective). Noradrenergic system (clonidine which ↓ the quantity of NE released may be helpful)
  - *Neuroimmunology*: PANDAS/ OCD seen as a sequela to Sydenham chorea (after β-hemolytic streptococcal infection)
- **Definition**: Recurrence of obsessions and/or compulsions that provoke severe distress (ego-alien), are time consuming (>1 hr/d), interfere with the pt's nl activities and relationships. Pts usually recognize them as being excessive, unreasonable, with a strong desire to resist them. They are not due to a substance or a medical condition. Insight in the condition may be present or not:
  - **Obsessions**: unwanted, intrusive, recurrent, inappropriate thoughts, impulses, images. The pt tries to suppress them with another thought or action. They are recognized as the product of the pt's own mind. (Fear of contamination by feces, urine, dust, germs; pathologic doubt such as about having turned off the oven; somatic, need for symmetry, aggressive; may be sexual, religious)
  - **Compulsions**: overwhelming, irresistible urges to engage in repetitive activities or mental acts that the pt recognizes as purposeless; done without pleasure and used to prevent distress or a dreaded event; may be observable (checking, washing, counting out loud, need to ask or confess, need for symmetry, hoarding) or be a private event (counting, praying). Trichotillomania (compulsive hair pulling), nail biting may be related.
- **Comorbidity**: depression, other anxiety disorders, Tourette disorder
- **Differential diagnosis**:
  - Medical conditions: neurologic disorders (trauma, status post encephalitis, temporal lobe epilepsy, focal lesions in basal ganglia or right parietal lobe, simple partial seizure), medications (clozapine, risperidone, olanzapine)
  - Other psychiatric disorders: schizophrenia (presence of more bizarre psychotic signs, no insight), obsessive-compulsive personality disorder (less impairment, no distress), phobias, depressive disorders (no OCD sx usually)
  - Related disorders: hypochondriasis, body dysmorphic disorder, kleptomania, pathologic gambling, compulsive sexual behavior), trichotillomania (compulsive hair pulling), nail biting
- **Course and prognosis**: mostly chronic with waxing and waning intensity.
- **Treatment**:
  - Behavior rx is the rx of choice (may be used alone if pt refuses medications): *exposure and response prevention* (more effective for compulsions than obsessions). Insight-oriented psychotherapy, supportive rx, family, group rx may be useful.

- Medications:
  - Start with an SSRI or clomipramine and move to other drugs if not effective.
  - Higher dosages than for depression are usually necessary. FDA-approved drugs for OCD are: fluoxetine (up to 40–60 mg/d), fluvoxamine (up to 100–300 mg/d), paroxetine (up to 60 mg/d), and sertraline (up to 50–200 mg/d). Non FDA-approved drugs are: citalopram (up to 10–40 mg/d), escitalopram (up to 5–20 mg). Most pts tolerate an SSRI better than clomipramine.
  - Clomipramine (150–300 mg/d) must be titrated over 2–3 wk to prevent SE (GI, orthostatic hypotension, sedation, anticholinergic effects), is dangerous in OD (give minimal amount at one time)
  - Other drugs if unsuccessful:
    - Augmentation with valproate, lithium, carbamazepine, or an antipsychotic (risperidone: 2–3 mg/d, or if a hx of tics, may use haloperidol: 5 mg/d)
    - Venlafaxine: start 37.5–75 mg po/d (XR), increase by 75 mg/d q wk up to 225 mg/d
    - Phenelzine (caution with the diet used in MAOI treatment)
  - Best outcome is with a combination of drug + behavior rx.

POSTTRAUMATIC STRESS DISORDER

- **Epidemiology**: 8% of gl population. Lifetime prevalence F : M is 10–12% : 5–6%. M (mostly combat experience); F (mostly assault, rape). In families with depression, ↑ risk of pt developing PTSD after trauma; more in singles, isolated, low socioeconomic groups.
- **Etiology**:
  - **Stressor**: not sufficient alone
  - **Risk factors**: extreme trauma, childhood trauma, personality disorders (borderline, dependent, antisocial, paranoid), no support system, alcoholism, genetic vulnerability, recent life change, subjective meaning of the stressor, poor coping skills, alexithymia (inability to identify, verbalize feeling states)
  - **Cognitive-behavioral factors**: (1) trauma (unconditioned stimulus) → fear that becomes paired with physical or mental reminder (conditioned stimulus) of the trauma (sights, smells, sounds); (2) the conditioned stimulus alone → fear; (3) pattern of avoiding conditioned + unconditioned stimuli
  - **Biology**:
    - Hyperactivity of the noradrenergic system: ↑ 24-hr urine conc. of epinephrine in veterans with PTSD, platelet α_2- and lymphocyte β-adrenergic receptors are down-regulated in PTSD
    - Hyperactivity of endogenous opiate system: low plasma β-endorphin conc. in PTSD; trials with naloxone (Narcan) and nalmefene (Revex)
    - HPA axis dysfunction: ↓ plasma and urinary free cortisol conc. in PTSD; Dexamethasone suppression test → cortisol ↓↓ in trauma-exposed pts with PTSD, compared to cortisol ↓ in trauma-exposed pts without PTSD. Possible role of hippocampus (↓ volume)
- **Definition**: Exposure to an extreme traumatic event, provoking intense fear with reexperiences of it in intrusive, repetitive ways (images, thoughts, flashback episodes, nightmares), presence of dissociative sx (numbness, loss of interest in surroundings, derealization, depersonalization, amnesia, feeling dead inside). Onset: immediate or delayed (>6 months or years post trauma). Avoidance of stimuli bringing memory of the trauma, ↑ arousal and anxiety (insomnia, irritability, lability, ↓ concentration, hypervigilance, ↑ startle response. Severe impairment in the pt's life. The duration of the **sx must be >1 month** (if <1 month: it is acute stress disorder).
- **Course**:
  - **Acute PTSD lasts <3 months and chronic is >3 months.**
  - Untreated: 30% recover completely, 50% will recover after 1 yr
  - Good prognosis: rapid onset, sx <6 months, good premorbid function, no other pathology, social support
  - Young children, elderly: more difficulties (often underestimated), comorbidity makes it worse
  - High risk of aggression, violence, depression, substance abuse
  - Particular areas: Gulf War syndrome (possible exposure to chemicals such as DEET, sarin, pyridostigmine, fumes, mustard, nerve gases), torture (mental, physical coercion), brainwashing, refugees (difficulties to readjust to normal life)
- **Comorbidity**: in two thirds: depression, substance abuse disorders, other anxiety disorders, bipolar disorders
- **Differential diagnosis**:
  - R/O head injury incurred during the trauma.

- R/O other mental disorders: depression, pain disorders, substance abuse, other anxiety disorders, borderline personality disorders, dissociative disorders, factitious disorders, malingering
- **Treatment**: education, pharmacology, psychotherapy needed
  - **Psychotherapy**:
    - Immediately after the trauma: use a model of crisis intervention (support, education, ↑ coping mechanisms)
    - Then use behavior-cognitive rx: exposure rx (imaging techniques, in vivo exposure) and teach stress management techniques
    - Eye movement desensitization and reprocessing (EMDR)
    - Individual, group, family rx
  - **Pharmacotherapy**: more useful for depression, anxiety, hyperarousal than for avoidance, numbness
    - First-line rx: sertraline (50–200 mg), paroxetine (20–50 mg), fluoxetine (60 mg); effective, safe
    - Buspirone may be used (adjunct)
    - Tricyclics: imipramine and amitriptyline (not always well tolerated)
    - Others: MAOIs (phenelzine), trazodone, anticonvulsants (valproate, carbamazepine)
    - Clonidine, prazosin, and propanolol may be useful as antiadrenergic agents (to decrease nightmares).
    - Antipsychotics may be used acutely to control aggression, agitation.
  - **Treat comorbidity**: substance use, self-destructiveness (prioritize interventions)

GENERALIZED ANXIETY DISORDER (GAD)

- **Epidemiology**: lifetime prevalence is 5%. F : M is 2 : 1.
- **Comorbidity**: exists in 50–90%: social phobia, panic disorder, depressive disorder, dysthymic disorders, substance abuse
- **Etiology**: some degree of anxiety is adaptive.
  - **Psychosocial factors**: cognitive-behavioral theories (selective attention to negative details, distortion in information processing, negative view of personal coping skills), psychoanalytic theories (anxiety due to unresolved unconscious conflict, hierarchy of anxieties: fear of annihilation or of fusion to another person → separation anxiety → castration anxiety → superego anxiety)
  - **Biologic factors**:
    - GABA: Benzo. (benzo. receptor agonists) ↓ anxiety; Flumazenil (benzo. receptor antagonist) ↑ anxiety
    - Serotoninergic system: buspirone (an agonist at the serotonin 5-HT1A receptor) ↓ anxiety
    - Other neurotransmitters may be involved: norepinephrine, glutamate, cholecystokinin
  - **Anatomy**: highest conc. of benzodiazepine receptors in the occipital lobe. Possible involvement of basal ganglia, limbic system, frontal cortex
  - **Genetic**: genetic relation between GAD and MDD in families: 25% in first-degree relatives. Concordance rate of 50% in monozygotic and 15% in dizygotic twins
- **Course and prognosis**: only one third seeks psychiatric rx. Chronic condition, high comorbidity. May be very disabling
- **Differential diagnosis**:
  - Dysthymia, depressive disorder (unipolar, bipolar): guilt, crying spells, fatigue, sadness, anhedonia with sx-free intervals. May coexist
  - Other anxiety disorders: phobias, PTSD, OCD, secondary anxiety (work-up: chemistry tests, ECG, thyroid panel)
  - Substance abuse (caffeine, stimulants intoxications; alcohol, sedatives, hypnotics, anxiolytics withdrawal)
  - Adjustment disorders, somatization disorder, personality disorders
- **Treatment**:
  - **Psychotherapy**: cognitive-behavioral (address cognitive distortions, relaxation techniques), supportive and insight-oriented rx (exploring the sources of the anxiety and ↑ its tolerance)
  - **Pharmacotherapy**:
    - Benzodiazepines: diazepam (15–25 mg/day), lorazepam (1–4 mg/day), alprazolam (1–4 mg/day); prn basis or for a limited time; are rapid acting; usually for 2–6 wk then to be tapered in 2 wk for discontinuation. Risk of tolerance and dependence

- Buspirone: pts treated previously with benzodiazepines may not respond. Effect in 2–3 wk. Doses: 45–60 mg/d in tid doses
- Antidepressants:
  - SSRIs: paroxetine (20–40 mg/d) and sertraline; Fluoxetine may transiently ↑ anxiety
  - Venlafaxine: (up to 225 mg/d), Duloxetine (Cymbalta: 60 mg/d up to 120 mg/d) may be used
  - Tricyclics: imipramine (150 mg/d)
- Clonidine: mostly in situational anxiety; ↓ the somatic manifestations

OTHER ANXIETY DISORDERS: SECONDARY ANXIETY DUE TO A MEDICAL CONDITION AND SUBSTANCE-INDUCED ANXIETY DISORDER

- **Epidemiology**: common for both
- **Etiology**:

TABLE 11.2.   Causes of Secondary Anxiety

• **Neurologic disorders**	• Tumors, traumas, strokes, infections, migraines, MS, Wilson disease, epilepsy (complex partial epilepsy), Huntington disease, Parkinson disease, Sydenham chorea
• **Cardiopulmonary conditions**	• Cardiac arrhythmias, MI, angina, pulmonary embolus, hypoxia, COPD, CHF, cardiomyopathy
• **Endocrine disorders**	• Pituitary, thyroid, parathyroid, adrenal disorders, pheochromocytoma, hypoglycemia
• **Inflammatory disorders**	• Lupus erythematous, temporal arteritis, rheumatoid arthritis, polyarteritis nodosa, Sjogren syndrome
• **Drugs**	• Intoxication (alcohol, amphetamines, vasopressors, caffeine, cannabis, hallucinogens like LSD or MDMA or PCP, cocaine, theophylline, yohimbine, antidepressants like SSRIs, tricyclics, MAOIs, buproprion). • Withdrawal (alcohol, benzodiazepines, nicotine, clonidine)
• **Miscellaneous**	• Anemia, vitamin B_{12} deficiency, porphyria, infections, uremia, carcinoid syndrome, chronic pain

- **Definition**: acute attacks or chronic anxiety; may exist with GAD or with panic attacks or with obsessive-compulsive sx. It is the direct consequence of the gl medical condition; not associated with a delirium; severe distress and impairment in functioning. If it is due to drugs, it develops during the use of the substance or within 1 month of cessation.
- **Differential diagnosis**: Anxiety exists also as a sx in other psychiatric illnesses. Primary anxiety disorders usually start <35 yo and are a diagnosis of exclusion. R/O personality disorders, malingering, and mood disorders.
- **Course and prognosis**: determined by the etiology
- **Treatment**: treat the underlying medical cause and/or substance use disorder. If anxiety persists: rx of specific anxiety disorders

MIXED ANXIETY-DEPRESSIVE DISORDER

- **Epidemiology**: Common: two third of pts with depressive sx have anxiety sx and one third has panic disorder. 20–90% of all pts with panic disorder have episodes of major depression. Prevalence in the general population is 1–10%.
- **Definition**: presence of both anxiety and depression with sx of autonomic nervous system hyperactivity.
- **Differential diagnosis**: other anxiety disorders, other depressive disorders, personality disorders (avoidant, dependent, obsessive-compulsive personality disorders), somatoform disorder
- **Course and prognosis**: anxiety and depression may alternate in their predominance.
- **Treatment**: depends on the sx and severity. Psychotherapy (cognitive-behavioral, supportive, insight oriented, in a time-limited manner) and pharmacology (antianxiety agents, antidepressants, or both). Alprazolam is frequently used (short term), as well as buspirone. Venlafaxine is approved by the FDA for depression and GAD. Many SSRIs are approved for MDD and GAD (fluoxetine, paroxetine, escitalopram, sertraline); SNRIs are also approved for both (Duloxetine).

RESOURCES

- APA practice guidelines for treatment of patients with acute stress disorder and posttraumatic stress disorder (November 2004) and Guideline Watch (March 2009)
- APA practice guidelines for treatment of patients with panic disorders, 2nd edition (published in January 2009)

12 ■ DISSOCIATIVE DISORDERS

Includes as per *DSM-IV*:

- **Dissociative amnesia (psychogenic amnesia)**
- **Dissociative fugue (psychogenic fugue)**
- **Dissociative identity disorder (multiple personality disorder)**
- **Depersonalization disorder**

GENERAL FEATURES

- loss of the sense of having one consciousness; lack of sense of identity; confusion about oneself; experiencing oneself as having multiple identities; abnormalities in integrating thoughts, feelings, and actions; partial or complete loss of the normal integration between memories of the past; awareness of identity and immediate sensations; and control of body movements
- Range from normal (state of hypnosis in normal people) to pathological
- M = F; sx ↓ with age; association with traumatic events (physical, sexual abuse); is a defense against trauma
- Differential diagnosis:

    Repression: material is transferred to the unconscious

    Splitting: anxiety tolerance and impulse control are impaired; in dissociation: memory and consciousness are affected. Both involve active separation of mental contents to ward off unpleasant effects associated with the integration of contradictory parts of the self.

    There is no evidence of a physical disorder explaining the phenomena.
- Course: if traumatic onset: few weeks to months, but may be slow to develop and chronic if ongoing problems.

Scales for dissociative disorders: Structured Clinical Interview for *DSM-IV* Dissociative Disorders (SCID-IV), Dissociative Experience Scale.

DISSOCIATIVE AMNESIA

Epidemiology: the most common; F > M; young > older adults; associated with stressful events; ↑ during wars and natural disasters

Etiology: learning theory (the memory laid down during an extraordinary emotional state is difficult to remember)

Diagnosis: the forgotten information is usually of a traumatic, stressful event.

Clinical features: rare spontaneous episodes; onset: usually abrupt after a trauma. **The amnesia is anterograde**; pts are aware of having lost their memory, upset or indifferent. Amnesia may provide a primary or secondary gain; depression and anxiety may be associated. Different forms: localized amnesia (loss of memory for the events of a short time; hours to days); generalized amnesia (loss of memory for a whole lifetime of experience); selective amnesia (failure to recall some but not all events that occurred during a short time)

Differential diagnosis: amnesia in dementia and delirium; postconcussion amnesia (head trauma, often retrograde amnesia, hx of unconsciousness, lasts usually <1 wk); epilepsy (sudden memory impairment with motor and EEG abnormalities; epileptic pts are prone to seizures during stress; hx of aura, head trauma, incontinence); anoxia; cerebral infections or tumors; substance-induced amnesia, post ECT; metabolic disorders; sleep-related amnesia (sleepwalking); transient global amnesia (acute and transient retrograde amnesia; recent > remote memory; pt may still perform complex tasks; lasts 6–24 hr; recovery is complete; most frequently due to transient ischemic attacks [TIAs] or migraines headaches, seizures, sedative-hypnotic drugs); other mental disorders (posttraumatic stress disorder [PTSD]; acute stress disorder; somatoform disorders; malingering, other dissociative disorders)

TABLE 12.1. Dissociative Amnesia vs Transient Global Amnesia (TGA)

Symptoms	Dissociative amnesia	TGA
Type of amnesia	No anterograde amnesia during the episode	Anterograde amnesia during the episode
Reaction to the episode	Upset or not	Very upset
Sense of personal identity	Lost	Retained
Selectivity of the memory loss	Selectivity of memory loss for certain areas Memory of remote events = memory of recent events	Generalized memory loss Remote events better remembered than recent events
Age	20s–40s	60s–70s (vascular problems)

Course and prognosis: stops abruptly; complete recovery

Treatment: hypnosis, or amobarbital interview, or benzodiazepines to restore memory; and psychotherapy

DISSOCIATIVE FUGUE

Epidemiology: rare; more during wars, natural disasters, and personal crises.

Etiology: desire to withdraw from emotional painful experiences; predisposing factors: mood disorders, personality disorders (borderline, histrionic, schizoid); stressors (marital, financial, work, depression, suicidal attempts, epilepsy, hx of substance abuse, hx of head trauma)

Diagnosis: confusion about identity or pt assumes a new identity after a fugue; onset is sudden; pt is unable to recall his past; not occurring only during the course of a dissociative identity disorder, or due to a general medical problem (epilepsy) or substance intoxication

Clinical features: wandering away from home with complete amnesia for past life and unawareness of the amnesia; the amnesia remains for the period of the fugue; pt may live a normal life in the new setting

Differential diagnosis: dementia, delirium, complex partial seizure; dissociative amnesia (where there are no episodes of purposeful travel or of assuming a new identity); malingering

Course and prognosis: hours to days, rarely months. Recovery is spontaneous, rapid; rare recurrences

Treatment: expressive-supportive psychodynamic psychotherapy

DISSOCIATIVE IDENTITY DISORDER (PAST MULTIPLE PERSONALITY DISORDER)

Epidemiology: very rare or underrecognized (particularly in men)? Adolescents and young adults (mean: 30 yo); co-exists with other disorders (anxiety disorders, mood disorders, somatoform disorders, sexual dysfunctions, substance-related disorders, eating disorders, sleeping disorders, PTSD); frequent suicide attempts.

Etiology: physical abuse, incest, death, witnessing trauma or death; poor external support. Frequency of abnormal EEG, differences in pain sensitivity?

Diagnosis: requires an amnestic component, the presence of >2 distinct personality states

Clinical features: often 2–3 personalities or more; transition from one to the other is often sudden; during each personality state (which has a fully integrated, complex set of characteristics, attitudes, relationship, behaviors), the pt is amnestic about other states but not always; the second personality may be spontaneous, frequently child-like; the personalities may be very different and opposite.

Differential diagnosis: dissociative amnesia; dissociative fugue (no shift in identity and no awareness of the original identity); psychosis with delusions; rapid cycling bipolar disorders (BPD); borderline personality disorders; malingering; complex partial epilepsy.

Course and prognosis: may develop in children (as young as 3 yo; may be accompanied by depression, amnestic periods, trance-like episodes, hallucinations, suicidal, self-injurious behaviors; boys > girls); in adolescents: more females; two patterns: chaotic life with promiscuity, drug use, suicide attempts (R/O: impulse control disorders, schizophrenia, rapid cycling BPD, personality disorders) or pattern of withdrawal and child-like behavior (R/O: mood disorders, somatoform disorder, generalized anxiety disorder [GAD]). Poorer prognosis if starts early; the most severe and chronic dissociative disorder; incomplete recovery.

Treatment: insight-oriented psychotherapy; hypnosis or drug-assisted interviewing. Consider safety issues for rx.

DEPERSONALIZATION DISORDER

Epidemiology: common phenomena if isolated experience (transient depersonalization in 70% population); F : M is 2 : 1.

Etiology: R/O endocrine disorders, epilepsy, brain tumors, sensory deprivation, trauma, substances use; frequently associated with anxiety disorders, depressive disorders, schizophrenia.

Diagnosis: persistent and recurrent episodes of depersonalization provoking distress and impairment in functioning

Clinical features: feelings of unreality and estrangement; parts or totality of the body and/or mental operations, behaviors may feel foreign; anxiety, distortions in sense of time or space; awareness of the disturbances in the sense of reality.

Differential diagnosis: mental disorders (depression, schizophrenia, manic episodes, conversion disorders, anxiety disorders, personality disorders); substance use; neurologic disorder (epilepsy, migraines, brain tumors, CV diseases, encephalitis), toxic, metabolic disorders (hypoglycemia, hypothyroidism, hypoparathyroidism), exhaustion, trauma.

Course and prognosis: acute onset; 15–30 yo; lasting condition with a steady course or occasional episodes; frequently associated with hyperventilation.

Treatment: treat underlying disorder; psychotherapy.

DISSOCIATIVE DISORDER NOS

- **Dissociative trance disorder**: Trance (transient alteration of consciousness or sense of identity with a narrowing of the immediate surroundings; or stereotyped movements experienced as being out of one's control; or a changed state of consciousness with a sense of a new identity, attributed to a spirit, power, deity, or another person; or experience of being controlled by an agent, with some amnesia for the event); not a part of an accepted collective cultural, religious practice; rare automatic writing or crystal gazing; related phenomena are highway hypnosis, pts on respirators for long periods of time, hypnosis.
- **Recovered memory syndrome**: memory distortion, retrospective falsifications, and external pressures.
- **Ganser's syndrome**: voluntary production of severe psychiatric sx (giving approximate answers representing the pt's sense of the illness); seen in schizophrenia, depression, toxic states, substance abuse, factitious disorders; with other dissociative disturbances (amnesia, fugue, conversion symptoms), personality disorders; frequent in male prisoners; previously classified as a factitious disorder.
- **Dissociated states**: in brainwashing, captivity by terrorists or cultists, survivors of concentration camps.

13 ■ FACTITIOUS DISORDERS

Pts intentionally produce sx of medical or mental disorders

These disorders may not be controlled but they are deliberate. **The disorder is on a continuum between somatoform disorders and malingering (to assume the sick role).**

Epidemiology: commonly seen in hospitals and in health care workers; F > M; more severe in ♀; physical sx more frequent than psychologic; factitious disorder by proxy: <1,000 of the 3 million cases of child abuse reported per year.

Comorbidity: frequent: mood disorders, personality disorders, substance-related disorders.

Etiology

- **Psychosocial factors**: childhood abuse, neglect, early hospitalizations, MD and RN seen as caring in contrast to the patient's family being rejecting, absent; masochistic personality features (the pain of medical procedures seen as a punishment for real or imagined sins, or to master past trauma); identification with a sick relative; pts with as-if personality (assuming identities of people around them)

- **Biologic factors**: impaired information processing? No evidence of genetic pattern or abnormal EEG

Diagnosis and clinical features: motivation is to assume the sick role (no external incentive for the behavior as in malingering); need multiple informants to reveal the false nature of the illness (a way of coping with psychologic problems).

- **Factitious disorder with predominantly psychologic sx**: feigned sx of mental disorders (bereavement, depression, PTSD, pain disorder, psychosis, dissociative disorder, eating disorder, amnesia, hypersomnia, paraphilias), not improving with regular rx; common; poorer prognosis if presents psychotic sx or borderline personality disorder. Suggestive of a factitious disorder: reported dramatic histories (pseudologia fantastica, impostorship)

- **Factitious disorder with predominantly physical sx (Munchausen's syndrome)**: feigned physical sx suggesting a disorder involving any organ system; pts are very versed and able to mislead very savvy physicians (believable medical hx, self-injuries/hematomas, skin problems, usage of medicines to produce sx such as bleeding, hypoglycemia, complaints of pain to receive narcotics, voluntary contamination of one's urine); frequent hospitalizations, tests, and surgeries; threatening litigation when confronted with negative results; pts may leave the hospital to repeat the cycle somewhere else. Predisposing factors: illnesses during childhood, past strong relationship with a physician, being a medical paraprofessional

- **Factitious disorder with combined psychologic and physical sx**: if neither type predominates

- **Factitious disorder NOS**: not meeting the criteria for a specific factitious disorder; Munchausen's syndrome by proxy (a person produces the sx in another person under their care: frequently mother–child dyad)

Pathology and laboratory examination: no specific test; psychologic testing useful (MMPI-2): frequent normal IQ, lack of thought disorder on the projective tests.

Differential diagnosis: eliminate any authentic illness, possible complications of past multiple surgeries

- **Somatoform disorders (or Briquet's syndrome)**: somatization disorder (unconscious and nonvolitional) vs factitious disorder (voluntary production of sx); conversion disorder (poor medical knowledge, sx related symbolically to specific conflicts); hypochondriasis (later age of onset, nonvoluntary production of sx, less willingness to get procedures and surgeries)

- **Personality disorders**: antisocial personality disorders (do not try to be in the hospital to get procedures); histrionic personality disorders with attention-seeking behaviors (factitious disorders may not be "dramatic"); borderline personality disorders (chaotic life, tumultuous relationships, self-injurious behaviors); schizotypal personality disorders (eccentric behaviors and thoughts)

- **Schizophrenia**: few pts with factitious disorders have severe thought disorder or bizarre delusions

- **Malingering**: pts seek hospitalization (financial compensation, to avoid police research), voluntary production of false physical or mental sx to avoid responsibilities, receive financial or material rewards, retaliate against someone or an organization.

    Epidemiology: frequent in jails, military, factories

    Symptoms: suspect if legal context, claimed disability vs objective findings discrepancy, poor cooperativeness with the medical evaluation and the recommended rx, antisocial personality disorder, possibility of self-inflicted injuries, drug-seeking behaviors, unprescribed drugs found in urine.

- **Differential diagnosis:** conversion disorder, other somatoform disorders (unconscious production of sx, no external incentives)

- **Treatment:** avoid confrontation, thorough observations, intensive rx approach to avoid having the pt lose face.

- **Substance abuse**: may co-exist

- **Ganser's syndrome**: prisoners who use approximate answers to questions to avoid punishment or responsibility; classified as a dissociative disorder NOS in *DSM-IV-TR*.

Course and prognosis: may start in early childhood after the beginning of a real illness or abandonment; pt becomes more knowledgeable about medical matters and more able to fake diseases. Repeated hospitalizations and rx may produce traumas, chaotic life, psychiatric hospitalizations, risk of death. Better prognosis: if no antisocial features, depression but no psychosis

Treatment: focus on management rather than cure; need for early recognition + good liaison between psychiatrists, medical and surgical staff; even though the patient lies and feigns the illness, the patient is still sick (do not act up on the countertransference); help other staff members to deal with the sense of being deceived and understand the patient's motivations; in Munchausen's syndrome by proxy, the legal and the child welfare services might need to be involved.

14 ■ CONSULTATION-LIAISON PSYCHIATRY

(1) Psychologic factors affecting medical conditions

- A gl medical condition is present and psychologic factors adversely affect it.
- The psychologic factors may be:
  - Mental disorder associated with the medical condition
  - Psychologic sx delaying the recovery or precipitating a medical crisis
  - Personality features affecting the medical condition due to poor coping skills
  - Unsafe behaviors affecting the medical condition
  - Stress-related physiologic response affecting medical conditions
  - Interpersonal, religious, cultural factors affecting the medical condition

TABLE 14.1. Management of Personality Styles in the Hospital

Traits	Management
Histrionic (dramatic, anxious, involved)	Supportive approach: appreciation of courage, qualities, ventilation of fears, no detailed explanations
Obsessive (orderly, anxious, involved)	Using detailed scientific explanations, intellectualization, making the pt a partner in the therapeutic decisions
Narcissistic (self-involved, controlling)	Support strength, make the pt an equal
Oral (clinging, demanding, attention seeking)	Support but give also firm limits on undue neediness and manipulativeness
Masochistic (depressed, help-rejecting, long-suffering)	Appreciate the pt's courage without undue reassurance or optimism, appeal to altruism
Schizoid (unsociable, remote)	Respect need for privacy and distance
Paranoid (suspicious, blaming, hypersensitive)	Be honest, repeat explanations, reorient to reality as much as possible

Hierarchy of adaptive ego defenses as a way of coping: some are more healthy than others but all help the pt cope with painful affects (see Vaillant, G. E. [1971]. Theoretical hierarchy of adaptive ego mechanisms. *Archives of General Psychiatry, 24*, 107–118).

TABLE 14.2. Ego Defenses and Coping with Distress

Hierarchy	Description
• **Narcissistic**: in "healthy individuals before age 5 and in adults dreams and fantasy"	• **Delusional projection**: paranoid attribution of internal feelings as if coming from outside "reality" • **Psychotic denial**: ignoring some aspects of external reality • **Distortion**: reshaping of external reality to suit inner needs
• **Immature**: in "healthy individuals between ages 3 and 16 and in personality disorders and affective disorders"	• **Projection**: attribution of one's own undesirable feelings to others • **Schizoid fantasy**: retreat into autistic daydreams for conflict resolution and gratification • **Hypochondriasis**: transformation of reproach toward the self or others into somatic symptoms • **Passive-aggression**: overt compliance but covert hostile behavior to punish others • **Acting out**: behavioral expression of unconscious conflicts to avoid consciousness of the affect that accompanies the conflict

Continued

TABLE 14.2.   Ego Defenses and Coping with Distress   Continued

Hierarchy	Description
● **Neurotic**: in "healthy adults with neurotic disorders or adults mastering acute distress"	● **Intellectualization**: removal of feelings linked to an event and overattention to detail ● **Regression**: forgetting some aspect of reality while keeping symbolic behavior suggesting that the repressed idea is not completely forgotten ● **Displacement**: conflicted feelings are redirected toward a different object than the person or situation arousing the feelings ● **Reaction-formation**: affect or behavior opposite to the unconscious, unwanted sexual or aggressive wish ● **Dissociation**: temporary modification of the sense of personal identity to avoid emotional distress
● **Mature**: in "healthy adults during optimal functioning"	● **Altruism**: vicarious gratifying service to others ● **Humor**: overt expression of feelings releasing tension, gratifying for the user and the beholder ● **Suppression**: conscious decision to postpone paying attention to a conflict ● **Anticipation**: realistic planning for possible future discomfort ● **Sublimation**: indirect or partial expression of sexual and aggressive needs without adverse consequences
● **Regression and progression**	● Are shifts in levels of defenses

(2) **Examples of psychosomatic disorders**: acne, allergic reactions, angina pectoris, arrhythmias, asthma, chronic pain syndromes, diabetes mellitus, duodenal ulcer, headache, hypoglycemia, irritable colon, migraine, mucous colitis, nausea, neurodermatitis, obesity, dysmenorrhea, pruritus, psoriasis, rheumatoid arthritis, tachycardia, tension headache, ulcerative colitis, urticaria

　　Etiology: stress, underlying psychophysiologic factors (hormonal, autonomic nervous system, immune system), genetics, organ vulnerability, specific personality; nature of unconscious emotional conflicts may interact to produce diseases.

　　Five steps to deal with somatic complaints

TABLE 14.3.   Tips to Deal with Somatic Complaints

● Listen to the complaints: without interrupting or offering solutions. All illnesses have a physical basis; ask about prior workups
● Be nonverbally attentive: undivided attention given
● Encourage the pt to find solutions: discuss prior ways of coping and results. Empathize with pt's frustrations
● Provide suggestions that appear reasonable to the patient
● If patient is not receptive to the suggested intervention: refer to a specialist or ↑ frequency of visits

　　Diagnoses producing somatoform complaints

TABLE 14.4.   Medical and Psychiatric Causes of Somatoform Complaints

● Physical diseases
● Affective disorders
● Anxiety disorders
● Substance use disorders
● Psychotic disorders
● Organic brain syndromes
● Voluntary symptom production (malingering; factitious disorders)
● Somatoform disorders
● Personality disorders

(3) **Consultation-liaison psychiatry**
Definition:
　　Is the study and practice of the relation between medical and psychiatric disorders
　　The **psychiatrist is a consultant to his or her medical colleagues**

○ The psychiatrist needs to understand the medical + the psychiatric aspects of the case
○ The psychiatrist needs to differentiate mental disorders and psychologic responses to physical illness, to identify personality features and the pt's coping techniques to recommend appropriate therapeutic interventions

Reasons for consultations

TABLE 14.5.   Reasons for Consulations and Interventions

● **Suicide threat or attempt**	● If risk, transfer to a psychiatric unit or provide 24-hr supervision on a 1 : 1
● **Depression**	● Assess suicidal risk and need for stronger supervision ● R/O dementia if presence of cognitive deficits ● Assess substance abuse (alcohol, cocaine, amphetamines) ● Check if pt on depressant medications (reserpine, methyldopa, thiazides, spironolactone, clonidine, oral contraceptives, steroids, cimetidine, barbiturates, benzodiazepines, propanolol, metoclopramide) ● Use antidepressant with special precautions (ECG)
● **Agitation**	● Assess presence of cognitive disorder ● Check for drug withdrawal ● R/O psychotic process, agitated depression ● R/O toxic reaction to medication ● R/O medical causes of anxiety (endocrine, drug related, cardiovascular and circulatory, respiratory system, metabolic, neurologic, GI, infectious disease, renal, nutritional, malignancies) ● Evaluate danger to self and others, need for restraints (physical or chemical) to control aggression; identify staff-pt dissonance, educate pt and staff to reduce it; prepare a disposition plan adequate for the pt's medical and psychiatric needs
● **Hallucinations and psychosis**	● Check for delirium tremens ● Sensory isolation in ICU ● R/O psychotic disorder. Check for all diagnostic possibilities (psychiatric, neurologic, endocrine, metabolic, deficiency states, postoperative states, systemic illnesses, drug withdrawal, intoxications, effects from medications) ● Check any acute change in blood work-up (sugar, electrolytes, CBC, blood arterial gas, fever) and vital signs ● Explain the pt's reality to the staff to better cope with the pt's behavior
● **Sleep disorder**	● R/O pain, depression, anxiety, substance withdrawal
● **Disorientation**	● R/O delirium, dementia, metabolic disorder, neurologic disorder, substance abuse, sensory deprivation
● **Poor compliance**	● Negative transference toward the treating doctor, denial of the illness, poor judgment, independency issues
● **Refusal to consent to treatment**	● Fear of the rx, cognitive disorder ● Assess for competency issues and need for a court hearing (incompetence can only be declared by a judge)

● **Wanting to sign out against medical advice**	● **It is a two-way transaction**:
	  The pt feels that he has been wronged, mistreated, misunderstood, misinformed or mismanaged
	  It is a disturbance in the doctor–patient relationship: may be due to inadequate preparation of the pt and the family by the staff (length of stay, procedures, change of rx without knowledge). It is the last desperate act of a pt, worsened by the staff pride to admit any error
	  May be link with alcohol or drug abuse; anger and anxiety are disguises for a sense of helplessness
	● **3 basic factors** involved: (1) *fear* of what is going to happen, (2) *anger* at fate, at the medical establishment, at the caretakers, and (3) *psychotic reactions and/or depression*
	● **Tasks** involved: ally with the pt to find out what is wrong, get the parties together for a reconciliation, give the pt a sense of autonomy, let the pt know that he has the freedom to leave assuming that the pt's judgment is sound, that the pt is not suicidal or homicidal, to allow the pt to come back, and allow for out-pt rx
	● **Exceptions**: pts with organic brain disease, psychotic pts who threaten to leave as a result of delusions or hallucinations

Continued

TABLE 14.5. Reasons for Consulations and Interventions   Continued

● Personality issues	● **Dependent patient**: not all the pt's needs can be realistically met; allow the staff to say "no" to the pt's excessive demands
	● **Rejecting patient**: give the pt some distance and autonomy
	● **Manipulative patient**: set firm limits on the manipulations; serve as a buffer for the staff, helping them to articulate their feeling toward the pt but to behave nonsadistically
	● **Guidelines for management of pts with borderline personality disorders**:
	    Acknowledge the pt's stressful situation
	    Avoid breaking down needed defenses; prevent primitive defenses (splitting, denial, primitive idealization or devaluation of the staff, projective identification on the staff, sense of omnipotence in the self or sense of impotence)
	    Avoid stimulating the pt's need for closeness
	    Avoid stimulating the pt's rage
	    Avoid confrontating the narcissistic entitlement

● Factitious disorders	● R/O malingering, factitious disorder, somatization disorder, conversion disorder

TABLE 14.6. How to Motivate a Patient with "Psychogenic Symptoms" to Accept Mental Health Assistance

- Empathic statements about what it must be like to have a psychiatric consultation
- Maintain compassionate stance
- Convey confidence in value of mental health rx
- Reassurance that the sx are seen as real
- Receiving mental health assistance will help to manage better the symptoms
- If available, provide pt with pt education material
- Clarify the connection between sx and stress or unpleasant effect
- Explain how everyone reacts physiologically to stress in his or her own manner
- State that emotional factors need to be treated since they make the sx worse, though they may not cause the sx
- Reassure that the pt's own doctor will still follow to assist with the physical aspects of the sx
- Explain as needed the influence of feelings or thoughts on the sx

Adapted from Goldsmith, S. (1983). A strategy for evaluating psychogenic symptoms. *International Journal of Psychiatry in Medicine, 13,* 167–172.

Legal aspects

TABLE 14.7. Legal Aspects of Consultation: Good Faith, Common Sense, and the Highest Standard of Care for the Patient are the Safest Haven

Physician's rights and obligations	● A physician is responsible for failure to adhere to the accepted standard of medical practice if the result is a compensable injury. A deviation from it must be justified ● Confidentiality is demanded and protected, unless this endangers the life of the pt or others ● Good Samaritan laws exist in most states ● Refusal to treat pts: is a right but must be clarified at the outset; does not apply to urgent medical problems; any effort to provide an alternative course to avoid claims of abandonment and assure continuity of care must be made ● The dying pt: see Chapter 24
Civil rights of the patient	see Chapter 27 on forensic psychiatry
Consent and competency	There can be no consent unless there is first competency. Competency is specific and depends here on 3 things: understanding the illness, the treatment, and the consequences of the decision, with a grasp of the risk–benefit ratio of what is proposed. Consider incompetency for psychiatric reasons (severe depression, psychosis, fluctuation in mental alertness, delirium, agitation). Clarify if the decision to refuse rx is a sx of the psychiatric disorder. A physician may not pronounce a pt "incompetent" in the legal sense

Adapted from Goldsmith, S. (1983). A strategy for evaluating psychogenic symptoms. *International Journal of Psychiatry in Medicine, 13,* 167–172.

SPECIFIC DISORDERS

CARDIOVASCULAR SYSTEM

- Risk factors for coronary heart disease: Type A behavior pattern ↑ risk by 2 (esp. the hostility component, acute stress)
- Psychiatric disorders may be a complication or comorbidity: depression (↑ suicide), anxiety, delirium, sleep problems, cognitive disorders. Uncertain relation between panic disorders and mitral valve prolapse. After coronary artery bypass surgery: memory and cognitive impairments, depression (if persists: ↑ mortality). In HBP: ↑ in anxiety, ↑ in aggressive pts

- Cardiovascular presentations of psychiatric disorders (seen in ER): palpitations, chest pains in somatization disorders, panic disorders, anxiety, depression

TABLE 14.8. Drug Interactions Between Psychiatric Drugs and Commonly Used Drugs in CV Disorders

Drugs	Comments	Drug interactions
Diuretics • **Thiazides** • **Potassium sparing** (amiloride, triamterene, aldosterone agonists) • **Loop** (bumetanide, ethacrynic acid, furosemide, torsemide) • **Osmotic**: mannitol, urea • **Xanthine**: aminophylline, caffeine, theophylline • **Carbonic anhydrase inhibitors**: acetazolamide		**Thiazides**: risk of lithium toxicity **Potassium sparing**: may ↑ lithium conc. Lithium may ↓ blood K+ level **Loop**: may ↑ lithium conc. **Osmotic**: ↓ lithium conc. **Xanthine**: ↓ lithium conc.; may ↓ antipsychotic effects Carbonic anhydrase: ↓ lithium conc.
Angiotensin converting enzyme (ACE) inhibitors: benazepril, captopril, enalapril fosinopril, lisinopril, moexipril, perindopril, quinapril, ramipril, trandolapril	Angioedema; swelling of the tongue, glottis, larynx; rare jaundice	↑ level of lithium (↑ toxicity) Risk of hypotensive crisis with antipsychotics
AT1 angiotensin II receptor blockers (ARBs): candesartan, eprosartan, irbesartan, losartan, olmesartan, telmisartan, valsartan	Cases of angioedema and rhabdomyolysis	Losartan, irbesartan do not alter lithium conc. Risk of hypotension with antipsychotics
Calcium channel blockers (CCBs): nifedipine, nimodipine, isradipine, amlodipine, nicardipine, nisoldipine, nitrendipine, diltiazem, felodipine, verapamil	Neurotoxicity Used to treat HTN, angina, cardiac arrhythmias Used also for mania and rapid mood-cycling types of BPD	**Verapamil**: ↑ carbamazepine neurotoxicity **Nifedipine**: no report of carbamazepine toxicity Caution if CCBs associated with: • cimetidine (↑ level of nifedipine and diltiazem) • lithium (may ↑ toxicity) **Diltiazem**: may ↑ level of buspirone
β-Adrenergic receptor antagonists: acebutolol, atenolol, betaxolol, bisoprolol, carvedilol, esmolol, labetalol, metroprolol, nadolol, penbutolol, pindolol, propanolol, sotalol, timolol	Used for lithium tremor, anxiety disorders Contraindicated in asthma/COPD	**All**: • Slight ↑ lithium conc. • DC β-blocker a few days prior to DC clonidine to ↓ risk of rebound HTN • Risk of bradycardia with some CCBs • Contrary to folk wisdom, β-blockers do not cause depression • SSRIs may ↑ blood levels of β-blockers **Carveditol**: do not use alcohol **Metroprolol** may ↑ levels of: bupropion, diphenhydramine, fluoxetine, paroxetine, thioridazine **Pindolol**: do not give with thioridazine **Propanolol**: do not give with thioridazine. Alcohol ↑ propanolol level Antipsychotic inhibits metabolism of propanolol → risk of hypotension

Continued

TABLE 14.8. Drug Interactions between Psychiatric Drugs and Commonly Used Drugs in CV Disorders   Continued

Drugs	Comments	Drug interactions
Antiarrhythmic drugs: adenosine, amiodarone, atropine, bicarbonate, digoxin disopyramide, dofetilide flecainide, ibutilide, isoproterenol, lidocaine, mexiletine, moricizine, propafenone, Quinidine		**Amiodarone:** half-life (25–50 days); DDI may persist after DC; ↑ levels of drugs metabolized by CYP450 enzymes; caution with β-blockers and calcium channel blockers; may ↑ QTc with trazodone; ↑ phenytoin level **Digoxin:** many DDIs **Disopyramide:** anticholinergic **Dofetilide:** monitor QTc (if used with verapamil, prochlorperazine, phenothiazines, antidepressants) **Flecainide:** caution with verapamil **Lidocaine:** monitor CNS SE if prolonged use **Mexiletine:** CNS SE, monitor levels if + phenytoin, phenobarbital, fluvoxamine **Propafenone:** ↑ β-blockers, desipramine, haloperidol, imipramine, venlafaxine levels. Risk of ↑ QTc if given with desipramine, paroxetine, sertraline (which ↑ level of propafenone) **Quinidine:** do not give with ziprasidone (QRS widening, ↑ QTc), interactions with phenytoin, phenobarbital, verapamil
Nitrates	Headaches	Risk of hypotension (if + psychotropics producing hypotension)
Pressors/inotropes: dobutamine, dopamine, ephedrine, epinephrine, inamrinone, mephentermine, metaraminol, midodrine, milrinone, norepinephrine, phenylephrine	Used in emergency May produce paranoid feelings	Antipsychotics antagonize pressor effect: risk of hypotension
Pulmonary arterial hypertension: bosentan, epoprostenol, iloprost, treprostinil		May ↑ hypotensive effects of other drugs CYP2C9 inhibitors and CYP3A4 inhibitors ↑ levels of bosentan
Thrombolytics: alteplase, reteplase, streptokinase, tenecteplase, urokinase	Contraindicated in prior cerebral hemorrhage, dementia, cerebral aneurysm, brain tumor, prior ischemic stroke	**SSRIs** may ↑ risk of bleeding in pts on anticoagulants, platelet inhibitors, thrombin inhibitors, thrombolytic agents, or agents that cause thrombocytopenia **Ginkgo** may ↑ effects of anticoagulants, platelet inhibitors, and thrombolytic agents, possibly ↑ the risk of bleeding **Clomipramine** is also a strong SSRI
Antiplatelet drugs: abciximab, aspirin + dipyridamole, clopidogrel, dipyridamole, eptifibatide, ticlopidine, tirofiban		May produce anxiety, depression, insomnia SSRIs may alter platelet function and induce bleeding. Caution with clomipramine, Ginkgo
Antiadrenergic agents: Clonidine, doxazosin, Guanfacine, Methyldopa, guanabenz, prazosin, reserpine, terazosin	Clonidine used in Tourette syndrome, opioid withdrawal, alcohol withdrawal, smoking cessation, ADHD, menopausal flushing Guanfacine used in ADHD Prazocin has been used in PTSD	• **Clonidine:** antipsychotic ↑ hypotensive effect. Clonidin may ↑ CNS depression due to barbiturates, alcohol, and sedative-hypnotics; if use of clonidine + β-adrenergic receptor antagonists: risk of severe rebound phenomena. Clonidine + verapamil: risk of hypotension and A-V cardiac block; some death attributed to use of clonidine + Ritalin • **Guanfacine:** less sedation and hypotension than clonidine • ↑ **depression as a group** (esp. reserpine): some controversies
Antihyperlipidemics • **Bile acid sequestrants:** cholestyramine, colesevelam, colestipol • **Statins and combinations:** lovastatin + niacin, atorvastatin, amlodipine + atorvastatin, fluvastatin, lovastatin, pravastatin, simvastatin, ezetimibe + simvastatin • **Others:** ezetimibe, fenofibrate, gemfibrozil	Monitor LFTs, creatinine-kinase if muscle pains	• **Colesevelam:** ↓ level of verapamil • **Atorvastatin, lovastatin, simvastatin:** not to use with inhibitor of CYT P450 (nefazodone) →↑ risk of myopathy, rhabdomyolysis • **Caution with atorvastatin + verapamil** • **Fluvastatin, pravastatin:** less metabolized by CYP450 → ↓ interactions

TABLE 14.9.   Risk Factors for Prolonged QT Interval +++

High doses of an antipsychotic
Thioridazine > ziprazidone > quetiapine > risperidone > olanzapine > haloperidol:+++
Newer antipsychotics also may ↑ QTc intervals: asenapine (Saphris), paliperidone (Invega)
Iloperidone (Fanapt is known to increase QTc at regular doses; Caution +++)
Treatment with droperidol, pimozide, sertindole, or thioridazine
Coadministered drugs that prolong the QT interval (see Table 14.10) particularly: Class 1A antiarrhythmics (e.g.,
   quinidine, procainamide) or Class 3 antiarrhythmics (e.g., amiodarone, sotalol), other antipsychotic medications (e.g.,
   ziprasidone, chlorpromazine, thioridazine), and antibiotics (e.g., gatifloxacin, moxifloxacin); other drugs known to ↑ QTc
   (e.g., pentamidine, levomethadyl acetate, methadone)
Heart disease:
   Myocardial ischemia
   Left ventricular dysfunction or hypertrophy
   Previous torsade de pointes
   ECG abnormalities (including bradycardia, ventricular extrasystole, heart block)
   Hx of cardiac arrhythmias
   Congenital prolongation of the QT interval
Hepatic or renal failure
Alcoholic liver disease
Low plasma K+, Ca_{2+}, or Mg_{2+}
Advanced age
Female gender

TABLE 14.10.   Selecting Safe Antidepressants in CVD and CHF

SSRIs: safe and effective for MDD in CVD and congestive heart failure
Venlafaxine: at doses >300 mg/d may ↑ BP (caution in depressed pts with hypertension)
Desvenlafaxine (Pristiq): found to ↑ BP and heart rate (avoid in pts with preexisting hx)
Duloxetine: may ↑ BP
Bupropion or mirtazapine in pts with CVD: unknown safety and efficacy
Tricyclic antidepressants: contraindicated for 6 months post-MI (↑ arrhythmias). Avoid in depressed pts with CVD or
   conduction defects (quinidine-like effects on conduction)

RESPIRATORY SYSTEM

30% of pts with asthma have panic disorder or agoraphobia. Emotional lability, sensitivity to rejection, severe anxiety ↑ use of antiasthma drugs, ↑ rates of hospitalizations.

TABLE 14.11.   Drug Interactions Between Psychiatric Drugs and Commonly Used Drugs in Pulmonary Disorders

Drugs	Indications	Drug interactions
Beta-agonists: albuterol, arformoterol, formoterol, levalbuterol, metaproterenol, pirbuterol, salmeterol, terbutaline	Acute asthma	Caution in pts on MAOIs or TCAs; ↑ CV side effects Risk of tolerance with continued use of short-acting β-agonists
Combinations: fluticasone + salmeterol, albuterol + ipratropium, budesonide + formoterol (*Symbicort*)	Chronic asthma	CYP 3A4 inhibitors ↑ fluticasone conc. (risk of adrenal suppression) Symbicort is long acting (↑ asthma-related deaths)
Inhaled steroids: beclomethasone, budesonide, flunisolide, fluticasone, mometasone, triamcinolone	Not for rx of acute asthma	CYP 3A4 inhibitors ↑ conc. of fluticasone, budesonide, mometasone (risk of adrenal suppression)
Leukotriene inhibitors: montelukast, zafirlukast, zileuton	Not for rx of acute asthma	Montelukast: phenobarbital ↓ level of montelukast Zileuton potentiates propanolol
Others: cromolyn, theophylline	Chronic asthma	Theophylline: DDI with carbamazepine, phenytoin, life-threatening overdose

Adapted from Sadock, B. J., & Sadock, V. A. (2002). *Kaplan and Sadock's Synopsis of Psychiatry: Behavioral Sciences/Clinical Psychiatry* (9th ed.). Baltimore, MD: Lippincott Williams & Wilkins.

GASTROINTESTINAL SYSTEM

Stress, anxiety ↑ physiologic response of the GI system, severity of GERD, ulcer vulnerability in peptic ulcer disease (↓ immune responses, ↑ vulnerability to *H. pylori* infection). In ulcerative colitis: pts have ↑ obsessive-compulsive traits. In Crohn disease: pts have ↑ in preexisting panic disorders, ↑ depression, anxiety, family conflicts.

TABLE 14.12. Psychiatric Effects and Drug–Drug Interactions Between Psychiatric Drugs and Commonly Used Drugs in GI Disorders

Drugs	Psychiatric effects	Drug interactions
Histamine 2-receptor antagonists (used for peptic ulcers): • Nizatidine (*Axid*) • Famotidine (*Pepcid*) • Cimetidine (*Tagamet*) • Ranitidine (*Zantac*)	Cimetidine: can cause delirium All may produce delirium (it is safer to use sucralfate/Carafate)	Cimetidine: ↑ levels of TCAs, carbamazepine, valproate, SSRI
Proton pump inhibitor (used in peptic ulcers) • Omeprazole (*Prilosec*) • Lansoprazole (*Prevacid*)		↑ Level of carbamazepine
Antiemetics • Prochlorperazine (*Compazine*) • Dronabinol (*Marinol*) • Ondansetron (*Zofran*)	Prochlorperazine: is a phenothiazine → EPS Dronabinol: dizziness, euphoria	Prochlorperazine: ↑ TCAs Ondansetron: SSRIs?
GI stimulant (used for GERD) • Metoclopramide (*Reglan*)	Akathisia, dystonia, depression	↑ Cyclosporine and ethanol absorption
Antiacids (*Maalox, Mylanta*)		Changes absorption of other drugs
Anti-infection • Interferon α (*Intron*): used for Hepatitis C • Metronidazole (*Flagyl*): used for Giardiasis • Tetracycline • Clarithromycin (*Biaxin*)	Interferon α: depression, suicidal behaviors, anxiety, confusion, aggressivity	Flagyl interacts with lithium, barbiturates, phenytoin, disulfiram (do not give flagyl within 2 wk of disulfiram) Tetracycline: may cause pseudo-tumor cerebri. Doxycycline levels may be decreased with barbiturates, carbamazepine, phenytoin Biaxin: do not use with cisapride, pimozide; ↑ carbamazepine level; has many drug interactions
Other antiulcer • Misoprostol (*Cytotec*) • Sucralfate (*Carafate*)	Carafate usually does not produce delirium	Carafate: interaction with phenytoin

Adapted from Sadock, B. J., & Sadock, V. A. (2002). *Kaplan and Sadock's Synopsis of Psychiatry: Behavioral Sciences/Clinical Psychiatry* (9th ed.). Baltimore, MD: Lippincott Williams & Wilkins. p. 829.

MUSCULOSKELETAL SYSTEM

Rheumatoid arthritis: stress → immune suppression. Rx: rest vs exercise, psychotherapy, rx of joints' pain, inflammation.

Systemic lupus erythematosus: psychiatric sx in 50% cases (depression, mood instability, psychosis, delusions, and hallucinations), sometimes caused by steroid rx. Medical sx: fever, photosensibility, butterfly rash, joint pains, fatigue. Lab: ANA +, + lupus erythematosus test, anemia, ↓ platelets, pericarditis.

Low back pain: careful physical exam with neurologic exam. MRI may be needed. Psychoeducation, symptomatic rx (aspirin, muscle relaxants/diazepam), physical rx, relaxation techniques, biofeedback. ↓ prognosis if comorbid psychiatric illness, or pt on disability or welfare roles.

Fibromyalgia: medical or psychologic phenomena? Is it a somatoform disorder or a pain disorder?
- **Pain and stiffness of soft tissues with trigger points**: **>3 months duration**, left and right side of the body, above and under the waist, axial pain in at least three segments of the body, with **at least 11 tender points of the possible 18 points** on digital examination (occiput, lower cervical areas, trapezius, supraspinatus, 2nd rib, lateral epicondyle, gluteal, greater trochanter, knee). *Trigger points* (tenderness upon palpation, twitch response upon stimulation, ↓ range of motion, muscle weakness, skin changes,

autonomic dysfunction, and taut bands within muscle); ↑ with stress; F > M; life-long disorder with significant disability. No pathognomonic laboratory findings

- **Differential diagnosis**: rheumatologic conditions, skeletal pain, hypothyroidism, infection, chronic fatigue syndrome (may be associated with it and with depression)
- **Rx**: avoid narcotics. Provide pt's education, sleep hygiene, analgesic (aspirin, acetaminophen), relaxation, muscle relaxants (baclofen, dantrolene, α2-agonists such as tizanidine/Zanaflex), exercises, massage, SSRIs, SNRIs such as Duloxetine (Cymbalta) and Milnacipran hydrochloride (**Savella**); Pregabalin (**Lyrica**); treat restless legs if present with dopamine agonists such as: ropinirole, pramipexole, or carbidopa/levodopa (sinemet 10/100 hs), or clonazepam (0.5–1 mg hs); *treat comorbidity* (irritable bowel symptoms with antispasmodics such as belladonna/Donnatal, and dicyclomine); treat affective disorders (antidepressant, anxiolytics, mood stabilizers); treat irritable bladder symptoms (antispasmodics such as oxybutynin); treat neurally mediated hypotension (fludrocortisone/Florinef, liberal salt intake); avoid TCAs, β-blockers, anticholinergic agents; use psychotherapy, rehabilitation approach

Chronic fatigue syndrome: puzzling disorder; ⅓–⅔ of CFS have psychiatric disorders; R/O: anxiety, depression, somatoform disorders, infectious causes. **Diagnosis: fatigue** that ↓ level of functioning, starting sometimes with flu-like sx, of **>6 months duration with at least four symptoms** *among the following: poor memory and concentration, sore throat, tender glands, myalgia, joint pain, headache, insomnia, tiredness*. There are no obvious medical or psychiatric causes; may be associated with fibromyalgia, irritable bowel disorder. *66% pts have one or more psychiatric comorbidities* (anxiety disorder, panic disorder, depression, and somatoform disorder). Psychiatric rx: CBT, exercise, build therapeutic alliance, supportive rx. No medication. International Association for Chronic Fatigue Syndrome: *http://www.aacfs.org.*

HEADACHES

↑ with stress, depression, anxiety, hypochondriasis. R/O organicity (CT scan with contrast or MRI; if normal head CT scan: consider LP to R/O subarachnoid hemorrhage, meningitis, or pseudo-tumor cerebri).

TABLE 14.13.   Indications for Neuroimaging in Patients with Nonacute Headaches +++

Focal neurologic exam
Sudden onset of "the worst headache of my life"
Headache exacerbated by coughing, sneezing, or straining
Headache with early AM worsening or awakening the pt at night
New headache starting after 40 yo or in young children
Progressively worsening daily headaches
Presence of altered mental status, nuchal rigidity, fever, or papilledema
New headache in HIV+ pts or those with known cancer

- **Migraine (vascular) and cluster headaches**

Sx: paroxysmal, recurrent headaches with or without visual sx (photophobia) and GI sx (nausea, vomiting); often familial, ↑ in obsessional personalities. Cluster headaches are related to migraines, unilateral; occur up to 8 times/d, associated with miosis, ptosis, and diaphoresis.

Rx:

- **Migraine headaches**:
  - **Abortive agents**:
    - **Mild headaches**: aspirin 800–1,000 mg po/day or NSAIDS (Ibuprofen, Naproxen sodium) or combinations containing caffeine
    - **Moderate headaches**:
      - Use migraine-specific agents (triptans, dihydroergotamine [DHE]) in pts with moderate or severe migraine or those not responding to NSAIDs or combinations such as aspirin + acetaminophen + caffeine. Failure to use an effective tx promptly may ↑ pain, disability
      - DHE nasal spray is safe, effective for the tx of acute migraine attacks: consider in pts with moderate to severe migraine (1 spray in each nostril q 15 min × 2 prn; max 6 sprays/d)
      - Select a nonoral route of administration for pts with migraine + severe N/V. Nausea itself is one of the most aversive and disabling sx of a migraine attack; it should be treated. Pts with N/V may be given intranasal or subcutaneous sumatriptan.
      - Consider a self-administered rescue medication for pts with severe migraine failing other tx (butorphanol nasal spray or acetaminophen + codeine combination).
      - Medication-overuse headache ("rebound headache"; "drug-induced headache"): with ergotamine (not DHE), opiates, triptans, simple analgesics, mixed analgesics containing butalbital, caffeine, or isometheptene. Limit acute tx to 2 headache days per week on a regular basis. Pts with medication overuse should use preventive tx.

Severe headaches: Triptans (5-HT1receptor agonists) are the first choice. Triptans cannot be given within 24 hr of ergots or other triptans; risk **of serotonin syndrome with SSRIs and MAOIs +++**. The most frequent triptans used are almotriptan, eletriptan, frovatriptan, naratriptan. Rizatriptan may be the best oral tryptan for aborting migraine headache, sumatriptan, zolmitriptan. They are contraindicated if ischemic heart disease, uncontrolled HTN, or focal neurologic findings +++.

Prophylaxis: indicated if ≥3 attacks/month, incapacitating or complicated migraines:

Highest efficacy: propanolol (40–120 mg po bid), timolol 20–30 mg po daily; amitriptyline 25–150 mg po q hs; divalproex sodium 250–750 mg po bid; gabapentin 100–1,200 mg po tid

Moderate efficacy: metoprolol 100–200 mg po daily; atenolol 50–200 mg po daily, nadolol 20–160 mg po daily; topiramate 50–200 mg po bid; nortriptyline 10–60 mg po q hr or riboflavin (vitamin B$_2$) 400 mg po daily; calcium channel blockers (Verapamil, Nimodipine)

Psychotherapy, biofeedback

- **Cluster headaches**:

  Have pt breathe 100% oxygen at 7–10 L/min by mask for 15–20 min

  Abortive agents: dihydroergotamine 1 mg IM or 0.5 mg nasal spray bilaterally; sumatriptan 6 mg SC or 20 mg intranasally; zolmitriptan 5–10 mg po or 1 mL of 10% lidocaine placed in each nostril using a cotton swab for 5 min

  Prophylactic agents: verapamil: 120–160 mg po tid; valproic acid 250–1,000 mg po bid; lithium 300 mg po bid–tid; topiramate 25–200 mg po daily; prednisone 50–80 mg po/d × 5 d, ↓ over 10–12 days

■ **Tension headaches**
↑ with stress, depression, anxiety, type A personalities. Rx: relaxation techniques, acetaminophen or NSAIDs, biofeedback, antidepressants (nortriptyline or amitriptyline 10–75 mg po q hs prophylactically), psychotherapy. Avoid ergots, caffeine, butalbital, opiates (abuse and dependence).

■ **Temporal arteritis**
Prednisone 40–60 mg po daily × 2–4 wk and ↓ dose 10% q 1–2 wk to min effective dose (duration may be 1–2 yr). Follow sx and erythrocyte sedimentation rate q month; Methylprednisone 1 g IV/d × 3 d for impending visual loss.

■ **Trigeminal neuralgia**
MRI/angiogram focusing on the cerebellopontine angle to R/O a mass or MS if: age <40, sensory loss, bilateral sx or poor response to medical rx. Rx options: carbamazepine 200–600 mg po bid (most effective); valproic acid 300–600 mg po bid; lamotrigine 200–400 mg po daily; baclofen 10–20 mg po tid; oxcarbazepine 300–600 mg po bid; gabapentin 300–1,200 mg po tid; topiramate 100–200 mg po bid; clonazepam 1–2 mg po tid; tiagabine: 12–56 mg po/d. If exacerbation: phenytoin 1 gm IV or lidocaine 1.5 mg/kg IV over 30 min. Surgical options if refractory.

■ **Analgesic rebound headaches**
Completely eliminate analgesics; use temporary dihydroergotamine; consider starting gabapentin or topamax to blunt the pain of rebound HA; in severe cases, inpatient rx for detoxification.

TABLE 14.14. Headache Syndrome Tracking

Headache syndromes	Location	Characteristics	Duration	Associated symptoms	Exacerbating factors	Relieving factors
Tension	Global bilateral	♀ > ♂ M. band-like pain or bilateral tightness	Variable min–hrs	Fatigue, unaffected by activity, nausea rare	Stress	Relaxation Biofeedback
Cluster	Retroorbital beriorbital bnilateral	Abrupt onset, M. F deep and stabbing, people are restless	5–80 min. Headache clusters	Ipsilateral lacrimation rhinorrhea, eye redness, miosis, ptosis, and sweating	Alcohol or nitroglycerin use	None
Migraines	70% unilateral	Rarely starts . 40 years, gradual onset, pulsating quality F . M, positive family history and migraine triggers	4–72 hrs	Nausea, vomiting, photophobia, phonophobia, and/or aura (classical)*	Activity, exertion, bright light, loud noise, and valsalva	Rest Darkness Quiet
Temporal arteritis	Temporal frontal	Tender temporal artery (33%) and age . 50	Variable severity	Fever, myalgias, fatigue, weight loss, ipsilateral blindness, ESR > 50, jaw claudication, and polymyalgia rheumatica		None
Trigeminal neuralgia	Trigeminal nerve area	Paroxysms of shock-like or stabbing pain in cheeks and jaw	Seconds—up to 2 min	Usually . 50 years	Brushing teeth Touching face Wind on face	None
Subarachnoid hemorrhage	Global	Sudden onset of "worst headache of my life"	Constant and severe	+/– Loss of consciousness vomiting, meningismus, and photophobia	Bright light	Darkness
Medical rebound	Global	Chronic analgesic overuse > 3x/week	Hours	Analgesic abuse mood disorders	Not applicable	Stopping medication

* Aura 5 fully reversible visual scotomata, fortification spectra, or oscillating lines, focal numbness or paresthesias, dysphasia, dysphasia, epigastric discomfort, fear or a bad smell developing gradually over 5 min. ESR = erythrocyte sedimentation rate (mm/hr)

ENDOCRINE SYSTEM

■ **Hyperthyroidism (thyrotoxicosis)**

- **Causes**: most frequently: exophtalmic goiter (Graves disease) and toxic nodular goiter
- **Medical sx**: sweating, diarrhea, tachycardia, weight loss, vomiting, fine tremor
- **Psychiatric sx**: insomnia, mood lability, ↓ concentration, hyperactivity, anxiety, dysphoria, pressured speech, short attention span, possible hallucinations, paranoia, and delirium
- **Lab**: ↑ Free T4, ↑ T3, ↓ TSH, ECG changes (atrial fibrillation, tachycardia, P and T wave changes)
- **R/O**: amphetamine or cocaine intoxication, anxiety, mania, CV disease
- **Rx may be**: Propylthiouracil (*PTU*), methimazole (*Tapazole*); radioactive iodine (*RAI*): sodium iodide I-131 (*Iodotope*), surgery. B-adrenergic receptor antagonists give sx relief. If needed, avoid low-potency antipsychotics (↑ pulse). Avoid TCAs. If depression, use SSRIs. Rx of the cause resolves the psychiatric sx. *Watch out for overtreated hyperthyroidism and appearance of hypothyroidism sx.*

■ **Hypothyroidism (myxedema)**

- **Medical sx**: cold intolerance, dry skin, constipation, ↑ weight, hair loss
- **Psychiatric sx**: depression, apathy, impaired memory, psychosis, paranoia, ↓ concentration; risk of refractory depression (will respond to the addition of liothyronine)
- **Lab**: ↑ TSH (unless due to pituitary disease), ↓ free T4, ECG (bradycardia)
- **R/O**: lithium therapy, pituitary or hypothalamic disease, MDD, bipolar I disorder (depressive type)
- **Rx may be**: Levothyroxine (*L-Thyroxine, Levolet, Levo-T, Levothroid, Levoxyl, Synthroid, T4*); Liothyronine (*T3, Cytomel, Triostat*); Levothyroxine + liothyronine (*Thyrolar*) = T4 + T3. *Watch out for overtreated hypothyroidism with appearance of hyperthyroidism sx.*

■ **Diabetes mellitus**

- **Ketoacidosis**:
  - Medical sx: polyuria, anorexia, dehydration, vomiting, acetone breath
  - Psychiatric sx: violence, confusion, agitation, delirium, possible seizures
  - Lab: ↑ glucose, urine ketones, acidosis, glycosuria
  - **Complex medical management** and supportive rx needed. Insulin may be involved in learning and memory. ↑ depression in pts with diabetes. Antipsychotics deregulates insulin metabolism

- **Hypoglycemia**:
  - Medical sx: sweating, drowsiness, tachycardia, tremor, possible seizures, coma
  - Psychiatric sx: anxiety, confusion, agitation
  - Lab: hypoglycemia, tachycardia
  - R/O: insulinoma, postictal states, agitated depression, paranoia

■ **Cushing syndrome**

- **Causes**: ↑ ACTH (pituitary adenoma); adrenal pathology
- **Medical sx**: central obesity, osteoporosis, proximal muscle weakness, purple striae, bruises
- **Psychiatric sx**: depression to manic sx with or without psychosis, suicidality, insomnia, delirium, agitation, ↓ energy, ↓ concentration
- **Rx**: tumors respond to surgery or irradiation. Medications (cause drowsiness): metyrapone (*Metopirone*) or cyproheptadine (*Periactine*)

■ **Addison disease**

- **Medical sx**: nausea, anorexia, ↓ BP, stupor, hyperpigmentation, coma
- **Psychiatric sx**: lethargy, depression, psychosis, delirium, fatigue
- **Lab**: ↓ Na+, ↑ K+, eosinophilia. ECG: ↓ QTc

■ **Hyperparathyroidism**

- **Medical sx**: nausea, constipation, polydipsia
- **Psychiatric sx**: depression, confusion, paranoia
- **Lab**: ↑ Ca

■ **Hypoparathyroidism**

- **Medical sx**: headache, tetany, carpopedal spasms, laryngeal spasm, abdominal pain, low BP
- **Psychiatric sx**: anxiety, depression, confusion, ↓ memory
- **Lab**: ↓ Ca ++; ECG: ↑ QTc, ventricular arrhythmias

■ **Hyperprolactinemia**: all antipsychotics ↑ prolactin (except clozapine, and olanzapine), as well as TCAs, SSRIs; hypothyroidism, pregnancy, breastfeeding, stimulation of the nipples ↑ prolactinemia.

TABLE 14.15. Endocrine Complications of Psychopharmacologic Agents

Impaired functions	Responsible agents	Recommendations
Thyroid function	Lithium: ↓ T3, ↓ T4, ↑ TSH which ↑ thyroid growth and nodularity Valproic acid: modest ↑ in TSH Quetiapine: ↓ T4 sometimes If above drugs are combined: synergistic inhibitory effect on thyroid function	Pts on lithium: baseline TSH then at 1, 6, 12 months after starting and q yr. If pt becomes hypothyroid: start thyroxine after medical consultation
Growth	Stimulants: slow growth in children with ADHD, usually for the first several years then regularize (due to ↓ appetite). Growth hormone secretion is normal	Height and weight at baseline and q 6 months while on stimulants. If height ↓ by more than 1 SD while on rx, obtain pediatric endocrine consultation
Hyperprolactinemia	Antipsychotics: Risperidone > Haloperidol > Olanzapine > Ziprasidone > Quetiapine > Clozapine > Aripiprazole Aripiprazole: has partial D2-DA agonist activity and ↓ prolactin level below baseline levels Effects are variable: prolactin → ↓ GRH → ↓ LH and FSH (hypogonadism, amenorrhea, puberty failure, ↓ libido, osteoporosis), ↑ lactation (galactorrhea, breast enlargement), inhibits penile erection, stimulates adrenal androgens (hirsutism) Antipsychotics do not seem to induce PRL-secreting pituitary tumors	Ask about menstruation, nipple discharge, sexual functioning, and puberty. If problems, check prolactin level. If ↑: pregnancy test, TSH, creatinine Management: ● **PRL <200 ng/mL**: ↓ dose of antipsychotic, or switch to a more PRL-sparing drug ● **PRL >200 ng/mL** or stays high after switch: MRI scan of sella turcica to R/O pituitary adenoma or para-sellar tumor. If MRI normal: treat hypogonadism, osteoporosis ● Rarely rx with dopamine antagonists such as cabergoline (*Dostinex*) or amantadine (*Symmetrel*): (risk of ↑ psychosis). Some suggesting evidence that aripiprazole is efficacious in treating iatrogenic and tumorogenic hyperprolactinemia
Metabolic syndrome (hyperinsulinemia due to insulin resistance)	Adults: ≥3 of the following criteria: ● **Waist circumference** > 40 inches (102 cm) in ♂ or >35 inches (88 cm) in ♀ ● **Fasting serum triglycerides** ≥150 mg/dL ● **Fasting HDL-C** <40 mg/dL in ♂ or <50 mg/dL in ♀ ● **BP** ≥130/85 mm Hg ● **Fasting blood glucose** ≥110 mg/dL Children: BMI is age and gender specific Risks of atypical antipsychotics: Clozapine = olanzapine > risperidone = quetiapine > aripiprazole = ziprasidone	**Diabetes monitoring**: all pts: FBS at baseline and q 6 months. High-risk pts (obese, rapid weight ↑, family hx of DM, blacks, pts on clozapine or olanzapine): FBS q month or q 3 months. If possible, use alternative drug choices. Diabetes may remit when drugs are stopped **Lipid monitoring**: fasting lipid panel at baseline then at 3 months then q yr for all pts. If high-risk pts, q 3 months. Rx: diet, fibrates, fish oil, statins, niacin, switch to lower-risk antipsychotic **Obesity monitoring**: each visit: weight and BMI, waist circumference at umbilicus, counseling on diet and exercise. If gain > 5%: switch drug. In resistant cases: Orlistat (Xenical), sibutramine (Merida), Metformin (Glucophage), topiramate (Topamax), amantadine (Symmetrel)
Polycystic ovary syndrome (PCOS) (chronic anovulation and hyperandrogenism, with or without polycystic ovaries, linked to insulin resistance, dyslipidemia, obesity)	Valproic acid: ↑ risk of PCOS, possible direct ovarian androgen synthesis	Ask: about menstruation, hirsutism, advice on diet and exercise, refer to endocrinologist, gynecologist if needed, consider other mood stabilizers

Growth charts: www.cdc.gov/growthcharts. Resources for diagnosis of metabolic syndrome in children and adolescents: www.kidsnutrition.org/bodycomp/bmiz2.html. Cook, S. (2004). The metabolic syndrome: Antecedent of adult cardiovascular disease in pediatrics. *Journal of Pediatrics, 145*(4), 439–444.

CHRONIC PAIN

See End of life care chapter in electronic addendum.

NEUROLOGIC CONDITIONS PRESENTING WITH PSYCHIATRIC SYMPTOMS

■ Head trauma

See also Chapter 9 (dementia due to head trauma.)

Pathophysiology: common, M > F, > in 15–25 yo; neuropsychiatric sequelae; 50% due to MVA but also falls, violence, sports-related. Blunt trauma involves actual trauma and "crashing + stretching" of the brain (back and forth violent movements) → hemorrhage + edema; many acute and chronic clinical pictures; duration of disorientation is an approximate guide to prognosis.

Symptoms: cognitive impairments (↓ attention, ↓ speed of information processing, ↓ problem-solving skills, ↑ distractibility, memory and learning problems) and behavioral sequelae (depression, agitation, ↑ impulsivity, ↑ aggression, personality changes); possibility of psychosis, delirium.

Course: depends on mental constitution, premorbid personality, epilepsy, environment, litigation, response in intellectual losses, amount and location of brain damage.

Treatment: treat sx; caution with medications' SE; psychotherapy.

■ Seizure disorders

Definition: involuntary activity, perception or behavior as a result of abnormal neuronal discharges in the cerebral cortex. It is epilepsy if the condition is chronic with recurrent seizures. The ictus is the seizure itself. The nonictal periods are preictal, postictal, or interictal.

Two categories:

- **Generalized seizures** (loss of consciousness, generalized tonic-clonic movements of limbs, tongue biting, incontinence, and postictal state with progressive clearing delirium): involve the entire brain. **Absence seizure or petit mal seizure is a type of generalized seizure** (no true loss of consciousness; no convulsive movement and has a characteristic pattern on EEG (*3/s spike and wave activity*)

- **Partial seizures:** epileptiform activity is in localized brain regions; may be **simple without alteration in consciousness, or complex,** *also called temporal lobe epilepsy, psychomotor seizures, limbic epilepsy,* **with an alteration in consciousness.** A nl EEG cannot exclude the diagnosis (needs: long-term recording, use of sphenoidal or anterior temporal electrodes, and sleep-deprived EEG)

Preictal symptoms (auras): jerking movements, autonomic changes (epigastric discomfort, blushing, respiration changes) fear, bad smell, focal sensory or psychic symptoms (fear, panic, depression, elation), cognitive sensations (déjà vu, jamais-vu, forced thinking, dreamy states), automatisms (facial grimacing, gesturing, lip smacking, finger snapping, walking, undressing).

Ictal symptoms: usually disorganized, brief, and uninhibited behaviors with amnesia during seizure and a period of resolving delirium after the seizure.

Interictal symptoms may be:

- **Personality disturbances: particularly in TLE** (religiosity, viscosity, quality of personality/slow, ponderous, pedantic, circumstantial quality with hypergraphia, changes in sexual behavior, heightened experience of emotions)

- **Psychotic sx: mostly with TLE** (> if left-sided lesions, ♀, left-handedness); paranoid delusions and hallucinations (normal affect, no thought blocking or looseness of associations vs Schizophrenia)

- **Violence:** mostly if temporal or frontal lobe origin, but very rare

- **Mood disorder sx:** if origin is temporal lobe of the nondominant cerebral hemisphere; depression or mania tend to be episodic; ↑ attempted suicide in epileptic pts

TABLE 14.16.   Seizures: Generalities

- All seizures may be convulsive or nonconvulsive
- May be partial, primary generalized, or secondary generalized
- Partial: can be simple without impairment of consciousness and may not have associated EEG changes
- Complex partial seizures have impairment of consciousness at onset
- Simple partial seizures may progress to complex partial seizure with or without secondary generalization
- Primary generalized seizures initially involve both hemispheres: can be absence, typical or atypical, myoclonic seizures, tonic, clonic, tonic-clonic, and atonic (astatic seizures)
- Secondary generalized seizures have a focal onset with secondary generalization
- An aura is a simple partial seizure
- May be frontal, parietal, or occipital seizures
- Stereotypicity in seizures

TABLE 14.17.   Classification of Seizures

Seizure Type G: generalized P: partial	Impaired consciousness	Tongue biting or incontinence	Aura	Hyperventilation triggers	Automatisms	Postictal duration
Simple partial seizure (P)	No	No	Yes	No	No	Seconds
Complex partial seizure (P)	Yes	No	Yes first	No	Yes (after aura)	Minutes–hours
Secondary generalized partial seizure (G)	Yes	Yes	Yes first	No	Possibly	Minutes–hours
Absence seizure (petit mal seizure) (G)	Yes	No	No	Yes	No	Seconds
Grand mal seizure (G)	Yes	Yes	In 50%	No	No	Minutes–hours

Some particular generalized seizures: (there is a loss of consciousness; affect both cerebral hemispheres from the beginning of the seizure).

- **Myoclonic seizures**: rapid, brief contractions of muscles, occurring at the same time on both sides of the body. Occasionally, they involve one arm or a foot.
- **Atonic seizures**: abrupt loss of muscle tone. Other names; drop attacks, astatic or akinetic seizures. They produce head drops, loss of posture, or sudden collapse; may result in injury of head and face
- **Infantile spasms**: clusters of quick, sudden movements that start between 3 months and 2 yr. If a child is sitting up, the head will fall forward, and the arms will flex forward. If lying down, the knees will be drawn up, with arms and head flexed forward.

Etiologies: posttraumatic, low Na+, low Mg++, hypoglycemia, hypocalcemia, congenital brain malformation, hyper or hypothyroidism, dialysis equilibrium syndrome, porphyria, severe hypoxia, CO_2 poisoning, meningitis, stroke, alcohol or benzodiazepine withdrawal, medications' SE, idiopathic. **Seizure triggers**: strong emotions, intense exercise, flashing lights, fever, menses, lack of sleep, stress.

History: + family hx, head trauma, febrile seizures, birth complications, substance abuse, sinusitis or otitis media, fever/headache/stiffness, HIV+, hx of cancer.

Work-up: chemistry panel, drug screen, EEG, TSH, LP for meningismus.

Imaging: noncontrast head CT scan for head trauma, new severe headache, anticoagulated pts. MRI preferred for focal neuro deficits, persistently altered mental status, hx of cancer, possible AIDS.

Differential diagnosis: migraines, syncope, TIA, pseudo-seizures, sleep disorder, conversion disorder, movement disorder.

TABLE 14.18.   Epilepsy vs Pseudoseizures

Features	Epilepsy	Pseudo-seizure (may exist alone or with a seizure disorder)
Clinical features	Common nocturnal seizure Presence of stereotyped aura Common self-injury Common incontinence Postictal confusion present Tonic or clonic (or both) body movements Nonaffected by suggestion	Uncommon nocturnal seizure No stereotyped aura Rare self-injury Rare incontinence No postictal confusion Nonstereotyped body movements Affected by suggestion
EEG	Spike and wave activity during seizure Postictal slowing	No spike and wave activity No postictal slowing
Prolactin level	↑ in primarily or secondarily generalized tonic-clonic seizures and partial complex seizures: ↑ up to 3–20×; Simple protocol: check serum prolactin level 20 min and 12 hr postictally (24 hr in outpatient settings) in pts whose seizure frequency is <1 in 12 hr	No change (or less than 2×) Cannot be used to differentiate simple partial seizures or absence seizures from nonepileptic seizures

Risks for recurrent seizures: hx of closed head injury, structural brain lesion, focal neuro exam, cognitive impairment, partial seizures, abnormal EEG, positive family hx.

Indications for chronic antiepileptic drug (AED) use:

Start after first seizure + 2 risk factors or start after second seizure

Discontinuation of rx: wean AED 25% every 2–4 wk; can attempt once seizure-free for at least 2–3 yr; ↑ risk of seizures if risk factors present, abnormal EEG, or abnormal imaging

Special precautions in pregnant women (risk of birth defects **(NAAED) Pregnancy Registry**: toll free number 1-888-233-2334)

TABLE 14.19.   Treatment

Medication	Pt age (yr)	AS	PS	GS	Starting po dose (mg)	Therapeutic dose (mg)	SE/monitoring
Carbamazepine*	≥6		+		200 bid	400 tid[†]	Hyponatremia, osteopenia, hepatitis, rash, leucopenia; follow levels, LFTs, CBC
Clonazepam‡	>10			+	0.5 tid	1.5 mg tid	Sedation, confusion, anemia, leucopenia
Ethosuximide*	>6	+			250 daily	250–750 bid[†]	GI upset, rare depression, psychosis, leucopenia
Ethotoin			+	+	≤ 1 g/d in 4–6 divided doses	0.5–3 g/d	Therapeutic levels; GI upsets
Felbamate*	≥2		+		400 tid	400–1,200 tid	GI upset, insomnia, hepatitis, aplastic anemia/ CBC
Gabapentin‡	≥3		+		300 q hr	300–1,200 tid	Somnolence, dizziness, weight gain, fatigue
Lamotrigine*	≥2		+	+	50 daily	200 bid	Rash, headache, tremor, vomiting, insomnia, diplopia
Levetiracetamil‡	≥16		+		500 bid	500–1,500 bid	Somnolence, asthenia, headache, agitation, anxiety, may produce behavioral problems, mood problems
Methsuximide		(Refractory AS)			300 mg daily; ↑ weekly	1,200 mg/d	CBC, UA, LFTs, suicidal thoughts and behaviors, rash, Steven-Johnson syndrome
Oxcarbazepine*	≥4		+		300 bid	600 bid	Dizziness, diplopia, nausea, ataxia, hyponatremia
Phenobarbital*	>12		+		60 daily	150 daily[†]	Rash, sedation, cognitive delays/follow levels
Phenytoin*	>16		+	+	1 gm load	300 daily[†]	Rash, gingival hyperplasia, mild hirsutism, hepatitis, osteopenia; follow drug levels and LFTs
Pregabalin	Not approved in children		As adjunct in adults		150 mg/d (divided bid or tid)	Max 600 mg/d in divided doses	Changes in visual acuity, muscle pains, ↑ CPK, peripheral edema if used with thiazolidinediones, withdrawal sx (taper off)

Continued

TABLE 14.19.   Treatment   Continued

Medication	Pt age (yr)	AS	PS	GS	Starting po dose (mg)	Therapeutic dose (mg)	SE/monitoring
Primidone‡	≥8		+		100 q hr	250 tid–qid	Rash, sedation, cognitive delays; follow levels
Tiagabine‡	≥12		+		4 mg daily	4–8 mg bid–qid	Dizziness, tremor, hair loss; follow levels
Topiramate‡	≥2		+	+	25 daily	200 bid	Ataxia, confusion, dizziness, fatigue, paresthesias, acidosis, nephrolithiasis, weight loss, ocular symptoms
Valproic acid*	>10	+	+	+	250 tid	500–750 tid†	Weight gain, tremors, hair loss; follow levels
Zonisamide‡	≥16		+	+	100 daily	200 daily	Fatigue, paresthesias, nephrolithiasis, anorexia, dizziness, ataxia, hyperhydrosis

Approved as monotherapy.

†Adjust based on serum drug levels.

‡Used as an adjunctive medication.

AS, absence seizures; GS, generalized seizures including tonic-clonic, clonic, myoclonic, atonic seizures; PS, partial seizures including partial complex seizures with secondary generalization.

Sources: Beyenburg, S., Bauer, J., Reuber, M. (2004). New drugs for the treatment of epilepsy: A practical approach. Postgraduate Medical Journal, 80(948), 581–587; LaRoche, S. M., & Helmers, S. L. (2004). The new antiepileptic drugs: Scientific review. Journal of the American Medical Association, 291(5), 605–614; LaRoche, S. M., & Helmers, S. L. (2004). The new antiepileptic drugs: Clinical applications. Journal of the American Medical Association, 291(5), 615–620; Vazquez, B. (2004). Monotherapy in epilepsy: Role of the newer antiepileptic drugs. Archives of Neurology, 61(9), 1361–1365; Bazil, C. W., & Pedley, T. A. (2003). Clinical pharmacology of antiepileptic drugs. Clinical Neuropharmacology, 26(1), 38–52.

■ **Demyelinating disorders**

Multiple sclerosis (MS): multiple episodes of sx with remission and exacerbations (sudden transient motor and sensory disturbances, impaired vision, slurred speech, incontinence); multifocal white matter lesions of the CNS (slow viral infection; immunological disturbances, CSF with ↑ gamma globulines, CT with degenerative patches in brain and spinal cord); prevalence: 50/100,000; more in cold and temperate climates; W > M; onset: 20–40 yo. Cognitive sx: mild in 30–50%, severe in 20–30% (mostly memory impairments). Behavioral sx: euphoria; depression: 25–50% (↑ suicide in ♂ and if onset <30 yo; recent diagnosis); personality changes (20–40%, irritability or apathy); rare psychosis.

Amyotrophic lateral sclerosis: progressive asymmetric muscle atrophy and sx of pyramidal tract; begins in adulthood; all muscles except cardiac and ocular muscles. Prevalence: 1.6/100,000; possible dementia; Death usually in 4 yr.

- **Encephalopathy**: for example, hepatic encephalopathy (euphoria, disinhibition, psychosis, or depression)

- **Strokes, TIA, subarachnoid hemorrhage**: infarction in cortical or subcortical areas may produce focal neurologic deficits including cognitive and emotional changes; diagnosis: clinical sx, MRI scans; depression is frequent and may cause pseudo-dementia; possible vascular dementia. *MDD will occur in 60% of pts with a left hemispheric lesion* and in 15% of pt with a right lesion (if untreated, the depression will last 8–9 months). *The closer the insult to the left frontal pole, the more depressed the pt will be. In right hemisphere lesions, the closer it is to the occipital pole, the more likely the pt is to be depressed* (however, if the lesion is in the right anterior location: ↑ apathy + inappropriate cheerfulness). In right hemisphere injury: differentiate "aprosodia/lack of inflection, rhythm and intensity of expression and depression," as a pt may have both

■ **Brain tumors**

50% have mental sx particularly if tumors are located in the frontal or limbic brain regions (rather than in parietal or temporal regions). Most frequently, *meningiomas → focal sx and gliomas (40–50% in 40–50 yo) → diffuse sx*; cerebellar tumors are most common in children. *Slow developing tumors give more personality changes as rapid tumors give more cognitive changes*. Delirium appears if rapidly growing or large or metastatatic tumors. Steroids used in the rx may produce behavioral and psychiatric sx. *Suspect frontal lobe tumor if incontinence and a temporal lobe tumor if abnormal memory or speech*. Sx are: headache, vomiting, papilledema, seizures, visual loss, focal finding, CT scan. Personality changes, mood changes, irritability, hallucinations are possible.

TABLE 14.20. Psychiatric Symptoms in Brain Tumors

Frontal lobe tumors	Depression, inappropriate affect, disinhibition, dementia, impaired coordination, psychotic symptoms
Temporal lobe tumors	Anxiety, depression, hallucinations (esp. gustatory and olfactory), TLE symptoms, schizophreniform-like psychosis
Parietal lobe tumors	Less psychiatric sx with anosognosia, autopagnosia, apraxia, aphasia

For effects depending on the specific location of the tumor in the brain, see Chapter 3, Psychiatric and neurologic assessment (Tables 3.2–3.10).

AUTOIMMUNE DISORDERS

Systemic lupus erythematosus: autoimmune multisystemic disease. Sx: fever, photosensitivity, butterfly rash, headache, joint pains; psychiatric sx (in 50%): depression, mood disorders, psychosis; diagnosis: + ANA, positive lupus erythematosus test, anemia, ↓ platelets; pleural effusion, pericarditis; steroids may produce psychiatric sx.

GENETIC DISORDERS

- Acute intermittent porphyria: autosomal dominant; may be precipitated by many drugs; medical sx: abdominal pain, fever, GI upsets, peripheral neuropathy, paralysis; psychiatric sx: depression, agitation, psychosis; lab: leukocytosis, ↑ delta aminolevulinic acid, ↑ porphobilinogen, tachycardia

- Wilson's disease: autosomal recessive disorder of copper metabolism with hepatolenticular degeneration; present in adolescence; medical sx: Kayser-Fleisher corneal ring, hepatitis, choreoathetoid movements, gait disturbance, rigidity; psychiatric sx: mood disorders, psychosis; lab: ↓ serum ceruloplasmin, ↑ copper in urine

- Huntington disease: autosomal dominant; medical sx: rigidity, choreoathetoid movements; psychiatric sx: depression, euphoria (see dementias in Chapter 9)

INFECTIONS

- Neurosyphilis: onset 10–15 yr after primary infection; affects frontal lobes; medical sx are: skin lesions, leukoplakia, periostitis, arthritis, progressive respiratory, cardiovascular distress; psychiatric sx: personality changes, poor judgment, irritability, delusions of grandeur (10–20%), dementia, tremor, paresis: Argyll-Robertson pupils (small, irregular, unequal with light-near reflex dissociation), tremor, dysarthria, hyperreflexia, CSF (↑ lymphocytes, ↑ protein) and VDRL is +

- AIDS: see Chapter 15.

- Herpes simplex encephalitis: focal encephalitis; affects frontal and temporal lobes; sx: anosmia, olfactory, gustatory hallucinations, personality changes, memory loss, psychosis; possible complex partial epilepsy

- Rabies encephalitis: rapidly fatal

- Chronic meningitis: more seen because of AIDS; due to *Mycobacterium tuberculosis*, Cryptococcus and Coccidioides; sx: headache, memory loss, fever, confusion

- Subacute sclerosing panencephalitis: after measles; in childhood; death in 1–2 yr

- Lyme disease: due to spirochete *Borrelia burgdorferi* (bite of deer tick); sx: bull's-eye rash at the site of the bite followed by flulike sx, cognitive and mood changes (↓memory, ↓concentration, irritability, depression); possible seropositve test for the spirochete; may become chronic if untreated (rx: Doxycycline/*Vibramycin* for 14–21 days); support groups exist

- Prion diseases: caused by transmissible infectious protein (prions that lack nucleic acid are mutated proteins coming from the human prion protein gene or PrP located on the short arm of chromosome 20; PrP mutates in different ways producing specific prion diseases; prenatal testing for abnormal PrP gene is available); include Creutzfeldt-Jakob disease (CJD), Gerstmann-Straussler syndrome (GSS), fatal familial insomnia (FFI), and kuru. The "mad cow disease" is a variant of CJD (transmission of bovine spongiform encephalopathy from cattle to human) (see dementias in Chapter 9)

- Tuberculosis: INH (inhibits monoamine oxidase) may produce memory impairment, confusion, euphoria, acute psychosis; Rifampin: possible memory problems, confusion; Ethionamide and cycloserine: possible depression and confusion; Cycloserine: possible toxic psychosis

NUTRITIONAL PROBLEMS

- Thiamine deficiency (vitamin B_1): beriberi (neuropathy, cardiomyopathy; Asia, famine areas) or Wernicke-Korsakoff syndrome (confabulation, confusion; due to chronic alcohol abuse); sx: apathy, depression, irritability, poor concentration, memory loss; lab: low thiamine level

- Niacin deficiency (nicotinic acid): pellagra seen in alcohol abuse, vegetarian diets, extreme poverty, starvation. Sx: apathy, irritability, insomnia, depression, stocking-glove dermatitis, diarrhea, delirium, dementia, death ("5 Ds")

- **Cobalamin deficiency (vitamin B$_{12}$)**: the lack of secretion by gastric cells of intrinsic factor prevents absorption of vitamin B$_{12}$ in the ileum; sx: macrocytic megaloblastic anemia (pernicious anemia); changes in peripheral nerves, spinal cord, and brain (80% of pts), apathy, depression, and encephalopathy (megaloblastic madness: delirium, paranoid delusions, hallucinations, and dementia). Lab: low B$_{12}$ level, Schilling test, megaloblastic anemia
- **Pyridoxine deficiency (vitamin B$_6$)**: caused by INH rx; Sx: apathy, irritability, memory disturbances, muscle weakness, seizures and peripheral neuropathies

CANCER/PSYCHO-ONCOLOGY

Cancer's impact on psychologic functions; role of psychologic variables on cancer risk and survival; reactions to the diagnosis and to the rx of cancer are important. Half of all cancer pts have mental disorders (adjustment disorders in 68%, MDD in 13%, delirium in 8%). Suicidality is frequent.

TABLE 14.21. Reasons for Consultations of Cancer Patients

Depression: 20% with MDD; see drugs implicated in following table; think also about infections

Delirium: often mislabeled depression

Psychosis: R/O steroid psychosis

Altered cognition: R/O meningitis, brain abscess

Weakness: drugs implicated (steroids, vincristine); combined chemo and radiations, bed rest; rx: physical rx, specific to etiology, may be due to progressing cancer

Treatment-resistant pain: see End of life care chapter in electronic addendum

Anticipatory nausea: 50% of chemotherapy pts have GI toxicity after 4–5th session; rx: systematic, desensitize, hypnosis, relaxation techniques, benzodiazepines

TABLE 14.22. Causes of Delirium in Cancer Patients

(Second common consultation problem in cancer pt: delirium can be hyperactive, hypoactive, or mixed); see delirium in Chapter 9)

Metabolic encephalopathy; hypoglycemia, hyperglycemia

Organ failure: liver, kidney, respiratory failure, pancreas

Electrolyte imbalance, dehydration, hypercalcemia, hyponatremia

Hypoxia

Radiations: delayed radiation encephalopathy

Nutritional deficiencies (thiamine, folic acid, B$_{12}$, malnourishment)

Infections ($\uparrow$ if immunosuppression), UTI, pneumonia, sepsis

Vascular disorders (coagulopathies), ischemia

Endocrine and hormonal abnormalities

Medications:
- Hormones: steroids, tamoxifen, diethylstilbestrol, chlorotrianisene
- Biologicals: interferon, interleukins, cytokines
- Chemotherapy agents: asparaginase, fluorouracil, cysplatin cytarabine, methotrexate, procarbazine, vincristine, vinblastine, chlorotrianisene, ifosfamide, bleomycin
- Medications: anticholinergic drugs, opioids, amphotericin B, quinolones, antiemetics, acyclovir, psychostimulants, benzodiazepines, NSAIDs, antihistaminics, TCAs (caution with combination of drugs)

Paraneoplastic limbic encephalitis

Brain metastases (from lung and breast cancers)

Advanced cancers

TABLE 14.23. Causes of Mood Disorders in Cancer Patients

Frequent SI but incidence of suicide only slightly greater than in the gl population

Medications:
- **Chemotherapy**: prednisone, dexamethasone, procarbazine, vincristine, vinblastine, L-asparaginase, interferon, methotrexate high IV dose, 5-Azacytadine, cytarabine, hormones (aminoglutethimide, tamoxifen, testosterone)
- **Opiates**
- **Drugs inducing depression**: antihypertensives, benzodiazepines, antiparkinson drugs, β-adrenergic receptor antagonists, steroids

Specific tumors:
- Hormone-secreting tumors
- Pancreatic cancer
- Central nervous system tumors

Associated medical conditions:
- Uremia and electrolyte imbalances
- Viral encephalopathies and other infections
- Cerebrovascular accidents
- Cancer pain
- Previous psychiatric disorders (substance abuse, mood disorders)

SKIN DISORDERS

Atopic dermatitis (atopic eczema, neurodermatitis): ↑ in anxious, depressed pts.

Psoriasis: Stress ↑ psoriasis and psoriasis → stress in interpersonal relationships (depression, anxiety, personality disorders, alcohol abuse).

Psychogenic excoriation (psychogenic pruritus): lesions due to scratching or picking with postinflammatory ↓ or ↑ of pigmentation.

Localized pruritus of the anus or the vulvae: starts with a local irritation or gl systemic disease (nutritional deficiencies, drug intoxication); perpetuated by scratching and inflammation; difficult to treat.

Hyperhidrosis: stress-induced ↑↑ sweating (palms, soles, axillae) leads to rashes, blisters, infections; R/O: drug-induced hyperhidrosis.

SPECIFIC PROBLEMS LINKED TO SPECIALIZED UNITS

Hemodialysis units: depression; suicide; sexual problems; **dialysis dementia** after many years, was due to ↑ exposure to aluminum salts;. Dealing with x issues (debilitating disease, dependency, disruption of life; depends on personality styles, previous experiences, social factors, support system, preparation, prior dialysis, expectations, location of rx).. If psychiatric drugs are needed: use more hepatically metabolized drugs at lower doses with ↑ dosage intervals.

Surgical units: delirium, depression, anxiety weaning from respirator

Transplantation units: help waiting to receive transplants, anxiety about the procedure, fear of death, organ rejection, life after transplant, aftercare of transplant. Treat MDD, adjustment reactions (20% of pt after 1 yr), suicidal thoughts, PTD, issues about the origin of the transplant (cadaver donor vs living donor), ethical issues.

Obstetric-gynecologic units: at risk pregnancies; difficult deliveries; premature babies in PICU.

ICUs: suicide attempt, overdose, depression, character disorder, delirium, drug and/or alcohol abuse, anxiety. R/O: delirium (more likely if severe illness), toxic reactions to medications, substance withdrawal. Review metabolic status, neurologic findings. R/O pain, anxiety, sensory isolation. R/O dementia; use physical restraints with caution; assess reasons for noncompliance with rx (pt–doctor relationship, negative transference, fears of medications or procedure, R/O cognitive disorder).

Burns unit: risk factors: drug and alcohol abuse, dementias, mental illness (schizophrenia, BPD), children from disadvantaged families (lack of supervision, abusive household). Caring for a burn victim:

- *Acute phase:* surgical care; delirium in 30–70% of pts (stress-induced metabolic disturbances, severity, and extent of the burns), hallucinations + agitation (risk for the recent grafts, caution with schizophrenic pts), pain (during dressing changes, pain medications must be available), SE from analgesics; two issues to deal with: denial + need for explanation (nature of the injury, degree of disfigurement, nature of rx, consequences): work to be done with the pt + family

- *Reconstitutive phase:* time of facing the injury, beginning to accept losses, of painful dressing changes, physical rx, loneliness; reevaluate premorbid psychologic status, coping skills, self-esteem, family support; grief work and venting of feelings if loss of family member in the fire; wound healing is done by small increments (realistic expectations, small goals, positive attitude, group rx); management of regression

- *Long-term adjustment phase:* avoid social withdrawal (if facial deformities); great need for psychotherapy

15 ■ NEUROPSYCHIATRIC ASPECTS OF HIV INFECTION AND AIDS

AIDS Clinical Trials Information Service: http://www.actis.org

AIDS Treatment News Online: http://www.immunet.org/atn

AIDS Treatment Guidelines: www.aidsinfo.nih.gov

CDC's National Center for HIV, STD, and TB Prevention Web site: http://www.cdc.gov/nchstp/od/nchstp.html

CDC National AIDS Hotline in English: (800) 342-2437

CDC National AIDS Hotline in Spanish: (800) 344-7432

CDC's National Prevention Information Network: http://www.cdcnpin.org **or (800) 458-5231 (information available in English and Spanish)**

HIV/AIDS Treatment Information Service: http://www.hivatis.org **or (800) 448-0440 (information available in English and Spanish)**

National Clinicians' Post-Exposure Prophylaxis Hotline: http://pepline.ucsf.edu/PEPline **or (888) 448-4911**

TRANSMISSION

- Brain involvement in 75–90% of autopsies of pts who had AIDS; HIV infection in 3.1% of the mentally ill (0.3% of gl population); 50% of pts have neuropsychiatric complications (HIV encephalopathy: in 10% of those pts, it is the first manifestation of the disease).

- **HIV**: a ribonucleic acid (RNA) containing retrovirus (ability to make DNA from RNA) infects cells of the immune and nervous systems. **HIV carries three enzymes** responsible for its life cycle (**reverse transcriptase, protease, and integrase** → treatments with transcriptase inhibitors and protease inhibitors).

- **Mechanism**: infection of T4 (helper) lymphocytes produces impaired cell-mediated immunity (infections and neoplasm). Infections of cells (primarily astrocytes) within the CNS causes neuropsychiatric syndromes to appear, complicated by opportunistic infections, neoplasms, antiviral treatments, independent psychiatric disorders, social stresses, and substance abuse

- **HIV is present in** blood, semen, saliva, cervical, vaginal secretions, tears, breast milk, and CSF. Transmission is either through sexual intercourse (anal, vaginal, and rarely oral) or contaminated blood.

- **Infection possible after one exposure**: unprotected vaginal sex (0.05–0.15%), unprotected receptive anal intercourse (0.8–3.2%), HIV-contaminated needle puncture (0.32%), contaminated needle to use drugs (0.67%). Risk ↑ with higher viral load, other STDs present (herpes, syphilis), skin disorders.

- **Only 50% of regular sexual partners of people with HIV** become infected themselves; ↑ in gay, bisexual ♂, and IV substance abusers. ♀ are infected through heterosexual contact more than through IV drug use. There is a link between crack cocaine use and HIV infection in ♀.

- **Children** may be infected in utero or from breast milk (prevented in >95% of HIV-infected pregnant ♀ if they are treated with Zidovudine and protease inhibitors).

- **AIDS** develops 8–10 years after HIV infection, if not treated.

TABLE 15.1. Diagnosis

- **Serum testing**: enzyme-linked immunosorbent assay (ELISA) and the Western blot assay. Seroconversion occurs usually between 2 and 6 wk after infection, sometimes up to 12 months
- **Viral load testing**: number of viral copies per unit of blood. If <20 copies: considered undetectable but does not mean that the virus is absent; *level ≥100,000 copies is the most powerful predictor of AIDS*
- **CD4-T cells**: a marker for the extent of the immunosuppression. *Cell counts ≤200 cells/μL is a risk for opportunistic infections*. If one or the other is present, the diagnosis is AIDS, and prophylaxis medications (sulfamethoxazole) are given

TABLE 15.2. Psychiatric Workup of HIV Patients

• **Perform initial exams**: to differentiate primary psychiatric disorder from HIV-related CNS pathology (HIV-associated dementia, HIV-associated minor cognitive disorder, or opportunistic infections)	• **Cognitive workup**: look for attention, memory, and orientation deficits, sensorium state, mood, anxiety, psychotic symptoms (MMSE, HIV-Dementia scale) • **Physical workup**: look for secondary infection, neurological sx (meningitis; motor, sensory, cranial nerves focal signs due to intracranial mass lesions/CNS neoplasms or infections)
• Evaluate lab results: treatment started if: 　**Pt is symptomatic** 　**CD4 count < 500/mm₃** 　(normal values > 1,000/mm³) 　**If pt's viral load > 5,000 copies/mL**	• CBC, electrolytes, kidney and liver function, VDRL, CSF analysis (special stains to detect different organisms responsible for AIDS), CD4, viral load
• Neuroimaging	• MRI > CT scan to R/O cerebral atrophy, lesions (*lymphoma, intracranial toxoplasmosis*)
• Neuropsychological testing	• Which of the **brain functions** are compromised? (Will differentiate HIV dementia which is a subcortical dementia from Alzheimer's which is a cortical dementia)
• Make the diagnosis	• Psychiatric sx secondary to HIV • Psychiatric disorders independent of HIV • Psychiatric sx due to the HIV treatment • Psychiatric sx due to concomitant infection • **SE of psychotropic medications in AIDS pts with neurologic sx**: these pts are more sensitive: ↑ EPS, dystonia, parkinsonism, NMS, delirium. Amantadine may be better than anticholinergic agents to treat extrapyramidal effects

Source: Bradley, M., & Muskin, P. R. (2007). 5-step psychiatric workup of HIV patients. *Current Psychiatry, 6*(12), 11–17.

TABLE 15.3. Factors Associated with HIV and AIDS

• **Nonneurological factors** associated with AIDS	• **Pneumocystis carinii pneumonia**: the most common infection • **Kaposi's sarcoma**: frequency ↓ • **Retinopathy** • **Marantic endocarditis**
• **Neurological factors** associated with HIV infection	• **HIV-associated CNS infections**: 　**Common**: Cryptococcus neoformans meningitis, progressive multifocal leukoencephalopathy, toxoplasma gondii, neurosyphilis 　**Less common**: Aspergillosis, coccidioidomycosis, cytomegalovirus, herpes simplex or varicella-zoster encephalitis, histoplasmosis, leptomeningeal tuberculosis, candida, aspergillosis • **Encephalopathy HIV-related**: in 50% of infected pts; is a subacute encephalitis resulting in a progressive subcortical dementia. R/O: depression. May result in a delirium • **Lymphoma (primary or metastatic)** • **Peripheral neuropathy** • **Cerebral hemorrhage**

TABLE 15.4. CNS Infectious Complications of AIDS

- • **Viral**: Cytomegalovirus, herpes simplex I and II, Herpes Zoster, Papovavirus (progressive multifocal leukoencephalopathy), HTLV-III dementia
- • **Bacterial**: *Mycobacterium avium* intracellulare, *M. tuberculosis* hominis, Nocardia, *Listeria monocytogenes*
- • **Fungal**: Candida, *Cryptococcus neoformans, Histoplasma capsulatum*, Coccidioides immitis, Aspergillus, Blastomyces dermatitidis
- • **Protozoa**: Toxoplasma gondii

Concomitant mental illnesses: ↑ mortality, ↑ **suicide;** schizophrenia and MDD are risk factor for HIV (lack of judgment).

HIV pts are at high risk to develop depression, anxiety, psychotic disorders, or PTSD.

TABLE 15.5.   Comorbid Mental Illnesses with HIV

● Depression	● **Diagnostic challenge**: fatigue, ↓ appetite, ↓ libido, poor memory. Risk of nonadherence to rx ● **Precaution choosing the antidepressant**: antivirals such as didanosine (DDI/Videx), zalcitabine (DDC/HIVID) may give peripheral neuropathy. If pt has peripheral neuropathy: may choose TCAs. If diarrhea from HAART, consider an anticholinergic antidepressant ● **DDIs**: many anti-HIV agents act on CYP450 system: avoid antidepressant that inhibit or induce these enzymes (Paroxetine, fluvoxamine, fluoxetine → ↑ levels of antiretrovirals and ↑ their SE). Also some retrovirals (ritonavir/Norvir, delaviridine/Rescriptor) may inhibit or induce enzymes and ↑ levels of antidepressants. Nevirapine (Viramune) may induce the CYP system → ↓ level of psychotropic agents ● **TCAs**: may be used (follow drug levels); SE may be problematic (anticholinergic SE; orthostatic hypotension) ● **Antidepressants**: may cause delirium, confusion, ↑ dementia (looks like a subcortical dementia) ● **Low dose of methylphenidate** may improve cognitive and affective status
● Schizophrenia	● **HIV may affect basal ganglia**: choose antipsychotics with less EPS SE ● **Avoid clozapine** (immunocompromised pt with an ↑ risk of agranulocytosis) ● **Protease inhibitors** may ↑ weight, dyslipidemia, and glucose dysregulation (avoid clozapine, olanzapine). Olanzapine may be good if loss of weight and pt is not on protease inhibitors. **Caution with ritonavir**: ↑ metabolism of olanzapine (higher dosage of olanzapine may be necessary). Ritonavir + indinavir (Crixivan) + risperidone: ↑ risk of EPS and NMS. **Monitor for overlapping toxicity between antipsychotics and antiretroviral medications** ● **Psychosis as an adverse event from HIV medication**: efavirenz (Sustiva) to be given 3 hr prior to sleep to avoid vivid dreams or hallucinations
● Bipolar disorder	● **HIV pts may respond better to antipsychotics than to mood stabilizers**: use atypical antipsychotics (aripiprazole, olanzapine, risperidone, quetiapine, ziprasidone). Caution when pt is taking ritonavir ● **Risks with valproic acid**: anemia with zidovudine + valproic acid (by ↑ level of zidovudine). *Valproic acid may ↑ the replication of the virus* ● **Lithium's advantages**: avoids hepatic metabolism, blood levels available, may be neuroprotective ● **Carbamazepine is to be avoided**: induces the CYP system and may ↓ levels of antiretroviral agents; may contribute to rx resistance
● Anxiety disorders	● **In HIV + population**: GAD (15.8%), panic disorder (10%), PTSD(30–50%) ● **Benzodiazepines**: if used, choose short-acting (acronym LOT for lorazepam/Ativan, oxazepam/Serax, temazepam/Restoril) ● **Antidepressant**: useful, caution with DDI ● **Buspirone**: used if pt has a substance abuse hx but caution with ritonavir (CYP pathway)
● Delirium and dementia	● **Antiretroviral agents with CNS permeability**: didanosine, stavudine (Zerit), zidovudine, efavirenz, nevirapine, indinavir ● **Treat depression and apathy**: stimulating antidepressants and psychostimulants ● **Lithium**: useful as a neuroprotectant but caution with SE (lower doses used) ● **Avoid highly anticholinergic agents** (aminotriptyline): worsening of cognition ● **Acetylcholinesterase inhibitors** (donepezil/aricept, rivastigmine/exelon, galantamine/reminyl): not clearly useful; ↑ GI risks of antiretrovirals ● **Delirium**: R/O metabolic or medications causes (steroid-induced psychosis, hypoxia): treat first, then may use antipsychotics (haloperidol, olanzapine, or ziprazodone IM). Avoid benzodiazepines, anticholinergic drugs. Molindone: more effective to treat psychosis and delirium here
● Substance use/ abuse	● ↑ Risk of HIV in pts with schizophrenia

Neuropsychiatric side effects of antiretroviral medications and interactions with psychotropic medications

See also: Panel on Antiretroviral Guidelines for Adults and Adolescents. (2009, December). *Guidelines for the use of antiretroviral agents in HIV-1-infected adults and adolescents* (p. 1–168). Department of Health and Human Services. Retrieved September 2, 2010, from http://www.aidsinfo.nih.gov/ContentFiles/AdultandAdolescentGL.pdf

TABLE 15.6. Neuropsychiatric Side Effects of Antiretrovial Medications and DDIs with Psychotropics

Antiretroviral medications for HIV/AIDS	Generic Names	Commercial names (typical daily dosage: mg/d)	Drug–drug interactions (DDIs)	Neuropsychiatric side effects
• Nucleoside analog reverse transcriptase inhibitors	• Abacavir	• (ABC) Ziagen	• Phenobarbital ↓ level of Ziagen • Phenytoin ↓ level of Ziagen • Interacts with valproic acid, morphine, naloxone, oxazepam, chlorpromazine, doxepin, imipramine, lamotrigine	• Depression, anxiety, psychosis
	• Didanosine	• (ddI) Videx • Videx EC (400 mg/d)	• Interacts with disulfiram (Antabuse) • With phenytoin: ↑ risk for neuropathy and pancreatitis • Methadone ↓ conc. of ddI	• Lethargy, nervousness, anxiety, confusion, mood disorders, psychosis, sleep problems
	• Stavudine	• (d4T) Zerit (80 mg/d)	• Methadone ↓ conc. of d4T	• Sleep disorder, mood disorders, delirium
	• Zalcitabine	• (ddC) Hivid (2.25 mg/d)	• Interacts with disulfiram (antabuse), with phenytoin	• Somnolence, poor concentration, mood disorders, delirium
	• Zidovudine	• (AZT) Retrovir (600 mg/d)	• ↑ plasma levels of methadone • ↓ plasma levels of phenytoin • Phenytoin ↑ level of Retrovir • Valproic acid ↑ levels of Retrovir	• Sleep problems, vivid dreams, agitation, mania, depression, psychosis, delirium
	• Lamivudine	• (3TC) Epivir (300 mg/d)		
• Combinations	• Lamivudine + Zidovudine	• (AZT+3TC) Combivir		
	• Abacavir + Lamivudine + Zidovudine	• (AZT+3TC+ABV) • Trizivir		
	• Abacavir + Lamivudine (once/day)	• Epzicom		
• Nucleotide analog reverse transcriptase inhibitor	• Tenofovir	• (TDF) Viread		
	• Emtricitabine (once/day)	• (FTC) Emtriva	• Does not affect CYP 450 enzyme, no advantage over lamivudine	

Continued

TABLE 15.6. Neuropsychiatric Side Effects of Antiretrovial Medications and DDIs with Psychotropics   Continued

Antiretroviral medications for HIV/AIDS	Generic Names	Commercial names (typical daily dosage: mg/d)	Drug–drug interactions (DDIs)	Neuropsychiatric side effects
● **Nonnucleoside reverse transcriptase inhibitors** (inducers of CYT P450 → ↓ methadone conc.)	● Adefovir	● Preveon	● ↓ Methadone levels	
	● Delavirdine	● (DLV) Rescriptor (1,200 mg/d)	● Benzodiazepines:↑ level of alprazolam (Xanax) ● Interacts with fluoxetine ● Life threatening with amphetamines ● Carbamazepine ↓ level of Rescriptor ● Phenobarbital ↓ level of Rescriptor ● Phenytoin ↓ level of Rescriptor ● ↓ methadone conc.	
	● Efavirenz	● (EFV) Sustiva	● ↓ Methadone conc.	● Agitation, depersonalization, hallucinations, vivid dreams, mood disorders, suicidality, psychosis, catatonia, delirium
	● Nevirapine	● (NVP) Viramune (400 mg/d)	● Phenytoin ↓ level of Viramune ● Viramune ↓ level of phenytoin ● ↓ methadone conc.	● Depression, cognitive impairment, psychosis
● **Protease inhibitors** 　Inhibitors of P450 ↑ plasma conc. of PI 　Inducers of P450 ↓ plasma conc. of PI (→ less efficacy and resistance) 　HIV protease inhibitors inhibit cytochrome P450 enzymes **(ritonavir > the others): risk of toxic drug interactions**	● Amprenavir	● (APV) Agenerase		● Mood changes
	● Atazanavir (once/day)	● (ATV) Reyataz	● Not to be used with indinavir (↑ bilirubinemia) ● Efavirenz, tenofovir, rifampin, H2 receptor antagonists, proton pump inhibitors, antiacid, St. John's wort: ↓ action of atazanavir	
	● Darunavir	● Prezista		
	● Tipranavir	● Aptivus		
	● Fosamprenavir	● Lexiva		
	● Indinavir	● (IDV) Crixivan (2,400 mg/d)	● ↑ level of midazolam (Versed) ● Interacts with triazolam (Halcion) ● Phenobarbital, phenytoin ↓ levels of indinavir	● Mood changes
	● Nelfinavir	● (NFV) Viracept	● ↑ Levels of sedative–hypnotics	

Continued

TABLE 15.6. Neuropsychiatric Side Effects of Antiretrovial Medications and DDIs with Psychotropics Continued

Antiretroviral medications for HIV/AIDS	Generic Names	Commercial names (typical daily dosage: mg/d)	Drug–drug interactions (DDIs)	Neuropsychiatric side effects
	• Ritonavir	• (RTV) Norvir (1,200 mg/d)	• ↑ Levels of sedative-hypnotics, bupropion, disulfiram, meperidine, phenobarbital, phenytoin, valproic acid, thioridazine (risk ventricular arrhythmia) • Avoid with zolpidem, TCAs, venlafaxine, trazodone, sertraline, risperidone, benzodiazepines • ↓ Levels of hydromorphone, morphine, lamotrigine, temazepam • Phenobarbital, phenytoin: ↓ level of ritonavir	• Anxiety
	• Saquinavir	• (SQVsgc) Fortovase (soft gel cap) • (SQV-hgc) Invirase (hard gel cap) (1,800 mg/d)	• Carbamazepine, phenobarbital, phenytoin may ↓ level of saquinavir • May interact with nimodipine • Saquinavir may ↑ level of triazolam (Halcion)	• Depression, anxiety, sleep disturbances
• Combination	• Lopinavir + Ritonavir	• Kaletra		
	• Efavirenz + Emtricitabine + Tenovir	• Atripla		
	• Emtricitabine + Tenofovir (once/day)	• Truvada		
• Fusion inhibitor (inhibits fusion of the HIV virus to the CD4 cell)	• Enfuvirtide	• (T-20) Fuzeon		

Highly active antiretroviral therapy (HAART): to avoid resistance: drug regimen contains at least three agents (2 nucleoside reverse transcriptase inhibitors [NRTIs] combined with either a third NRTI or a protease inhibitor (PI). Side effects to HAART: hypersensitivity reactions, mitochondrial toxicity (hepatic steatosis, lactic acidosis with NRTIs, neuropsychiatric sx, hepatitis with NNRTIs, osteopenia, hyperlipidemia, hyperglycemia, lipodystrophy syndrome with the PI).

TABLE 15.7.   HIV Counseling

• Principles	• Protect confidentiality of pts • Obtain informed consent before HIV testing • Provide pts the option of anonymous HIV testing • **Provide information regarding the HIV test to all who are recommended or** are to receive the test, regardless of whether prevention counseling is provided • Adhere to local, state, and federal regulations and policies that govern provision of HIV services • Provide services that are responsive to pt and community needs and priorities • Provide services that are appropriate to the pt's culture, language, sex, sexual orientation, age, and developmental level

• Information	• All pts who are recommended or who request HIV testing should receive information, even if the test is declined:
	  ◦ **Information regarding the HIV test, its benefits and consequences**
	  ◦ **Risks for transmission and how HIV can be prevented**
	  ◦ **The importance of obtaining test results and procedures for doing so**
	  ◦ **The meaning of the test results in understandable language**
	  ◦ **Where to obtain further information and HIV prevention counseling**
	  ◦ **Where to obtain other services**

• Elements of HIV prevention counseling	• Keep the session focused on HIV risk reduction • Include a personalized risk assessment • Acknowledge and provide support for positive steps already made • Clarify critical misconceptions • Negotiate a concrete, achievable behavior-change step that will ↓ HIV risk • Be flexile in the prevention approach and counseling process • Provide skill-building opportunities • Use explicit language when providing test results
• Additional counseling considerations for special situations	• Persons with newly identified HIV infection • Persons with a single, recent nonoccupational HIV exposure • Persons with indeterminate HIV test results • Persons seeking repeat HIV testing • Persons who use drugs • Sex or needle-sharing partners of HIV-infected persons • Health care workers after an occupational exposure • Participants in HIV vaccine trials • Pregnant women, children, and adolescents, partners of people affected by the disease
• Factors that influence HIV risk behavior change	• **Knowledge about risk**: practical advice on behavior changes needed to ↓ risk, taking into account the realities of the client's lifestyle • **Perceived personal vulnerability**: accurately communicate the client's risk level, encourage the client's self-appraisal of risk • **Behavior change intent**: assess with the client the readiness for change; set achievable risk-reduction goals • **Self-efficacy**: assign incremental risk-reduction "tasks" for a sense of competency and success • **Skill training**: self-management, patterns identification, habits that ↑ risk; developing alternative plan to address these behaviors • **Reinforcement of behavior changes**: contracts that ↑ change efforts, discuss problems encountered, ↑ self-praise in risk-reduction changes • **Environmental barriers**: discuss the barriers to risk-reduction behaviors; use strategies to overcome those

Source: Branson, B. M., Handsfield, H. H., Lampe, M. A., Janssen, R. S., Taylor, A. W., Lyss, S. B., et al. (2006). Revised recommendations for HIV testing of adults, adolescents, and pregnant women in health-care settings. *MMWR Recommendations and Reports, 55*(RR-14), 1–17. Retrieved September 2, 2010, from http://www.cdc.gov/mmwr/preview/mmwrhtml/rr5514a1.htm.

16 ■ EARLY-ONSET DISORDERS

National organizations:

American Association on Mental Retardation (AAMR): http://www.aamr.org/

American Association on Intellectual and Developmental Disabilities (AAIDD): http://www.aaidd.org

The ARC Web: http://wwwthearc.org

Tests: Wechsler Intelligence Scales (for adults: WAIS-III, for children: WISC-III) (Psychological Corp.); Kaufman Brief Intelligence Test (K-BIT) (American Guidance Service); Stanford-Binet (SB: FE) (Riverside Publishing); Vineland Adaptive Behavioral Scales (American Guidance Service); McCarthy Scales of Children's Abilities (MSCA) (Psychological Corp.); Bayley Scales of Infant Development (BSID-III) (Pearson Education); Wechsler Preschool and Primary Scale of Intelligence (WPPSI). **IQ is rather stable normally after 4–6 yo.**

Prevalence: 2.5 million in the United States (2.3% of population) M : F = 1.5 : 1.

Onset: before age 18.

Definition: IQ ≤ 70, deficits in ≥2 areas: communication, self-care, interpersonal skills, academic, work, social skills.

TABLE 16.1. Classification

Mild MR: IQ 50–55 to 70 (85%), max grade level (4–6), developmental level of 7–11 yo, appear immature, need supervision during stress, may live independently and do simple work
Moderate MR: IQ 35–40 to 50–55 (10%), max grade level (2), developmental level of 3–7 yo, poor social skills, may be able to live in supervised group homes and very simple work
Severe MR: IQ 20–25 to 35–40 (4%), max grade level (preschool), developmental level of 1–3 yo, need ongoing supervision in very structured group homes
Profound MR: IQ <20 or 25 (1%), no speech, developmental level <1 yo, need institutionalization

Causes:

(1) **Biologic (50–80%):**

- **Chromosomal:** Down syndrome (trisomy 21: the most common), Fragile X syndrome (2nd most common, males, 1 : 2,000), Cri du chat syndrome (5p deletion), Klinefelter syndrome (XXY), Turner syndrome (XO/XX), Williams syndrome (mutation of chromosome 7), Angelman syndrome (abnormality on chromosome 15q11–13), Bardet-Biedl syndrome (problems on chromosome 3), Laurence-Moon syndrome, Cockayne syndrome (defective CSA and CSB genes on chromosome 5), Brachman-De Lange syndrome (defective NIBL gene on chromosome 5), Rubinstein-Taybi syndrome, Prader-Willi syndrome (malfunction of chromosome 15), Rett syndrome, Smith-Magenis syndrome (deletion of 17p11.2), Lesch-Nyhan syndrome (X linked), adrenoleukodystrophy (X linked)

- **Other genetic diseases:** neurofibromatosis (Von Recklinghausen disease), Huntington chorea, Sturge-Weber syndrome, tuberous sclerosis

- **Inborn errors of metabolism and other metabolic disorders:** *lipid metabolism* (Niemann-Pick disease, Infantile Gaucher disease, Tay-Sachs disease, generalized gangliosidosis, Krabbe disease, metachromatic leukodystrophy, Farber's lipogranulomatosis), *mucopolysaccharide metabolism* (Hurler disease), *glycoprotein and oligosaccharide metabolism*, *amino acid metabolism* (phenylketonuria [PKU], hemocystinuria, maple syrup urine disease, urea cycle disorders), *galactosemia*, *Wilson disease*, hypothyroidism, hypoglycemia, hyperparathyroidism

- **Prenatal insults:** maternal rubella (1st trimester), herpes simplex, cytomegalovirus, chicken pox, herpes zoster, syphilis, toxoplasmosis, diabetes, maternal alcohol abuse (fetal alcohol syndrome), toxic medications (thalidomide, phenytoin, radiation), toxemia, maternal malnutrition, erythroblastosis fetalis

- **Birth trauma:** prematurity, anoxia

- **Brain diseases:** tumors, infections (encephalitis, meningitis), trauma, poisons (lead, mercury), hydrocephalus

(2) **Social: deprivation, childhood abuse and neglect, lack of education**

Differential diagnosis: pervasive developmental disorder (PDD), dementia, schizophrenia, borderline IQ (IQ 70–79), mixed expressive-receptive language disorder with normal IQ, profound deprivation.

Associated disorders: neurologic diseases (frequent seizure disorders), psychiatric syndromes (behavioral problems, low frustration tolerance, impulsivity, aggressiveness, depression, schizophrenia). Stereotypies, self-injurious behaviors are frequent.

Course: chronic or progressive like in Tay-Sacks disease.

A comprehensive newborn screening testing is now required (CNBS): biochemical testing includes a total of 20 disorders or more depending on state regulations.

Treatment: special education, supportive environment, reality-oriented psychotherapy, genetic counseling, behavioral rx, rx of associated psychiatric or neurologic disorders, pharmacology (risperidone: 0.02–0.06 mg/kg/d; lithium or propanolol may ↓ self-abuse or aggression; clomipramine for self-injurious behaviors; naloxone).

LEARNING DISORDERS (LDs)

National organizations:

    Learning Disabilities Association of America: www.ldanatl.org

    National Center for Learning Disorders (NCLD): www.ncld.org

Diagnosis: The achievement in that LD is significantly lower than expected for age group, intelligence, and education level, and the LD interferes with academic achievements or daily life.

Comorbidity: ADHD, communication disorders, conduct disorders, depressive disorders, lead poisoning, fetal alcohol syndrome, in utero drug exposure. R/O: hearing, visual impairments.

Prognosis: drop out of school, unemployment, poor social adjustments.

Four types of learning disorders

TABLE 16.2.   Learning Disorders

Types	Reading disorder (developmental dyslexia)	Mathematical disorder (developmental dyscalculia)	Disorder of written expression (developmental dysgraphia)	Learning disorder NOS
Epidemiology	4% of school-age children, greater in boys	1–6% of school-age children, greater in girls	Uncommon, greater in boys	
Etiology	Is a language deficit genetic factor; prenatal exposure to a maternal infection in winter? Pregnancy, prenatal, perinatal injuries	Familial (50%), genetic: some cases associated with Fragile X syndrome; deficit in the right cerebral hemisphere? maturational, cognitive, emotional, educational?	Familial?	
Symptoms	Reading and usually writing difficulties (apparent 1–6 grades), poor reading comprehension	Difficulty learning numbers, mathematical terms, symbols, manipulation of spatial and numerical relations Apparent between ages 6 and 10 Comorbidity: reading, writing, and language disorders	Poor writing skills (spelling, grammatical, punctuation errors, poor handwriting) Apparent between ages 7 and 10 Ability to express ideas verbally may also have mathematics disorder	Not meeting the criteria for specific learning disorder, but causing impairment
Comorbidity, complications	ADHD, behavior disorders, depression, difficulties in language or written expression, frustration, behavioral problems, social difficulties	Other learning, language disorders, developmental coordination disorder. Embarrassment, frustration, depression	Other learning, language disorders (expressive and receptive), ADHD	
Course	May improve	From chronic to remission	Chronic; depends on the severity, the age of remediation	
Differential diagnosis	Inadequate schooling, partial blindness, MR (all cognitive abilities), rare loss of a prior ability to read	Inadequate schooling, MR, acquired dyscalculia (rare, lesions of the left parietal lobe)	Poor penmanship, isolated poor spelling, acquired pure dysgraphia, ADHD, depression	
Tests	Standardized spelling test, written composition, design copying, Woodcock-Johnson Psychoeducational Battery-Revised, sentences completion	Measures of intelligence, the Keymath diagnostic arithmetic test	Intelligence tests (WISC-III or the revised Wechsler Adult Intelligence Scale: WAIS-R), standardized expressive writing tests (TOWL, the DEWS, and TEWL)	
Treatment	Remedial education	Remedial education	Remedial education	

DEVELOPMENTAL COORDINATION DISORDER
(DEVELOPMENTAL CLUMSINESS, CLUMSY CHILD SYNDROME)

6% of school-age children; poor balance, gross motor, fine motor, and hand–eye coordinations; rx: remedial gym classes, sensory-integration programs.

COMMUNICATION DISORDERS

National organizations:

National Institute on Deafness and Other Communication Disorders: http://www.nidcd.nih.gov

The American Speech-Language-Hearing Association (ASHA): http://www.asha.org

The Stuttering Foundation: http://www.stutteringhelp.org/

Two types of communication disorders

- **Language disorders**: expressive and mixed expressive-receptive language disorders
- **Speech disorders**: phonologic disorder and stuttering

TABLE 16.3.   Communication Disorders

Language disorders (LDs)	**Expressive language disorder (developmental expressive aphasia)**	3–5% of school-age children, more in boys; difficulty speaking by age 3 or later Comorbidity: receptive language disorders, phonologic disorder, developmental coordination disorder, LD, communication disorders, ADHD, soft neurologic signs, abnormal EEG, anxiety disorders, ODD, conduct disorders, left-handedness or ambilaterality R/O: hearing loss, acquired expressive aphasia, MR, autism, selective mutism, phonologic disorder, mixed expressive-receptive LD (difficulty in following complex spoken sentences) Rx: remedial education
	Mixed receptive-expressive language disorder (developmental sensory aphasia)	3% of school-age children, more in boys. If severe, apparent by age 2 Sx: difficulty understanding spoken language, associated with difficulty in speaking Chronic, severe if identified in a young child; academic and social failures, LD R/O: acquired mixed receptive-expressive dysphasia (loss of acquired language skills; causes may be infarctions, tumors, encephalitis, Landau-Kleffner syndrome), MR, autism, deafness, deprivation Rx: remedial education
Speech disorders	**Phonologic disorder (developmental articulation disorder, developmental dysarticulation)**	3% of children Familial, maturational delay, soft neurologic sx, rare neurologic impairments Sx: delay or failure to produce expected speech, apparent by age 2–6; substitutions, omissions, distortions seen in speech Comorbidity: expressive language disorder, mixed receptive-expressive language disorder, reading disorder, developmental coordination disorder, delay in starting speech, ADHD, other LD R/O: cleft palate, dental malocclusion, cerebral palsy, MR, autism, deafness, expressive or mixed expressive-receptive language disorder Rx: speech rx
	Stuttering	3–4% of population. M : F is 3–4 : 1. Peak onsets: 2–3½ and age 5–7; genetic and environmental, ↑ with stress, cognitive dysfunction? Appears progressively between ages 2 and 7, with grimacing, blinking, movements of the head and neck, ↑ when stress 75% remit fully by age 16; 25% have partial remission Comorbidity: speech and language disorders, anxiety disorders, ADHD, abnormal motor movements R/O: normal speech dysfluency in preschool, spastic dysphonia (presence of an abnormal breathing pattern), cluttering (erratic speech patterns of jerky spurts of phrases), brain lesions (infarctions, tumors); medications (tricyclics, SSRIs, neuroleptics); neurologic diseases (Parkinson disease, progressive supranuclear palsy). In these cases, onset of stuttering is >10 yo, acute Rx: speech rx, relaxation techniques, individual and family rx. Clomipramine (150 mg/d in adults) or low doses of neuroleptics (haloperidol, risperidone)

PERVASIVE DEVELOPMENTAL DISORDERS

National organizations:

The National Autism Association: http://www.nationalautismassociation.org

US Autism and Asperger Association (USAAA): http://www.usautism.org

Autism Society of America: http://www.autism-society.org/site/PageServer

MAAP: *M*ore advanced individuals with *A*utism, *A*sperger's syndrome, and *P*ervasive developmental disorder (PDD): http://www.maapservices.org/What_Is_Maap.asp

AUTISTIC DISORDER

Epidemiology: lifetime prevalence: 0.05%, M : F is 3–5 : 1.

Sx: **onset prior to 3 yo**, **qualitative impairment in social interactions** (impairment in nonverbal behaviors: poor eye contact, body postures, facial expressions; failure to develop age-appropriate peer relationships, lack of interest in other people and social or emotional reciprocity, lack of emotional contact, fascination with inanimate objects), **qualitative impairment in communication and language** (delay in or lack of speech; inability to initiate or sustain a conversation; stereotyped, idiosyncratic language; lack of normal symbolic or imaginative play), **restricted interests and activities** (repetitive, stereotyped), **mannerisms, compulsive and repetitive behaviors, catastrophic reactions** (if routines are transgressed), **unusual responses to sensory stimuli** (sound, pain, vestibular stimulation), **hyperkinesis MR is seen in 75% of pts.** Some may have superior abilities in particular areas (memory, music performances). **Seizures are seen in 20%.**

Etiology: is a developmental behavioral disorder, primary or idiopathic (inherited, concordance for siblings is 5%, for DZ twins is 20%, for MZ twins 60–90%), or secondary (in Fragile X syndrome, Down syndrome, tuberous sclerosis, Rett syndrome, neurofibromatosis or Von Recklinghausen disease, phenylketonuria, CMV encephalitis, congenital rubella, perinatal complications). MRI: possible enlargement in occipital, parietal, temporal lobes. Autopsy studies: ↓ number of Purkinje cells (role on attention, arousal, and sensory processes), neuronal migration defect. One third has ↑ plasma serotonin concentrations (nonspecific).

Course: chronicity. Two thirds need supervision, some are capable of independent living. Persistent sx: aloofness, awkwardness in social setting.

Differential diagnosis: childhood onset schizophrenia (>6 yo, hallucinations and delusions), deafness, blindness, mixed receptive-expressive language disorder, isolated MR, psychosocial deprivation.

Rx: behavior modification (to ↑ socially acceptable behavior, ↓ odd behaviors, improve verbal and nonverbal communication), special education, family counseling; low doses of neuroleptics (haloperidol or risperidone) for withdrawn and stereotyped behaviors, to ↓ aggressive or self-injurious behaviors. Clomipramine (3–4 mg/kg/d) may also be useful. Clonidine (transdermal: 0.005 mg/kg/d, methylphenidate: to ↓ hyperactivity. Naltrexone: to ↓ self-injurious behaviors. SSRIs: to ↓ obsessive-compulsive, stereotyped behaviors. Amantadine (Symmetrel) may improve irritability, hyperactivity, aggressivity. Risperidone (5–16 yo) and aripiprazole (6–17 yo) are now FDA approved for tx of irritability in autistic children. Rett syndrome (Rett disorder)

Epidemiology: rare (<1/15,000), **mostly females**

Sx: appears in four stages:

- Stage1: **Period of normal development, then, around 10 months, slowing in development**
- Stage 2: **around 18 months**: **loss of previous abilities** (withdrawal, appearance of autistic features with loss of acquired speech, midline hand stereotypies and biting, licking, tapping, slapping, irregular respiration, ↓ in head growth → microcephaly with severe MR)
- Stage 3: **around 3 yo, partial restitution of lost abilities. In 80% of pts, seizures appear**
- Stage 4: scoliosis, dystonia, poor muscle coordination, abnormal gait, **choreoathetosis may appear only in adolescence or early adulthood**

Etiology: **genetic** (mutations in the gene MECP2 on the X chromosome?), **metabolic** (deficiency in enzyme metabolizing ammonia?). The rare male cases are usually lethal. Autopsies of children: hypoplasia without gliosis, ↓ of melanine in the substantia negra. In autopsies of adults: presence of some gliosis.

Course: **chronic after stage 4 and then static**. After 10 yr, pts become wheelchair-bound with rigidity, no language.

Complications: same as MR.

Differential diagnosis: other causes of MR and autism. In Rett syndrome, there is a *characteristic course with the partial remission of stage 3.*

Rx: rehabilitation. Rx of seizures: carbamazepine, divalproex, lamotrigine. Naltrexone may ↑ sx. Bromocriptine may be tried to ↓ the autistic sx.

CHILDHOOD DISINTEGRATIVE DISORDER (HELLER SYNDROME OR DISINTEGRATIVE PSYCHOSIS)

Epidemiology: 1 : 100,000 boys, M : F is 4–8 : 1.

Etiology: frequently associated with seizure disorders, tuberous sclerosis, metabolic disorders.

Sx: **normal development for 2–4 yr.** Onset is slow or abrupt with loss of language, of social skills, of motor skills, enuresis or encopresis, regression in reciprocal interactions, onset of stereotyped movements, restricted interests, decrease in play.

Course: deterioration with MR.

Differential diagnosis: autism (language is very limited before the diagnosis), Rett disorder (earlier deterioration, characteristic hand stereotypies).

Rx: same as in autism.

ASPERGER DISORDER

Etiology: possibly related to autistic disorder.

Sx: **impairment in social interaction** (abnormal nonverbal communication, failure of developing peer relationships, no social or emotional relatedness, lack of interest in others) rigid, stereotyped, repetitive, restricted patterns of behaviors, interests, activities. **No significant delays in language, cognitive development, or in acquiring age-appropriate self-help skills, presence of curiosity about the environment +++.**

Differential diagnosis: autism (language delay and impairment), PDD NOS, schizotypal personality disorder, schizophrenia, OCD, attachment disorder of childhood.

Course and prognosis: good if normal IQ and good social skills.

Rx: techniques used for autism.

PERVASIVE DEVELOPMENTAL DISORDER NOS

Sx: severe pervasive disorder, not meeting the criteria for specific PDDs, schizophrenia, schizotypal and schizoid personality disorders. Represented by "atypical autism" (late age onset, atypical sx)

Course: better than autism.

Rx: same as autism.

ATTENTION DEFICIT/HYPERACTIVITY DISORDER

Clinical guidelines:

http://pediatrics.aappublications.org/cgi/reprint/105/5/1158 (2000)

http://www.aacap.org/galleries/PracticeParameters/StimMed.pdf (2002)

National organizations

   Children and Adults with ADD (CHADD): http://www.chadd.org/; National Office: 305-587-3700/305-384-6869/303-792-8100

   Attention Deficit Disorder Association (ADDA): http://www.add.org/; 800-487-2282

   Attention Deficit Disorder Advocacy Group (ADDAG): 303-690-7548

Scales: Vanderbilt ADHD Diagnostic Parent Rating Scale (VADPRS) and Vanderbilt ADHD Diagnostic Teacher Rating Scale (VADTRS); Adult ADHD Self-Report Scale (ASRS); Conners Comprehensive Behavior Rating Scales (Conners CBRS); SNAP Scale; SWAN Scale; Child Behavior Checklist (CBCL); Brown ADD Scale.

Epidemiology: 3–7% of school-age children, M : F is 2–10 : 1. In first-degree relatives: ↑ ADHD, disruptive behavioral disorders, anxiety disorders, depressive disorders. In siblings: ↑ LD. In parents: ↑ ADHD, antisocial personality disorder, alcohol use disorders, conversion disorders.

Sx: usually **apparent by age 7**: hyperactivity, distractibility, impulsivity.

ADHD in adults: underdiagnosed (pts are not asked, unable to recall sx before age 7, other diagnoses are assumed such as: hypomania, depression, anxiety). Sx may ↓ or be < in adulthood (↓ hyperactivity, impatience, emotional reactivity, boredom, restlessness, difficulty initiating, completing tasks or multitasking, procrastination, avoidance of tasks demanding attention, poor executive and adaptive functioning, ↑ unemployment, ↑ divorces, few friends, ↑ moves and ↑ arrests), high comorbidities (↑ STD, ↑ psychiatric disorders: ↑ mood, anxiety, substance abuse, impulse control, personality disorders, ↑ suicide).

Course: gradual ↓ to remission of sx in two thirds of pts by adulthood. One third continues to have restlessness, distractibility, poor concentration, irritability (quick temper, intolerance of stress, poor interpersonal relations, poor job stability); frequent LD; hyperactivity ↓ with age.

Complications: academic failure, antisocial personality disorder (> in ♂), somatization disorder (> in ♀), alcoholism, drug abuse.

Etiology: genetic (mutations in genes for DRD4, MZ twins > DZ twins); MRI: posterior vermal hypoplasia. Secondary cases: lead encephalopathy, hypothyroidism, early insults to the brain (↑ soft neurologic signs), exposure to winter infections during the first trimester of gestation (↑ in September births)? Dysfunction in adrenergic (Locus ceruleus's role in attention, containing mostly noradrenergic neurons) + dopamine (DA) systems? Stimulants affect both DA and NE (by ↑ release and ↓ reuptake of catecholamines). NE agonist (Clonidin) treats hyperactivity.

Differential diagnosis: chaotic homes, medications (phenobarbital), MR, mania in BPD (directed hyperactivity, mood changes, sleep problems, family hx), agitated depression (↓ appetite, sadness, fatigue, ↓ sleep), cyclothymic disorder, intermittent explosive disorder.

TABLE 16.4.   Mania or ADHD

Symptom	ADHD	Bipolar
Elation	Transitory, rarely impairing	Outrageous behavior
Grandiosity	Brags to boost self-esteem	Truly believing in own specialness
Decreased need for sleep	Never needed much sleep or difficulty falling asleep due to medications	Needs 2+ hr less than usual and is fully rested
↑ Pleasurable activities, potential for painful consequences	Less search for pleasurable activities	Frequent deviation from social norms (substance abuse, gambling, promiscuity,...)
Racing thoughts	If low IQ or LD, can be difficult to follow	Usually with elevated mood; causes interference
Increase in goal-directed activity	Chronic and unfocused hyperactivity	Hyperactivity, engagement in elaborate schemes
Pressured speech	Chronic	Loud, hard to interrupt, patient is intrusive
Depression/suicidal thoughts/ affective family history	Usually less severe Suicidal thoughts are rare Rare affective family hx	May be severe; bipolar disorder may first present as a MDD Frequent family hx of affective disorders
Murderous rage	Not seen	Possible
Psychosis	Not seen	Possible
Hypersexuality	Not seen	Frequent if mania
Overlapping symptoms	• Inattention • Hyperactivity • Impulsivity	• **Inattention**: associated with racing, tangential thoughts, psychosis, shifting mood, disorganization, excessive energy • **Hyperactivity**: associated with ↑ energy and activity, pressured speech • **Impulsivity**: associated with impulsive, pressured speech, grandiosity, impatience, irritability

Adapted from Youngstrom, E. (2008). How can you tell when it's bipolar disorder in children and adolescents? [PowerPoint handout], Harvard CME Course on Bipolar Disorders.

Treatment:

- Special education, behavioral programs, supportive individual rx, family rx.
- Pharmacology:
  - **Stimulants**: (may be divided in an AM and noon dose, not to be given after 6 PM for risk of insomnia). In children: start with a low dose, increase q/wk until control, SE, or max dose. When stable, can switch to 1×/d with a long-acting preparation.
  - **Starting treatment**: Physical exam with weight, height, blood pressure, ECG, routine lab work including thyroid and liver functions, CBC.

TABLE 16.5.   Medications for ADHD

Group	Medication	FDA approval	Starting dose	Mean doses, Max	Risks	Benefits
	Dextroamphetamine (DEX) (half-life: 11 hr) • **SA** (4–6 hr): *Dexedrine, Dextrostat* (onset of action: 20–60 min) • **LA** (6–9 hr): *Dexedrine spansules* (onset of action: 60–90 min)	Approved for children 3 yo	**<25 kg:** 2.5 mg in AM **25–35 kg:** 5 mg bid **>35 kg:** 10 mg bid	**<25 kg:** 7.5 mg tid **25–35 kg:** 10 mg tid **>35 kg:** 15 mg tid *Max daily dose of 45 mg* (7.15 mg–15 mg tid) Max: 1.5 mg/kg/d DEX: 0.15–0.5 mg/kg/dose	See risks of stimulants	Work on concentration, attention span, motor hyperactivity, impulsiveness
Stimulants (Schedule II prescribing rules) **SA:** short acting (3–5 hr), given bid or tid **IA:** intermediate acting (3–8 hr), given once/d or bid **LA:** long acting (8–12 hr), given once/d (OROS, bead, patch, spheroidal oral drug absorption system [SODAS], technologies)	**Methylphenidate/MPH** (half-life: 3–5 hr) • **SA** (3–5 hr): *Ritalin, Equasym, Methylin, Metadate* (onset of action: 20–60 min) • **IA** (3–8 hr): *Metadate ER, Methylin SR, Ritalin SR, Equasym XL* (onset of action: 60–90 min) • **LA** (8–12 hr): • *Metadate CD, Concerta, Ritalin LA* (onset of action: 30 min–2 hr)	Children >6 yo and adults	**<25 kg:** 2.5 mg bid **25–35 kg:** 5 mg bid **>35 kg:** 10 mg bid	Max: 25 mg/dose if multiple doses/d Total daily doses: 10–65 mg (adults up to 90 mg) **MPH:** 0.3–0.7 mg/kg/dose Max: 2 mg/kg/d **Concerta:** 18–72 mg once/d Max: 2 mg/kg/d	See risks of stimulants	Best cognitive effect: 0.3 mg/kg Best behavioral response: 1 mg/kg
	Methylphenidate transdermal: (*Daytrana*) (12 hr) • 12.5 cm² = 10 mg patch strength • 18.75 cm² = 15 mg patch strength • 25 cm² = 20 mg patch strength • 37.5 cm² = 30 mg patch strength	Children 6–12 yo	**4 sizes** (mg equiv. of oral MPH) 12.5 cm² (27.5 mg) 18.75 cm² (41.3 mg) 25 cm² (55 mg) 37.5 cm² (82.5 mg)	9 hr wear time max	Sensitization to methylphenidate (papules + erythema)? vs local allergy?	Nonoral form Bypasses the liver Optimal dose may be lesser compared to oral MP Placed on the hip Will continue to work 2–3 hr after removal

Dexmethylphenidate: • *Focalin* (6 hr) • *Focalin XR*	XR approved: children >6 yo, adolescents, and adults	Start 5 mg/d in children Start 10 mg/d in adults (once in AM if XR form or divided doses for the immediate release form)	Doses: half those of MPH **Focalin**: given bid: 5–20 mg/d **Focalin XR**: Max for adults: 40 mg/d Max for children: 30 mg/d	See risks of stimulants	Work on concentration, attention span, motor hyperactivity, impulsiveness
Mixed amphetamine salts/AMP • **SA** (4–6 hr): *Adderall* (onset of action: 30–60 min) • **LA** (10–12 hr): *Adderall XR* (onset of action: 1–2 hr)	Approved for children 3 yo Adderall XR approved for adults ADHD	Adderall **<25 kg**: 2.5–5 mg in AM **25–35 kg**: 5–10 mg in AM **>35 kg**: 10 mg in AM Adderall XR: start 10–20 mg/d up to 0.5–1.5 mg/kg/d, given q day	Adderall <25 kg: 10 mg in AM or bid 25–35 kg: 10–15 mg in AM or bid >35 kg: 20–40 mg in AM or bid Max 45 mg/d or 1 mg/kg/d Mean optimal weight-adjusted dose: **4–7 yr**: 0.38 mg/kg/dose **8–10 yr**: 0.30 mg/kg/dose **11–17 yr**: 0.18 mg/kg/dose	See risks of stimulants	
Methamphetamine hydrochloride (*Desoxyn*) (4–6 hr); action-onset: 30 min	>6 yo	5 mg once or 2×/d	20–25 mg divided in 2 doses	See risks of stimulants	
Prodrug stimulant: **Lisdexamfetamine dimesylate (LDX) (*Vyvanse*)** Half-life 9 hr	ADHD children age 6–12	Start: 30 mg/d ↑ by 20 mg q 3–7 days Half-life 9 ½ hr, max conc. in 3 1/2 hr Given once/d	Max: 70 mg/d	Possible ↑ QTc	Undergoes biotransformation before therapeutic effects; converts into l-lysine (active d-amphetamine). Is not a controlled-release drug, not affected by GI pH ↓ abuse potential (less euphoria)

Continued

TABLE 16.5.   Medications for ADHD   Continued

Group	Medication	FDA approval	Starting dose	Mean doses, Max	Risks	Benefits
Antidepressant (**warning box**: ↑ suicidal ideations in children or adolescents)	**TCAs: nortriptyline (*Pamelor*), imipramine (*Tofranil*), desipramine (*Norpramine*)** Half-life 24–36 hr	FDA: no	Imipramine: divided dose of 1 mg/kg/d May start at 10–25 mg/d in adults Desipramine: may start at 10–25 mg/d in adults	Nortriptyline: up to 2 mg/kg/d Imipramine: max up to 5 mg/kg/d Desipramine: 5 mg/kg/d (dosage: ~150 mg/d) ↑ slowly	**Cardiac side effects**: ECG **Risk of overdose**: TCA–marijuana interactions Latency of response DDI Sedation, Anticholinergic effects ↓ seizure threshold Sudden death with desipramine	May be used if tics Check therapeutic levels No rebound Desipramine and imipramine generally work better than other TCAs
	Bupropion (*Wellbutrin, Wellbutrin SR, Wellbutrin XL*) Half-life 10–27 hr	FDA: no	Start at 37.5 mg/d in adults	XL form: 450 mg/d (once/d) SR form: 400 mg/d (2×/d)	↓ **Seizure threshold**	Helpful if comorbidity (substance abuse, mood, or anxiety disorder) Less effective than TCAs
	Venlafaxine (*Effexor, Effexor XR*) Half-life 5 hr	FDA: no	12.5–37.5 mg bid if needed	50–150 mg/d 2–5 mg/kg divided bid or tid Max: 225 mg/d (Effexor ER); 375 mg/d (Effexor)	Insomnia, irritability, GI sx, BP changes	Less established effectiveness

Others				
Atomoxetine (*Strattera*): is a selective NE reuptake inhibitor Half-life 5 hr	Children >6 and adults	**Children:** 0.5 mg/kg/d in the first wk (taken with food) **40–62 lb: 18 mg** **63–93 lb: 25 mg** **94–126 lb: 40 mg** **Adults:** 40 mg/d the first wk Given q d or bid	**Children:** target dose: 1.2 mg/kg/d Max: 1.4 mg/kg/d **40–62 lb: 25 mg** **63–93 lb: 40 mg** **94–126 lb: 80 mg** **Adults:** target dose: 80 mg/d Max:100 mg/d Better tolerated in PM, better efficacy in AM	↑ Suicidal ideations in children or adolescents Slow titration, or time change, or splitting the dose if dry mouth, dyspepsia, constipation, urinary retention, sex. problems, ↑ seizures, ↑ QTc, ↑ BP) Metabolized through CYP 2D6 (check: **liver enzymes**, bilirubin) Mild ↑ BP and pulse	Pts with ADHD all day long, ADHD + anxiety, ADHD + substance abuse (is not a controlled drug), ADHD + tics or Tourette syndrome, ADHD + depression Improvement is gradual: evaluate efficacy after 6 wk of target dose Can be added to a stimulant. If switch from a stimulant to atomoxetine, overlap until atomoxetine takes effect ATX may be added to an antipsychotic if comorbidity Long-term rx well tolerated
Modafinil (*Provigil*) Half-life: 10–15 hr	FDA: no	lower doses may be better (50–200 mg/d)	tablets of 100 and 200 mg	**Cases of erythema multiform and Stevens-Johnson** Safety not established <16 yo Case reports of mania, delusions, hallucinations, and suicidal ideation	Lower risk of abuse than stimulants Schedule IV drug No discontinuation syndrome Less activating than stimulants Improves attention Check liver function; many DDIs

Continued

TABLE 16.5. Medications for ADHD   Continued

Group	Medication	FDA approval	Starting dose	Mean doses, Max	Risks	Benefits
	Clonidine (*Catapress*) (α2 adrenergic agonist) Half-life: 8–12 hr in children 12–16 hr in adults	FDA: no	**Oral: start slow:** *0.025–0.05 mg at hs, then bid; titrate over 2–4 wk slowly (by 0.1 mg/d/ each wk)* **Transdermal clonidine:** given q 5–7 days (Catapres-TTS): 0.1–0.3 mg/d Do not start with transdermal Start in PM For sleep: 0.025–0.05 mg at bed time Change location with each application	Usually 0.05 mg–4 mg/ d max	**Very sedative, hypotension,** ↓ **pulse,** ↑ **blood sugar** Taper off gradually Caution: **sudden death reported in combination: methylphenidate + clonidine Multiple drug interactions Rebound** effects (short action) Slow response (2 wk.–3 months) Not effective for inattention **Withdrawal:** ↑ **BP** (taper by 0.05 mg/d or q 3rd day if prescribed >4 wk) Depressive reaction	Used in ADHD + Tourette or tics (may be combined with stimulants) Used for aggression No risk of abuse Works well on hyperactivity Some death reports in children taking methylphenidate with clonidine together (cardiac monitoring)
	Guanfacine (*Tenex*) (α2-adrenergic agonist) Half-life:17 hr in adults 1/10 the potency of clonidine **Guanfacine Extended-release form (*Intuniv*)**	FDA: no	0.5 mg bid Intuniv: once/d (do not give with high-fat meals)	Doses titrated up to 1–3 mg/d 0.5–2 mg up to tid	Check BP and pulse Taper off gradually	Used if tics Results + on hyperactivity and inattention Little rebound or sedation or hypotension, less sedative than clonidine

Max dose guideline only. May give higher doses if no or limited SE.

TABLE 16.6.   Risks of Stimulants

Contraindications	• **Do not give if serious heart problems**: "black box" safety warning due to ↑ risk for severe cardiovascular problems in adults and children (**heart attack, stroke, high blood pressure, and arrhythmia**). See http://www.aap.org/pressroom/aap-ahastatement.htm • **Do not give with MAOIs** • **Lower the seizure threshold**: if seizure hx, monitor EEG, use with antiseizure drug if absolutely necessary • Caution if comorbid disorder (eating, sleeping disorder, **motor tics**, depression, anxiety disorder) • **Abuse potential** (d-amphetamine peaks sooner than lisdexamfetamine: ↑ euphoria) • **Do not give if**: sensitivity to stimulants; **glaucoma**; hyperthyroidism; unstable bipolar disorder • **Psychosis, marked anxiety, agitation, severe depression, mania** • **Liver disorder** (pemoline/Cylert was removed from the market) • **Hx of Tourette syndrome, severe motor tics** • **Breastfeeding mothers, pregnancy**
Side effects of stimulants	• ↓ **Appetite, weight loss**: give after meals, give snack in late PM; ↑ calorie foods in AM and PM, nutrition shakes; ↓ dose or change medications • **Cardiovascular**: palpitations, tachycardia, ↑ BP • **Insomnia**: ↓ last dose of the day (do not give after 4 PM), give earlier during day, give clonidine: 0.1–0.2 mg at hs (caution) or guanfacine: 1–2 mg at hs. Mirtazapine (7.5 mg at hs may ↑ sleep and appetite), no caffeine or TV in room, routine before bed; use < duration stimulant • **Irritability**: if just after medication is given (due to peak), if late in PM (due to rebound): ↓ dose. Dysphoria, mild social withdrawal if MPH > 0.5 mg/kg. Evaluate comorbidity • **Sadness**: reevaluate diagnosis, ↓ dose, change to long acting • **Abdominal pain, headache, nausea, vomiting**: ↓ dose may go away after 4 wk • **Growth suppression (DEX > MPH)**: drug holiday, switch to a nonstimulant • **Rare cognitive impairment or perseverative behaviors** (↓ dose, drug holidays) • **CNS**: psychosis, tics, abnormal involuntary movements • **Behavioral rebound** (↑ original sx, after sudden discontinuation, or 5–20 hr after last dose): overlap the stimulant dosing pattern, or switch to longer-acting, or combine short-acting + sustained-release or add bupropion • **Other**: leukopenia, jaundice, anemia, ↑ liver enzymes
If abuse potential (misuse, abuse, diversion)	• Limit, keep track of pills, urine toxicology screens to see if co-use of other substances, schedule frequent visits, use long-acting preparations, safe storage, use atomoxetine, antidepressant, clonidine • **Overdose**: CNS damage, CV damage, hypertension, paranoid hallucinations

TABLE 16.7.   Comorbidity in ADHD: >50% of ADHD Children Have Some Comorbidity

Secondary to ADHD sx and their impact	ODD, anxiety and mood disorders, LD
Risks of some disorders increased by ADHD	CD, impulsive disorders
Genetic variants of ADHD	ADHD + Tourette syndrome ADHD + CD ADHD + borderline or antisocial personality disorders
Disorders sharing environmental risks	Depression, CD, substance abuse

TABLE 16.8.   Stimulants–Drug Interactions

• **With antidepressants**:
  - **TCAs**: risk of arrhythmia, ↑ level of TCA (?)
  - **SSRIs**: no interaction
  - **Bupropion**: no known problems
• **Do not use within 14 days of using MAOI**
• **Inhibits metabolism of warfarin**
• **With anticonvulsants**: MPH may inhibit their metabolism: ↑ side effects
• **With α2-agonists**: with **guanethidine**: rebound hypertension and sedation; with **clonidine**: death reports, do not use if hx of sudden death, repeated fainting or arrhythmias in family members. If clonidine used, start with 0.05 mg at hs, and ↑ very slowly (max: 0.3 mg/d); if used to control aggression, divide into 4×/d
• **With sympathomimetic drugs**: ephedrine, pseudoephedrine, cocaine are potentiated

TABLE 16.9.   Age-Specific Use of Stimulants

Preschool children	MPH: doses < 0.5 mg/kg/dose. Given 1–2×/d. Start: 1.25 mg. Crush pills if problem swallowing; parent training, structured preschool, behavior rx
Older children	MPH: doses 0.3–0.8 mg/kg/dose. Given often 2–3×/d. Do not stop in teen years (ADHD continues into adulthood)
Adolescents	Long-acting drugs indicated (Concerta), cannot be ground up or snorted. May need to add an immediate-release form in the afternoon before homework
Adults	Respond well to stimulants (Focalin XR, Vyvanse are FDA approved for adults). If not, use other drugs: fluoxetine, atomoxetine, bupropion). (SSRIs are not useful. Atomoxetine is approved for adult ADHD (particularly if + substance abuse). MAOIs may be used; but risk of hypertension crisis (severe dietary restrictions). Preliminary support for nicotinic analogs and donepezil

TABLE 16.10.   Treatment of ADHD with Comorbid Disorders

Depression, anxiety disorders	If severe MDD, treat first with antidepressants. If ADHD is primary, treat ADHD first. Bupropion and TCAs are good for adults but may not be for pediatric depression. Strattera may be more effective in ADHD + anxiety. If anxiety does not respond to nonpharmacologic treatment, may add SSRI to the stimulant
Manic episode	**Use neuroleptic or mood stabilizer first.** May combine both with stimulant or clonidine. **Risk factors for stimulant-induced mania when ADHD and bipolar symptoms overlap:** ● Family hx of bipolar disorder ● Early onset of mood disorder ● Comorbid substance use disorder ● Hx of rapid cycling or antidepressant-induced mania ● Multiple antidepressant trials
Tic disorders	In majority of pts, tics do not increase with stimulants. Get proper consent before a trial of stimulant. Try to ↓ dose. If tics remain, may try TCA, clonidine, guanfacine, bupropion, atomoxetine. If stimulant is the only effective drug but ↑ tics: may add α2-agonist. If unsuccessful, consider stimulant + atypical neuroleptic
Conduct disorders and aggression	May add a neuroleptic (risperidone) or a mood stabilizer (divalproex) Clonidine may be used
Substance use disorders	● If stimulants necessary: use long-acting stimulants or stimulant prodrug: LDX (Vyvanse) ● Or use nonstimulants (atomoxetine, bupropion) ● Always with psychosocial interventions (cognitive-behavior rx, motivational interviewing, contingency management, family rx, 12-step approaches, and specific SUD interventions)
Childhood stimulant treatment and risk for later substance abuse	● *Stimulant rx are not associated with ↑ risk of adolescent substance use* (severe conduct problems are +++) ● Stimulant rx in high school may be a protector against hallucinogen abuse disorder in adulthood

○ **Response to treatment:** combination of medication + behavioral rx better than medication alone better than behavioral rx alone.
○ **Attention-deficit/hyperactivity disorder NOS**
○ Pts have sx of inattention or hyperactivity—impulsivity but do not meet criteria for ADHD.

DISRUPTIVE BEHAVIOR DISORDERS

OPPOSITIONAL DEFIANT DISORDER (ODD)
Epidemiology: oppositional behavior may be adaptive (terrible twos, search for identity formation and autonomy in adolescence); if prolonged, becomes ODD. Prevalence is 2–16%; onset ~8 yo; > in boys prior to puberty.

Etiology: temperament (genetic, familial), struggle against authority, negative attention seeking (learned behaviors), defense mechanism (for conflicts resolution or against helplessness, anxiety from trauma, chronic illness, MR).

Symptoms: >6 months of defiant behaviors that cause significant impairment in social, school, or work functioning (temper tantrums, arguments with adults, defiance of rules, provocative behaviors, not taking responsibility, anger, resentment).

Differential diagnosis: conduct disorder, antisocial personality disorder, reaction to stress.

Complications: poor relationships, school failure, depression, temper outbursts, substance abuse, conduct disorder (esp. if + fighting, bullying; if starts <age 12; if + ADHD).

Prognosis: 25% improve, depends on family functioning and comorbidity.

Treatment: family rx (behavior rx), individual rx, eliminate punitive parenting (physical and emotional abuse), ↑ positive parent–child interactions.

CONDUCT DISORDER (CD)

Organization: National Runaway Switchboard: 1-800-RUN-AWAY

Epidemiology: 1–10% of the population. Onset is earlier in boys (10–12 yo) than in girls (14–16 yo). M : F is 3–5 : 1.

Etiology: parental factors (punitive parenting, chaotic home, lack of supervision, domestic violence or conflicts, neglect, parents' substance abuse, *x* removals from home, parents' serious mental illnesses or antisocial personality disorders), physical and sexual abuse, depression, prior poor school performances, neurobiologic factors (ADHD, brain damage, ↓ noradrenergic functioning: low plasma level of dopamine β-hydroxylase, ↑ serotonin levels in the blood, ↓ 5-HIAA levels in CSF).

Symptoms: persistent, frequent aggressivity (bullying, cruelty to people, animals, physical violence, use of weapons), hostility, defiance, abusiveness, persistent lying, oppositionality against peers and adults, stealing, breaking into someone's property, shoplifting, forgery, forceful sexual acts, destruction of property, fire setting, severe violation of rules (running away, truancy, staying out at night, promiscuity, gang participation, use of drugs, alcohol, blaming others to get out of trouble, deceitfulness), superficial emotional attachments (superficial charm, lack of trust, no real remorse or guilt); impairs social, school, and work functioning.

Three types: childhood-onset, adolescent-onset, unspecified.

Differential diagnosis: ODD (no severe violation of others' rights), mood and substance abuse disorders, ADHD, LD, MR.

Prognosis: poor if: early onset, pt is a loner, comorbid disorders (mood disorders, substance use disorders, low IQ). 50% will improve in adulthood.

Complications: academic failure, incarceration ↑ if aggressive behaviors and parents' criminal behaviors.

Treatment: structure with consistent rules and expectations in the community (multimodality rx with family rx, social skills training, school remediation, community resources such as in-home services, involvement of the legal system if needed, individual and group rx). Removal from home if the family is abusive or too chaotic (foster homes, therapeutic foster homes, group homes, residential rx facilities). Medications for aggressivity: antipsychotics (haloperidol/*Haldol*, risperidone/*Risperdal*, olanzapine/*Zyprexa*), lithium (*Eskalith*); anticonvulsants (carbamazepine/*Tegretol*); clonidine/*Catapress*. SSRIs (fluoxetine/*Prozac*, sertraline/*Zoloft*, paroxetine/*Paxil*, citalopram/*Celexa*) may help with the irritability, impulsivity. Treat all comorbidities.

DISRUPTIVE BEHAVIOR DISORDER NOS

Conduct and oppositional behaviors that do not meet the full criteria but produce significant impairments.

FEEDING AND EATING DISORDERS OF INFANCY OR EARLY CHILDHOOD

TABLE 16.11.   Feeding and Eating Disorders of Infancy or Early Childhood

Types	Pica	Rumination disorder	Feeding disorder of infancy or early childhood
Epidemiology	Persistent (>1 month) eating of nonfood items Onset: 12–24 months (any time if MR, if pregnant pts, postpartum)	Usually between 3 months and 1 yo. More in severe or profound MR (3–10%). M > F	15–30% of infants and young children have feeding difficulties; failure to thrive in 3%. Onset <6 yo
Etiology	Lack of supervision, neglect, iron, zinc deficiencies	Self-stimulatory behavior, mother–infants negative interactions, GERD, hiatal hernia, bulimia nervosa, anorexia nervosa	
Symptoms	Eating of paint, clay, starch, plaster, string, hair, cloth, dirt, feces, stones, paper, sand, tobacco, trash, wood, ice (pagophagia). Pts eat regular food as well (no weight loss)	Repeated regurgitation and rechewing of the food (then swallowed or spit out), of >1 month duration after nl functioning, voluntary induced, pleasurable	Persistent (>1 month) failure to eat adequately, failure to gain weight, or loss of weight, not due to a medical or mental disorder, or lack of food
Laboratory	CBC, lead levels ↑ if ingestion of lead-based paint, iron-deficiency anemia	Thyroid function tests, CBC, serum electrolytes	Thyroid function tests, CBC, serum electrolytes
Differential diagnosis	Cultural in Australian aborigines; also in schizophrenia, anorexia nervosa, autism, dementia, delirium, **Klein-Levin syndrome** (hypersomnolence + hyperphasia + hypersexuality), **Kluver-Bucy syndrome** (psychic blindness + hypermetamorphosis or irresistible impulse to notice and react to everything within sight, + hyperorality + hypersexuality), psychologic dwarfism (form of severe failure to thrive), precocious puberty	GERD, hiatal hernia, bulimia nervosa, anorexia nervosa, pyloric stenosis (projectile vomiting prior to 3 months)	GI disorders
Course	Stops usually in adolescence, may be limited during pregnancy. May be chronic in MR	Stops by age 12 months, tends to be chronic if MR	Most pts with feeding problems during the 1st yr will do well. If onset is at age 2 or 3: risk ↑ for growth and development problems
Complications	Lead poisoning, intestinal parasites (toxoplasmosis, toxocariasis), anemia, zinc or iron deficiencies, intestinal occlusion, constipation	Dehydration, failure to thrive, developmental delays, may be fatal (25%), malnutrition, aspiration pneumonia, ↓ resistance to disease, caries, and halitosis, parent's alienation	Failure to thrive
Treatment	Supervision, education, behavior rx, ↓ stressors, rx of medical complications	Education, behavioral rx (lemon juice put in the mouth when rumination occurs). Treat medical complication, anatomic abnormalities. If necessary use psychotherapy for both parents	Improving mother–infant interactions during feeding time, helping to recognize child's patterns

TIC DISORDERS

Definition: tics are repetitive, rapid, involuntary muscle contractions that result in movements or vocalizations; usually begin during childhood or adolescence. Can be suppressed for minutes/hours; may be irresistible, produce discomfort. May ↓ during sleep, activity, relaxed states.

Types:

- **Simple tics**: Motor (eye blinking, brow wrinkling, neck jerking, shoulder shrugging, facial grimacing); vocal (coughing, throat clearing, grunting, sniffing, snorting, barking, hissing); sensory tics (tickles, itches)

- **Complex tics**: motor (smelling of objects, touching objects or people, imitating, hopping, throwing, clapping, obscene gestures); vocal (repeating words, coprolalia, or use of obscene phrases: 10%; repetition of own or others' words); sensory (premonitory urges appearing just before motor tics)

Four categories of tic disorders:

■ **Tourette disorder (Gilles De La Tourette syndrome)**

Epidemiology: lifetime prevalence: 0.05%; M : F is 3 : 1. Average onset is 7 yo (usually a single motor tic).

Etiology: **genetic** (autosomal pattern intermediate between dominant and recessive); some relation between Tourette's and ADHD (50% have ADHD), Tourette's and OCD (40% have OCD); **immunological** (strept infections? Some are sequelae to Sydenham chorea); **neurochemical**: dopamine (antagonists like antipsychotics ↓ tics; agonists like amphetamines or cocaine ↑ tics); endogenous opioids (antagonists like naltrexone) ↓ tics in Tourette's.

Diagnosis: multiple simple or complex motor and vocal tics, ×/d, but intermittently for >1 yr. No free-tic period for more than 3 months. Motor tics may progress in a rostral-caudal sequence. Sensory tics are common. Obsessions or compulsions may appear within 2 yr of the onset of tics.

Differential diagnosis: dystonias, choreiform, myoclonic, hemiballismic, tremors, mannerisms, stereotypies (head banging, body rocking).

TABLE 16.12.   Types of Abnormal Involuntary Movements

Athetosis	Sinuous writhing movement of the fingers and hands
Chorea	Continuous jerky movements; each movement is sudden; the resulting posture is held for a few seconds. Usually affects head, face, or limbs. The focus may move from one part of the body to another at random
Dystonias	Muscle spasms contracting the neck, limbs, and trunk into typical postures
Hemiballism	Wild flinging/throwing movements of one arm or leg
Myoclonus	Rapid muscle jerks, frequently repetitive
Spasmodic torticollis	Presents in middle age or elderly with torticollis or sometimes retrocollis or anticollis. Can be repetitive causing tremulous torticollis. Often has a compensatory lordosis
Tardive dyskinesia	At least 6 months rx with neuroleptics; more frequent in elderly; in 20% of pts on chronic rx; persists in 40% of cases after DC of rx. Characterized by orofacial mouthing with lip-smacking and tongue protrusion, body rocking, and distal chorea. In younger pts may cause axial and cranial dystonia
Tics	Repetitive stereotyped movements. Pt can initiate voluntarily and intentionally suppress for a short time. Can be simple or complex
Tremor	Rhythmic movement of part of the body. Three types of pathologic tremor: static, postural, or action tremors

Etiology

Due to substances: gasoline inhalation, carbon monoxide poisoning, stimulants (methylphenidate, amphetamines, pemoline, cocaine), tardive dyskinesia (TD; prolonged neuroleptic exposure). Antipsychotics may hide preexisting abnl movements like tics. If they reappear after DC or during rx, differentiation from TD will be difficult. Stimulants may ↑ tics (predisposition? caution).

Due to infections: Sydenham chorea, encephalitis lethargica, postinfectious (strept), herpes simplex encephalitis

Genetic disorders: Hallervorden-Spatz disease, dystonia musculorum deformans, Huntington disease, Wilson disease, neuroacanthocytosis, XYY genetic disorder, Duchenne muscular dystrophy, Fragile X syndrome, hyperreflexias

> **Posttraumatic**: brain trauma, developmental and perinatal disorders, postangiographic complications

Transient tics of <1 yr or chronic isolated tics (minor form of Tourette's?).

Comorbidity: behavioral (ODD, CD), mood disorders (MDD, BPD), ADHD. May exist with autism and MR.

Course: chronic with ↑ and ↓. If severe: risk of depression, social, academic, and occupational problems, motor tics provoke joint damages, sensory tics may cause excoriations.

Treatment of the tics

- **Neuroleptics**: very effective, start with low doses, ↑ q wk. Educate pts and families about dystonic reactions, parkinsonism, tardive dyskinesia, neuroleptic syndrome, metabolic syndrome.

    - Haloperidol (Haldol): start with 0.25–0.5 mg, average dose is 3–4 mg, max is 10 mg (↑ akathisia). Not approved for children <3 yo, max 3 mg/d for children 3–12 yo (0.05–0.075 mg/kg divided in 2 or 3 doses/d)

    - Olanzapine (Zyprexa): start with 5 mg, average dose is 10 mg, max is 15 mg (↑ metabolic syndrome)

    - Risperidone (Risperdal): start with 0.5 mg, average dose is 2–4 mg, max is 6 mg (↑ akathisia, ↑ prolactinemia, ↑ dysphoria)

    - Ziprazidone (Geodon): start with 5 mg, average dose is 20–30 mg, max is 40 mg (less studied)

    - Pimozide (Orap) is a second choice due to risk of arrhythmia and ↑ QT intervals: start with 1–2 mg/d in divided doses, average is <0.2 mg/kg/d or 10 mg/d, max is 0.3 mg/kg/d or 20 mg/d. Avoid if child <12 yo. Check ECG regularly.

- **Alpha-2 blockers**: less effective, SE: drowsiness, headache, irritability, hypotension.

    - Clonidine (Catapress): start with 0.05 mg bid, average dose is 0.25 mg bid, max is 1 mg/d. Is not FDA approved for use in Tourette disorder, but ↑ attention span, ↓ tics and tension

    - Guanfacine (Tenex): start with 0.5 mg/d, average dose is 1 mg bid, max is 4 mg/d

- **Desipramine (Norpramin)**: not in children or adolescents. For adults: start with 25 mg/d, ↑ every few days to 100 mg/d

- **Clonazepam (Klonopin)**: risk of dependence, start with 0.5 mg/d, ↑ q wk, average dose is 1 mg bid, max is 2 mg bid

Treatment of comorbidity:

- **OCD**: SSRIs with or without antipsychotics
- **ADHD**: methylphenidate may not increase rate and intensity of the tics (still debated). Buproprion (*Wellbutrin* ↑ the tics in some children with Tourette disorder + ADHD). Be careful of cardiac risks of the TCAs

■ Chronic motor or vocal tic disorder

Epidemiology: chronic tic disorder; > in boys, may be 1–2% of population. Onset in early childhood

Etiology: familial

Diagnosis: chronic presence of motor or vocal tics, not both

Differential diagnosis: other motor movements (choreiform, myoclonus, restless legs syndrome, akathisia, dystonias), other tic disorders (Tourette disorder, transient tic disorder), SUD, general medical condition.

Course: usually stops in adolescence. Poorer prognosis if tics involve limbs or trunk

Treatment: varies with the severity and the pt's distress. Psychotherapy, behavioral rx. Haloperidol if severe tics (risks of tardive dyskinesia).

■ Transient tic disorder

Epidemiology: common, 5–25% of children. Onset before 18 yo

Etiology: organic may progress to Tourette disorder; psychogenic tics may disappear; ↑ with stress

Diagnosis: single or complex motor or vocal tics, occurring many ×/d, >1 month but <1 yr

Course: single episode or recurrent during stress. Rarely chronic

Differential diagnosis: Tourette disorder, chronic motor or vocal tic disorder, substance intoxication, gl medical condition

Treatment: depends on the severity. Behavioral techniques effective

■ Tic disorder NOS

Does not meet criteria for a specific tic disorder.

ELIMINATION DISORDERS

TABLE 16.13.   Elimination Disorders

Types	Encopresis (functional encopresis)	Enuresis
Epidemiology	1–1.5% of children age 5–8 yr, M : F is 3 : 1	Develops between ages 5 and 7. Frequency is: 5% at age 5, 1% at age 18. M : F is 2 : 1. Primary or secondary (after normal continence >6–12 months); ↑ if stress, low social status, family hx
Etiology	Initial constipation following anxiety, acute stress, diet change, travel, dehydration → anxiety about defecation, ↑ external sphincter activity → ↑ constipation and overflow incontinence; primary or secondary	Bladder and urinary tract abnormalities (gI development delays; 3% of obstructive lesions?), R/O bladder infections. Sleep studies: problems with arousability. Possible inability to concentrate urine at night: DDAVP efficacy. Genetic research: chromosomes 13q, 12q, 8 and 22? Is most frequently not associated with any style of toilet training
Symptoms	NI continence exists by age 4. Soiling with feces occurs >1×/ **month and for > 3 months duration** Retentive (leakage around the fecal mass) or nonretentive encopresis (no control of bowel movement)	Diurnal or nocturnal or mixed voiding of urine into the bed or the clothes, **>2×/wk and >3 months**, causing significant distress, if **age >5 yo**
Differential diagnosis	Stress related; associated with MR, with ADHD; voluntary soiling. Medical causes: Hirschprung disease, rectum stenosis, smooth muscle disease, hypothyroidism, medications (anticholinergics, antihistamines)	R/O drug-induced enuresis (diuretics, clozapine, sedating drugs), medical condition: UTI, polyuria (diabetes mellitus, diabetes insipidus, cystic medullary disease, sickle cell disease), anatomic lesions (bladder outlet obstruction, urethral valves, meatal stenosis), spastic bladder (cerebral palsy, spina bifida), nocturnal seizures, pressure on the bladder (pelvic masses, impacted stool), obstructive sleep apnea UA and culture; more invasive studies if enuresis occurs during the day time, signs of voiding disturbance
Course	Poor prognosis if inability to relax the anal sphincter, rare in adolescents (spontaneous remissions), good response to rx (85%)	High rate of spontaneous remissions between 5 and 7 yo and >12 yo
Complications	Shame, family conflicts	Poor self-esteem

Continued

TABLE 16.13.   Elimination Disorders   Continued

Types	Encopresis (functional encopresis)	Enuresis

Treatment	• **Educational, psychologic, behavioral** (bowel training with daily scheduled times to go to the toilet, 20 min after meals, rewarded if successful, putting soiled clothes away properly)
	• **Initial digital disimpactation or enema** if required, oral laxatives, high fiber diet, stool softener
	• **Biofeedback training** if abnormal defecation dynamics
	• **Pharmacology:** Imipramine (Tofranil: 25–75 mg/d for a few days to a few weeks), amitriptyline?
		• **Behavioral rx:** Restrict fluids >1 hr before bedtime; empty bladder at q hs. Prohibit caffeine. Place rubber undersheet on the bed. Avoid diapers. If fails, use enuresis alarm, bell and pad method with reward contingencies (75% improvement), retention-control training, or with an alarm clock set to go off after 2–3 hr of sleep, or a monitoring system attached to an abdominal belt signaling the bladder reaching a specific capacity. Continue at least for 3 months of continuous continence, then discontinue. Reinstitute the program if needed. The Bedwetting Store (*www.bedwettingstore.com*); Pediatrics Warehouse (*www.pediatricswarehouse.com/enuresisalarms.html*); Wet Busters (*www.wetbuster.com*); *The Bedwetting Handbook* (*www.bedwettinghandbook.com*)
		• **Medications:**
		  Imipramine: start at 25 mg at bedtime, with 4–7 days dosages increment of 10–25 mg, average dose is 75–125 mg/d (max: 5 mg/kg/d). Baseline ECG; regularly if higher doses (sudden death reported). When remission, taper slowly and DC q 3 months to reevaluate need. Restart if needed. Effect not related to the antidepressant action but to the renal tubular antidiuretic one
		  DDAVP: more successful if >age, >bladder capacity, <wet nights. Nasal form SE: nasal stuffiness, headache, epistaxis, abdominal pain, cases of hyponatremia when fluids were not restricted in the evening. Dosage: start at 5 µg q hs, max is 20–40 µg q hs (intranasal); 86% improvement. Oral form: 200–600 µg/d **(20 µg nasal = 200 µg oral form)**
		  Experimental rx: acupuncture, oxybutynin hydrochloride, mesterolone (synthetic androgen), hypnosis, diclofenac, carbamazepine
		• **Combination of behavioral rx and medication**

OTHER DISORDERS OF INFANCY, CHILDHOOD, AND ADOLESCENCE

SEPARATION ANXIETY DISORDER
Epidemiology: 2–5% of school-age children; onset at 6–7 yo.

Etiology: childhood equivalent to panic disorder with agoraphobia?

Symptoms: extreme lasting fear (+ autonomic arousal) upon separation from the parents, inappropriate for the child's age + developmental level; school refusal.

Differential diagnosis: is *normal from 8–24 month up to 6 yo;* parental overprotectiveness; school bullying; schizophrenia; autism; medications SE (haloperidol, risperidone, pimozide); other anxiety disorders (OCD, GAD, specific phobia).

Course: ↑ and ↓ with good prognosis. Chronic (if comorbidity with other psychiatric disorders, family psychopathology, >1 yr of school absence)

Complications: absenteeism from school, depression, somatic complaints, ↓ time spent with friends, panic disorder, agoraphobia.

Treatment:

- CBT: individual, family, group rx; remedial school work; psychodynamic psychotherapy (issues of separation-individuation, self-esteem, assertiveness). CBT techniques: exposure (gradual exposure, desensitization with relaxation), contingency management (positive reinforcement, shaping, extinction), cognitive strategies (problem solving, self-talk), modeling
- Medications: as an adjunct. Imipramine: start 10–25 mg/d, ↑ slowly up to a max dose of 3 mg/kg/d, or limiting SE, observe for 6 wk. Alprazolam (0.5–2 mg/d, keep for 1 month if pt asymptomatic before tapering down over a few months). SSRIs are also helpful.

SELECTIVE MUTISM (ELECTIVE MUTISM)
Epidemiology: 0.06–0.7% of school-age children, onset between 3 and 6 years (insidious or acute).

Etiology: temperament, parental overprotectiveness.

Symptoms: the child speaks when alone with a family member or a friend but becomes mute with strangers or in school, associated with shyness.

Differential diagnosis: normal adjustment to a new situation (1% of children keep quiet at the beginning of the school year), language disorder (problems speaking at home as well), immigrant children not yet bilingual.

Course: less than a few months.

Complications: school refusal, academic failure.

Treatment: behavior rx, SSRIs (fluoxetine: 0.6 mg/kg/d).

REACTIVE ATTACHMENT DISORDER OF INFANCY OR EARLY CHILDHOOD

Epidemiology: uncommon, onset in first few years of life.

Etiology: neglect, severe abuse, institutionalization.

Symptoms: young children: lack of smile, of eye contact, of interest in others, poor grasp, apathy, malnourishment. Older children: inhibition (withdrawal, hypervigilance), or disinhibition (indiscriminate in relationships or overfriendly with anyone).

Differential diagnosis: autism, severe MR, failure to thrive.

Course: death from malnutrition, poor relationships.

Treatment: consistent nurturing must be done early on, if not: risk of hospitalizations, foster placement, or residential treatments.

STEREOTYPIC MOVEMENT DISORDER AND DISORDER OF INFANCY, CHILDHOOD, OR ADOLESCENCE NOS

Epidemiology: prevalence of self-injurious behaviors is 2–3% of children and adolescents, M > F, 10–20% of pts with MR, frequent in genetic syndromes (Lesch-Nyhan syndrome), Tourette disorder, pts with blindness, deafness.

Etiology: genetic factors (Lesch-Nyhan syndrome: sx are: MR, hyperuricemia, spasticity, self-injurious behaviors); autism; deprivation; DA? Dopamine agonists ↑ stereotypic behaviors and dopamine antagonists ↓ them; possible role of endogenous opioids.

Symptoms: compulsive, repetitive motor behaviors interfering with normal activities; are voluntary and usually comforting; may produce self-injuries:

- Head banging: M : F is 3 : 1; usually begins in infancy, has a rhythmic, monotonous pattern
- Nail biting: may be associated with severe MR, schizophrenia; ↑ with anxiety; risk of infections

Differential diagnosis: OCD, tic disorders, trichotillomania, PDD.

Course: ↑ and ↓; duration and course vary: may disappear by age 4, or become chronic (esp. in MR and PDD).

Complications: eye poking, severe bites, infections, bleeding.

Treatment:

- Behavioral: adjust environment, use behavioral rx to ↑ positive safe behaviors and ↓ self-injurious behaviors; sometimes physical restraints, helmets
- Pharmacology: neuroleptics, opiate antagonists, fenfluramine (*Pondimin*), clomipramine (*Anafranil*), fluoxetine (*Prozac*). Buspirone (*Buspar*) and trazodone (*Desyrel*) have been tried.

17 ■ EATING DISORDERS

National organizations:
  National Eating Disorders Association: www.nationaleatingdisorders.org
  Academy of Eating Disorders: www.aedweb.org
  Eating Disorders Awareness and Prevention (EDAP): www.edap.org
  Anorexia Nervosa and Associated Disorders (ANAD): www.anad.org
  Bulimia Anorexia Nervosa Association (BANA): http://www.bana.ca/

Readings:
  Lock, J., Le Grange, D., Agras, W. S., & Dare, C. (2005). *Treatment manual for anorexia nervosa: A family-based approach.* New York: Guilford Press.
  Practice guidelines for the treatment of eating disorders, *American Journal of Psychiatry* (2006), *163*(7 suppl), 1–54.

Scales for eating disorders: Eating Disorders Examination (EDE; better than the SCID-I for purging behaviors).

High prevalence, more pts are seen in outpatient clinics, by pediatricians and primary care physicians, limitation of pharmacotherapy or psychotherapy alone, multidisciplinary team is more effective; if untreated: high morbidity and mortality rates.

TABLE 17.1. Men and Eating Disorders

- 10% of eating disorders (46% have bulimia nervosa [BN] and 22% have anorexia nervosa [AN])
- ↑ family members with mood disorders, OCD, anxiety, alcohol dependence
- Risk factor: sexual and physical abuse
- ↑ steroid use
- Later onset, low stress tolerance, ↑ in gay communities?
- Men with AN have ↑ risk for psychotic disorders
- Men with BN have ↑ risk for personality disorders

TABLE 17.2. Evaluation Components in Eating Disorders

- Psychiatric evaluation
- Medical work-up
- Records/consultation with other involved parties (therapists, school, coaches/ trainers, ministry)
- Presenting problem (dieting, restricting, bingeing, purging, exercise, drive for thinness)
- Weight history: highest, lowest, current, ideal
- Typical food day
- Family/social hx
- Medical/psychiatric hx
- Assess distorted attitudes: striving for perfection, asceticism superior to self-indulgence, feeling fat
- Goals for rx: assess motivation, denial, resistance

TABLE 17.3. Laboratory Studies in Eating Disorders

● All eating disorders	● Electrolytes, glucose, albumin, liver and renal function, CBC with diff., U/A, ECG, TSH
● Anorexia nervosa	● Serum magnesium, phosphate, calcium; creatinine clearance; chest X-ray, estrogen in ♀, testosterone in ♂, bone density scan, sometimes brain MRI, drug screen
● Bulimia and purging	● Serum magnesium, phosphate, calcium, bone density scan if also AN, amylase (fractionated), fecal occult blood, urine for electrolytes and laxatives, drug screen
● Binge eating	● FBS, lipid panel

ANOREXIA NERVOSA (AN)

Definition: refusal to maintain a normal weight (often to the point of starvation), intense fear of gaining weight, disturbance of body image.

Criteria: must have less than 85% of normal body weight and in post-menarchal ♀, absence of at least three consecutive menstrual cycles. Denial of sx, secrecy, resistance to seek rx are usual.

Two types:

- **Restrictive**: no loss of appetite, refusal to eat with others in public, only food intake restriction. Possible ↑ exercise, more in cluster C personality disorders.

- **Binge eating/purging**: secretive binges followed by self-induced vomiting, misuse of laxatives, diuretics, enemas; overexercising, particular behaviors about food (hiding food, collecting recipes, cooking for others). Some common features with pts who have BN without AN, obesity in the family, sometimes with substance abuse, impulse control disorders, personality disorders (cluster B and C), depression, social isolation. Loss of control indicators: faster eating than normal, until uncomfortably full, eating large amounts even when not hungry, eating alone (shame), self-disgust, guilt after overeating.

Medical changes in AN

TABLE 17.4.   Medical Complications of AN

● Cachexia	● ↓ Fat and muscles, ↓ thyroid metabolism, intolerance to cold, hypothermia
● CV	● Arrhythmias, ↑ QT interval, bradycardia, low BP, edema of extremities, risk of sudden death
● GI	● Constipation, abdominal pain, ↑ liver enzymes
● Reproduction	● Amenorrhea, ↓ levels of FSH, LH, GnRH; delayed psychosexual development, normal prolactin, ↑ cortisol
● Skin	● Lanugo, skin dryness, yellowish palms and soles, hair loss; optic hyperesthesia; zinc deficiency (poor skin healing)
● Blood changes	● Leucopenia, electrolyte changes, dehydration (↑ BUN), shock, low FBS, rare↓ platelets, late anemia
● Psychiatric	● Depression, cognitive disorder, abnormal taste sensation (zinc deficiency), OCD, rigidity, perfectionism
● Bones	● Osteoporosis, hypomagnesemia, ↑ calcemia

Epidemiology: 0.5–1% of adolescent girls; F : M is 10–20 : 1; onset (85%: ages 13–20; age of onset is becoming younger: ♀ and ♂ ages 8–9); all ethnic groups.

Etiology:

- **Biology**: ↓ NE activity in some pts with AN (↓ MHPG in urine and CSF), disturbances in DA function (↑ dopamine D2 and D3 receptor activity in the dorsal caudate), role of endogenous opioids in the denial of hunger; changes during starvation (↑ cortisolemia, suppression of thyroid function, amenorrhea with ↓ LTH, FSH, GRH hormones, enlarged sulci and ventricles in brain on CT scans) are corrected after realimentation.

- **Social factors**: society's role, emphasizing thinness and exercise; ↑ hostility, chaos, marital difficulties in families.

- **Genetics**: genes may be greater than culture or environment. Frequent anxiety disorders (OCD, social phobias).

- **Psychologic factors**: conflicts about autonomy, assertiveness, self-control, womanhood, unacceptable oral needs, problems with parents.

Differential diagnosis: R/O: medical illness (brain tumor, cancer), mental illnesses (depression: loss of appetite, no fear of obesity, normal body image; somatization disorders: less weight loss, less body image distortion, no amenorrhea; schizophrenia: delusions such as food being poisoned, no fear of being obese; bulimia nervosa: episodes of bingeing followed by self-induced vomiting, weight in a normal range, but may coexist with AN).

Course: varies; restrictive types recover less than binge-purging type. Mortality rates: 5–18%; poor outcome: parental conflicts, bulimia nervosa, comorbidity (OCD, depression). Many pts with AN have also bulimia nervosa. In AN: 50–70% get better, 30% stay chronically ill, 10% will die. Men: poorer prognosis.

Treatment: comprehensive, individualized rx plan (medical, behavioral, individual, family rx, sometimes medications), long term. Treat comorbidity (anxiety, depression, OCD, psychosis, PTSD are less frequent in AN than in BN, but greater in AN with binge eating/purging than in the restrictive type). Depression and anxiety may improve with weight restoration alone.

- **Goals**

TABLE 17.5.   Goals of Treatment

- Restore healthy weight (return of menses/ovulation)
- Treat medical complications
- Improve motivation to change
- Provide education on healthy nutrition
- Correct dysfunctional cognitive processes about thoughts, attitudes, and feelings
- Address individual issues (mood, self-esteem) and family issues
- Prevent relapses

- ## Challenges

TABLE 17.6.   Treatment Challenges

- **Challenge the pt's resistance:**
  - Rx threatens the artificially constructed world perpetuating the safe illusion of personal control and exposes the pt to realities
  - Rx exposes the body-image distortions, the lack of psychologic insight
  - Rx may be forced
- **Address the pt and the family's resistance over successive phases:** stages are similar to those in the rx of addictions (precontemplation, contemplation, preparation, action, maintenance, relapses)
  - Develop a therapeutic alliance by being absolutely honest about the rx
  - Validate the sx brought up by the pt (fatigue, insomnia, intolerance to cold, ↓ efficiency of thinking, loneliness)
  - Acknowledge the differences of opinions between pt and therapist
  - Explain that the therapist will intervene to save the pt's life even if it is unacceptable by the pt
  - Review all steps of rx (medical evaluation, strategy, team meetings)
  - Provide cognitive restructuring, supportive rx, psychodynamic approach (adaptive functions of the disorder, coping strategies, developmental arrest of the pt, understanding the obsessive-compulsive personality style), reconnect to peers and family, health-diet education, ↑ assertiveness skills
- **Provide strategies for dealing with relapses:** sx are markers of unmanaged conflicts

Adapted from Sansone, R. A., Levitt, J. L., & Sansone, L.A. (2005). A primer on psychotherapy treatment of anorexia nervosa in adolescents. *Psychiatry, 2,* 40–46.

TABLE 17.7.   Levels of Care for Eating Disorders

Hospitalization	Partial hospitalization or day program	Outpatient treatment
Reasons: ○ Weight <75% of the minimum weight for health, dehydration ○ Heart rate <45, cardiac arrhythmias, QTc > 0.444 ms ○ Temperature < 97.3°F (36.3°C) ○ ↓ Systolic BP (lying to standing) of 10 mm Hg or more ○ ↑ HR from lying to standing of 35 bpm or more ○ K+ level <3 mEq/L, ↓ Na+, hypophosphatemia ○ Psychotic depression, suicide attempt, incapacitating obsessions and compulsions, personality disorder, or out of control substance abuse ○ Pts who have relapsed or ill for more than 6 months, with hx of repeated hospitalizations for AN and not functioning in the community ○ Acute food refusal ○ Acute medical complications: syncope, seizures, cardiac failure, pancreatitis **Procedures:** ○ Commitment may be needed if refusal to eat and risk of death from malnutrition ○ Monitor daily weight, input and output serum electrolytes, supervision for 2–3 hr after meals (prevent vomiting), small regular feedings, liquid food supplements ○ The first goal is restoration of weight (slow refeeding). The second goal is preventing relapse	• Transition from inpatient program for pts with hx of *x* hospitalizations • Severe chronic AN • Pts with repeated relapses • Pts with severe comorbid personality disorders or substance abuse • Recent relapse, causing severe impairment in function • Out of control bingeing or purging with no major medical consequences	• First episode • No previous treatment • Relapse after resuming nl weight • Relapse after abstinence from bingeing and purging • Continuing rx after partial hospitalization or hospitalization

Adapted from Halmi, K. A. (2005). A complicated process: Diagnosing and treating anorexia nervosa and bulimia. *Psychiatric Times, XXII*(6), 59–62.

- **Psychotherapy**: individual and family dynamic psychotherapies, also CBT, CAT, Internet-facilitated group sessions (?). The family-based Maudsley treatment (FBT) appears effective (vs "parentectomy!") early in the illness and for adolescents greater than adults (work on rigidity, enmeshment, conflict avoidance, overprotectiveness); early weight gain and alliance predict better outcome.

- **Medications**: medications are adjunct and not effective as sole or primary tx; caution in their use for comorbid conditions such as MDD or OCD (may resolve with weight gain alone). Avoid drugs that ↑ QTc interval in pts with borderline/prolonged QTc. Note: drugs that ↑ QTc interval include antipsychotics, TCAs, macrolide antibiotics, and some antihistamines. If they are essential, monitor ECG. Insufficient evidence to use the following drugs: cyproheptadine (*Periactine*: 4–8 mg tid up to 32 mg/d) in nonpurging type; amitryptyline (*Elavil*: up to 160 mg/d), clomipramine (*Anafranil*), pimozide (*Orap*), chlorpromazine (*Thorazine*: 10 mg tid, max 50 mg tid), fluoxetine (*Prozac*). SSRIs may prevent relapse, treat anxiety, depression, OCD. Avoid TCAs if low-weight and risk of hypotension, cardiac arrhythmias; rarely ECT (AN + severe MDD). Modest improvement with low doses of antipsychotics (olanzapine: 2.5 mg/d up to 10–15 mg/d; risperidone; quetiapine). Estrogens do not offer protection against bone loss but weight restoration does.

BULIMIA NERVOSA (BN)

Web site: www.bulimiaguide.org

Standard growth charts, National Center for Health Statistics. CDC and Prevention: www.cdc.gov/growthcharts

Definition: recurrent episodes of binge eating frequently triggered by mood states (sweet, high-calorie food, eaten secretly, rapidly in large quantities), sense of lack of control, self-induced vomiting, misuse of laxatives, diuretics, excessive exercise to prevent weight gain. In BN, weight may be normal or ↑ or ↓; presence of body-image disturbances. Pts are usually more sexually active than in AN. Feelings of guilt, depression, self-disgust are present.

Criteria: pt binges >2×/wk for at least 3 months.

Two types:

- **Purging type**: regularly purging during an episode.
- **Nonpurging type**: pt uses compensatory behaviors to prevent weight gain but not purging (fasting, exercise)

Medical complications of purging: laboratory findings will vary if bulimia alone, bulimia with vomiting, if bulimia with vomiting and laxative or diuretic abuse.

TABLE 17.8. Medical Complications of Purging

● **Metabolic changes**	● ↓ K+, hypochloremic alkalosis, ↓ Mg++, dehydration, changes in calcium, magnesium, phosphates levels, ↑ cholesterol, thiamine or niacin deficiencies
● **GI and dental sx**	● Large salivary glands, ↑ amylase, abdominal pain, esophagitis (Barrett's esophagus), diarrhea, lacerations of palate and posterior pharynx, callus on dorsum of the hands (Russell sign), gum diseases. Loss of enamel and decays of front teeth
● **Neurologic sx**	● Seizures, neuropathy, cognitive disorders, cramps
● **Psychiatric sx**	● Depression, anxiety
● **CV sx**	● Hypotension, bradycardia, arrhythmias, shortness of breath, hypokalemic cardiopathy, QT and T-waves changes
● **Reproductive sx**	● Irregular menses

Etiology:

- **Biology**: role of serotonin in satiety; role of NE, endorphin?
- **Social factors**: high achievers, societal pressures, ↑ family depression, conflicts, past neglect, or sexual abuse.
- **Psychologic factors**: difficulties with autonomy, lack of super-ego control, poor ego strength, poor impulse control, past trauma (rape). Frequent in cluster B personality disorders.

Differential diagnosis: seizures, Kluver-Bucy syndrome (visual agnosia, compulsive licking and biting, hypersexuality, hyperphagia), Klein-Levin syndrome (episodes of hypersomnia and hyperphagia, more in men), and borderline personality disorder.

Course: better prognosis than AN, chronic, variable course; poor prognosis if severity of purging, onset >16 yr, association with AN; some spontaneous remissions. 40–50% are cured.

Treatment: individualized rx with **CBT** (20 sessions/5 months, targets food restriction and body image concerns; 50% of patients in CBT have full recovery), **intensive group**, **individual psychotherapy**, **IPT** (targets maladaptive interpersonal context), family rx, pharmacology. Benefit of combined tx. Hospitalization (if binges are out of control, outpatient rx has failed, suicidality, substance abuse). Nutritional rehabilitation is needed prior to treatment of any comorbidity; relaxation techniques.

- Long-term rx (6–12 months) with antidepressants (even nondepressed bulimics respond): **SSRIs are the first line (fluoxetine: start low and ↑ up to 60–80 mg/d, the only FDA-approved drug for BN)** useful to ↓ binge eating and purging and ↑ satiety; sertraline (50–200 mg/d); citalopram (20–60 mg/d); fluvoxamine (50–300 mg/d). Others: imipramine (*Tofranil*), **desipramine** lowers binge frequency about 50% (*Norpramine*: 100–300 mg/d), trazodone (*Desyrel*). SNRIs: little experience (duloxetine: 120 mg/d); venlafaxine: *Effexor*). **Bupropion is contraindicated by FDA due to ↑ seizures risk** in this population (if purging). Avoid MAOIs due to diet restrictions.

- **Topiramate**: linked to appetite suppression and ↓ weight (*Topamax*: start dose: 25 mg/d, ↑ up to 250 mg/d, max 600 mg/d), **Zonisamide (*Zonegran*:** 100 mg/d up to 600 mg/d). Ondansetron (*Zofran*; 24 mg/d): antiemetic, multiple daily dosing (?). Start slow and go slow with topiramate or zonisamide

- Other drugs (naltrexone: *Revia* at 200–300 mg/d; concerns with liver toxicity); weight neutral antipsychotics: ziprazidone or aripiprazole, used as adjunct for antidepressants (in severe, chronic, refractory BN)

- Phototherapy: tried with some success

- Appetite suppressants not indicated

- Treat comorbid disorders (PTSD in 13% of pts with BN, *MDD is more common in the purging type*, alcohol dependence, borderline personality disorders, social phobia); process countertransference

TABLE 17.9.   CBT Principles for Treating Binge-Eating Disorders (CBT, IPT, and DBT are Equally Effective)

• Self-monitor	• Keep detailed records of all dietary intake • Note antecedents to and consequences of binges • Look for patterns in timing, type, amount of food eaten
• Eat regularly; ↑ dietary restraint	• Only 3 planned meals and 2 snacks/d; modest calorie restriction
• Substitute other behaviors for bingeing	• Alternate pleasant activities • Recognize urges to binge and use a substitute activity
• Identify and revise erroneous thinking patterns (cognitive restructuring)	• Have realistic expectations in weight loss/ideal body size • Minimize self-criticism, negative thoughts • Develop new domains of self-worth (not body shape or weight)
• Limit vulnerability to relapse	• Have realistic expectations • Treat self-esteem, depression, anxiety • Create plan for encountering high-risk scenario

Adapted from Fairburn, C. G. (1995). *Overcoming Binge Eating*. New York: Guilford Press; Cloak, N. L., Powers, P. S. (2006). Beating obesity: Help patients control binge eating disorder and night eating syndrome. *Current Psychiatry*, 5(6), 25. Also see: Fairburn, C. G. (1997). Interpersonal psychotherapy for bulimia nervosa. In: D. M. Garner & P. E. Garfinkel (Eds.), *Handbook of Treatment for Eating Disorders* (2nd ed., p. 278–294). New York: Guilford Press.

EATING DISORDERS NOS

Residual category that does not meet previous criteria (e.g., purging disorder without large binge-eating episodes, and not during the course of AN).

OBESITY

National organizations:

American Obesity Association: www.obesity.org

eDiets.com: www.ediets.com

Food and Nutrition Information Center: www.nal.usda.gov/fnic

Obesity Surgery: www.obesitysurgery.com

Overeaters Anonymous: www.oa.org

Partnership for Healthy Weight Management: www.consumer.gov/weightloss

Shape Up America! www.shapeup.org

Take Off Pounds Sensibly (TOPS): www.tops.org

Weight Control Information Network (WIN): http: win.niddk.nih.gov

Reading:

Clinical guidelines on the identification, evaluation, and treatment of obesity in adults: http://www.nhlbi.nih.gov/guidelines/obesity. Retrieved September 4, 2010.

Definition: body weight exceeds by 20% the standard weight listed in the height–weight tables. Currently body mass index (BMI) is used.

BMI = (body weight in kg)/(height in m)^2. A normal BMI is 20–25. Obesity: BMI > 30.

Epidemiology: *intake of energy > energy output*. Genetic factors (80% of obese pts have overweight family members, twin studies), developmental factors (early weight gain involves ↑ number and size of adipocytes), hormones (leptin), physical activity, CNS (lateral and ventromedial hypothalamus), clinical disorders (Cushing disease, hypothyroidism, Frohlich syndrome, depression), medications (antipsychotics, SSRIs, some mood stabilizers), and psychologic factors (hyperphagia as a means to coping with stress) may be involved.

TABLE 17.10.   Psychiatric Medications Less Associated with Weight Gain +++

● **Mood stabilizers**	● Lamotrigine (*Lamictal*), oxcarbazepine (*Trileptal*), topiramate (*Topamax*)
● **Antipsychotics**	● Molindone (*Moban*), ziprasidone (*Geodon*), aripiprazole (*Abilify*)
● **Antidepressants**	● Bupropion (*Wellbutrin*), nefazodone (*Serzone*), venlafaxine (*Effexor*)

Differential diagnosis: R/O BN (binge eating); night eating syndrome (NES: where awakenings and eating are seen; NES is related to affective disorders. R/O sleep-related eating disorder [SRED], where pts eat unusual things in a confused state); Pickwick syndrome (obesity + respiratory + CV pathology); body dysmorphic disorder.

Course: illnesses, risk of premature death. Prognosis for ↓ weight is poor with relapses, progression. **Childhood obesity**: more resistant and severe. Psychosocial consequences: ↓ self-esteem, poor quality of life, low employments, lower education, discrimination, ↓ marriage in ♀. In obesity with binge eating: > 6-fold for MDD, > 8-fold for panic disorder, >13-fold for borderline personality disorder compared with obesity alone. In obesity with NES: ↑ depression, anxiety, substance use disorders.

Medical problems in obesity

TABLE 17.11.   Medical Problems in Obesity

● **Cardiovascular**	● Coronary disease, ventricular arrhythmias (sudden death), CHF, hypertension, brain disorders (infarction, hemorrhage), legs edema, varicose veins
● **Respiratory**	● Obstructive sleep apnea, Pickwickian syndrome, polycythemia
● **Hepatobiliary**	● Cholelithiasis, liver steatosis, GERDs
● **Metabolic**	● Diabetes mellitus, gout, hyperlipidemias
● **Renal**	● Proteinuria
● **Muscular-skeletal**	● Osteoarthritis, osteoarthrosis
● **Cancers**	● In ♀ : ↑ endometrium, breast, ovary, cervix, gallbladder cancers ● In ♂ : ↑ colon, rectum, prostate cancers

Treatment: weight reduction may be life saving.

- **Diet**: ↓ intake calories below optimal: low-calorie diet (1,200 calories), vitamins (iron, folic acid, zinc, vitamin B$_6$). Weight watchers behavioral weight loss program or equivalent
- **Exercise**: obese pts expend more calories for the same amount of activity than pts with normal weight. Exercise helps keep weight loss.
- **Treat cause if possible**: NES with melatonin, antidepressants, appetite suppressants, light therapy; treat SRED as a parasomnia.
- **Pharmacotherapy**:
  - Appetite suppressors (risk of tolerance)

TABLE 17.12.   Medications Used in Obesity Treatment

● Amphetamine, dextroamphetamine: 12.5–20 mg/d
● Methamphetamine (*Desoxyn*): 10–15 mg/d
● Benzphetamine (*Didrex*): 75–150 mg/d
● Phendimetrazine (*Bontril, Plegine, Prelu-2, X-Trozine*): 105 mg/d
● Phentermine hydrochloride (*Adipex-P, Fastin, Oby-trim*): 18.75–37.5 mg/d
● Phentermine resin (*Ionamin*): 15–30 mg/d
● Diethylproprion hydrochloride (*Tenuate*): 75 mg/d
● Mazindol (*Sanorex, Mazanor*): 3–9 mg/d
● Phenylpropanolamine (*Dexatrim, Acutrim*): 75 mg/d
● **Orlistat (Xenical)**: ↓ fat absorbed by 30%, to be used with low-fat diet (risk of oily spotting); 120 mg tid. Add vitamin supplement. Some pts misuse it to compensate for the binge eating
● **Sibutramine (Meridia)**: 5–15 mg/d (start low), is a *controlled drug (schedule IV)*; is an SNRI: do not use with MAOIs or serotoninergic agents (risk of serotonin syndrome), monitor BP, do not use if coronary heart disease, stroke, CHF, arrhythmias. Some report of psychosis

Dexfenfluramine (Redux) and fenfluramine (Pondimin) have been removed from the market because of reports of aortic and mitral regurgitation.

Options for binge-eating disorders with obesity and mood disorders:

Depression:

Mild: first line (topiramate), second line (SSRI or venlafaxine), third line (bupropion or zonis-amide/*Zonegran* or add orlistat)

Moderate to severe: first line (venlafaxine or SSRI or bupropion/caution risk of seizures particularly in BN, or topiramate), second line (zonisamide or add orlistat)

Bipolar disorders: minimize antidepressants and appetite suppressants if unstable bipolar disorder

Mild: first line (topiramate), second line (zonisamide or lithium, or lamotrigine, or other mood stabilizer), third line (add orlistat or add antidepressant)

Severe: first line (lithium + topiramate), second line (lamotrigine + topiramate, or lithium + zonisamide), third line (topiramate, or zonisamide + other mood stabilizer or add orlistat or add antidepressant)

Note: in **olanzapine-treated pts who gained weight**: some strategies (poor controlled studies): Nizatidine (Axid): 300 mg bid or Amantadine (Symmetrel): 100–300 mg/d or metformin (Glucophage): 500–2,550 mg/d or topiramate (Topamax).

- **Bariatric surgery**: gastric bypass (the Roux-en-Y gastric bypass, bilio-pancreatic bypass), gastroplasty (stapling, adjustable gastric banding):

    ↑ Vomiting, electrolyte imbalances, food malabsorption, obstructions; changes the absorption of drugs not exposed to gastric acid. One third of bariatric candidates take psychiatric medications (use immediate-release forms), crush oral medications in the immediate post-op period; monitor serum levels; postoperative ↓ weight (mostly adipose tissue) affects lipid-soluble drugs (fluoxetine, oxcarbazepine). After weight loss: ↓ glomerular filtration → less lithium needed. Psychiatric contraindications: active psychosis, *x* suicide attempts in past 5 yr, substance abuse, poor compliance with rx.

- **Psychotherapy**: insight oriented, CBT (develop new eating habits, recognize hunger cues, keep a diary of food consumed), group rx

PICA

Definition: pathologic craving for and eating of nonnutritive items (e.g., clay, paper, metals, foam rubber, hair, egg shells, foreign objects, toothpaste, chalk, sand, soil, blood) or food ingredients (e.g., flour, raw potatoes, baking soda). This behavior must be **repeated for >1 month** and be developmentally inappropriate. 50% of normal children aged 18–36 months have pica but this ↓ with age.

TABLE 17.13.   Examples of Pica

- Pagophagia: ice
- Geomelophagia: raw potatoes
- Plumbophagia: lead, painted chips
- Geophagia: clay
- Mylophagia: laundry starch
- Cautopyreiophagia: burnt matches
- Trichophagia: hair
- Lithophagia: stones
- Coprophagia: feces

Etiology: developmental (age, cognitive level, MR), psychologic (maternal deprivation, neglect, disorganized family, poor parent–child interactions), sociocultural (ethnicity such as sedentary aborigines in Australia, historic, geographic like in Turkey: eating clay to ↑ fertility), nutritional (deficiency in iron, zinc, calcium; dietary habits; lead intoxication); mostly in children and pregnant ♀, pts with severe psychiatric disorders (psychosis), pts with CNS congenital anomalies, deafness, seizures, neuroleptic use. CNS neurochemical iron-dependent appetite regulation possible (iron loss may promote pica).

Complications: lead poisoning (lead levels must be <25 mg/dL), LD, ↓ attention span, impulsivity, MR, seizures, peripheral neuropathy, behavioral disturbances (stereotypic behaviors, self-abuse). Absorption of paper; risk of mercury poisoning; ingestion of soil: risk of parasitic infections.

Treatment: behavioral, pt's education, iron supplement, lead levels, pharmacologic rx (SSRIs, atypical neuroleptics, dopaminergic drugs: bromocriptine, methylphenidate), bupropion, buprenorphine, chlorimipramine.

18 ■ NORMAL SLEEP AND SLEEP DISORDERS

National organizations:
American Academy of Sleep Medicine: http://www.aasmnet.org/
Sleep Research Society: http://www.sleepresearchsociety.org/
Scales: Functional Outcomes of Sleep Questionnaire (FOSQ), Verran and Snyder-Halpern Sleep Scale, Epworth Sleepiness Disorder Scale, Sleep Disturbance Scale for Children (SDSC).

NORMAL SLEEP

Normal sleep is cyclic (45 cycles/night), active, and has a restorative function.

Two states:
- *Nonrapid eye movement* **(NREM)**: stages $1 \rightarrow 4$, $\downarrow$ physiologic functions, episodic movements present, good muscle tone. Stage 4 mostly occurs in the 1st third of the night (arousal from stage 3 or $4 \rightarrow$ disorganization/like in sleepwalking, night terrors).
- *Rapid eye movement* **(REM)**: $\uparrow$ brain activity and physiologic functions, $\downarrow$ muscle tone, penile erection +, dream is common, EEG (low voltage, fast, "sawtooth" waves), REM latency of 90 min in adults, REM cycles occur q 90–100 min, lasting 10–40 min each. In the last third of the night: REM periods lengthen, stage 4 disappears, lighter sleep.

Life span:
- Neonatal period: REM >50% of total sleep time.
- Adulthood: NREM (75% with stage 1 made of 5%, stage 2 of 45%, stage 3 of 12%, stage 4 of 13%), REM (25%).

EEG: *waking* (*alpha* waves: 8–12 cps), stage 1 (low voltage, theta waves: 3–7 cps), stage 2 (sleep spindles: 13–15 cps and high spikes: K complexes), stage 3 (delta waves, high voltage: 0.5–2.5 cps), *stage 4* (*delta waves*: 0.5–2 cps).

Sleep regulation: *x* centers in brainstem, role of serotonine (L-tryptophan deficiency $\rightarrow$ $\downarrow$ REM sleep), role of locus ceruleus ($\uparrow$ in noradrenergic activity $\rightarrow$ $\uparrow$ in wakefulness), role of cholinergic system ($\downarrow$ REM sleep in Alzheimer disease), melatonin (role of hypothalamus and pineal gland in the circadian patterns), DA (arousal effect).

Sleep–wake rhythm: natural body clock follows a 25-hr cycle; external factors (light-dark cycle, meals, jet lag), biologic rhythms (neonatal vs adult patterns, menstrual cycles).

TYPES OF SLEEP DISORDERS

Generalities:
- **Definition**: may need to be studied in the sleep laboratory.
  - **Insomnia**: difficulty initiating or maintaining sleep. 40% of adults
  - **Hypersomnia**: excessive amounts of sleep, excessive daytime sleepiness (somnolence: sleepiness + tendency to fall asleep suddenly in the waking state). 5% of adults
  - **Parasomnias**: unusual phenomena appearing suddenly during sleep or at the limit of wake and sleep. Usually in stages 3 and 4, associated with amnesia
  - **Sleep–wake schedule disturbance**: inability to sleep or being awake at regular times but ability at other undesired times:
- **Risks**: if sleep >8.5 hr or <3.5 hr $\rightarrow$ 15% $\uparrow$ mortality

Primary sleep disorders:
- Not caused by another mental illness, a physical condition, a substance
- **Dyssomnias**: primary insomnia, primary hypersomnia, narcolepsy, breathing-related sleep disorder (obstructive sleep apnea syndrome, central alveolar hypoventilation), circadian rhythm sleep disorder (sleep–wake schedule disorder such as delayed sleep phase type, jet lag type, shift work type), dyssomnias NOS (nocturnal myoclonus or periodic limb movements, restless legs syndrome, Klein-Levin

syndrome, menstrual-associated syndrome, sleep disturbance in pregnancy, insufficient sleep, sleep drunkenness)

- **Parasomnias**: nightmare disorders, sleep terror disorder, sleep-walking disorders, parasomnias NOS (bruxism, REM sleep behavior disorder, sleep-talking, sleep-related head banging, sleep paralysis)
- **Insomnia and hypersomnia related to Axis I or Axis II disorder (another mental disorder)**: >1 month, severe → distress and ↓ in functioning

Other sleep disorders:

- **Sleep disorders due to a general condition**: epileptic seizures (disrupts REM sleep), cluster headaches (REM sleep), abnormal swallowing (with coughing, choking), asthma, cardiovascular symptoms, GERD, paroxysmal nocturnal hemoglobinuria (AM urine is brownish red)
- **Substance-induced sleep disorder**: during or within 1 month of substance intoxication or withdrawal but not only during a delirium

INSOMNIA

Etiology:

TABLE 18.1.   Causes of Insomnia

• **Related to another mental disorder**	• Depressive episode of major depression or bipolar disorder, mania or hypomania • Dysthymia • Schizophrenia • Generalized anxiety disorder, PTSD
• **Related to general medical condition**	• Circadian rhythm sleep disorder (jet lag, night shift work) • Sleep apnea • Restless legs syndrome • Syndrome of painful legs and moving toes • Nocturnal myoclonus • Chronic pain or distressing condition (GERD, arthritis, CHF) • Aging • CNS lesions • Endocrine and metabolic disorders • Infectious, neoplastic diseases
• **Related to substances**	• Caffeine, stimulants (cocaine, nicotine, amphetamines, hallucinogens, ephedrine, corticosteroids, theophylline), alcohol withdrawal, chronic use of alcohol (fragmented sleep), opioid withdrawal, sleeping-pill insomnia due to tolerance or withdrawal. Medications: cancer drugs, thyroid hormones, ACTH-like drugs, oral contraceptives, α-methyldopa, anticonvulsants, antidepressants
• **Related to environmental conditions**	• Major stress (illness, divorce, family problems) → may become self-perpetuating, conditioned insomnia

Adapted from Moore, D. P. (2006). *The Little Black Book of Psychiatry*, (3rd ed). Sudbury, MA: Jones & Bartlett Learning. p. 267.

Diagnosis: *nonrestorative sleep, difficulty in initiating or maintaining sleep (frequent or early awakening), >1 month.*

- **Questions to ask the pt**: sleep attacks or naps during the day? Poor concentration during the day? Trouble falling asleep? Pattern of sleep (hour of sleep, frequency of spontaneous or provoked awakenings), how long has it been going on? Precipitant (pains, worries, shift work, travels)? Morning awakening (time, feeling rested or no)? Substances use (alcohol, coffee, tea)? Prescription and nonprescriptions medications used? Mental illness? Medical problems? Snoring? In conditioned insomnia, pt's daytime function is nl, pt worries excessively about not being able to sleep, sleeps better away from home, cannot clear his mind at bedtime, has muscular tension.
- **Questions to ask the sleep partner about the pt**: snoring? Stop breathing? Kicking, jerking of limbs? Seizure?

Course: usually chronic in primary insomnia (rare, onset in childhood), may resolve in months (10% in gl population).

Treatment:

- R/O and treat specific syndromes
- Sleep hygiene

TABLE 18.2. Advice for Sleep Hygiene

(1) Maintain a regular bedtime and awakening time schedule including weekends. No day nap
(2) Establish a regular, relaxing bedtime routine (warm bath or shower, aroma therapy, reading, or listening to soothing music). Practice evening relaxation techniques
(3) Sleep in a room that is dark, quiet, and cool in a comfortable bed
(4) Use bedroom only for sleep and sex. Have work materials, computers, and TVs in another room. Avoid daytime naps. If not asleep after 5–10 min, get up, go to another room and do something else
(5) Finish eating at least 2–3 hr prior to going to bed. Eat at regular times; avoid large meals prior to going to sleep
(6) Discontinue caffeine, alcohol, and smoking
(7) Exercise regularly but stop a few hours before bed time

- Relaxation techniques: progressive muscular relaxation, meditation, biofeedback, satisfying sex, psychotherapy (cognitive rx?)
- Pharmacotherapy:
  - Hypnotic drugs: caution with the elderly (start with lower doses; risk of falls; DDIs to be checked in particular if the pts are on multiple medications and/or have dementia, or other disabilities)
  - **Benzodiazepine and benzodiazepine-like drugs**: use for <2 wk (risk of tolerance and withdrawal with rebound insomnia)
    - **Short-acting for problems falling asleep**, like triazolam (*Halcion*: 0.125–0.250 mg hs), zolpidem (*Ambien*: 5–10 mg hs; *Ambien-CR*: 12.5 mg po q hs, CR form may be used chronically), zaleplon (*Sonata*: 5–10 mg hs). Rebound insomnia may be associated with them if long-term use
    - **Short and intermediate action**: nonbenzodiazepine hypnotic eszopiclone (*Lunesta*: 1–3 mg q hs); benzodiazepines such as temazepam (*Restoril*: 7.5–30 mg po q hs up to 7–10 days), or estazolam (*Prosom*: 1–2 mg po q hs up to 12 wk)
    - **Long-acting for middle of the night insomnia**, like flurazepam (*Dalmane*: 15–30 mg at hs), lorazepam (*Ativan*: 2–4 mg hs)
  - **Melatonin receptor agonist**: ramelteon (*Rozerem*: 8 mg hs)
  - **H1 antihistamines**: diphenhydramine (25–50 mg hs), hydroxyzine (50–100 mg hs): caution in the elderly (DDIs and anticholinergic effects)
  - **Antidepressants**: mirtazapine (15–30 mg hs), trazodone (50–200 mg hs)
  - Dietary supplements: Melatonin (risk of eosinophilic myalgia), L-tryptophan (risk of serotonin syndrome if used with an SSRI)
- Light therapy.

HYPERSOMNIA

Etiology:

TABLE 18.3. Causes of Hypersomnia

● Related to a mental disorder	● Depressive episode of a major depression or bipolar disorder
● Related to a medical disorder	● Narcolepsy ● Sleep apnea ● Circadian rhythm sleep disorder ● Klein-Levin syndrome (recurrent form of primary hypersomnia) ● Pickwickian syndrome (central alveolar hypoventilation syndrome) ● Respiratory failure ● Myotonic muscular dystrophy ● Endocrinologic, metabolic, toxic conditions ● Post head trauma ● Focal brain lesions (cerebral hemispheres, thalamus, hypothalamus, brain stem) ● Encephalitis
● Related to substances	● Alcohol, sedative-hypnotics, antidepressants, neuroleptics, opioids (acute use or withdrawal), withdrawal from stimulants
● Related to the environment	● Sleep deprivation, avoidance reactions

Diagnosis: primary hypersomnia: excessive sleepiness (prolonged or daytime sleep episodes, >1 month, q day). Recurrent type: >3 days at a time, × times/yr, for >2 yr. Can be primary (diagnosis of exclusion) or secondary.

- **Narcolepsy**:
  - Lifetime prevalence: 0.1%, onset in late teens or early adulthood, attacks occur for >3 months; abnormality of the REM-inhibiting mechanisms in brain stem; sporadic or hereditary cases
  - **Four symptoms**:
    - **Narcoleptic attacks**: overwhelming desire to sleep followed by REM sleep of a few seconds up to 30 min; pt is easily awakened, feels refreshed, and remembers vivid dreams. Other causes of sleep attacks: brain stem, diencephalic, temporal lobe lesion, postencephalitis lethargica, idiopathic recurrent stupor (attacks are gradual at onset and termination, and last hours to days)
    - **Cataplectic attacks**: sudden bilateral weakness, generalized (fall, slumping over) or focal (jaw drop, neck, hand, knees), precipitated by a strong emotion, clearing in <1 min; if, longer, may be + visual hallucinations. Pt is alert during attack. Other causes of cataplexia: idiopathic, dominantly inherited, simple partial seizure, mesencephalic or pontine lesions
    - **Sleep paralysis**: upon falling asleep or awakening, usually pt is alert, may have visual hallucinations. Few seconds or more
    - **Hypnagogic hallucinations**: (visual > auditory), vivid, occurring when pt falls asleep
  - **Diagnosis**: polysomnographic recording (characteristic sleep-onset REM period with appearance of REM sleep within 10 min of sleep onset). In daytime: presence of multiple sleep-onset REM periods
  - **HLA-DR2** (type of human leukocyte antigen) was found in 90–100% of pts with narcolepsy. It is falsely + in 20% of the normal population. ↓ levels of hypocretin in CSF and hypothalamus
  - **Treatment**: no cure, chronic disease, may be life threatening
    - Forced regular naps sometimes sufficient, lifestyle adjustment, psychotherapy
    - Medications:
      - **Only effective on narcolepsy**:
        - Stimulants: methylphenidate (Ritalin: 20–60 mg/d)
        - Modafinil (Provigil: 200 mg 1×/d)
      - **Effective on narcolepsy and cataplexy**: Clomipramine (Anafranil: 25–75 mg/day, risk of sedation), Desipramine (Norpramin: 25–75 mg/day), Protriptyline (Vivactil: 10–40 mg/day), Imipramine (Tofranil: 75–300 mg/day), Selegiline (Emsam patch: 6–12 mg/d) but dietary restrictions, DDIs

- **Obstructive sleep-apnea (breathing-related sleep disorder)**
  - **Lifetime prevalence**: 1–10%, M : F is 3 : 1. Onset: middle years, ♀ after menopause. Hypersomnia during the day. Chronic
  - An apneic period (no airflow through mouth and nose), lasts 10–120 s and 30–300 may happen in one night, each followed by an arousal. **Pathologic: >5× in 1 hr or >30/night**. Interrupted with a loud gasping snort. Normal arterial blood gas (ABG) levels during the day.
  - **Three types**:
    - **Obstructive apneic episodes**: airflow stops but respiratory effort ↑ during apnea. Obstruction in the airway (micrognathia, tonsillar or adenoidal hypertrophy, lingual hypertrophy in acromegaly, hypothyroidy, obesity)
    - **Central apneic episodes**: airflow stops with no respiratory effort during apnea (usually no gasping snort). Causes are obesity, defective brain stem, respiratory mechanism
    - **Mixed apneic episodes**
  - **Risks**: crib deaths, pulmonary and cardiovascular deaths in adults, elderly (arrhythmias, ↑ pulmonary blood pressure, changes in BP, daytime accidents, morning headaches, mood changes)
  - **Diagnosis**: polysomnography; Oximetry; 24 hr ECG
  - **Treatment**: treat obesity, surgery if severe obstruction (tonsillectomy, uvulopalatopharyngoplasty, or tracheostomy), nasal continuous positive airway pressure (**nCPAP**), medications to ↓ REM sleep (paroxetine: 20 mg/d, tricyclics like protriptyline: 20 mg/d), theophylline. Avoid all sedative medications, alcohol. Pts should sleep on their side.

- **Pickwickian syndrome (central alveolar hypoventilation syndrome)**
  - **Common**: gradual onset with obesity, drowsiness, day somnolence, confusion. No significant apneic episode
  - **Lab**: ↑ CO_2, ↓ O_2, erythrocytosis

- **Complications**: obstructive sleep apnea, pulmonary hypertension, poor functioning. Severe hypercapnia → ↑ intracranial pressure (papilledema). Death may occur during sleep.
- **Treatment**: weight loss, mechanical ventilation

- **Klein-Levin syndrome (recurrent form of primary hypersomnia)**
  - Recurrent periods of prolonged sleep, with periods of normal sleep and alertness. The episodes last 1–2 wk, with hypersomnolence (>18 hr/d), hyperphagia, hypersexuality (sexual disinhibitions). Affective changes may exist (mania, depression, with or without psychosis), withdrawal, disorientation, poor memory
  - Rare, onset between 10 and 21 yo. Occurs at the beginning q 3–6 months, then ↓ and ceases
  - **Differential diagnosis**: bulimia nervosa (no somnolence, shorter episodes)
  - **Etiology**: thalamus, brain stem damages? Some cases preceded by a flu-like illness?
  - **Treatment**: Lithium? Stimulants?

CIRCADIAN RHYTHM SLEEP DISORDER

Epidemiology: common

Etiology: role of the hypothalamic suprachiasmatic nucleus. Not due to a mental illness, another sleep disorder, medical condition, or a substance.

Definition: misalignment between the endogenous sleep–wake and the environmental demands. Four types:

- **Delayed sleep phase**: spontaneous presence of delayed sleep onset and delayed awakening times, familial
- **Jet lag**: sleepiness and alertness appearing after travels to several time zones, usually eastward
- **Shift work**: somnolence while working at night and insomnia when attempting to sleep during the day associated with night shift work or x changes in shift work
- **Unspecified**: advanced sleep phase syndrome (not interfering with work), or disorganized sleep–wake pattern (irregular pattern of sleep and alert times but total amount of sleep in 24 hr is normal)

Complications: accidents, ↓ work performance, ↑ peptic ulcers, ↑ cardiovascular diseases.

Course: the advanced sleep phase type appears chronic. The delayed sleep phase may normalize after a few years. The jet lag and the shift work types usually reset within 1–2 wk.

Treatment: Resetting the endogenous clock (adhere to the new environmental schedule; expose to bright light if needs wakefulness).

Jet lag may need a number of days = the number of time zones traversed. Short-acting hypnotics for a few nights (zolpidem: 10 mg hs, or zaleplon: 5–10 mg hs). Melatonin: 5 mg 2 hours before bedtime in the delayed sleep phase type.

RESTLESS LEGS SYNDROME (EKBOM SYNDROME)

Epidemiology: prevalence: 2–10%. Family hx + in 50–90%, ↑ with age. 20% have onset < age 10.

Definition: need to move legs; uncomfortable feeling like itching, crawling, burning, tingling (mostly in the calves); ↑ at rest, ↓ with walking, prevents sleep, frequently + nocturnal myoclonus (periodic limb involuntary movement during sleep).

Differential diagnosis: akathisia due to neuroleptics, due to Parkinson disease, peripheral neuropathy, nocturnal leg cramps.

Etiology: primary (autosomal dominant/related to CNS iron metabolism disturbances) or secondary (peripheral neuropathy, low iron anemia, pregnancy, uremia, chronic hemodialysis, rheumatoid arthritis, peripheral vascular disease).

Complications: fatigue, irritability.

Course: chronic, ↑ and ↓ or progressive.

Treatment: treat cause if secondary. May be useful (as 1st choice: *gabapentin* or clonazepam).

- Dopaminergic drugs like levodopa (50–250 mg/day), pramipexole (Mirapex; 0.125–0.75 mg/day), bromo-criptine (1.25–7.5 mg/day): sx may appear earlier during the day and may become more severe
- Antiepileptic drugs like gabapentin (600 mg in the early PM and 1,200 mg q hs), carbamazepine, valproate
- Benzodiazepines like clonazepam (0.5–2 mg q hs)
- Opioids: oxycodone (15 mg hs), propoxyphene (65 mg hs)

- Clonidine (0.025–0.05 mg hs)
- Others: quinine, propanolol

PERIODIC LIMB MOVEMENTS OF SLEEP (NOCTURNAL MYOCLONUS)

Epidemiology: 40% > age 65.

Definition: sudden jerking limb movement of one or both lower extremities (ankle, knee, thigh), lasting 0.5–10 s, occurring in episodes (each lasting minutes to an hour or greater), in an unaware pt, frequent awakenings and fatigue. Sometimes associated with restless legs syndrome. Usually during NREM sleep.

Etiology: primary inherited (disturbances in DA transmission in the basal ganglia) or secondary (spinal cord lesions, renal failure, acid folic deficiency, CHF, pregnancy)

Differential diagnosis: hypnic jerks when pt falls asleep only, movement due to antidepressants, encephalopathy (hepatic, uremic).

Course: chronic.

Complications: fatigue, irritability.

Treatment: like restless legs syndrome.

PARASOMNIAS

(1) **Nightmare disorder**: *during REM sleep*, recurs weekly or more; ↑ with stress, fatigue, fever, frightening stories. No confusion or disorientation during awakening. Dream → distress. Remits in adulthood. R/O: night terrors (during NREM), nocturnal panic attacks (NREM, daytime associated panic attacks). Rx: avoid precipitating factors; suppression of REM with TCAs (nortriptyline or imipramine) or a Benzo (paradoxical action, ↑ nightmares)

(2) **Sleep terror disorder (pavor nocturnus)**: *NREM sleep in the 1st third of the night*; behavioral sx of intense fear, loud scream, blank staring, disorientation, autonomic arousal; no response to attempts to be awakened or comforted. May develop into sleepwalking. There is amnesia of the episode. Attacks appear q few weeks or months, sometimes during a daytime nap. 1–4% of children. More in boys. Resolves in adolescence. May be the first sx of temporal lobe epilepsy. R/O: nightmares (REM sleep, end of the night, recall of the dream, lack of motor activity, rapid alertness), nocturnal panic attacks, nocturnal complex partial seizures (presence of other seizure types at other times). Rx: reassurance. Imipramine (25–50 mg hs) or diazepam (2.5–5 mg at hs) may prevent the attacks

(3) **Sleepwalking disorder (somnambulism)**: complex behaviors; *NREM sleep; in the 1st third of the night*, without consciousness or later memory of the event. Episodes last 15–30 min. Familial. Risk of injuries. Resolves in adolescence. Late-onset cases may become chronic. 2–3% of children. R/O: nocturnal complex partial seizures, sleep-drunkenness (upon morning awakening), SE from antidepressants, neuroleptics, sedative-hypnotics. Rx: safe environment (locked doors and windows, no hazardous materials), benzodiazepines: diazepam (5–10 mg hs) or clonazepam (0.5–1 mg hs). Imipramine (10–50 mg hs), paroxetine (20 mg hs) may be effective.

(4) **Parasomnia NOS**:

- **Sleep-related bruxism**: tooth grinding, throughout the night (stage 2). 10% of the population. Damages the teeth, the jaw. Rx: dental bite, corrective orthodontics

- **REM sleep behavior disorder**: chronic, mostly in men; loss of atonia during REM sleep (pts can act up their dreams). Risk of injury to the bed partner. Reported in pts treated with stimulants, tricyclics, fluoxetine. Rx: clonazepam (Klonopin: 0.5–2 mg/d), carbamazepine (100 mg tid)

- **Sleep talking (somniloquy)**: in all sleep stages. No secret revealed! May be associated with night terrors and sleepwalking. Alone: no rx.

- **Sleep-related head banging (jactatio capitis nocturna)**: before and during light sleep. Prevent injuries.

- **Sleep paralysis**: sudden paralysis just at the onset of sleep or on awakening. Benign.

19 ■ IMPULSE-CONTROL DISORDERS

ETIOLOGY

- **Psychodynamic factors**: to master painful effects by means of action; weak ego and super-ego, incomplete sense of self; fixation at the oral stage?
- **Biologic factors**: abnormal function of the limbic system? Role of testosterone? Role of temporal lobe epilepsy, hx of head trauma? Mixed cerebral dominance? ADHD? MR, organic brain syndromes? Role of serotonin neurotransmitter system ($\downarrow$ levels of 5-HIAA in CSF of people who have committed suicide); role of the dopaminergic and noradrenergic systems in impulsivity; role of stress, fatigue, past trauma, past deprivation
- **Psychosocial factors**: learning theories (violence in the home, alcohol abuse, promiscuity, antisocial tendencies)

TYPES

TABLE 19.1.   Shared Features by All Types

- Patients do not resist the impulses
- Patients may not plan the behaviors
- Before the act: sense of tension or arousal
- Postaction: feeling of pleasure or relief or satisfaction
- Possible, but not always, sense of remorse or guilt
- Acts are ego-syntonic

INTERMITTENT EXPLOSIVE DISORDER

Definition:

- Several episodes of loss of control with aggressivity out of proportion with the stressor (if no other mental disorder, substance use, or medical condition)
- Often soft neurologic signs, nonspecific EEG findings, abnl neuropsychologic testing, and abnl prefrontal cortex (?)
- Frequency of job losses, trouble with the law, marital problems

Etiology: defense against narcissistic injuries; $\male$ with poor sense of masculinity, identification with aggressor, violent childhood environment, predisposing factors (perinatal trauma, seizures, head trauma, ADHD, encephalitis); $\downarrow$ serotoninergic transmission, $\downarrow$ control of violent tendencies; $\uparrow$ CSF testosterone found in some violent men (antiandrogenic agents$\downarrow$ aggression); familial and genetic factors.

Epidemiology: M > F.

Comorbidity: $\uparrow$ rates of fire setters, other disorders of impulse control, substance use, mood, anxiety, eating disorders.

Differential diagnosis:

- In personality disorders (antisocial or borderline personality disorder), ADHD, and conduct disorders, aggressiveness and impulsivity are present between outbursts.
- In psychosis and in mania: possible response to delusions and hallucinations, poor reality testing
- In substance abuse: mostly with intoxications (alcohol, barbiturates, hallucinogens, amphetamines)
- In medical condition: head trauma, dementia, epilepsy, brain tumors, endocrine disorder

Course: usually starts in the 20s and 30s and then ↓.

Treatment:

- Psychotherapy (group and family)
- Pharmacology: anticonvulsants (mixed results), antipsychotics, antidepressants (may be effective, risk if underlying seizure disorder), benzodiazepines (may ↑ dyscontrol), lithium, carbamazepine, phenytoin, valproex, gabapentin are used. Sometimes: propanolol, buspirone, and trazodone. Fluoxetine and other SSRIs are used to ↓ aggressivity and impulsivity. Surgery is controversial.

KLEPTOMANIA

Definition: recurrent, irresistible impulses to steal unneeded objects (in the absence of conduct disorder, mania, antisocial personality disorder). Usually presence of relief at the time of the theft and later on guilt or shame.

Etiology: expression of aggressive or libidinal impulses, need to restore the mother–child relationship, a means of seeking punishment, symbolism (of the act of stealing, the stolen object, and the victim of the theft), role of stresses, losses, separations; changes in serotonin metabolism, brain diseases, MR, ↑ OCD, and mood disorders in family members.

Comorbidity: other impulses disorders, mood and anxiety disorders, OCD, bulimia nervosa, personality disorders.

Epidemiology: prevalence is 0.6%; F : M is 3 : 1; 5% of identified shoplifters.

Differential diagnosis: ordinary stealing is planned for the object's value; conduct disorder or antisocial personality disorder or mania; MR or demented patients who forget to pay.

Course: onset is usually in late adolescence. ♂ start later than ♀. Chronic with ups and downs; ↑ with losses. Legal consequences; possible good prognosis if treated.

Treatment: psychotherapy, CBT (systematic desensitization, aversive conditioning), medications (SSRIs, tricyclics, trazodone, valproate, lithium, naltrexone), ECT.

PYROMANIA

Definition: fascination in fire and its paraphernalia, pleasure in watching or deliberately setting fires (usually > 1×) with satisfaction, or indifference to the consequences; no remorse; not done for monetary gain or political reasons, or to conceal a criminal activity, or for revenge, or secondary to a mental illness (dementia, psychosis, MR, intoxication, conduct disorder, mania, personality disorder). Some fire setters are sexually aroused by the fire.

Etiology: fire (sexual excitation), pyromania (craving for power, recognition, venting rage and despair), absent father in childhood, female fire setters: fewer but ↑ delinquency (↑ kleptomania, promiscuity); possible serotonergic and adrenergic involvement.

Comorbidity: MR, alcohol use disorders, antisocial traits, enuresis, animals cruelty, ADHD, adjustments disorders.

Epidemiology: M > F.

Differential diagnosis: simple fascination of young children with fire, lighters, matches; arson (done for political, retaliation, or monetary reasons), deliberate fires in CD and antisocial personality disorders, poor judgment in pts with brain dysfunction (MR, dementias, intoxications) or psychosis.

Course: starts in childhood, ↑ destructiveness, episodic; prognosis is good for treated children but poor in adults.

Treatment: multimodal, supervision to prevent repetition of the behavior, possible incarceration for safety, behavior rx, family rx.

PATHOLOGIC GAMBLING

Definition: recurrent and persistent gambling causing economic, personal, social, occupational problems; inability to control and stop; need to ↑ the amounts of money for same levels of excitement; preoccupation with gambling, use of gambling to escape from problems; lies to conceal its extent; illegal acts (forgery, embezzlement, fraud) to finance the habit.

Etiology: predisposing factors (death of a parent, divorce, inappropriate parental discipline, gambling activities in adolescence, emphasis on financial symbols); unconscious desires to lose, gambling to ↓ guilt, omnipotent fantasies; neurobiology of risk-taking behaviors: abnormalities in serotonergic receptor systems (low platelet monoamine oxidase activity) and in noradrenergic receptor systems (↑ urinary output of NE, ↑ MHPG conc. in the CSF).

Comorbidity: other impulse-control disorders, substance use, mood disorders, ADHD, antisocial, borderline, narcissistic personality disorders, anxiety disorders.

Epidemiology: 3% of the population; 2–8% of the adolescents; M > F; rate ↑ if gambling is legal, if a parent has a gambling problem or alcohol dependence.

Differential diagnosis: social gambling (with friends; acceptable losses; on special occasions), mania.

Course: starts later for ♀, becomes chronic; four phases taking up to 15 yr (winning phase → progressive-loss phase → desperate phase → hopeless stage).

Treatment: Gamblers Anonymous; in rare cases: hospitalization; insight-oriented psychotherapy, family rx, CBT. Some success with fluvoxamine, lithium, clomipramine. Treat any comorbidity.

TRICHOTILLOMANIA

Definition: recurrent pulling out of hair, preceded by ↑ sense of tension, followed by a sense of relief (not due to another mental illness, a gl medical illness); causes significant distress or impairment in gl functioning; all areas of the body (mostly scalp, but also eyebrows, eyelashes, beard, or pubic hair, trunk, armpits); mixture of healthy hair and broken strands, with nl skin underneath (sometimes pruritus); possible trichophagy (risks: trichobezoars, malnutrition, intestinal obstruction); evidence of trichomalacia (changes in the hair follicle in biopsy).

Etiology: stress, disturbed mother–child relationship, fear of being alone, objects loss. Contributing factors: substance abuse, depression, may be biologically determined.

Epidemiology: F > M; family hx of alopecia; associated disorders: OCD, obsessive compulsive personality, borderline personality disorder, MDD.

Differential diagnosis: OCD (obsessive thoughts and multiple compulsions in OCD), factitious disorders and malingering (pt does not acknowledge the self-inflicted nature); stereotyped movements (not distressing to the pt); dermatologic disorders (biopsy).

Course: variable with ↑ and ↓.

Treatment: topical steroids, antihistaminics, antidepressants (SSRIs), antipsychotics. Some reports of response to lithium, SSRI + pimozide, buspirone, clonazepam, fenfluramine, naltrexone. Biofeedback, insight-oriented rx, hypnosis, behavior rx.

IMPULSE-CONTROL DISORDER NOS

Such as compulsive buying, Internet addiction, cellular phone compulsion, repetitive self-mutilation, and compulsive sexual behavior.

National organizations:

Drug information: http://www.usscreeningsource.com/druginformation.htm **US Screening Source: Toll free: 1-866-323-7336**

National Institute on Drug Abuse (NIDA): http://www.nida.nih.gov/; 301-443-1124 (240-221-4007 en Español)

Drug Enforcement Administration (US-DEA): http://www.usdoj.gov/dea/index.htm

National Institute on Alcohol Abuse and Alcoholism (NIAAA): http://www.niaaa.nih.gov/

Substance Abuse and Mental Health Services Administration (SAMHSA): http://www.samhsa.gov/; has a 24-Hour Helpline at 1-800-662-HELP (1-800-662-4357)

American Academy of Addiction Psychiatry (AAAP): http://www.aaap.org/; (401) 524-3076

American Society of Addiction Medicine (ASAM): http://www.asam.org/; 301-656-3920

Partnership for a Drug-Free America: http://www.drugfree.org; 212.922.1560

Self-help groups: http://www.mentalhelp.net/selfhelp/

See also federal laws about confidentiality of substance abuse treatment (more strict than most other confidentiality rules); state laws might be more restrictive. Need for strict medical documentation.

GENERALITIES

Substance dependence and abuse: there are a number of definitions, like the one below:

- **Dependence (or "addiction"):** behavioral dependence (substance-seeking activities and pathologic use patterns) and physical dependence (physiologic effects of the multiple episodes of substance use). Possible common neurochemical and neuroanatomical substrates among all addictions (substances, gambling, sex, stealing, eating), with similar effects on specific rewards areas of the brain (ventral tegmental area, locus ceruleus, nucleus accumbens)

- **Psychologic dependence (or "habituation"):** continuous or intermittent craving for the substance to avoid a dysphoric state

- **Substance abuse:** presence of at least one specific sx indicating that substance use has interfered with the person's life; there is substance abuse for a particular substance only if the pt meets the criteria for dependence on the particular substance.

Codependence: behavioral patterns of family members affected by another family member's substance use or dependence (enabling, denial).

Diagnostic criteria

TABLE 20.1.   Some Criteria

Substance intoxication	• **Reversible substance-specific syndrome due to recent exposure** to a substance • **Maladaptive or psychological changes** due to the effect of the substance on the CNS (aggressivity, labile mood, poor judgment, impaired functioning) and developing during or shortly after use of the substance. Heavy use can cause poisoning and death (alcohol and opioids causing respiratory depression; cocaine causing heart attacks)
Substance withdrawal	• **Substance-specific syndrome due to the cessation or ↓ in heavy and prolonged substance use** • Causes significant distress and impairment in *x* areas of functioning; life-threatening risks (alcohol causing severe withdrawal and delirium tremens, benzodiazepines causing seizures)
Substance abuse	• **Maladaptive pattern of substance use that leads to significant impairment or distress occurring within a 12-month period** (not fulfilling obligations at work, school, home; recurrent use in situations that could be physically dangerous; recurrent legal problems related to the substance abuse; continued use despite social or interpersonal problems due to the effects of the substance) • **Sx never met the criteria for dependence** for that class of substance

Continued

TABLE 20.1.   Some Criteria   Continued

Substance dependence	**Maladaptive pattern of substance use (>1 yr)** that lead to *3 or more of the following*: • **Tolerance**: a need for increased amounts of the substance to achieve intoxication or the desired effect • **Withdrawal**: as defined in substance withdrawal; or if the same or closely related substance is taken to relieve the withdrawal sx • The substance is taken in **larger amounts or for a longer period of time than intended** • **Inability to cut down or stop** • **Much time spent** (compulsive use) in obtaining or using or recovering from the effects • Important ↓ **in social, occupational, recreational activities due to the use** • **Continued use despite recognition of the negative** physical and psychologic problems due to the use **May be with or without physiologic dependence (tolerance and withdrawal)**
Polysubstance abuse	• If criteria for abuse is met for each substance, the diagnosis needs to be recognized for each substance

Substance abuse history

TABLE 20.2.   Taking a History

- **History of drug use**: first substance used, age at first use, drugs used, context of introduction, describe the experiences, the situations. When was the second attempt at use? Ask about all psychoactive substances. For adolescents: ask about cigarettes, cannabis (types and presentations, preferences), alcohol, OTC medications such as antihistamines, cough medications (dextrometorphan), party drugs (ecstasy), amphetamines, prescription misuse or abuse, caffeine, cocaine, hallucinogens, inhalants opioids, phencyclidine (PCP), sedatives, anxiolytic-hypnotics (Ativan, Xanax), and others
- **Effects of the drugs over time**: pattern of use of each substance, frequency, amount, route(s), progression of sx, social context(s) of use, continued use despite concerns of family and friends, attempts to cut down or control use; taken more amounts of drugs or over a longer period than intended; time using, use before or soon after school, missing on schoolwork or sports due to use, obtaining drugs, or recovering from use? Blackouts, shakes, withdrawal sx, compulsivity of use, and/or craving? IV use?
- **Tolerance, intoxication, withdrawal, overdose?** For each drug ever used, explore tolerance, intoxication, and withdrawal sx. Focus on opioid-related syndromes. For cannabis: possible clear-cut hx of dependence and withdrawal sx
- **Relapse or attempts at abstinence; addiction treatment hx**: what is the patient's relapse hx? In the past year, past 5 yr, and lifetime? Switch from one addicting substance to another? Rx is most frequently enforced, and the adolescent is difficult to engage and remains in rx
- **Psychiatric hx**: very frequent before the onset of drug use (ODD or CD and ADHD); sx can also appear during or after substance use: substance-induced psychotic disorder, mood disorder, anxiety disorder, persisting perceptual disorder, persisting amnestic disorder, persisting dementia, or sexual dysfunction? **Persistent psychiatric sx more than or what could be accounted for by the offending drug(s) point to the comorbid or newly emergent psychiatric disorder**
- **Family hx**: immediate, extended relatives, intergenerational issues (like heroin, cocaine), alcoholism, "drinking problems," legal problems, psychiatric conditions, suicide, medical consequences of drug abuse
- **Medical hx**: DTs, withdrawal complications, or ODs; **tuberculosis, HIV infection, viral hepatitis** (A, B, C, D), syphilis, STDs, endocarditis, pericarditis, cardiomyopathy, liver, kidney problems? Infections, pregnancy, addicting prescription drugs, pain or neurologic problems; trauma, accidents, and hospitalizations? *Think about preventive care*
- **Prescriptions**: from several physicians? "Lost," forged, stolen, misused prescriptions for medications?
- **Cost/consequences of drug use**: compulsivity or craving, loss of control over drug use, do others (family, friends, employers, physicians, or others) think differently about the pt's use?
- **Social and recovery environment**: insight, motivation, readiness to change? Is rx coerced or voluntary? Families enabling continued use (denial, lack of skills, limited access to rx, high crime high drug neighborhoods)

Course: six possibilities, *the first 12 months following dependency is a high-risk time for relapse.* Recovery: consider the length of time since the last use, the total duration of disturbance, the need for continued evaluation.

- **Early full remission**: no criteria of dependence or abuse for >1 month after cessation but <12 months
- **Early partial remission**: no criteria of dependence or abuse for >1 month after cessation but one or more criteria for dependence or abuse (but not full criteria for dependence) have been met in less than the following 11 months.
- **Sustained full remission**: no criteria for dependence or abuse for >12 months after cessation
- **Sustained partial remission**: full criteria for dependence or abuse have not been present for >12 months after cessation, but one or more have been met during that period of time.
- **Pts on agonist therapy**: no criteria of dependence or abuse for >1 month after cessation but possible tolerance to or withdrawal from the agonist.
- **Pts in a controlled environment**: no criteria for dependence or abuse for >1 month specified if pts are closely supervised (jail, therapeutic communities, locked hospital units, juvenile detentions).

Types:

The substance-related disorders include substance-induced disorders and substance-related disorders. Substance-induced disorders are: substance intoxication delirium, substance withdrawal delirium, substance-induced persisting dementia, substance-induced persisting amnestic disorder, substance-induced psychotic disorder, substance-induced mood disorder, substance-induced anxiety disorder, substance-induced sexual dysfunction, and substance-induced sleep disorder.

Epidemiology: 40% of the population use one or more illicit substances in their lifetime and 15% in the past yr. Lifetime prevalence: 20%; all age groups, both genders; peak prevalence of SUD: 18–29 yr of age.

Results of the survey of 2000 are available at www.samsha.gov.

- **Patterns**: recreational use, iatrogenic "addiction," chronic drug abuse
- **Predictive factors**: lower educational, low income levels (not race, ethnicity, or urban environment), lifetime dependency rate of particular substances (opioids: 23%; tobacco: 32%; cocaine: 17%; alcohol: 17%, more in ♂ than ♀; hallucinogens: 5%); peer influence role on continued drug use after rx. *A major decision is to cultivate new friends who are sober.*
- **Differences in age group**: more illicit drugs in people aged 18–25 yr, then 26–34 yr
- **Current illicit drug use** (*>30 days*): M > F, more are unemployed (in 2000: 15.4% of unemployed adults vs 6.3% of FT employed adults), blacks, western states. Rates unchanged since 1999. Some ↓ of use in the youngest age group. Most frequent illicit drug is marijuana (59% used only marijuana, 17% used marijuana + another drug, 24% used an illicit drug other than marijuana). Americans > age 12: 29% use a tobacco product and 46.6% are alcohol drinkers.

Etiology:

- **Psychodynamic factors**: for orgasm, defense against anxiety, poor social skills, lacking friends, for approval, oral regression, depression, disturbed ego functions, need to self-medicate, unstable childhood, personality disorders, relationship with family and society, drug culture
- **Behavioral theories**: positive reinforcing qualities of the first use, ability to discriminate the substance of abuse from other substances, cues connected with the substance-taking experience, use to avert dysphoric withdrawal sx
- **Genetic factors**: the level of response to alcohol is genetically controlled and determines a risk factor for alcohol dependence.
- **Neurochemical factors**: opioids acting on opioid receptors; modulation of the receptor systems due to prolonged use of a particular substance (development of tolerance within CNS); effects of substances on the second-messenger system and on gene regulation; *dopaminergic system (ventral tegmental area + the nucleus accumbens: responsible for the sensation of reward/possibly for amphetamines and cocaine); adrenergic system (locus ceruleus/possibly for opiates)*

Comorbidity: cooccurrence of two or more psychiatric disorders in a single pt:

- Antisocial personality disorders (35–60%)
- Depression (35–50% of pts with opioid abuse/dependence, 40% of pts with alcohol abuse/dependence)
- Suicide: 20× more than in the gl population; 15% of pts with alcohol abuse/dependency commit suicide.

Selecting a treatment

Variety of substances means different interventions (**legal vs illicit drugs**).

Five stages of change (Prochaska, DiClemente, & Norcross, 1992): **precontemplation, contemplation, preparation, action, maintenance with relapse prevention**. Start with the pt's level of readiness to change. *Motivational interviewing* acknowledges these stages; the intervention is aimed at moving the individual to the action stage.

Length of rx: depends on the substance, the characteristics of the pts: brief interventions for smoking and drinking but longer for illicit drugs (>3 months); *longer treatment retention supports longer term sobriety.*

High rate of drop out: "Cold turkey" withdrawal from drugs as a "detox" practice was traditional but in fact does not support continued engagement in rx and sobriety (higher dropouts even during rx).

Different programs: out-patient programs, in-patient unit (detoxification), residential communities; legally enforced or not, different philosophies of rx (NA, AA), public vs private sector.

Rx of comorbidity: *integrated rx more effective* than parallel or sequential treatment.

ALCOHOL-RELATED DISORDERS

National organizations:

- **Alcoholics Anonymous**: http://www.aa.org
- **Al-Anon groups and Alateen**: http://www.ola-is.org/ and http://www.al-anon.alateen.org/english.html
- **National Institute on Alcohol Abuse and Alcoholism (NIAAA)**: http://www.niaaa.nih.gov/

Epidemiology: 68% of Americans drink, 12% are heavy drinkers; 30–45% of all adults in United States had more then one transient episode of alcohol-related problem (blackout, DIU, missing a day of school or work); M : F is 2 : 1 (♂: more binge and heavy drinkers); 10 millions have alcohol abuse problems. Lifetime risk: 13%; alcohol-related: 50% of homicides, 50% of automotive deaths (75% in the late evening), 25% of suicides; ↑ risk for: urban blacks (even though whites have the highest rate: 56%), some Indian tribes, bartenders, musicians; mixed abuse with other drugs is common; alcohol abuse ↓ life expectancy by 10 yr. Higher the education achieved, the more likely the current use of alcohol (but heavy alcohol use in pts who completed college is 4% vs 7% in pts who didn't complete high school); ↑ school dropouts, truancy, delinquency, anti-social personality.

Comorbidity: antisocial personality disorders (may not be causally related), mood disorders (30% have MDD during lifetime, higher in ♀, ↑ risk of suicide, ↑ other substance-related disorder, may be treated only after 2–3 wk of sobriety with antidepressant drugs, risk of alcoholism ↑ in bipolar I disorders), anxiety disorders (25–50% of alcoholics have anxiety disorders, mostly phobias and panic disorders), suicide (prevalence of suicide is >10–15%, particularly if MDD present, lack of psychosocial support + medical condition, unemployment, living alone).

Etiology: *predisposing heritable biologic brain function* (neurocognitive testing deficits, low amplitude of the P300 wave on evoked potential testing, abnormal EEG), *personality disorders* (shy, isolated, impatient, anxious, sexually repressed); *psychodynamic theories* (aphorism: "the superego is soluble in alcohol," self-punitive attitude, fixation at the oral stage; alcohol may ↓ tension, psychic pain, and ↑ sense of power and self-worth); *social expectation* (college, military; Asians and conservative Protestants drink < liberal protestants and Catholics); *learning factors* (familial drinking habits, positive reinforcing effects/feelings of euphoria, ↓ fear and anxiety); *genetic theories* (close family members have 4× ↑ risks; risk is higher in identical twin of an alcoholic than in fraternal twin; adoption studies: adopted children of alcoholics have ↑ risk); low conc. of serotonin, DA, GABA, or metabolites, in CSF of pts with alcohol-related disorders.

Patterns of use:

TABLE 20.3.   Patterns of Alcohol Use

Category	Definition
● Moderate drinking	M: ≤2 drinks/d; W: ≤1 drink/d; elders >65 yr of age: ≤1 drink/d
● At-risk drinking	M: >14 drinks/wk or >4 drinks/occasion; W: >7 drinks/wk or >3 drinks per occasion
● Hazardous drinking	At risk for adverse consequences
● Harmful drinking	Causing physical or psychologic harm
● Alcohol abuse	See criteria for substance abuse
● Alcohol dependence	See criteria for substance dependence

Effects of alcohol:

- ● Usual drinks

TABLE 20.4.   Ethanol Equivalency

One drink is equal to 12 g of ethanol (= ethyl alcohol = $CH_3\text{-}CH_2\text{-}OH$)
(1) **1½ oz. of 80-proof liquor (40% ethanol)**: whiskey or gin
(2) **12 oz. of regular beer** (7.2 proof, 3.6% ethanol in the United States); beers vary in their alcohol content, vary in the quantity absorbed (cans vs mugs)
(3) **5 oz. of table wine (or 3–4 oz of fortified wine)**: size of glasses vary from 2 to 6 oz.
(4) Mixed drinks may contain 2–6 oz. of liquor each
One drink ↑ blood level of alcohol of a 150-lb man by 15–20 mg/dL
The body can get rid of 1 drink/hr: mean elimination of ethanol is 20 mg/dL/hr (range: 16–25)

- ● **Absorption**: peak conc. reached in 45–60 min (varies with food or empty stomach), more rapid if beverages contain 15–30% alcohol (30–60 proof). 10% is absorbed in the stomach and the rest through the small intestine. High conc. in the stomach may close the pyloric valve → nausea and vomiting. Intoxication effects ↑ when blood conc. is rising.

- ● **Metabolism**: 90% through the liver (oxidation), 10% is excreted unchanged by the kidneys and lungs. Two enzymes involved: alcohol dehydrogenase (alcohol → acetaldehyde which is toxic) and aldehyde dehydrogenase (acetaldehyde → acetic acid). Disulfiram (Antabuse) inhibits the aldehyde dehydrogenase.

- ● **Effects of alcohol**:

TABLE 20.5.   Pathologic Effects of Alcohol on Different Organs

Brain	Alcohol changes the fluidity of cellular membranes: ● ↑ Ion channel activities associated with nicotinic, acetylcholine, serotonin 5-HT3, GABA type A receptors ● ↓ Ion channel activities associated with glutamate receptors and voltage-gated calcium channels **Alcohol is a depressant** (*cross-tolerance and cross-dependence with barbiturates and benzodiazepines*) **Alcohol blood levels**: ● 0.05%: ↓ thought, ↓ judgment, ↓ restraint ● 0.1%: clumsiness ● **0.1–0.15%: legal intoxication in most states** (if impaired driving or commercial drivers: level of 0.4% can result in DIU) ● 0.2%: depression of motor and emotions in related areas of the brain ● 0.3%: confusion, stupor ● 0.4–0.5%: coma ● Higher levels: respiratory depression, death **Women** may have a higher level of alcohol blood level in drinking the same quantity: ↑ risk for abuse or dependence **Sleep**: ↓ sleep latency, ↓ REM (dream) sleep, ↓ stage 4 (deep sleep), ↑ sleep fragmentation (↑ episodes of awakening)
Liver	Fat liver, alcoholic **hepatitis**, alcoholic **cirrhosis**
GI	Esophagitis, gastritis, achlorhydria, gastric ulcers, **esophageal varices** (*rupture is a medical emergency*), pancreatitis, pancreatitic cancer, **vitamin deficiencies** (B vitamins)
Other systems	↑ Risk for myocardial infarctions and CV diseases ↑ Risk for cancer (head, neck, esophageal, stomach, liver, colon, lung) ↑ **Risk of hypoglycemia in acute intoxications** ↑ Estradiol blood levels in women, impotence ↑ Muscle weakness
Laboratory tests	↑ γ-**glutamyl transpeptidase levels**, ↑ mean corpuscular volume (MCV), possible ↑ in uric acid, triglycerides, AST and ALT, hypomagnesemia, megaloblastic anemia, thrombocytopenia, ketoacidosis
Drug interactions	Competition for the same metabolism system (risk of toxicity): Phenobarbital (Luminal), other sedatives, and hypnotics Synergy of effects with other CNS depressants such as: sedatives (e.g., benzodiazepines), hypnotics (e.g., chloral hydrate), antipain, antiallergy, antimotion sickness, narcotics. **Caution: combination of CNS depressants and alcohol when driving or operating machinery**

Disorders:

(1) Alcohol dependence and alcohol abuse:

- ● Symptoms:
  - ◉ Need for daily use of large amounts of alcohol for adequate functioning
  - ◉ Regular heavy drinking during weekends

- Periods of sobriety interspersed with binges of heavy drinking for weeks or months
- Inability to cut down or stop
- Amnestic periods (blackouts)
- Continuation of drinking despite serious physical disorder exacerbated by alcohol
- Impaired social or occupational functioning, legal difficulties, problems with entourage due to the drinking
- **Subtypes**:

TABLE 20.6. Subtypes of Alchohol Abusers

Type A	Late onset, few childhood factors, **mild dependence**, few alcohol-related problems, little psychopathology, respond to interactional psychotherapies
Type B	Many childhood risk factors, **severe dependence, early onset** of alcohol-related problems, high level of psychopathology, family hx of alcohol abuse, frequent polysubstance abuse, severe life stresses, long hx of alcohol rx, may respond better to coping skills training

(2) **Alcohol intoxication**: legal intoxication is 100 mg (%)

- **Recent ingestion of alcohol** with clinically significant behavioral or psychologic changes appearing during or shortly after the ingestion.
- **Symptoms**: (which are not due to a general medical or another mental disorder) are one or more:

TABLE 20.7. Symptoms of Alcohol Intoxication

- **Slurred speech**
- **Incoordination**
- **Unsteady gait**
- **Nystagmus**
- **Poor attention or memory**
- **Stupor or coma**: may lead to respiratory arrest or aspiration of vomitus

The severity of the sx parallels the blood conc. of alcohol

- **Medical complications**: cardiac ($\uparrow$ HR, $\downarrow$ BP, atrial fibrillation, ventricular arrhythmias), respiratory (aspiration, bradypnea), GI (vomiting, bleeding), metabolic ($\uparrow$ or $\downarrow$ temp, alcoholic ketoacidosis), falls **with subdural hematomas, fractures,** facial hematomas. **Alcoholic coma is an emergency (levels above 250–400 mg/100 mL)**: check alcohol level, presence of other drugs; intubation; CPR; rehydrate, correct electrolyte disturbances, any medical problem (hypoglycemia, infections, toxic psychosis of other etiology)
- **Differential diagnosis**: schizophrenia, mania, depression, hysteria, medical problems, alcohol idiosyncratic intoxication (controversial, marked aggressiveness or emotional lability following ingestion of small quantities of alcohol in a normal person, with the same pattern for life, may last hours or days with amnesia for the episode afterward), temporal lobe epilepsy.
- **Management**: nonpharmacologic management (quiet room, support) but sedation may be needed (cautious of oversedation). Decide if pt needs to "sleep it off," is at risk for withdrawal, or is becoming comatose. Can the pt go home with family to be observed overnight or needs hospitalization? Be familiar with community resources.

(3) **Alcohol withdrawal**:

- **Diagnosis**: is due to the cessation or $\downarrow$ of alcohol that has been used in a heavy and prolonged way; sx cause significant distress or impairment in functioning and are not due to a gl medical or another mental condition. $\uparrow$ risk in debilitated, medically ill pts
- **Symptoms**: develop a few hours or days after cessation of alcohol and are ≥ 2:

TABLE 20.8. Symptoms of Alcohol Withdrawal

- Autonomic activity (sweating or pulse >100, mydriasis, $\uparrow$ BP, facial flushing)
- $\uparrow$ Hand tremor, tremulousness (develops after 6–8 hr), hyperreflexia
- Nausea or vomiting
- Insomnia
- Agitation
- Transient hallucinations or illusions (starts after 8–12 hr), possible alcohol withdrawal delirium (may start after 72 hr)
- Anxiety, hypervigilence
- Grand mal seizures (may start after 12–24 hr, usually >1, rare status epilepticus, consider other causes as well/head injuries, CNS infections or tumors, other CV diseases, electrolytes imbalances). If seizure is focal, suspect CNS pathology (e.g., subdural)

The Clinical Institute Withdrawal Assessment of Alcohol, Revised (CIWA–Ar) (Foy et al., 1988; Sullivan et al., 1989). This instrument rates 10 withdrawal features, takes only a few minutes to administer, and can be repeated easily when necessary. A total score of 15 or more points indicates that the patient is at increased risk for severe withdrawal effects.

TABLE 20.9. Alcohol Withdrawal Assessment Scoring Guidelines (CIWA-Ar)

Nausea/vomiting: rate on scale 0–7 0: None 1: Mild nausea with no vomiting 2 3 4: Intermittent nausea 5 6 7: Constant nausea and frequent dry heaves and vomiting	**Tremors**: have patient extend arms and spread fingers. Rate on scale 0–7 0: No tremor 1: Not visible, but can be felt fingertip to fingertip 2 3 4: Moderate, with patient's arms extended 5 6 7: Severe, even w/arms not extended
Anxiety: Rate on scale 0–7 0: No anxiety, patient at ease 1: Mildly anxious 2 3 4: Moderately anxious or guarded, so anxiety is inferred 5 6 7: Equivalent to acute panic states seen in severe delirium or acute schizophrenic reactions	**Agitation**: Rate on scale 0–7 0: Normal activity 1: Somewhat normal activity 2 3 4: Moderately fidgety and restless 5 6 7: Paces back and forth, or constantly thrashes about
Paroxysmal sweats: rate on scale 0–7 0: No sweats 1: Barely perceptible sweating, palms moist 2 3 4: Beads of sweat obvious on forehead 5 6 7: Drenching sweats	**Orientation and clouding of sensorium**: Ask, "What day is this? Where are you? Who am I?" Rate scale 0–4 0: Oriented 1: Cannot do serial additions or is uncertain about date 2: Disoriented to date by no more than 2 calendar days 3: Disoriented to date by more than 2 calendar days 4: Disoriented to place and/or person
Tactile disturbances: Ask, "Have you experienced any itching, pins and needles sensation, burning or numbness, or a feeling of bugs crawling on or under your skin?" 0: None 1: Very mild itching, pins and needles, burning, or numbness 2: Mild itching, pins and needles, burning, or numbness 3: Moderate itching, pins and needles, burning, or numbness 4: Moderate hallucinations 5: Severe hallucinations 6: Extremely severe hallucinations 7: Continuous hallucinations	**Auditory disturbances**: Ask, "Are you more aware of sounds around you? Are they harsh? Do they startle you? Do you hear anything that disturbs you or that you know isn't there?" 0: Not present 1: Very mild harshness or ability to startle 2: Mild harshness or ability to startle 3: Moderate harshness or ability to startle 4: Moderate hallucinations 5: Severe hallucinations 6: Extremely severe hallucinations 7: Continuous hallucinations
Visual disturbances: Ask, "Does the light appear to be too bright? Is its color different than normal? Does it hurt your eyes? Are you seeing anything that disturbs you or that you know isn't there?" 0: Not present 1: Very mild sensitivity 2: Mild sensitivity 3: Moderate sensitivity 4: Moderate hallucinations 5: Severe hallucinations 6: Extremely severe hallucinations 7: Continuous hallucinations	**Headache**: Ask, "Does your head feel different than usual? Does it feel like there is a band around your head?" Do not rate dizziness or lightheadedness 0: Not present 1: Very mild 2: Mild 3: Moderate 4: Moderately severe 5: Severe 6: Very severe 7: Extremely severe

The CIWA-Ar is in the public domain. Source: Mayo-Smith, M. F., Beecher, L. H., Fischer, T. L., Gorelick, D. A., Guillaume, J. L., Hill, A.,...American Society of Addiction Medicine. (2004). Management of alcohol withdrawal delirium. An evidence-based practice guideline. *Archives of Internal Medicine, 164*(13), 1405–1412.

Procedure:

(a) Assess and rate each of the 10 criteria of the CIWA scale. Each criterion is rated on a scale of 0 to 7, except for "Orientation and clouding of sensorium," which is rated on a scale of 0 to 4. Add up the scores for all 10 criteria. This is the total CIWA-Ar score for the patient at that time. Prophylactic medication should be started for any patient with a total CIWA-Ar score of 8 or more (i.e., start on withdrawal medication). If started on *scheduled* medication, additional prn medication should be given for a total CIWA-Ar score of 15 or more.

(b) Document vitals and CIWA-Ar assessment on the withdrawal assessment sheet. Document administration of prn medications also on the assessment sheet.

(c) The CIWA-Ar scale is the most sensitive tool for the assessment of a patient experiencing alcohol withdrawal. Nursing assessment is vitally important. Early intervention for CIWA-Ar score of 8 or more provides the best means to prevent the progression of withdrawal.

TABLE 20.10.   Assessment Protocol Form for CIWA-Ar

Assessment Protocol	Date											
a. Vitals, assessment now	Time											
b. If initial score ≥8 repeat q 1 hr × 8 hr,	Pulse											
then if stable q 2 hr	RR											
× 8 hr, then if stable q 4 hr	O$_2$ sat											
c. If initial score <8, assess q 4 hr × 72 hr. If score <8 for 72 hr, d/c assessment. If score ≥8 at any time, go to (b) above	BP											
d. If indicated, (see indications below) administer prn medications as ordered and record on MAR and below												
Assess and rate each of the following (CIWA-Ar scale): refer to reverse for detailed instructions in use of the CIWA-Ar scale												
Nausea/vomiting (0–7)												
0: none; 1: mild nausea, no vomiting; 4: intermittent nausea; 7: constant nausea, frequent dry heaves, and vomiting												
Tremors (0–7)												
0: no tremor; 1: not visible but can be felt; 4: moderate w/arms extended; 7: severe, even w/arms not extended												
Anxiety (0–7)												
0: none, at ease; 1: mildly anxious; 4: moderately anxious or guarded; 7: equivalent to acute panic state												
Agitation (0–7)												
0: normal activity; 1: somewhat normal activity; 4: moderately fidgety/restless; 7: paces or constantly thrashes about												
Paroxysmal sweats (0–7)												
0: no sweats; 1: barely perceptible sweating, palms moist; 4: beads of sweat obvious on forehead; 7: drenching sweat												

Continued

TABLE 20.10. Assessment Protocol Form for CIWA-Ar   Continued

Orientation (0–4)														
0: oriented; 1: uncertain about date; 2: disoriented to date by no more than 2 days; 3: disoriented to date by >2 days; 4: disoriented to place and/or person														
Tactile disturbances (0–7)														
0: none; 1: very mild itch, pins and needles, numbness; 2: mild itch, pins and needles, burning, numbness; 3: moderate itch, pins and needles, burning, numbness; 4: moderate hallucinations; 5: severe hallucinations; 6: extremely severe hallucinations; 7: continuous hallucinations														
Auditory disturbances (0–7)														
0: not present; 1: very mild harshness/ability to startle; 2: mild harshness, ability to startle; 3: moderate harshness, ability to startle; 4: moderate hallucinations; 5: severe hallucinations; 6: extremely severe hallucinations; 7: continuous hallucinations														
Visual disturbances (0–7)														
0: not present; 1: very mild sensitivity; 2: mild sensitivity; 3: moderate sensitivity; 4: moderate hallucinations; 5: severe hallucinations; 6: extremely severe hallucinations; 7: continuous hallucinations														
Headache (0–7)														
0: not present; 1: very mild; 2: mild; 3: moderate; 4: moderately severe; 5: severe; 6: very severe; 7: extremely severe														
Total CIWA-Ar score:														

Prn med: (circle one) Diazepam Lorazepam	**Dose given (mg)**:													
	Route:													

Time of prn medication administration:														
Assessment of response (CIWA-Ar score 30–60 min after medication administered)														
RN initials														

Scale for scoring: Total score = 0–9: absent or minimal withdrawal; 10–19: mild to moderate withdrawal; more than 20: severe withdrawal	Indications for prn medication: a. Total CIWA-Ar score 8 or higher if ordered prn only (symptom-triggered method) b. Total CIWA-Ar score 15 or higher if on Scheduled medication. (Scheduled + prn method) *Consider transfer to ICU for any of the following*: total score above 35, q 1 hr assess. × more than 8 hr required, more than 4 mg/hr lorazepam × 3 hr **or** 20 mg/hr diazepam × 3 hr required, or respiratory distress

Patient identification (Addressograph)				
Signature/title		Initials	Signature/title	Initials

Treatment:

TABLE 20.11. Treatment Using the CIWA-Ar 1

Treatment approach	Treatment component
Monitoring	• Monitor the pt by administering the CIWA-Ar1 test q 4–8 hr until the score has been less than 8–10 points for 24 hr • Use additional assessments as needed
Symptom-triggered regimens	• Perform the CIWA-Ar q hr to assess the pt's need for medication • Administer one of the following medications q hr when the CIWA-Ar score is ≥8–10 points: 　○ Chlordiazepoxide (50–100 mg) 　○ Diazepam (10–20 mg) 　○ Lorazepam (2–4 mg)
Fixed-schedule regimens	• Administer one of the following medications q 6 hr: 　○ Chlordiazepoxide (4 doses of 50 mg, then 8 doses of 25 mg) 　○ Diazepam (4 doses of 10 mg, then 8 doses of 5 mg) 　○ Lorazepam (4 doses of 2 mg, then 8 doses of 1 mg) • Provide additional medication if these regimens do not control the sx (CIWA-Ar score remains ≥8–10 points)

TABLE 20.12. Other Possibilities for Alcohol Detoxification

Use of Benzodiazepines	**Standard treatment**: Benzodiazepines given po or IM. **Avoid IM of diazepam (Valium) and chlordiazepoxide (Librium) due to inconsistent absorption** • Monitor for withdrawal sx q 4 hr • Give thiamine 100 mg IM or po initially (then 50 mg po qd) • Give multivitamin qd • Folic acid 1 mg po qd **If withdrawal sx emerge (see above table)**: monitor q 2 hr and give: 25–100 mg of chlordiazepoxide q 2 hr prn (max 600 mg/24 hr) or lorazepam 1–3 mg q 2 hr prn (max 15 mg/24 hr) Use the total mg received in first 24 hr, **then taper** on day 2 by 25% and then 25% per day **Extreme agitation**: Chlordiazepoxide IV (0.5 mg/kg at 12.5 mg/min) until calm, then titrate **Hallucinosis**: Lorazepam orally (2–10 mg q 4–6 hr) **Seizures**: Diazepam IV (0.15 mg/kg at 2 mg/min)
Other possibilities (monotheraphy or adjunct)	• **Carbamazepine**: 600–800 mg/d × 5–7 days, then 1–2 wk taper. If needed >1,200 mg/d: high rates of discontinuation due to adverse effects. Effective in monotheraphy or as an adjunct to benzo • **Divalproex**: 500 mg bid–tid × 5–6 days, then taper over 2–4 wk. If needed >1,500 mg/d: high rates of discontinuation due to SE. Used as an adjunct to benzo • **Gabapentin**: 400 mg tid–qid × 3–5 days, then taper over 2–4 days: used as an adjunct to benzo • **Propanolol**: may be used as an adjunct to benzo • **Acupuncture**: as an adjunct to benzo • **Clonidine** (Catapress) used to ↓ autonomic activity but does not work on seizures or delirium

(4) **Delirium tremens (DT)**: **usually develops on the third day after admission to the hospital,** usually after 5–15 yr of heavy drinking (typically binge type). 5% of hospitalized pts with alcohol-related disorders develop DTs. ↑ if associated medical illness (hepatitis, pancreatitis, and malnourishment)

DT is a medical emergency

• **Diagnosis**: significant morbidity and mortality (20% if untreated: pneumonia, renal disease, hepatic failure, heart failure), pts may be assaultive, suicidal, or acting on hallucinations or delusions; must be prevented; may or may not be preceded by seizures

TABLE 20.13. Symptoms of DT

• **Delirium**: appearing within 1 wk after stopping alcohol • **Autonomic hyperactivity** (tachycardia, diaphoresis, fever, anxiety, insomnia, ↑ BP) • **Perceptual disturbances** (visual, tactile hallucinations) • **Fluctuating psychomotor activity** (hyperexcitability to lethargy)

TABLE 20.14.   Treatment of Delirium Tremens (DT)

Prevention	Benzodiazepines: such as chlordiazepoxide (25–50 mg q 2–4 hr)
Treatment	Constant observation Record pulse, BP, temp q 30 min initially. Treat shock with fluids, vasopressors as needed Benzodiazepine: Chlordiazepoxide (50–100 mg q 2–4 hr) Correct dehydration: correct hypokalemia (slowly over 24 hr or more via IV) and hypomagnesemia (may ↑ seizures; give magnesium sulfate 2–4 mL of 50% solution IM q 6 hr × 2 days) Check for and treat: hypoglycemia, prolonged PT (give vitamin K: 10 mg IM), fever (aspirin, sponge baths, R/O superimposed infection) Give Thiamine: 100 mg IM then 50 mg po tid for 4 days Need for seclusion if severe agitation (pt will fight restraints) Avoid antipsychotics which may ↓ seizure threshold Focal neurological sx: lateralizing seizures, ↑ intracranial pressure, skull fracture must R/O any additional neurologic disease Treat withdrawal seizures: if they persist, consider 5–10 mg of diazepam slowly by IV or 100–150 mg of phenobarbital IM. If a primary seizure disorder exists: begin diphenylhydrantoin (Dilantin) Supportive psychotherapy needed for these frightened pts. Antianxiety agents may be of use for 1–2 wk

(5) **Alcohol-induced persisting dementia**: role of alcohol, poor nutrition, multiple trauma, multiple organs dysfunction (liver, kidney, pancreas)

(6) **Alcohol-induced persisting amnestic disorder**:

- **Blackouts**: transient global amnesia associated with intoxication; intact remote memory + specific short-term memory deficit; can perform complicated tasks; pt may appear normal to others (role of the hippocampus + related temporal lobes).

- **Disturbance in short-term memory caused by heavy and prolonged use of alcohol** (pts >35 yr); poor nutrition and malabsorption → **thiamine deficiency**; symmetrical and paraventricular lesions (mammillary bodies, thalamus, hypothalamus, midbrain, pons, medulla, fornix, cerebellum)

  Wernicke's encephalopathy: is a medical emergency, *usually reversible* alcoholic encephalopathy, acute disorder with ataxia, vestibular dysfunction, confusion, bilateral ocular motility abnormalities (horizontal nystagmus, lateral orbital palsy, gaze palsy), sluggish reaction to light, anisocoria (unequal size of pupils); responds to high doses of thiamine (start with 100 mg po 2–3×/d and continue for 2 wk, may be added in IV glucose solution: 100 mg/L)

  Korsakoff syndrome: *chronic* amnesic syndrome following Wernicke's encephalopathy with impaired recent memory, anterograde amnesia in an alert pt, confabulation; 20% may recover somewhat; rx: thiamine 100 mg po 2–3×/d up to 12 months

(7) **Alcohol-induced psychotic disorder**: during intoxication or withdrawal, common auditory hallucinations lasting <1 wk with impaired reality testing, temporal relation with alcohol withdrawal, R/O schizophrenia (full history of previous mental disorder with long-lasting hallucinations) and DTs (delirium).

(8) **Alcohol-induced mood disorder**: onset during intoxication or withdrawal; manic, depressed, or mixed features, causal relation.

(9) **Alcohol-induced anxiety disorder**: onset during intoxication or withdrawal; GAD, panic attacks, OCD, phobias.

(10) **Alcohol-induced sexual/dysfunction**

(11) **Alcohol-induced sleep disorder**

(12) **Alcohol-related use disorder NOS**: such as idiosyncratic alcohol intoxication (intolerance to small amounts of alcohol, R/O complex partial epilepsy, forensic interest)

(13) **Other alcohol-related neurologic disorders**: peripheral neuropathy (vitamin B deficiencies), alcoholic cerebellar degeneration, central pontine myelinolysis, Marchiafava-Bignami disease, cerebral atrophy, alcoholic myopathy (and cardiomyopathy), alcoholic pellagra encephalopathy (deficiency in niacin: to be given 50 mg po 4×/d or 25 mg IM 2–3×/d), systemic diseases due to alcohol with neurologic complications (liver: hepatic encephalopathy, chronic hepatocerebral degeneration; GI: malabsorption syndromes, pancreatic encephalopathy; CV: cardiomyopathy, arrhythmias, abnormal BP; blood: hemorrhagic CV disease; infections: meningitis; hypoxia, toxic encephalopathies, confusional states due to electrolyte imbalances, ↑ **incidence of trauma**: epidural, subdural, intracerebral hematoma, spinal cord injury, posttraumatic seizure disorders, compressive neuropathies and brachial plexus injuries, posttraumatic normal pressure hydrocephalus).

(14) **Fetal alcohol syndrome**

National Organization on Fetal Alcohol Syndrome (NOFAS): http://www.nofas.org/faqs.aspx

Fetal alcohol syndrome is the leading cause of MR, due to exposure of the fetus to ethanol and metabolites. Alcohol-related neurodevelopmental disorder (**ARND**) refers to the mental and behavioral impairments due to fetal exposure to alcohol. Alcohol-related birth defects (**ARBDs**) refer to the physical defects due to fetal alcohol exposure.

Symptoms

TABLE 20.15. Symptoms of Fetal Alcohol Syndrome

- Microcephaly (small head circumference and brain size)
- Mental retardation and delayed development, learning disorders
- Craniofacial malformations with distinctive facial features: small eyes, an exceptionally thin upper lip, a short, upturned nose and a smooth skin surface between the nose and the upper lip
- Vision and hearing problems
- Limb defects (deformities of joints, limbs, fingers)
- Poor coordination
- Heart defects
- Short adult stature (slow physical growth before and after birth)
- Maladaptive behaviors (ADHD, poor impulse control, extreme nervousness, and anxiety)
- Sleep problems

Treatment and rehabilitation: 10–40% of alcoholics enter rx. Good prognostic factors predicts > 60% chances of ≥1 yr of abstinence.

- **Good prognosis**: no antisocial personality disorder, no other substance abuse or dependence, stable life, no legal problems, good motivation and participation in rx

- **Bad prognosis**: severe drug problems (IV cocaine or amphetamine dependence), preexisting psychiatric disorders (schizophrenia, bipolar I disorder, antisocial personality disorder; will need concomitant rx)

- **Interventions**

  Recognize the disorder, develop a personal rapport with the pt (warm, supportive but firm, insist on abstinence, on maintaining employment and social involvement), treat medical complications, treat any psychiatric illness (caution: TCAs ↑ the CNS depressant effect of alcohol, alcohol ↑ lithium toxicity); then three steps: intervention, detoxification, and rehabilitation.

  - *Maximize the motivation*: break through denial with confrontation to recognize the consequences of drinking, convincing the pts of their own responsibilities and reminding how alcohol has created the life impairments

  - *Be persistent* but nonjudgmental with multiple interventions

  - *Enlist family* in rx (evaluate family contribution to the problems, may need family or marital rx), AA and Al-Anon groups

  - *Detoxification*: thorough H and P, varies with the severity of sx, rest, adequate nutrition, x vitamins including thiamine.

    - *Mild or moderate withdrawal*: may use any depressant to wean the pt off the alcohol over 5 days. For example: chlordiazepoxide, 25 mg po 3–4×/d (skip a dose if pt is sleepy), if pt has tremor or autonomic dysfunction; add 1 or 2 doses in the first 24 hr, then decrease progressively the daily dose by 20% each day.

    - *Severe withdrawal*: treat like DT

  - *Rehabilitation:* maintenance of motivation for abstinence, readjusting to a lifestyle free of alcohol, relapse prevention; inpatient settings (if severe medical or psychiatric sx, past failures of outpatient programs, must be followed by >3–6 months in outpatient care using combinations of individual, group, family rx, and self-help groups such as AA and 12-step programs), or only outpatient settings

  - *Counseling*: first 3–6 months of care: focus on ↑ motivation, day-to-day life issues, focus on here and now, exploring the consequences of drinking and the improvement expected with abstinence, provided for 1 month in individual or group sessions (>3×/wk), need for a sober peer group, plan for social and recreational events, ↑ communications with close ones

  - *Relapse prevention*: coping with craving, stress slips, identify high-risk situations, involve family members and friends. Recovery program lasts >12 months.

  - *Medications*:

    - Little evidence that antianxiety or antidepressant medications are useful (if no mood disorder, schizophrenia, or anxiety disorder)

    - **Disulfiram (Antabuse**: 250 mg tab): start 125–500 mg qd, usual dosage: 125–500 mg qd; alcohol-sensitizing agent produces uncomfortable physical reactions (N/V, burning sensation in the face and stomach); if pt resumes alcohol; risks: mood swings, rare psychosis, ↑ peripheral neuropathies, fatal hepatitis. Cannot be given if heart disease, cerebral thrombosis, diabetes

    - Opioid antagonist **naltrexone (ReVia**: tab 25, 50, 100 mg), given to ↓ craving and blunt the reward effect of alcohol; start dose 25 mg qd; usual dosage: 50 mg/d×12 wk

- **Acamprosate (Campral**: 333 mg delayed release tab): may act at GABA receptors and NMDA sites; start: 333–666 mg tid, usual dosage: 666 mg tid, ↓ emotional and physical discomfort after pt stops drinking.
- Topiramate?
- Buspirone (Buspar): antianxiety, inconsistent effects
- *Self-help groups*: available 24×7, variety of groups with different combinations of members, different philosophies

AMPHETAMINE (OR AMPHETAMINE-LIKE)-RELATED DISORDERS

FDA-approved indications for amphetamines: ADHD and narcolepsy.

Amphetamines are also used in obesity, depression, chronic fatigue syndrome, AIDS, neurasthenia, adjunct for resistant depression.

Preparations:

- Other names are analeptics, sympathomimetics, stimulants, and psychostimulants.
- Available are dextroamphetamine (Dexedrine), methamphetamine (Desoxyn), mixed dextroamphetamine-amphetamine salt (Adderall), methylphenidate (Ritalin)
- Street names: ice, crystal, crystal meth, speed
- Amphetamine-like substances: ephedrine, pseudo-ephedrine (nasal decongestants, sold over the counter), phenylpropanolamine (PPA); less potent, but abuse → life-threatening HBP, toxic psychosis, death
- **Methamphetamine ("ice"):** synthetic; inhaled, smoked, IV; very powerful
- **Designer amphetamines:** hallucinogens, structure close to amphetamines:
    - MDMA (3, 4-methylenedioxyamphetamine) is "ecstasy," "XTC," "Adam" (the most available) (Schedule I drug under the CSA along with LSD, heroin, and marijuana)
    - MDEA (N-ethyl-3, 4-methylenedioxyamphetamine) is "Eve"
    - MMDA or MDA (5-methoxy-3, 4-methylenedioxyamphetamine): peak 1 hr, disappears after 5 hr
    - DOM (2, 5-dimethoxy-4-methylamphetamine) is "STP" (serenity, tranquility, peace)
    - PMA (paramethoxyamphetamine) is "Death or Dr Death" (↑↑ body temperature)

Epidemiology: lifetime prevalence is 1.5%; M : F is 1 : 1. Methamphetamine abuse: second-most used illicit drug internationally after marijuana.

Neuropharmacology: taken orally, onset of action in <1 hr; **classic amphetamines release DA** (activation of reward circuit pathway, addictive); **designer amphetamines: release DA, NE, and serotonin** (mixed effect of amphetamines and hallucinogens).

Diagnosis:

(1) **Amphetamine dependence and abuse:** needs high doses for the usual high and physical effects; ↓ *weight and* ↑ *paranoia.*

(2) **Amphetamine intoxication:** similar to cocaine intoxication, usually *resolves in 48 hr.*

TABLE 20.16. Symptoms of Amphetamine Intoxication

Recent use of amphetamine or related substance, the sx are not due to a gl medical or another mental disorder
Behavioral or psychological changes during or shortly after the use:
• Euphoria or affective blunting
• Hypervigilance, anxiety, tension, anger
• Impaired judgment, possible psychosis
• Impaired social or occupational functioning
Physical changes: ≥2
• Pulse: ↑ or ↓
• Dilated pupils: +++
• BP: ↓ or ↑
• Sweating or chills
• Nausea, vomiting
• Weight loss
• Psychomotor retardation or agitation
• Respiratory deprezzsion, cardiac arrhythmias, muscular weakness, chest pain
• Confusion, seizures, dyskinesias, dystonias, coma
• Possible hallucinations
• Possible delirium (↑ if sleep deprivation, high doses, sustained use, combination of substances, prior brain damage)

(3) **Amphetamine withdrawal**: described as a *"crash," peaks in 2–4 days, resolves in <1 wk*

TABLE 20.17. Symptoms of Amphetamine Withdrawal

Cessation of heavy and prolonged use of amphetamine or related substance, sx are not due to a gl medical condition or another mental disorder and there is a significant ↓ in *x* areas of functioning
Dysphoric mood (risk of depression and suicidality)
Physiological changes: ≥2
• Fatigue
• Anxiety, tremulousness, headaches
• Profuse sweating
• Muscle cramps, stomach cramps
• Nightmares, rebound in REM sleep
• ↑↑ appetite
• psychomotor retardation or agitation

(4) **Other amphetamine-induced disorders**:

- **Amphetamine-induced psychotic disorder**: R/O schizophrenia (with amphetamines: paranoia, predominance of visual hallucinations, appropriate affect, no alogia, hypersexuality, confusion, no disordered thinking, no loose associations, positive urine drug screen, and ↓ sx in a few days). Rx: short-term use of antipsychotic (haloperidol)

- **Amphetamine-induced mood disorder**: intoxication: manic or mixed mood features; withdrawal: depressive features

- **Amphetamine-induced anxiety disorder**: sx such as OCD, panic disorder, phobias

- **Amphetamine-induced sexual dysfunction**: induces erectile disorder and other sexual dysfunctions

- **Amphetamine-induced sleep disorder**: intoxication → insomnia, withdrawal → hypersomnolence and nightmares

Clinical features:

(1) **Amphetamines**:

- **Physical**: cerebrovascular (ischemic or hemorrhagic stroke), cardiac (↑ HR, palpitations, SOB, myocardial infarction, severe HTN, cardiomyopathy), GI (nausea, vomiting, bruxism), flushing, pallor, cyanosis, fever, neurologic (twitching, tremor, ataxia, seizures, coma, death), fatal OD; IV use: risk of HIV, hepatitis, lung abscesses, endocarditis, necrotizing angiitis, unsafe sex practices; obstetrical complications of use during pregnancy: ↓ birth weight, ↓ head circumference, prematurity, growth retardation

- **Psychologic**: restlessness, dysphoria, insomnia, irritability, hostility, confusion, anxiety, psychosis

(2) **Substituted amphetamines**:

- Same as do classic amphetamines
- Others:
  a. *Short term*: sense of closeness with other people, trismus, tachycardia, bruxism, dry mouth, ↑ alertness, luminescence of objects, tremor, palpitations, diaphoresis, concentration problems, paresthesias, insomnia, hot or cold flashes, ↑ sensitivity to cold, dizziness, visual hallucinations, blurred vision, hyperthermia (↑ with excessive activity like in "raves")

  b. *Moderate term*: drowsiness, muscle aches, depression, trismus, headache, problem concentrating, dry mouth, anxiety, irritability

(3) **Other agents**:

- **MDMA/ecstasy**: 100–150 mg: ↑ mood, self-confidence, sensory sensitivity, ↓ appetite, dysphoria, psychosis, sympathomimetic effects (up to 8 hr), some tolerance, fatal OD, changes in the serotonergic pathways, possible long-term toxicity

- **Khat**: chewing of fresh leaves of *Catha edulis* (active ingredient: cathinone); used in Africa; quickly metabolized → ↑ BP, dependency; synthetic-related drug is methcathinone ("CAT," "goob," "crank"): Schedule I drug under the CSA

Treatment and rehabilitation: difficulty to remain abstinent (very reinforcing, much craving). Inpatient setting uses *x* modalities (individual, family, group rx); medications for specific disorders (psychosis, anxiety), usually for a few days. Treat depression: possibly bupropion (Wellbutrin) after withdrawal from the amphetamines (helps with the dysphoria).

CAFFEINE-RELATED DISORDERS

80% of adults consume caffeine, a psychoactive drug.

Sources of Caffeine

Table 20.18.   Sources of Caffeine

In drinks	In some medications (1 tablet)
1 cup (5–6 oz.) • of coffee:100–150 mg • of tea: 30–100 mg • of cocoa: 5–50 mg • of decaffeinated coffee: 2–4 mg 1 glass (8–12 oz.) • regular soft drink (Pepsi, Coke, …): 25–50 mg • caffeine-free: 0 mg	**Migraine medications**: Cafergot, Migralam (100 mg); Darvon, Fiorinal (32–50 mg) **Analgesics**: Exedrin (60 mg); Norgesic, dolor (30 mg); Advil, Aspirin, Midol 200, Nuprin **Appetite suppressants**: Caffedrine (250 mg); Anorexin (100 mg)

Epidemiology: adults in average consume 200 mg/d in the United States; 30% consume >500 mg/d; even young children.

Comorbidity: 2/3 use also sedative-hypnotic drugs.

Neuropharmacology: half-life is 3–10 hr; peak conc. in 30–60 min; caffeine is an antagonist of the adenosine receptors (which activate an inhibitory G protein and prevents the formation of c AMP); Caffeine intake → ↑ cAMP conc. in neurons with adenosine receptors. Caffeine ↑ DA activity (↑ psychosis in pts with schizophrenia) and affects noradrenergic neurons (role in caffeine withdrawal); possible genetic predisposition to continued coffee use after exposure; is a substance of abuse (100 mg → mild euphoria; 300 mg → anxiety, dysphoria; evidence of physical tolerance and withdrawal sx); provokes ↓ in cerebral blood flow by vasoconstriction (may be also in coronary arteries).

Differential diagnosis: GAD, panic disorders, bipolar II disorder, ADHD, sleep disorders, abuse of anabolic steroids, other stimulants (amphetamines, cocaine), pheochromocytoma, hyperthyroidism.

Diagnosis:

(1) **Caffeine intoxication**:

TABLE 20.19.   Symptoms of Caffeine Intoxication

Recent use of caffeine (>250 mg or >3 cups of coffee) with significant distress or impairment in functioning, not due to a gl medical condition or another mental disorder **≥5 signs** need to be seen during or shortly after the intake: • **restlessness or nervousness or excitement or psychomotor agitation** • **insomnia** • **flushed face** • **diuresis** • **muscle twitching** • **GI disturbance** • **rambling flow of thought and speech** • **tachycardia or cardiac arrhythmias** • **Periods of inexhaustibility**

(2) **Caffeine withdrawal**: reflects the tolerance and physiologic dependence with continued use.

TABLE 20.20.   Symptoms of Caffeine Withdrawal

Prolonged daily use needed with an abrupt cessation or reduction; sx cause significant distress or impairment in functioning and are not due to a gl medical condition or another mental disorder Starts with a **headache** followed by: • fatigue or drowsiness • marked anxiety or depression • nausea or vomiting

(3) **Other caffeine-induced disorders**:

• **Caffeine-induced anxiety disorder**: similar clinically to GAD, panic attacks
• **Caffeine-induced sleep disorder**: difficulty falling, staying asleep, early morning awakening
• **Caffeine-related disorder NOS**

Clinical features:

- 50–100 mg of caffeine → ↑ alertness, sense of well-being, ↑ verbal and motor performances, ↑ diuresis, intestinal peristalsis, ↑ gastric secretion, mild ↑ BP and cardiac muscle stimulation
- Adverse effects: cardiac arrhythmias, ↑ gastric secretion (risk in gastric ulcers), may be associated with fibrocystic disease of the breasts in ♀

Treatment: headaches: aspirin or other analgesics; rare use of benzodiazepines for withdrawal sx for a short time; make a diary to evaluate all caffeine intake and plan a fading schedule with a ↓ of 10% q few days.

CANNABIS-RELATED DISORDERS

National organization:

Marijuana anonymous: http://www.marijuana-anonymous.org/; 1-800-766-6779

Epidemiology: *Cannabis sativa*, hardy annual herb, the most used illicit drug, contains psychoactive cannabinoids (Δ9-tetrahydrocannabinol or Δ9-THC); common names: marijuana, grass, pot, weed, tea, Marie Jane. Other names: hemp, bhang, ganja, dagga, sinsemilla. M : F is 2 : 1; by age group: 12–17 yo (whites > blacks), 17–34 yo (whites = blacks), >35 yo (blacks, Hispanics).

Neuropharmacology: *Cannabis plant contains >400 chemicals*; in the body, Δ9-THC is converted into hydroxy-Δ9-THC, active in CNS. The cannabinoid *receptor is linked to the inhibitory G protein* and found in the basal ganglia, hippocampus, cerebellum, not in the brain stem (minimal effect on respiration and cardiac function). Cannabinoids affect monoamine and GABA neurons. When smoked: euphoric effects appear within minutes, peak in 30 min, last 2–4 hr; motor and cognitive effects may last 5–12 hr. If taken in food: 3× the quantity is needed; if chronically used, will **stay in urine up to 30 days. Currently, cannabis is an illegal, controlled substance with a high potential for abuse, with no medical use recognized by the DEA** (nausea secondary to chemotherapy, MS, chronic pain, AIDS, glaucoma).

Clinical features:

TABLE 20.21. Effects of Cannabis

Short-term effects	• Red eyes • Mild tachycardia • Orthostatic hypotension (high doses)
Long-term effects	• Chronic respiratory disease and lung cancer • Cerebral atrophy and risk of seizures • Chromosomal damages and birth defects • Impaired immune reactivity • Alteration in testosterone concentration and dysregulation of menstrual cycles

Diagnosis

(1) **Cannabis dependence and abuse**: tolerance, psychologic dependence but less support for physical dependence

(2) **Cannabis intoxication**

TABLE 20.22. Symptoms of Cannabis Intoxication

Recent use of cannabis with significant behavioral or psychologic changes (**impaired motor coordination, euphoria, sensation of slowed time, anxiety, impaired judgment, social withdrawal**) developing during or shortly after cannabis use, sx are not due to a gl medical condition or another mental disorder ≥2 signs **within 2 hr of use:** • **conjunctival injection** • **↑ appetite** • **dry mouth** • **tachycardia** • **possibility of perceptual disturbances, delirium**

(3) **Other cannabis-induced disorders**:

- **Cannabis-induced psychotic disorder**: rare, transient paranoia. Possible if long-term access to high potency drugs (hemp insanity), if preexisting personality disorder; a "bad trip" usually happens when cannabis is associated with a hallucinogen
- **Cannabis-induced anxiety disorder**: frequent in inexperienced users
- **Flashbacks**: persisting perceptual abnormalities after the short-term effects have disappeared (possible cannabis tainted with PCP?)
- **Amotivational syndrome**: with long-term heavy use

Treatment and rehabilitation:

- Abstinence: hospitalization or outpatient setting with strict monitoring (urine screen)
- Support with individual, family, group rx, education. Treat any comorbidity.

COCAINE-RELATED DISORDERS

National organization:

Cocaine anonymous: http://www.ca.org/; 310-559-5833

Narcotics anonymous (NA): http://www.na.org/

Epidemiology: *the most addictive substance abused;* other names: snow, coke, girl, lady; inhaled as a white powder; *freebase and crack cocaine are more potent,* are smoked or injected; alkaloid derived from leaves of a shrub (*Erythroxylon coca*) from South America; **classified as narcotic** in 1914; Approximately 36.8 million Americans ages 12 and older have tried cocaine at least once in their lifetimes; 0.7 million new male users each year, and 0.5 million new females each year. More than 400,000 infants are born addicted to cocaine each year in the United States; street prices: cocaine ($100–150 for 1 g vial), crack ($10 for a single dose of 50–100 mg); through a straw or a coke spoon: typically contains 5–20 mg of the drug, may be used to snort cocaine; 1-inch line typically contains 25–100 mg of the drug; crack may be smoked in a pipe bowl containing 50–100 mg or in a cigarette with as much as 300 mg; frequent cocaine users: 0.3% of population; mostly 18–25 yo (1.3%), less if > age 35 (0.4%).

Neuropharmacology: competitive blockade of DA reuptake by the DA transporter → ↑ conc. of DA in synapses and activation of DA, D1 and D2 receptors, possibly also D3; blocks also reuptake of serotonin and NE; cocaine ↓ cerebral blood flow; short-lived behavioral effects (30–60 min); may stay in **the blood and urine up to 10 days** (if chronic use). Very addictive: possible psychologic dependence after 1 dose, physiologic dependence is less than with opiates; during **cravings** for cocaine: ↑ activity in the mesolimbic DA system/amygdale and anterior cingulate (max after 3–4 wk of withdrawal: ↑ *risk for relapse; still apparent up to 18 months*).

Methods of use: snorting (or "tooting"), subcutaneously or IV, smoking (freebasing ↑ effects by mixing street cocaine with the freebase or pure cocaine alkaloid), smoking crack cocaine. IV and smoking are associated with CV diseases, cardiac abnormalities, and death. Crack is sold in "rocks" (very addictive, intense cravings); **"speedballs" is a combination of opioids + cocaine (risk of death).** In speedballing, heroin is injected or snorted, followed immediately by smoking of cocaine.

Comorbidity: MDD, bipolar II disorder, cyclothymic disorder, anxiety disorders, antisocial personality disorder, alcohol-related disorders.

Clinical features:

TABLE 20.23.   Effects of Cocaine

Common changes	• Irritability, ↓ concentration, compulsive behavior, severe insomnia, weight loss • ↑ Inability to do normal tasks at work and home • Frequent self-removal (q 30–60 min) from normal situations to use cocaine • Debts due to cost of cocaine
Adverse effects	• **Nasal congestion**, ulcerations, and perforation of nasal septa • Bronchial and lung damages with freebasing • IV use: **infections, embolisms, HIV** • Neurologic complications: acute dystonia, tics, headaches • **CV disease: nonhemorrhagic cerebral infarctions** > hemorrhagic infarctions > TIA > spinal cord hemorrhages • **Seizures**: (*cocaine > amphetamine*); usually single events, ↑ in pts with epilepsy using high doses of cocaine or crack; R/O partial complex status epilepticus if fluctuating course • **Cardiac effects: myocardial infarction, arrhythmias, cardiomyopathy,** cardioembolic cerebral infarction, QT prolongation, catecholamine toxicity, microvascular disease • **Death**: death from acute cocaine toxicity is relatively rare, seen in "body packers" or "body stuffers"; the only cocaine users likely to become seriously ill or die are the chronic users

Diagnosis

(1) **Cocaine intoxication:** low doses: elation, euphoria, ↑ sense of self-esteem, ↑ performance on mental + physical tasks; high doses: agitation, impulsive sexual behaviors, aggression, mania, tachycardia, **mydriasis**, hypertension. Delirium possible if high doses of cocaine use with rapid increases in the blood conc. or if mixed with other drugs (amphetamines, opiates, alcohol) or pts with preexisting brain damage

TABLE 20.24.   Symptoms of Cocaine Intoxication

Recent use of cocaine
Significant behavioral or psychologic changes and physical sx seen during or shortly after the use of cocaine and not due to a general medical condition or another mental disorder
Similar to those of amphetamine intoxication

(2) **Cocaine withdrawal**: postintoxication *"crash."* In mild use: withdrawal sx end within 18 hr; in heavy use: sx may last up to 1 wk, but peak in 2–4 days (intense cravings, self-medicating with alcohol, sedatives, hypnotics, antianxiety agents)

TABLE 20.25.   Symptoms of Cocaine Withdrawal

Cessation or reduction in prolonged and heavy use of cocaine
Dysphoric mood and physiologic changes appearing within a few hours to several days of the cessation
Sx not due to a gl medical condition or another mental disorder
Similar to those of amphetamine withdrawal

(3) **Other cocaine-induced disorders**:

- **Cocaine-induced psychotic disorder**: hallucinations, paranoid delusions (50% of cocaine users, mostly IV and crack users; M > F); sensation of bug crawling under the skin (**formication**)
- **Cocaine-induced mood disorder**: manic during intoxication and depression in withdrawal
- **Cocaine-induced anxiety disorder**: mostly OCD, panic disorders, and phobias
- **Cocaine-induced sexual dysfunction**: cocaine is used as an aphrodisiac, to delay orgasm, leading to impotency.
- **Cocaine-induced sleep disorder**: in intoxication: insomnia; in withdrawal: hypersomnolence, abnormal pattern of sleep

Treatment and rehabilitation: includes social, psychologic, biologic rx; *intense craving for the drug*: +++; frequent need for hospitalization or partial hospitals; *Frequent unscheduled testing*; **relapse-prevention**: necessary with CBT.

(1) **Individual, group, family rx**, including support groups such as **Narcotics Anonymous (NA)**.

(2) **Pharmacologic rx**: chronic use of cocaine induces a state of relative DA insufficiency.

- **Dopaminergic agonists**: Amantadine (*Symmetrel*: 100 mg bid); bromocriptine (*Parlodel*: 2.5 mg bid): of little use
- **Antidepressants**: Bupropion (*Wellbutrin*), MAOI (such as selegiline/*Eldepryl*), SSRIs (*fluoxetine*)
- **Mood stabilizers**: Carbamazepine (*Tegretol*), valproic acid (*Depakene*), phenytoin (*Dylantin*: 300 mg/d)
- **Methylphenidate**: (*Ritalin*): in pts + ADHD to withdraw from cocaine
- **New treatments in development**: such as cocaine-binding antibodies, butyrylcholinesterase (a selective cocaine hydrolyzer present in the body)?

HALLUCINOGEN-RELATED DISORDERS

Epidemiology:

- Natural or synthetic substances (psychotomimetics, psychedelics) producing hallucinations, expanded consciousness, no contact with reality
- Most frequent are:

  - **Natural: psilocybin** (found in mushrooms from southern United States and South America, dose of 5–10 mg of dried mushroom taken orally gives psychosis of 4–6 hr duration), **mescaline** (found in peyote cactus from south western United States, dose of 200–400 mg/or 4–6 cactus buttons taken orally may have an effect for 10–12 hr), **morning glory seeds** (similar to LSD, effects may last 3 hr; 7–13 seeds taken orally as infusion can produce a toxic delirium), **nutmeg** and **mace** (1 teaspoon or 5–15 g taken orally or as a snuff may produce atropinism with seizures, death), **toads** (skin contains bufotoxins)

  - **Synthetics: LSD** (lysergic acid diethylamide, usually taken orally at a dose of 100 µg, effects last 6–12 hr), **MDA** (3, 4-methylenedioxyamphetamine is a phenethylamine, taken orally at a dose of 80–160 mg, with effects lasting 8–12 hr), **MDMA** (3, 4-methylenedioxymethamphetamine is a phenethylamine taken orally at a dose of 80–150 mg with effects lasting 4–6 hr). **MDA and MDMA are called designer amphetamines** (see paragraph on amphetamines).

- 10% in United States have used them once or more; ratio white : black is 2 : 1; white : Hispanic is 1.5 : 1; higher in young white males; US western states > US southern states; substance-related ED visits: 1% for hallucinogens vs 40% for cocaine; lifetime prevalence: 0.6%

Neuropharmacology: LSD acts as a partial agonist at postsynaptic serotonin receptors; rapid absorption, orally, smoking, or IV; rapid tolerance after 3–4 days of continuous use but reverses in 4–7 days; no physical dependence or withdrawal signs.

Clinical features: onset of action of LSD is in <1 hr, *peaks in 2–4 hr.*

Diagnosis:
(1) **Hallucinogen dependence and abuse**: rare long-term use; *meth-mouth* (dry mouth, cracked teeth/due to clenching and grinding of teeth, neglect of oral hygiene)

(2) **Hallucinogen intoxication**: onset is generally 30–60 min with 4–8 hr duration; with sx of *sympathetic stimulation* (↑ pupils, diaphoresis, piloerection), hyperthermia, possible neuroleptic malignant syndrome (NMS; reported with LSD), rhabdomyolysis (esp. if pt is restrained), panic attacks with *cross-sensory hallucinations* (*tasting colors, seeing sounds*), ↑ DTRs, tachycardia, vomiting, and diarrhea (esp. mescaline, psilocybin), may produce delirium (esp. if mixed with other substances); risk of death due to poor judgment

  ● **Signs of hallucinogen intoxication**

TABLE 20.26.   Hallucinogen Intoxication: Symptoms

Recent use of a hallucinogen
Significant changes appearing during or shortly after use, not due to a gl medical condition or another mental disorder
● **Behavioral**
● **Psychological**: ↑ anxiety or depression, ideas of reference, paranoia, fear of going "crazy," impaired judgment, impaired functioning, philosophical or religious insight
● **Perceptual changes in a state of full alertness**: ↑ perceptions (unusually brilliant, intense), depersonalization, derealization, hallucinations, synesthesias (colors may be heard and sounds may be seen), intense labile emotions, awareness of internal organs, recovery of lost memories, reliving past events

● **Physical changes**: >2
  ○ **Pupillary dilatation**
  ○ **Tachycardia**
  ○ **Sweating**
  ○ **Palpitations**
  ○ **Blurred vision**
  ○ **Tremors, incoordination**

  ● **Differential diagnosis**: anticholinergic intoxication, cocaine intoxication, amphetamine intoxication, alcohol withdrawal

(3) **Hallucinogen persisting perception disorder (flashbacks)**: flashbacks of a perceptual sx (trails of images from moving objects, hallucinations, halos, time expansion, intense emotion, micropsia, macropsia) long after the use of the hallucinogen (R/O: migraine, seizure, PTSD); may be triggered by: stress, sensory deprivation, use of another substance (marijuana, alcohol); causing distress or impairment in functioning; not due to gl medical condition (brain lesion, infection, epilepsies) or another mental disorder (delirium, dementia, schizophrenia) or hypnopompic hallucinations

(4) **Others**:
  ● **Hallucinogen-induced psychotic disorders**: "bad trip" (resemblance to an acute panic reaction) usually ends when the effect of the hallucinogen wears off; may produce true psychotic sx (if chronic: difficult to R/O a nonorganic psychotic disorder; in schizophrenia: negative symptoms + poor interpersonal relatedness); may be prolonged in pts with preexisting schizoid personality disorder

  ● **Hallucinogen-induced mood disorder**: may resolve when the substance wears off; sx may be unpredictable (mixed sx of mania and depression with psychotic sx)

  ● **Hallucinogen-induced anxiety disorder**: ↑ panic sx with agoraphobia

Treatment and rehabilitation:
  ● **Intoxication**: talking down, reassuring that sx are drug induced and will resolve. If severe sx: haloperidol or diazepam (20 mg orally is very effective)

  ● **Flashbacks**: behavioral rx (avoid caffeine, alcohol, stress, marijuana); treat comorbidity (panic disorder, MDD, alcohol dependence), treat with long-acting benzodiazepines (clonazepam/Klonopin), rarely with anticonvulsant (valproic acid or carbamazepine). Do not use antipsychotics (risk of paradoxical effect).

  ● **Hallucinogen-induced psychosis**: antipsychotics, lithium, carbamazepine, ECT, antidepressants, benzodiazepines, anticonvulsants may be useful.

INHALANT-RELATED DISORDERS

Substances: Solvents, glues, adhesives, aerosol propellants, paint thinners, fuels (e.g., gasoline, varnish, lighter fluid, cleaning fluid, spray paint, correction fluid)

Epidemiology: available, legal, inexpensive; 1% of all substance-related deaths and <0.5% of all substance-related ER visits (20% in pts <18 yo); associated with CD or antisocial personality disorder; 5% in the United States have used inhalants more than once and 1% are current users; active components are: toluene, acetone, benzene, trichloroethane, perchlorethylene, trichloroethylene, halogenated hydrocarbons.

Neuropharmacology: are CNS depressants; tolerance may develop (mild withdrawal sx); absorbed through the lungs, with effects appearing in <5 min, lasting for 30 min up to several hours; conc. ↑ if used with alcohol; detectable in the blood for 4–10 hr; may enhance the GABA system and membrane fluidization.

Diagnosis:

(1) **Inhalant dependence and abuse**: rare

(2) **Inhalant intoxication**:

TABLE 20.27.   Symptoms of Inhalant Intoxication

Recent exposure to volatile inhalants, with sx not due to a gl medical condition or another mental disorder, appearing during or shortly after the exposure
Significant behavioral or psychological changes: apathy, assaultiveness, impaired judgment and functioning
Physical signs: >2
• Dizziness, incoordination, unsteady gait, nystagmus
• Slurred speech, lethargy, psychomotor retardation, depressed reflexes
• Generalized muscle weakness
• Tremor, blurred vision, or diplopia
• Euphoria
• May produce delirium, stupor, or coma

(3) **Inhalant-induced disorders**

- **Inhalant-induced persisting dementia**: likely to be irreversible
- **Inhalant-induced psychotic disorder**: frequent paranoia
- **Inhalant-induced mood disorder**: mostly depression
- **Inhalant-induced anxiety disorder**: mostly panic disorders, GAD

Clinical features:

TABLE 20.28.   Effects of Inhalants

Small initial doses	Euphoria, excitement, floating sensations
High doses	Fearfulness, sensory illusions, hallucinations, distortions of body size, slurred speech, ataxia, irritability, emotional lability, poor memory; if mild withdrawal sx: sleep disturbances, irritability, sweating, nausea, vomiting, psychosis, tachycardia
Adverse effects	**Risk of death**: respiratory depression, cardiac arrhythmias, asphyxiation, aspiration of vomitus, accident with injuries **Liver failure, renal failure** (toluene), **rhabdomyolysis** **Brain atrophy** (toluene), **temporal lobe epilepsy**, ↓ **IQ** (organic solvents copper, zinc, and heavy metals), **peripheral neuritis, headache, cerebellar signs, lead encephalopathy, paresthesia** **Chest pain, respiratory problems** **GI**: pain, nausea, vomiting, hematemesis **Abnormal fetal development** **Motor impairment** (toluene)

Treatment and rehabilitation: counseling and education; risks ↑ if associated with antisocial personality disorder or CD.

NICOTINE-RELATED DISORDERS

Epidemiology: very addictive; 1 billion smokers worldwide, smoking 6 trillions cigarettes/yr; kills >3million people/yr; ↓ in the United States but still 22–29% of the population smokes; used in cigarettes, pipes, cigars, snuff, and chewing tobacco; 3–6% use smokeless tobacco; heavy alcohol use in 12.6% of smokers vs 2.7% of nonsmokers; illicit drug use in 13.6% of smokers vs 3% in nonsmokers; about 29% of smokers between 12 and 17 yo; same rates in different ethnicities; smokeless tobacco: whites > blacks or Hispanics; M > F; higher in psychiatric pts; deaths ↑ (chronic bronchitis, emphysema, lung cancer, myocardial infarction, cerebrovascular diseases, cardiovascular diseases; multiple cancers: oropharyngeal, bladder, GI, kidney, liver).

Neuropharmacology: nicotine is an agonist at the nicotinic subtype of AC receptors; activation of DA reward system, ↑ circulating NE and epinephrine and release of vasopressin, ↑ β-endorphin, ACTH, cortisol (stimulatory effects); half-life is 2 hr. **One cigarette delivers 0.5 mg of nicotine (60 mg in an adult is fatal/leads to respiratory paralysis).**

Diagnosis:

(1) **Nicotine dependence**: social factors, genetic components?

(2) **Nicotine withdrawal**: within 2–48 hr of cessation, may last for weeks or months, after use of nicotine for several weeks; sx: dysphoric mood, tension, irritability, craving, poor concentration, drowsiness, restlessness, anxiety, ↓ HR, ↓ BP, ↑ appetite and weight

(3) **Nicotine-related disorder NOS**: intoxication, abuse, mood disorders, anxiety disorders

Clinical features:

TABLE 20.29.   Effects of Nicotine

Short-term effects	↑ Attention, learning, mood, ↑ cerebral blood flow (long-term exposure: ↓ CBF) ↓ Tension, muscle relaxation
Adverse effects	Nausea, vomiting, abdominal pain, diarrhea Dizziness, headache, tremor Cold sweats Tachycardia, ↑ BP Poor concentration, confusion, sensory disturbances ↓ Amount of REM sleep During pregnancy: low birth weight babies, ↑ newborns with pulmonary hypertension

Treatment and rehabilitation: smoking cessation with behavioral support programs, systemic nicotine (nicotine patch or gum or inhaler), and other pharmacologic agents: clonidine (Catapress), buspirone (BuSpar), antidepressants such as fluoxetine (Prozac), bupropion (Zyban).

OPIOID-RELATED DISORDERS

National organization:

Narcotics Anonymous (NA): http://www.na.org/; (818) 773-9999

Epidemiology: in 1991: 1.3% of the population had used heroin at some time; prevalence of lifetime heroin use: 0.7–1.5%.

Substances: **Opium** (juice of opium poppy, *Papaver somniferum*, contains >20 opium alkaloids); **natural opiates**: morphine, heroin (diacetylmorphine is *twice as potent as morphine*), codeine (3-methoxymorphine), hydrocodone (*Lortab, Vicodin*), hydromorphone (*Dilaudid*) oxycodone (*OxyContin, Percocet, Percodan*); **synthetic opioids**: fentanyl (*Actiq, Duragesic, and Sublimaze*), meperidine (*Demerol*), methadone (*Dolophine*), pentazocine (*Talwin*), propoxyphene (*Darvon*); **opioid antagonists**: naloxone (*Narcan*), naltrexone (*ReVia*), nalorphine, levallorphan, apomorphine; **mixed agonists and antagonists**: pentazocine, butorphanol (*Stadol*), buprenorphine (*Buprenex inj., Subutex tabs and SL*); can be taken po, intranasally and IV or subcutaneously.

Comorbidity: MDD, alcohol use disorders, antisocial personality disorder, anxiety disorders; 15% of opioid-dependent pts try to commit suicide and 90% have comorbid psychiatric disorders or substance use.

Neuropharmacology: effects on **opioid receptors**: μ-opioid receptors (analgesia, respiratory depression, constipation, dependence), μ-opioid receptors (analgesia, diuresis, sedation), Δ-opioid receptors (analgesia) and on **dopaminergic** (rewarding properties) and **noradrenergic** transmitter systems: heroin crosses blood–brain barrier faster than morphine (more dependency); codeine is transformed into morphine in the body; all opioids ↓ cerebral blood flow in some brain regions (locus ceruleus [LC]); *tolerance develops quickly*; long-term use of opiates results in changing the number and sensitivity of opioid receptors; short-term use: ↓ activity of noradrenergic neurons in LC (withdrawal → ↑ hyperactivity/clonidine ↓ the release of NE and is used in rx of withdrawal sx); long-term use: ↑ sensitivity of dopaminergic, cholinergic, and serotoninergic neurons.

Etiology: ↑ with poverty, families already affected by substance abuse, at risk adolescents (agitation, anxious depression, impulsiveness, poor coping skills, aggressivity, need for immediate gratification, substance-abusing peers); biologic and genetic predisposition? psychodynamic theories (regression to pregenital levels of psychosexual development, ego dysfunction, affective disturbances).

Diagnosis:

(1) **Opioid dependence and abuse**: physical dependency can occur after short periods of daily use (e.g., 2 wk)

(2) **Opioid intoxication**:

TABLE 20.30.   Symptoms of Opioid Intoxication

Recent use of an opioid with sx not due to a gl medical condition or another mental disorder
Significant behavioral or psychologic changes appearing during or shortly after the use: euphoria followed by apathy, psychomotor agitation or retardation, poor judgment, impaired functioning
Physical symptoms:
● Pupillary constriction +++
● Drowsiness or coma
● Slurred speech
● Problems in attention or memory
Possibility of perceptual disturbances or delirium

(3) **Opioid withdrawal**

TABLE 20.31.   Symptoms of Opiate Withdrawal

Cessation or reduction in heavy and prolonged use of an opioid, or use of an opioid antagonist after a period of opioid use, with sx not due to a gI medical condition or another mental disorder
Significant distress or impairment in functioning
Signs: ≥3 appearing within minutes to several days
• **Dysphoric mood (restlessness, depression, irritability)**
• **Nausea or vomiting, abdominal cramps**
• **Muscle aches, bone aches**
• **Tremor, weakness**
• **Rhinorrhea or lacrimation**
• **Pupillary dilatation, piloerection**
• **Sweating**
• **Diarrhea**
• **Yawning**
• **Fever or temperature dysregulation**
• **Hypertension, tachycardia**
• **Insomnia**
• **Craving**
Withdrawal may be spontaneous or precipitated (if administration of an opioid antagonist such as naloxone or naltrexone +++)

TABLE 20.32.   Timing of Withdrawal Symptoms

Morphine and heroin: starts 6–8 hr after last dose, peaks on day 2–3 and ↓ in 10 days, may persist >6 months
Meperidine: starts quickly, peaks in 8–12 hr and ends in 4–5 days
Methadone: starts 1–3 days after last dose and ends in 10–14 days (drugs with longer half-lives generally have less severe spontaneous withdrawal sx)

(4) **Others**:

- **Opioid-induced psychotic disorder**: may begin during intoxication
- **Opioid-induced mood disorder**: may begin during intoxication, usually mixed sx (irritability, expansiveness, depression)
- **Opioid-induced sleep disorder**: insomnia < hypersomnia
- **Opioid-induced sexual dysfunction**: mostly impotence

Clinical features:

TABLE 20.33.   Effects of Opioids

Short-term effects	Rush (initial euphoria, feeling of warmth, dry mouth, itchy nose, facial flushing), followed by sedation, nausea, or vomiting **Respiratory depression** **Pupillary constriction** **Smooth muscle contraction** **Constipation** **Changes in BP, pulse, body temperature**
Adverse effects	**Possible transmission of hepatitis and HIV (contaminated needles)** **Anaphylactic shock** **Pulmonary edema** **Death** **Severe drug interaction between meperidine and MAOIs: autonomic instability, agitation, coma, seizures, death** **MPTP-induced parkinsonism** (if opioid contaminated with N-methyl-4-phenyl-1, 2, 3, 6-tetrahydropyridine [MPTP], its metabolite concentrates in the substantia nigra neurons and destroys them → Parkinson sx)

TABLE 20.34.   Opioid Overdose: A Medical Emergency

Symptoms	Unresponsiveness, coma, slow respiration, hypothermia, hypotension, bradycardia (triad: pinpoint pupils, coma, respiratory depression); needle tracks on the body
Treatment	• Open airway • Vital signs maintained • Administration of an opioid antagonist: naltrexone (0.4 mg IV, to be repeated 4–5 times during first 30–45 min); caution due to short duration of action of naltrexone • Antagonist may precipitate a severe withdrawal reaction • Risk of grand mal seizures with meperidine overdose

Treatment and rehabilitation:

■ 1. Current state of opioid addiction treatment

Two main rx modalities: psychosocial approaches (such as residential rx communities, 12-step mutual programs such as NA and 12-step- or abstinence-based treatment programs) either as stand-alone interventions or in combination with pharmacotherapy; includes: (1) *agonist maintenance with methadone or LAAM,* (2) *antagonist maintenance using naltrexone,* and (3) *the use of antiwithdrawal or detoxification agents such as methadone, clonidine, and lofexidine* (*under investigation in the United States, alpha2-adrenergic-agonist,* commonly used for detoxification in the United Kingdom, not addicting, easy to use with a favorable safety profile).

TABLE 20.35.   Types of Opiates (Many Legal Requirements for Methadone Dispensing +++)

Full agonists: heroin, LAAM, methadone, morphine

Partial agonists: buprenorphine (may precipitate withdrawal under certain circumstances: more likely if high level of dependence, short time interval between administration of full agonist and partial antagonist, or if high dose of partial agonist/by displacing the full agonist and only partially activating the receptor → a net decrease in activation)

Antagonists: Naloxone, Naltrexone

- **Methadone**: long-acting μ agonist (duration of action: 24–36 hr), taken po, synthetic opioid, suppresses withdrawal sx; doses: 20–80 mg usually, may be up to 120 mg/d; once/d dosage; 30–40 mg will block withdrawal but not craving; 80 ± 20 mg is the average rx dose that will block abstinence sx and heroin euphoria; causes dependence on an opioid

- **Other opioid substitutes**:
  - **LAMM** (Levo-α-acetylmethadol) administered **3× wk as an alternative to methadone** (30–80 mg); minimal euphoria is an agonist with longer half-life (2–4 days), peak plasma conc. at 2 hr and 15 days to steady state; same regulations as methadone
  - **Buprenorphine**: **mixed agonist-antagonist** at the opiate receptor, synthetic opioid; **Subutex is buprenorphine**; **Suboxone is buprenorphine + naloxone** (*preferred for maintenance*); half-life: 37 hr for buprenorphine and 1.1 hr for naloxone; respiratory and CNS depression can occur if IV used; produces opioid dependence. The naloxone in Suboxone can cause opioid withdrawal if used IV or SL by opioid-dependent pts; cases of hepatic failure and allergic reactions. May be useful in adolescents

- **Opioid antagonists**:
  - **Naloxone (Narcan)** used in the rx of opioid OD, no narcotic effect, and no dependence. Give: 0.4–2 mg IV q 2–3 min prn or 0.4–2 mg IM/SC q 2–3 min prn; may repeat q 1–2 hr if sx recur; question the dx if no response after 10 mg
  - **Naltrexone (Revia)** blocks opioid euphoric effects, longer acting (>72 hr), needs to be taken regularly: dose: 50 mg daily, 100 mg every 2 days or 150 mg every third day. Frequent lack of adherence; hepatotoxicity

- **Clonidine**: **(α2 agonist)**, 0.1–0.3 mg tid or qid may be used for detoxification

■ 2. Detoxification

TABLE 20.36.   Opiate Detoxification

Using short-term methadone: +++	Follow VS: **at first sx of withdrawal, give 10 mg methadone po (liquid)** **Repeat VS** at 1 hr (baseline) and repeat at least q 4 hr **Give an additional 10 mg po methadone if** systolic BP is 15 mm Hg over baseline or if HR is 10–15 bpm over baseline, or if at least 2 of the following sx are present: dilated pupils, sweating, goose-flesh, runny nose Repeat methadone dosing as required × 24 hr. **Total mg in first 24 hr = stabilization dose (usually <40 mg).** Give the stabilization dose for the next 2 days in divided doses **Then taper methadone** by 5 mg/d or by 20% per day, whichever is less. When the dose is 10 mg/d, ↓ by 2 mg daily
Use of LAAM	Single doses of 30–60 mg block opiate withdrawal for 24–48 hr Induction: dosed 3×/wk (if more frequent, many accumulate and be toxic). Start: 20–40 mg 3×/wk or q other day, with successive doses ↑ by 5–10 mg (↑ dose too rapidly will produce sedation); 2 wk needed for steady state. If inadequate withdrawal suppression: ↑ 72 hr dose or change to q other day schedule or supplement with methadone dose **Risks: cardiac** (torsade de pointes, ↑ QTc: do not start in ♀ if QTc > 450 or in ♂ if QTc > 430 ms; discontinue if QTc > 480) **Contraindications**: bradycardia, cardiac diseases, rx for arrhythmias, rx with MAOIs, or drugs that ↑ QTc, electrolyte imbalance, other illicit drugs such as cocaine, pregnancy. Document risks/benefits after discussion with pt
Using clonidine (Catapress) as monotherapy or adjunct: +++	**Give 0.1–0.3 mg clonidine po q 4–6 hr, max 1 mg/d on day 1.** Monitor VS (risk of high sedation and low BP). **Max dosage: 2 mg/d (inpatients) and 1.2 mg/d (outpatients)** **At completion after day 5, reduce** 0.2 mg/d (give in divided doses; the night time dose to be reduced last) or ↓ total dosage by one-half q day, not to exceed 0.4 mg/d **Patch method**: patch comes in 3 strengths (#1, #2, #3), delivering over 1 wk the equivalent of a daily dose of oral clonidine (e.g., #2 patch = 0.2 mg oral clonidine, daily, etc.). One technique is to apply one #2 patch for pts <100 lb, two #2 patches for pts 100–200 lb and three #2 patches for pts >200 lb. On day 1 (the day the patch is applied), oral clonidine may be necessary: 0.2 mg q 6 hr for 24 hr, then 0.1 mg q 6 hr for the next 24 hr. Remove the patch if systolic pressure <80 mm Hg or diastolic pressure <50 mm Hg. Advantages: pts don't have to take pills ×/d, even blood levels of medication, prevention of withdrawal sx during night. Take BP before and 20 min after a dose of clonidine. Give adequate fluid
Use of clonidine for detoxification with Naltrexone (Revia) induction	For people who have failed detoxification before: Day 1: clonidine up to 1.2 mg; Days 3–5: taper clonidine with Day 1: Naltrexone: 12.5 mg; Day 2: Naltrexone: 25 mg and Day 3: Naltrexone: 50 mg
Useful medications for sx control during opiate withdrawal: +++	Provide medications the pt is allowed some control over: Lomotil, 2 tablets qid, prn diarrhea Kaopectate 30 cc prn after a loose stool Pro-Banthine, 15 mg or Bentyl 20 mg q 4 hr prn abdominal cramps Tylenol, 650 mg q 4 hr prn for headache Naprosyn, 375 mg q 8 hr for back, joint, and bone pain Mylanta, 30 mL q 2 hr prn for indigestion Phenergan suppositories, 25 or 50 mg, prn nausea Atarax, 25 mg q 4 hr prn nausea Librium, 25 mg q 4 hr prn for anxiety Benadryl, 50 mg or temazepam 30 mg hr prn sleep
Use of Buprenorphine: +++ (Subutex: buprenorphine; Suboxone: buprenorphine + naloxone)	**Subutex should be used for induction when sx of withdrawal are present** (better suppression than with clonidine). To avoid precipitating withdrawal, pts may be given 8 mg of Subutex on day 1 and 16 mg of Subutex on day 2. **On day 3 and thereafter, Suboxone at a dosage of 16 mg/d is recommended** (usual doses between 4 and 24 mg/d SL) Typical detoxification takes 3–5 days **Subutex should be administered at least 4 hr after use of heroin or other short-acting opioids** Combination of buprenorphine plus naloxone (Suboxone): ↓ abuse potential; sublingual naloxone has a bitter taste; **combination ratio is 4 : 1 (buprenorphine to naloxone)** **Office treatment:** **Day 1** ● **Pts dependent on short-acting opioids** (such as heroin): pt must abstain for 12–24 hr and be in mild withdrawal state for first dose (usually 4 mg); monitor in office for 2 + hr after first dose and if opioid withdrawal reappears, may be given a second dose (max 8 mg/d) ● **Pts dependent on long-acting opioids** (methadone): First ↓ until 30 mg of methadone or equivalent; start induction 24 hr after last dose of methadone or 48 hr after last dose of LAAM (start with lower dose: 2 mg of buprenorphine) and give no further methadone or LAAM once buprenorphine induction is started. Expect the first day dose to be 8 mg of buprenorphine **Day 2:** Adjust on pt's experience of the first day (higher dose if withdrawal sx after leaving the office; lower dose if sedation at the end of the first day) **Then, continue to adjust the dose by 4/1 mg increments until target dose (max 32/8 mg)**

TABLE 20.37.   Opiate Detoxification under Anesthesia

Ultra-rapid: 24–48 hr
The opiate withdrawal is precipitated by **naloxone 4 mg infusion (0.5 mg/kg) or naltrexone 150 mg**.
Deep sedation over 5–6 hr
Moderate withdrawal lasts several days after the procedure
Possible **complications**: pulmonary failure, renal failure, vomiting, ↑ BP
Frequent relapses: 40–80% over 6–9 months

TABLE 20.38.   Appropriateness for Office-Based Buprenorphine

Opioid dependence
Pt is interested in the office-based buprenorphine rx
Pt understands the risks/benefits of buprenorphine rx
Compliance is reasonable: pt agrees on rules and expectations (office rules, urine testing, problematic behaviors, full disclosure of nonprescriptive psychoactive substances, signed contract)
Pt will follow the safety procedures
The pt is psychiatrically stable
Good support system
Pt is not taking other medications that may interact with buprenorphine
No other drug dependence (benzodiazepines, alcohol, other CNS depressants)
No suicidal or homicidal ideations
No lack of previous response to buprenorphine
No multiple past relapses
No risk of severe withdrawal
No acute intoxication
No pregnancy
No severe medical condition

TABLE 20.39.   Treatment Facilities

Legal requirements for the drugs: the narcotic drug must be approved by the FDA for use in maintenance or detoxification rx of opioid dependence, be Schedule III, IV, or V; the practitioner (licensed MD, certified for such prescriptions by specific organizations, and registered at the **US Health and Human Services** for such practice: **(800) 729-6686 TDD: (800) 487-4889; Español: (877) 767-8432**), the facility (the program such as methadone program must be registered); if a practitioner wants to prescribe buprenorphine, his practice needs to follow the Buprenorphine practice guidelines as well **Laws and regulations vary from state to state. Federal laws may change over time**
Substance Abuse and Mental Health Services Administration (SAMHSA): http://www.samhsa.gov/. Has a 24-Hour Helpline at 1-800-662-HELP (1-800-662-4357)
Center for Substance Abuse Treatment for accreditation (CSAT)
Multiple courses given for physicians: contact American Society of Addiction Medicine (ASAM): **http://www.asam.org/** 301-656-3920 **or American Academy of Addiction Psychiatry (AAAP)**: http://www2.aaap.org/ (401) 524-3076

■ 3. Maintenance

Pharmacology

TABLE 20.40.   Pharmacology

Methadone maintenance	Pt is eligible if failed 2 detoxifications in 1 yr Dose is individualized Adequate dose to prevent withdrawal or craving over 24 hr Continued as long as desired by the pt, as continuing benefits derived from the rx Usual doses: 30–40 mg/d; may be constant for years or may need adjustments with stress, depression, work, … Methadone serum concentration when necessary Always with: counseling, toxicology reports (for other drug use, and confirmation of methadone ingestion), adjusting dose if heroin use/IDU continues, always a clinical judgment **Drug interactions**: ● ↓ Methadone conc.: phenytoin, carbamazepine, rifampin, efavirenz, nevirapine ● ↑ Methadone conc.: fluvoxamine, ciprofloxacin
LAAM maintenance	Maintenance doses 70–100 mg three times weekly will block heroin "high"; 15 days for steady state Convenient dosing and cost-effective Average dose is 1.2–1.3× methadone dose (not to exceed 120 mg to start) **Check ECG**
Buprenorphine maintenance (Subutex: buprenorphine; **Suboxone**: buprenorphine+ naloxone)	Use Suboxone and ↑ the dosage by 2–4 mg/d to suppress opioid-withdrawal sx; the range is 4–24 mg/d. Subutex should be administered at least 4 hr after use of heroin or other short-acting opioids **Combination of buprenorphine + naloxone (ratio is 4 : 1)**: ↓ abuse potential Onset of effects slower for the sublingual route (possible lower abuse potential); less respiratory depression and less physical dependence than other opioids Dose increase of 2/0.5 mg or 4/1 mg/d. Expect average daily dose to be between 8/2 mg and 32/8 mg of Suboxone. The pt should receive a daily dose until stabilized, then possible every other day Withdrawal from buprenorphine may be wilder than from other opioids if conducted over long periods (>30 days)

Psychotherapy: individual, behavioral, cognitive, family, support groups (NA), social skills trainings, **need for abstinence and education, safe-sex practices, free needle-exchange programs.**

Therapeutic communities: abstinence is the rule, needs high level of motivation, rigorous screening process, self-help groups with confrontation, isolation from outside world, long-term rx, effective, large drop-out rate (Phoenix House/12–18 months of rx).

■ **4. Special populations**
- **Opioid use in geriatric population**: illicit use exists; usual diagnostic criteria are less appropriate, medical comorbidity, use of other medications (DDI), rx with more gradual induction and closer monitoring.
- **HIV pts**: interaction with antiretroviral medications (*protease inhibitors* ↑ *levels of buprenorphine*), refer to specialized programs.
- **Acute and chronic pain pts**: acute pain is not addressed by the maintenance dose of the opioid; if pt needs opioid rx for chronic pain, it is better to use methadone or LAAM as rx for the opioid dependence. Many pain syndromes are treated with opioids.
- **Risks in pregnancy**:
  - **Neonatal withdrawal**: possible miscarriage, fetal death; *pregnant ♀ may be maintained with 10–40 mg methadone/d* (if high dose at the beginning of the pregnancy, must be decreased slowly: 1 mg every 3 days; if needs withdrawal, it is better done during the second trimester); mild neonatal withdrawal is treated with low dose of paregoric
  - **Fetal HIV transmission**: during pregnancy or breastfeeding
  - **Methadone maintenance during pregnancy** is the **gold standard** medication for rx of opioid dependence during pregnancy. Some limits of the rx: in the United States *x* regulations, pejorative attitudes, risk of loosing custody of infant if required to live in a "drug-free" residential tx setting with infant vs requiring methadone. Refusal should be documented as a decision against medical advice.
  - **Do not use Suboxone**

PHENCYCLIDINE (OR PHENCYCLIDINE-LIKE)-RELATED DISORDERS

Epidemiology: easy to synthesize, inexpensive, variable purity and strength; ↑ in men 20–40 yo, minorities in big cities (Washington, DC > Los Angeles, Chicago, Baltimore); national PCP-related-death is 3%.

Comorbidity: users of PCP also use alcohol, opiates, marijuana, amphetamines, and cocaine.

Neuropharmacology:
- **PCP (phencyclidine) is called Angel dust, crystal, peace, super grass (if mixed with cannabis, flake hog, rocket fuel, and horse tranqs)**.
- Developed first as an anesthetic. Related substance: ketamine (Ketalar) or **special K** may be abused; effects are similar to those of hallucinogens such as LSD.
- PCP: smoked: effects start in 5 min and plateau in 30 min, only 30% bioavailable; IV: 75% bioavailable; half-life is 20 hr (ketamine: half-life is 2 hr)
- Is an antagonist at the NMDA subtypes of glutamate receptors and activates dopaminergic neurons (reward system); tolerance and psychologic dependence occur but *usually no physical dependence.*

Diagnosis:
- **PCP dependence and abuse**: long-term users; sx: dull thinking, ↓ reflexes, ↓ memory, ↓ impulse control, depression, lethargy, poor concentration
- **PCP intoxication**:

TABLE 20.41. Symptoms of PCP Intoxication

Recent use of PCP or related substance, with sx not due to a gl medical condition or another mental disorder
Significant behavioral changes appearing during or shortly after use of PCP: aggressiveness, impulsiveness, unpredictability, agitation bizarre behaviors, poor judgment, impaired functioning
Physical signs: ≥2 appearing in <1 hr
- **Nystagmus**
- **Hypertension or tachycardia**
- **Numbness**
- **Ataxia**
- **Hyperacusis**
- **Muscle rigidity**
- **Dysarthria**
- **Decrease in responsiveness to pain**
- **Possible perceptual disturbances, delirium** (25% of PCP-related ER patients)

- **PCP-induced psychotic disorder**: average 4–5 days, may last up to 30 days; pts may arrive to ER in a comatose state or with intense behavioral disturbances (public masturbation, stripping off clothes, violence, urinary incontinence, inappropriate emotional displays), physical sx (↑ BP and nystagmus), physical injuries, frequent amnesia of the psychotic period; 6% of PCP-related ER pts
- **PCP-induced mood disorder**: more manic type; 3% of PCP-related ER pts
- **PCP-induced anxiety disorder**: frequent

Clinical features: PCP *may stay in the blood for up to 1 wk; 5 mg of PCP is a "low dose," 10 mg is a high dose.*

TABLE 20.42.   Effects of PCP

Short-term effects (3–6 hr), up to several days is possible	Speedy feelings, euphoria, bodily warmth, peaceful floating sensations, feelings of depersonalization, estrangement, auditory and visual hallucinations
	Alterations of body image, distortion of time and space, delusions
	Confusion, anxiety +++
	Dependency feelings, feelings of isolation
	Oversociability or hostility at other times
	Nystagmus
	Head-rolling movements, stroking, muscle rigidity
	Hypertension, hyperthermia
	Frequent vomiting
	Repetitive chanting speech
	Possible depression, irritability, paranoia, possible violence (homicidal or suicidal), unpredictability +++
Adverse effects	Are dose related: doses >20 mg may cause convulsions, coma, death
	Rhabdomyolysis (↑ CPK), renal failure
	Hypertension, ↑ pulse rate, nystagmus
	Low doses: dysarthria, ataxia, muscle rigidity, ↓ response to pain, ↑ DTRs
	High doses: fatal hyperthermia, agitation, athetosis, clonic jerking of extremities, opisthotonus, bilateral ptosis, hypersalivation, diaphoresis, drowsiness, coma, seizures, respiratory arrest, death

Differential diagnosis: other substance-related disorders, brief psychosis.

Treatment and rehabilitation: symptomatic, talking down is not useful; benzodiazepines and dopamine receptor antagonists (haloperidol) to control the behavior, monitor level of consciousness, BP, temp, muscle activity, toxic reactions. *Gastric lavage may induce laryngeal spasm and aspiration.* Treat muscle spasms, agitation, seizures with benzodiazepines (diazepam), *constant observation*; Phentolamine (Regitine) to treat severe high BP; *acidify the urine.* Even if pt took small dose, sx may worsen; prevent violence and suicide until full recovery.

SEDATIVE-HYPNOTIC-ANXIOLYTIC—RELATED DISORDERS

Substances:

- **Benzodiazepines: are schedule IV controlled substances by the DEA**; such as diazepam, flurazepam, oxazepam, chlordiazepoxide; flunitrazepam (Rohypnol, used outside of the United States; when used with alcohol, has been seen involved in promiscuous sex and rape); risk of dependence
- **Barbiturates**: *short acting* with half-life of 3–6 hr (pentobarbital/Nembutal, also called yellow jackets, yellows, nembies; secobarbital/also called reds, red devils, seggies, downers) or *intermediate acting* with half-life of 6–12 hr (amobarbital, also called reds and blues, rainbows, double-trouble and tooies when mixed with secobarbital), or *long acting* with half-life of 12–24 hr (barbital/Veronal; Phenobarbital/Lumictal); **amobarbital, secobarbital, pentobarbital are schedule II controlled substances and phenobarbital is a schedule IV controlled substance**
- **Barbiturate-like substances**: methaqualone (used at a dose of 300–600 mg to ↑ sexual pleasure, named mandrakes or soapers)

Epidemiology: F : M is 3 : 1; whites : blacks is 2 : 1; benzodiazepines: used to ↓ withdrawal sx of cocaine and to ↑ euphoric effects of opioids, as well as ↓ anxiety caused by other substances (stimulants, hallucinogens, PCP).

Neuropharmacology: *effects on GABA-A receptor complex* → influx of Cl into the neuron; has an inhibitory effect; with progressive attenuation of the receptor effect with long-term use.

Diagnosis:

(1) **Dependence and abuse**

(2) **Intoxication**: blood levels; benzodiazepines intoxication gives less euphoria, more behavioral disinhibition than barbiturates; frequently used with alcohol; sx depend on half-life of the abused substance.

TABLE 20.43.   Symptoms of Sedative, Hypnotic, Anxiolytic Intoxication

Recent use of sedative, hypnotic, or anxiolytic with sx not due to a gl medical condition or another mental disorder
Significant behavioral or psychological changes appearing during or shortly after such use: hostility, aggressivity, disinhibition of sexual impulses, mood lability, paranoia, suicidal ideations, poor judgment, impaired functioning
Physical signs:
- Sluggishness
- Incoordination
- ↓ DTRs, hypotonia
- Unsteady gait
- Poor memory and poor attention, difficulty in thinking
- Slurred speech
- Nystagmus, diplopia, strabismus
- Stupor or coma

(3) **Withdrawal**:
- **Benzodiazepines**: with short acting: starts 2–3 days after cessation of use; with long acting: 5–6 days; risk of seizures

TABLE 20.44.   Classification of Benzodiazepines

Short acting: <12 hr	Xanax, Serax, Halcion
Medium acting: 10–15 hr	Ativan, Prosom, Restoril
Long acting: 25–100 hr	Valium, Tranxene, Dalmane, Librium, Klonopin

- **Barbiturates**: sx (appear usually after 5–15 yr of heavy use), may be life threatening (hypotension, seizures, delirium, CV collapse, death); 75% of pts have withdrawal seizures (particularly if taking >800 mg/d of Phenobarbital; appearing on the second or third day, seizures precede delirium); psychotic disorder starts after third day up to the eighth day. Sx usually do not occur after 1 wk and if present, disappear in 2 wk.

TABLE 20.45.   Signs of Withdrawal from Sedative, Hypnotic, or Anxiolytic

Cessation or ↓ in heavy and prolonged use of sedative, hypnotic, or anxiolytic, with sx not due to a gl medical condition or another mental disorder
Significant distress or impairment in functioning
Signs: appearing within a few hours or days
- Autonomic hyperactivity (sweating, ↑ pulse rate)
- Hand tremor, muscle twitching
- Nausea or vomiting
- Insomnia
- Psychomotor agitation
- Anxiety, dysphoria, intolerance for bright lights and noises
- Transient hallucinations
- Grand mal seizures +++ (usually if use of >50 mg/d of diazepam)

(4) **Delirium**: in barbiturate withdrawal > benzodiazepines withdrawal; seen in both intoxications if high dosages
(5) **Persisting dementia**: controversial
(6) **Persisting amnestic disorder**: more with short half-life benzodiazepines (triazolam/Halcion)
(7) **Psychotic disorders**: develop after 1 wk abstinence, more with barbiturates (intoxications and withdrawal)
(8) **Other disorders**: mood disorders, anxiety disorders, sleep disorders, sexual dysfunctions

Clinical features:

TABLE 20.46.   Patterns of Abuse and Risks for Sedatives, Hypnotics, and Anxiolytics

Patterns of abuse	Oral use: • **Occasional pattern**: young people, used for recreation, mild euphoria • **Regular use**: middle age, middle class, obtained for anxiety, insomnia IV use: pleasant, warm, drowsy feeling; in barbiturates > opioids, risk of HIV, cellulitis, vascular complications, infections, allergic reactions → ↑ tolerance, dependence
Overdose	**Benzodiazepines**: large margin of safety, minimal respiratory depression; ↑ danger if with other sedative-hypnotics (risk of death); Flumazenil (Romazicon) is used in ER to reverse the effects of benzodiazepines (risk of seizures, do not give if associated OD with TCA, given IV very slowly 0.2 mg over 30 s, may be repeated up to cumulative dose of 3 mg administered at 30 s–1 min intervals) **Barbiturates**: lethality due to respiratory depression, effects additive to those of other sedative-hypnotics (alcohol, benzodiazepines); coma, respiratory arrest, CV failure, death; *effective dose vs lethal dose is 1 : 3; withdrawal needs to be done in hospital* **Barbiturate-like substances**: intermediary lethality between benzodiazepines and barbiturate; methaqualone rarely causes respiratory depression or CV failure, unless mixed with alcohol

Treatment and rehabilitation:

TABLE 20.47.   Treatment of Withdrawal of Sedative, Hypnotic, Anxiolytic

Benzodiazepines	• ↓ **Dosage gradually over several weeks**
	• **Determine required dose of benzodiazepine for stabilization**
	• **Detoxification from supratherapeutic dosages**:
	   ○ Hospitalize if poor social support, polysubstance dependence, if medical or psychiatric indications
	   ○ Stabilize on the drug used by the pt or switch to longer-acting benzo. (diazepam, clonazepam) or Phenobarbital
	   ○ Then, ↓ dosage by 30% on day 2 or 3, then q few days by 10–25% as tolerated (some do rapid tapering: 25% q 3 days: safe but uncomfortable; some do 25% q 7 days better tolerated; some do it very slowly particularly in stable outpatients: 10% q 7 days)
	   ○ Adjunctive medications: carbamazepine (Tegretol), β-adrenergic receptor antagonists, valproate, clonidine, sedative antidepressants
	• **Detoxification from therapeutic dosages**:
	   ○ Start with ↓ dose by 10–25% q few days if tolerated and adjust as needed
	• **Psychologic intervention** (immediate and longer term)
	• **Alprazolam (Xanax, Xanax XR) detoxification: taper more slowly** (e.g., by 0.125–0.25 mg q 3–7 days) to avoid severe withdrawal reactions. Some prefer to switch from alprazolam to a longer-acting benzodiazepine such as clonazepam (Klonopin). Use a liberal dosage conversion **(1 mg alprazolam = 1 mg clonazepam)** and then taper clonazepam

Barbiturates	• **Determine a pt's daily use (hx, challenge test)** • **Taper the daily dose by 10% after at least 2 days of being maintained at the usual dose equivalent** • **Use a long-acting barbiturate for the detoxification period (Phenobarbital)** • **Use 30 mg of Phenobarbital for every 100 mg of the short-acting substance** • **Follow-up with psychological, psychiatric, community treatments**

TABLE 20.48.   Test Dose with Pentobarbital for Barbiturate Withdrawal (Challenge Test)

• Give **200 mg pentobarbital po**: *observe after 1 hr* for signs of intoxication: sleepiness, slurred speech, nystagmus
• **If pt is not intoxicated**: give another 100 mg q 2 hr (max 500 mg over 6 hr)
• **Total dose given to produce mild intoxication is equivalent to daily abuse level of barbiturates**
• May substitute **Phenobarbital 30 mg** (longer half-life) for each 100 mg of pentobarbital:
   ○ **Level I**: pt is asleep but arousable: estimated 24-hr oral dose used of pentobarbital is 0 mg (Phenobarbital: 0 mg)
   ○ **Level II**: mild sedation (slurred speech, drowsy, nystagmus, ataxia): estimated 24-hr oral dose used of pentobarbital is 400–600 mg (Phenobarbital: 150–200 mg)
   ○ **Level III**: no evidence of sedation, fine nystagmus: estimated 24-hr oral dose used of pentobarbital is 800 mg (Phenobarbital: 250 mg)
   ○ **Level IV**: no drug effect: give additional 100 mg pentobarbital q 2 hr, until mild intoxication is produced (max of 500 mg)
• **Multiply milligrams required for mild intoxication by 4 to give total 24-hr pentobarbital dose**
• **Convert 24-hr pentobarbital estimate to Phenobarbital equivalent**
  Estimated 24-hr oral dose used of pentobarbital is 1,000–1,200 mg (Phenobarbital: 300–600 mg)
  Give Phenobarbital equivalent for 2 days
  After 2 days, taper Phenobarbital by 30 mg/d or 10% per day, whichever is less

TABLE 20.49. Treatment of Overdose of Sedative, Hypnotic, Anxiolytic

- Gastric lavage if not unconscious, activated charcoal to delay gastric absorption
- Monitoring of vital signs and CNS activity
- If comatose, IV fluid line, monitor VS
- Insert endotracheal tube to maintain airway, mechanical ventilation if necessary
- Move to ICU

TABLE 20.50. Therapeutic Equivalent Doses of Benzodiazepines

Generic name	Trade name	Dose (mg)
Alprazolam	Xanax	1
Chlordiazepoxide	Librium	25
Clonazepam	Klonopin	0.5–1
Clorazepate	Tranxene	15
Diazepam	Valium	10
Flurazepam	Dalmane	30
Lorazepam	Ativan	2
Oxazepam	Serax	30
Temazepam	Restoril	20
Triazolam	Halcion	0.25
Zolpidiem	Ambien	10

ANABOLIC STEROID ABUSE

Epidemiology: natural: testosterone; synthetic anabolic steroids are multiple, easily available: fluoxymesterone (such as Halotestin) and nandrolone (such as Durabolin) and the dietary supplement dehydroepiandrosterone (DHEA is not FDA approved). The body can turn DHEA into other steroid hormones, including testosterone, estrogen, and cortisol; most are used po, IM, or gel or cream rubbed on the skin; are *schedule III drugs* (*like narcotics*); are illegally used to increase physical performances in athletes; M : F is 50 : 1; many pts start <age 16 with peak age 18–25 and 26–35; 50–80% of body builders. Steroids are *addictive drugs*: possible iatrogenic addiction.

Forms:

Testosterone preparations: injections (25–200 mg/wk); abused doses: up to 3× the recommended use.

Steroids: usually by mouth (35–200 mg/wk); abused up to 4× the recommended dose.

Injection and oral forms are used during a 6–12 wk cycle.

Injectable preparations are less likely to cause liver problems. Oral forms are cleared from the body faster and preferred to avoid detection. "*Stacking*" is when *x* steroids are used at the same time. "*Pyramiding*" is when doses are ↑ through a cycle allowing for doses to be ↑ 10–40× the usual dose; these two methods ↓ the SE of steroids. Supplements (vitamins, proteins) are used to ↑ the steroid effects and Tamoxifen is used to ↓ breast enlargement. Gyms may procure them illegally (foreign mail orders, Internet). Quality of these drugs or even whether these are actual steroids cannot be ensured.

Neuropharmacology: low availability if taken po; metabolized in the liver.

Diagnosis: induce euphoria and hyperactivity, then anger, arousal, hostility, anxiety, crashes into depression; risk of hypomanic or manic episodes or psychotic sx; risk of violence (cases of committed murders and severe violence); pts seem to distort the view of their body.

Clinical features: rapid development of muscle bulk; acne, balding, gynecomastia, ↓ size of testicles and prostate, ↓ sperm count, ↓ growth in adolescents, sexual characteristic changes in women.

Treatment and rehabilitation: abstinence, urine tests, psychotherapy, correct body image distortions, change lifestyle.

Drug combinations: used frequently such as:

- Motivations: ↑ sexual performance (e.g., methamphetamine, poppers/amyl nitrates, sildenafil/Viagra); getting a "better high" with "party drugs" combinations (e.g., methamphetamine, GHB, ketamine/special K), or controlling the undesirable after effects of some drugs
- Polydrug users may use "speedballs" (heroin + cocaine, or methamphetamine + heroin injected in the same syringe), combinations of licit and illicit drugs such as "blunts" (nicotine and cannabis in a cigarette)

- Consequences vary with types of drug, routes of administration, dosage, purity, types of adulterants. Various medical outcomes (overdose mortality, nonfatal overdose, hypothermia, coma, anxiety, panic reactions). *Ecstasy + GHB or ecstasy + opiates give more comas; Ecstasy + cocaine give more panic attacks.*
- Increased risk for STD, HIV infection

21 ■ HUMAN SEXUALITY, PSYCHOSEXUAL DISORDERS, GENDER IDENTITY DISORDERS

NORMAL SEXUALITY

Generalities:

Anatomy, physiology, psychology, culture, relationship with others, developmental experiences are involved in the outcome of sexuality. Normal sexuality involves feelings of desire, behaviors bringing pleasure to oneself and sexual partner, stimulation of the primary sexual organs, coitus.

The term **psychosexual** describes personality development and functioning (as these are affected by sexuality).

The term **libido** means not only sexual desire, but also the instinct energy or force and the psychic energy.

Genital play in infants is a part of normal development.

Psychosexual factors:

- **Sexual identity**: pattern of a person's biologic sexual characteristics (chromosomes: XX or XY; differentiation results from the action of fetal androgens, starting at wk 6 of embryo and completed at the end of the 3rd month) → differentiated external, internal genitalia, gonads, secondary sex characteristics; role of endogenous or exogenous androgens for the masculinization of the brain

- **Gender identity**: a person's sense of maleness or femaleness (*by age 2–3 yo*); family environment, culture will help establish a sense of masculinity or feminity

- **Gender role**: not established at birth but *built up through learning*; is all the things that a person says or does that shows himself or herself as having the status of a man or a woman; usual outcome: congruence of gender identity and of gender role

- **Sexual orientation**: describes the object of a person's sexual impulses (hetero, homo, or bisexual)

- **Sexual behavior (physiologic responses)**:
  - **Stage I (desire)**: reflects motivation, drives, personality; characterized by sexual fantasies + desire to have sex
  - **Stage II (excitement)**: minutes to hours then ↑ excitement lasting from 30 s to a few minutes
    - **Males**: psychologic arousal, penile erection, enlargement and elevation of testes
    - **Females**: psychologic arousal, vaginal lubrication, nipple erection, ↑ breast size, enlargement of clitoris and labia minora, vasocongestion of the external genitalia
    - **Both**: myotonia, tachycardia, ↑ BP, ↑ respiration, sexual flush before orgasm, some secretions from local glands (males: Cowper's glands, females: Bartholin's glands)
  - **Stage III (orgasm)**: 3–15 s, peak of sexual pleasure, some cloudiness of consciousness
    - **Males**: ejaculation, involuntary muscular contractions (e.g., pelvis), followed by a refractory period (several minutes to several hours)
    - **Females**: contraction of the outer third of vagina, some involuntary pelvic thrusting; may be multiple; no refractory period
    - **Both**: loss of voluntary muscular control, rhythmic contractions of rectal sphincter, hyperventilation, tachycardia

Stage IV (resolution): 10–15 min; if no orgasm: 2–6 hr may be associated with irritability and discomfort

- **Males**: detumescence in 5–30 min, relaxation, sense of well-being.
- **Females**: detumescence in 5–30 min, relaxation, sense of well-being.

Role of hormones: ↑ DA levels mean ↑ desire; ↑ serotonin levels mean ↓ desire; testosterone ↑ libido in ♂ and ♀; estrogens ↑ lubrication and sensitivity to stimulation in ♀; progesterone, prolactin, and cortisol ↓ desire in ♂ and ♀; oxytocin ↑ after orgasm. There are gender differences in the baseline level of sexual desire, in erotic fantasies, and their stimuli.

Masturbation: normal precursor of object-related sexual behavior; common in infancy and childhood (**begins at about 15–19 months of age**); ↑ in teenagers (M > F) with presence of sexual fantasies; lifetime prevalence of masturbation: all ♂ and ¾ of ♀; continues in adulthood; moral taboos even though masturbation is mostly adaptive; pathologic if becomes compulsive.

Homosexuality: is not a pathologic disorder as per *DSM-IV* and is now considered a variant of human sexuality.

- **Definition**: **homosexuality** describes a person's overt behavior, sexual orientation, sense of personal and social identity; **gay and lesbian** refer to a combination of self-perceived identity and social identity; **homophobia** is a negative attitude toward or fear of homosexuality and homosexuals
- **Prevalence**: 1994 US survey showed a rate of 2–3% for ♂; attraction to same-sex partners is usual during pre- to early adolescence; 56% of lesbians had heterosexual intercourse prior to their first homosexual intercourse, comparing to 19% of gay ♂
- **Etiology**:
  - **Psychologic factors**: (arrest of sexual development, castration anxiety, fears of maternal engulfment, fixation on the mother, no effective fathering, inhibition of masculine development, regression to a narcissistic stage of development for ♂ homosexuals? lack of resolution of penis envy with unresolved oedipal conflicts in lesbians?)
  - **New formulations**: same-sex erotic fantasies appearing at 3–5 yr of age, centering on the father or father surrogate and identification with the mother to "attract father's love."
  - **Biologic factors**: role of prenatal androgens in organizing the CNS toward sexual orientation; genetic studies with monozygotic twins

Love and intimacy: mature love is marked by intimacy between two persons; sexual love is an expansion of tenderness, self-affirmation, loss of feeling of separateness during orgasm; sex + love become healthily fused

Laws: regulate abortion, pornography, prostitution, sex education, sex offenders, right to sexual privacy; other issues such as criminalization of oral or anal sex by consenting adults, or the need for parental consent for minors wanting an abortion vary from state to state

Taking a Sexual History

TABLE 21.1   Taking a Sexual History

● **Identifying data**	● Age, sex, occupation, relationship status, sexual orientation

● **Current functioning**	● **Satisfactory or not**, complaints, feelings about partner satisfaction
	● **Dysfunctions**:
	    Type (lack of desire, poor arousal, anorgasmia, premature or retarded ejaculation, pain)
	    Lifelong or acquired (onset with drugs, medications, life stresses, interpersonal difficulties)
	    Generalized or situational
	● **Libido**: sexual feelings, thoughts, fantasies, dreams
	● **Typical sexual interaction**: initiation, foreplay, coitus, verbalizations, afterplay, feelings after sex
	● **Sexual compulsivity?**

● **Past sexual history**	**Childhood sexuality** (parental attitudes about sex, nudity; learning about sex, viewing or hearing primal scene or sex play of others than parents, view of sex between animals) **Childhood sexual activities**: self-stimulation, sexual play with another child?
● **Adolescence**	**Puberty** **Sense of self as feminine or masculine** **Sex activities** **Dating, first crush, or first love** **Experiences of kissing, petting, necking** **Orgasm** **First coitus**

Continued

TABLE 21.1.   Taking a Sexual History   Continued

● **Adult sexual activities**	● **Premarital sex** (types of sex play experiences, contraception, first coitus, cohabitation, engagement) ● **Marriage** (types and frequency of sexual interactions, first sexual experience with spouse, honeymoon, effects of pregnancies and children on sex, extramarital sex, postmarital masturbation, extramarital sex by partner, swinging, conflicts in marriage)
● **Sex after loss (death, divorce, separation)**	● Celibacy, masturbation, intercourse, number of partners, orgasms
● **Special issues**	● History of rape, incest, molestation, physical abuse ● Domestic violence ● Chronic illness ● STDs ● Fertility problems ● Problematic pregnancies ● Gender identity problems ● Paraphilias

ABNORMAL SEXUALITY AND SEXUAL DYSFUNCTIONS

If source of distress only; lifelong or acquired types, generalized or situational types, due to psychologic or combined factors.

SOME NATIONAL ORGANIZATIONS

Sex Addicts Anonymous (SA): http://saa-recovery.org/ 1–800–477–8191

Sex and Love Addicts Anonymous (SLAA): http://www.slaafws.org/

SEXUAL DESIRE DISORDERS

- **Two types**: hypoactive sexual desire disorder (20% of population) and sexual aversion disorder (less frequent)
- **Etiology**: defense against fears about sex; Freud's concept of vagina dentata (fixation of some ♂ at the phallic state fearing castration by the vagina); unresolved oedipal conflicts; chronic stress, anxiety, depression; abstinence from sex for a long time; hostility in the relationship; biologic drive, self-esteem, self-acceptance as a sexual being, previous experiences, availability of a sex partner, age, health

SEXUAL AROUSAL DISORDERS

- **Female sexual arousal disorder**: persistent or recurrent failure to attain physiologic sexual excitement until completion of the sexual act (consider the focus, intensity, duration of the sexual act); role of hormones, medications (antihistaminic or anticholinergic action: ↓ lubrication)
- **Male erectile disorder**: recurrent and persistent failure to attain or maintain an erection (erectile dysfunction or impotence); 10–20% of ♂, ↑ with age; fear of impotence in all ♂ >40; 75% of ♂ are impotent at age 80 except if available sexual partner, consistent sexual activity, absence of vascular disease; mostly of nonorganic cause in young ♂ with spontaneous erections, AM erections, good erection with masturbation or with other partners; conflicting feelings between sexual desire and normal affection, punitive superego, inability to trust, feelings of inadequacy, feeling undesirable sexually, moral prohibition, anxiety, anger, poor relationship; is self-reinforcing

ORGASM DISORDERS

- **Female orgasmic disorder**: recurrent delay or anorgasmia after a normal sexual excitement phase (by masturbation, genital caressing, or coitus); 5% of married ♀ have never experienced orgasm; ↑ with age; often associated with lack of excitement; prevalence is 30%; psychologic factors: fears of pregnancy, vaginal damage, hostility toward men, guilt about sexual impulses, cultural expectations
- **Male orgasmic disorder**: persistent or recurrent delay or absence of orgasm after a normal excitement phase during coitus; differentiate orgasm and ejaculation; prevalence is 5%; lifelong type: rigid puritanical background, difficulty with closeness, incest wishes, sex is sinful, distractibility; acquired type: interpersonal difficulties
- **Premature ejaculation**: ejaculation happens before or shortly after entering the vagina and before the man's wish; not exclusively due to an organic cause or another psychiatric disorder; more in college-educated men; 35% of men treated for sexual disorders; etiology: sex anxiety, unconscious fears of the vagina, cultural, guilty or shameful prior sexual experiences, inexperience, poor intimate relationships

- **Other orgasm disorders**: multiple spontaneous orgasms in ♀ (cases of temporal lobe epilepsy, antide-pressant-induced while yawning: fluoxetine, clomipramine)

SEXUAL PAIN DISORDERS

- **Dyspareunia**: recurrent or persistent genital pain during intercourse (♀ and ♂); more in ♀: may be secondary to an organic cause, or vaginismus, or lack of lubrication; causes: hx of rape, childhood sexual abuse, tension about sex; in ♂: associated with organic conditions (herpes, prostatitis, Peyronie disease)
- **Vaginismus**: involuntary muscle constriction of the outer one third of the vagina, interfering with penile insertion; less frequent than anorgasmia; mostly in educated ♀; causes: past sexual trauma, first coital experience, feelings of sin, emotional abuse

SEXUAL DYSFUNCTION DUE TO A GENERAL MEDICAL CONDITION

- **Male erectile disorder due to a general medical condition**: 20–50% of men with erectile disorder

TABLE 21.2.   Medical Conditions Producing Male Erectile Disorder

• **Endocrine disorders**	• **Diabetes mellitus** +++ • Others (hyper- or hypothyroidism, Addison's disease, etc.)
• **Cardiovascular diseases**	• **Atherosclerotic disease** +++ • **Cardiac failure** • **Leriche syndrome** • **Aortic aneurysm**
• **Neurologic disorders**	• **Multiple sclerosis** • **Parkinson disease** • **ALS** • **Temporal lobe epilepsy** • **Spinal cord diseases and injuries** • **Tumors** • **Peripheral neuropathy**
• **Prescribed drugs**	• **Psychotropic drugs** +++ (TCAs, MOAIs, antipsychotics, lithium, amphetamines, SSRIs, SNRIs, anitianxiety agents) • **Hormones** • **Antihypertensive drugs** +++ (clonidine, methyldopa, spironolactone, hydrochlorothiazide, guanethidine) • **Others**: antiparkinsonians, clofibrate, digoxin, indomethacin, propanolol, glutethimide, phentolamine
• **Substances**	• **Alcohol** +++ • **Other dependence-inducing substances** (barbiturates, cannabis, cocaine, heroin, methadone, morphine) • **Lead** • **Poisons**
• **Surgical procedures**	• **Perineal prostatectomy, colostomy, cystectomy, sympathectomy**
• **Renal and urological disorders**	• **Peyronie disease** • **Renal failure** • **Hydrocele** • **Varicocele**
• **Hepatic disorders**	• **Cirrhosis**
• **Miscellaneous**	• **Genetic disorders (Klinefelter syndrome, congenital abnormalities of the penis)** • **Radiation therapy** • **Pelvic fracture** • **Malnutrition and vitamin deficiencies** • **Severe systemic diseases**

Adapted from Sadock, B. J., & Sadock, V. A. (2002). *Kaplan and Sadock's Synopsis of Psychiatry: Behavioral Sciences/Clinical Psychiatry* (9th ed). Baltimore, MD: Lippincott Williams & Wilkins. p. 708.

- **Dyspareunia due to a general medical condition**:
  - In ♀: surgical procedures of the genital area, irritated hymenal remnants, episiotomy scars, Bartholin's gland infection, vaginitis, endometriosis, ↓ lubrication, vulvar vestibulitis, interstitial cystitis
  - In ♂: Peyronie disease
- **Hypoactive sexual desire disorder due to a medical condition**: after mastectomy, hysterectomy, prostatectomy, colonostomy, severe depression, any debilitating illness

- Other male sexual dysfunction due to a general medical condition: for example, male orgasmic disorder: R/O: retrograde ejaculation (semen passes backward into the bladder during ejaculation; pleasurable sensation but orgasm is dry; harmless; after genitourinary surgery, medications with anticholinergic effects such as thioridazine/Melleril, antihypertensive drugs, tricyclics, SSRIs, other phenothiazines)

- Other female sexual dysfunction due to a general medical condition: for example, inhibited female orgasm: medical conditions: diabetes mellitus, hyperprolactinemia, hypothyroidism, medications such as antihypertensives, CNS stimulants, TCAs, SSRIs, MAOIs, antipsychotics

- Substance-induced sexual dysfunction: when fully explained by the substance use as the sx developed during or within a month of substance intoxication; impaired desire, impaired arousal, impaired orgasm, or sexual pain

TABLE 21.3.   Sexual Effects of Dependence-Inducing Substances

• Alcohol	• ↑ Initiation of sexual activity but ↓ performance • ↓ Testosterone levels in ♂ (→ erectile disorders) and may ↑ testosterone in ♀ (↑ libido, in small quantity)
• Cocaine, amphetamines	• ↑ Initiation of sexual activity but ↓ performance. May impair erection and ejaculation
• Sedative, anxiolytics, hypnotics	• ↓ Desire. Benzodiazepines may ↓ libido but may improve sexual functions if prior inhibition was due to anxiety. Buspirone is not associated with sexual dysfunction • Barbiturates: may ↑ sexual pleasure in some; sedation may ↓ libido
• Opioids and opiates	• ↓ Libido and → erectile failure
• Cannabis	• May ↑ sexual pleasure; prolonged use → ↓ testosterone levels
• Hallucinogens	• ↓ or ↑ sexual function

- Pharmacologic Agents Implicated in Sexual Dysfunction:
  - Antipsychotics: erectile dysfunction (not common), ↓ libido, retrograde ejaculation (mostly local anticholinergic effects) possible with thioridazine (Mellaril), trifluoperazine (Stelazine), chlorpromazine (Thorazine); rare cases of priapism. Sexual dysfunction with risperidone, haloperidol > quetiapine (less with quetiapine)
  - Antidepressants: anticholinergic effect interferes with erection and ejaculation (less with desipramine/Norpramin); TCAs may ↑ pleasurable sensitivity of the glans, delay ejaculation (which may be painful), impair erection; Clomipramine (Anafranil) was reported to ↑ sex drive as well as selegine (Deprenyl: an MAOI type B) and bupropion (Wellbutrin); Venlafaxine (Effexor) and SSRIs (paroxetine mostly) → ↑ in serotonin levels, may impair ejaculation, ↓ sex drive and ↓ orgasm (rx is cyproheptadine/Periactin with serotonergic effects and methylphenidate/Ritalin with adrenergic effects); Trazodone → priapism due to α2-adrenergic antagonism effects; MAOIs → impaired erection, delayed or retrograde ejaculation, vaginal dryness, inhibited orgasm (tranylcypromine/Parnate may have amphetamine-like properties and may be paradoxically sexually stimulating). Also, depression ↓ libido. Mirtazapine and bupropion (less associated with sexual SE) may alleviate sexual dysfunction if used to augment SSRIs
  - Lithium: may ↓ hypersexuality in manic states; may impair erection
  - Sympathomimetics: ↑ libido at first then loss of desire and ↓ erection
  - α-adrenergic and β-adrenergic receptor antagonists: cause impotence, ↓ volume of ejaculate, produce retrograde ejaculation, changes in libido
  - Anticholinergics: Amantadine (Symmetrel), benztropine (Cogentin) → dry mucous membranes and impotence
  - Antihistamines: diphenhydramine (Benadryl) may inhibit sexual function; cyproheptadine (Periactin) is a serotonin antagonist, may be used to treat delayed orgasm and impotence produced by SSRIs
  - Antihypertensive drugs: impaired erection (no impaired ejaculation for spironolactone and hydrochlorothiazide)
  - Antiparkinsonian drugs: impaired erection and ejaculation
  - Digoxin: impaired erection
  - Indomethacin: impaired erection
  - Carbamazepine, gabapentin, phenytoin: ↓ libido, erectile dysfunction, retarded ejaculation (effects not seen with oxcarbazepine or lamotrigine); possible less sexual SE with valproate

SEXUAL DYSFUNCTION NOS

- **Female premature orgasm**: rare cases of *x* spontaneous orgasms without sexual stimulation (temporal lobe epilepsy, antidepressant)
- **Postcoital headache**: may last for several hours, in occipital or frontal areas, throbbing pain
- **Orgasmic anhedonia**: organic causes (sacral or cephalic lesions), guilt over sexual pleasure, dissociative response
- **Masturbatory pain**: R/O vaginal tear, Peyronie disease
- **Compulsive masturbation**: risk of damage to the genital area
- **Autoerotic asphyxiation**: masturbating while hanging by the neck (mild hypoxia ↑ erotic sensation, ↑ orgasmic intensity); > in ♂; 500–1,000 deaths/yr, seen in transvestism, in adolescence, severe mood disorders, schizophrenia

Treatment

- **Identify causes**: manage medical etiologies (diabetes, HTN, hyperlipidemia, smoking) in 80% cases; if due to a psychotropic: maintain the regimen for 6–8 wk to see if pt builds a tolerance to the sexual SE; may lower dosage (SSRI, TCA); schedule 1–2 day drug "holidays"; switching psychotropics or add a drug to restore sexual function
- **Psychotherapy**: rx of unconscious conflicts and interpersonal difficulties
- **Rx of the sx of sexual dysfunction with behavioral techniques**
- **Outcome**: ↑ success in couples who regularly practice assigned exercises, have a flexible attitude, younger couples with inhibitions, fears of performance failure; difficult if severe marital discord
- **Dual-sex therapy**: (*the marital unit is the object of rx*; Masters & Johnson, 1974): sex education with the couple and ♀ + ♂ therapists; specific sexual activities as homework to reestablish the communications, the relatedness, ↓ performance fears, ↑ open communication about sexual needs
- **Specific techniques and exercises** (vaginismus: gradual vaginal dilatation; premature ejaculation: squeeze technique, or the stop-start technique; ♂ erectile disorder: masturbation; ♂ orgasmic disorder: extravaginal ejaculation followed by gradual vaginal entry after stimulation; ♀ orgasmic disorder: masturbation, use of vibrator, areas of sexual stimulation)
- **Hypnotherapy and relaxation techniques**
- **Behavior rx**: desensitization, assertiveness training, graduated sexual exercises, cooperative partner
- **Group rx**: members with the same problem or of the same sex with a variety of sexual problems; as an adjunct to other forms of rx; or married couples with sexual dysfunction; offer role playing, psychodrama, education, behavioral technique discussion; contraindicated when one partner is uncooperative, severe mental illness
- **Analytically oriented sex rx**: longer time period of rx; usually combined approach
- **Biologic approaches**:
  - **Pharmacology of the sexual dysfunction**
    - **Sildenafil (*Viagra*)**: nitric oxide enhancer; ↑ blood in the penis → erection; effect 1 hr after ingestion (50–100 mg given 30–60 min before sex), lasts up to 4 hr; needs sexual stimulation; SE: headaches, flushing, dyspepsia; **contraindicated with nitrates** (*risk of fatal hypotension*); ineffective in 50% of postradical prostate surgery, chronic diabetes, nerve damages; DDI: nitrates, dihydrocodeine, drugs active on CYP-2C9 and 3A4
    - **Tadalafil (*Cialis*), Vardenafil (*Levitra*)**: similar to the above
    - **Oral phentolamine (*Vasomax*)**: not approved in the United States; hypotension, tachycardia
    - **Apomorphine**: Uprima discontinued in the United Kingdom, risk is sweating, nausea, not effective.
    - **Injectable alprostadil (*Caverject*)**: form of prostaglandin E; no need for sexual stimulation; direct injection in the corpora cavernosa; erection in 2–3 min lasting up to 1 hr; risk of penis bruising, changes in liver function test, priapism, sclerosis of the small veins of the penis, burning sensation
    - **Transurethral alprostadil (*MUSE*)**: risk of burning sensation
    - **Creams incorporating alprostadil and other ingredients**: for mild erectile dysfunction; also tried in ♀ sexual arousal disorder
  - **Other pharmacology agents**: antianxiety agents; SSRIs and TCAs used for rx of premature ejaculation; antidepressants for pts who are phobic of sex or with PTSD; Bromocriptine (*Parlodel*) used in hyperprolactinemia; Bethanechol (*Urecholine*): cholinergic agent may ↓ TCA-induced erectile dysfunction (given at 20 mg 1–2 hr before sex; many contraindications). Amantadine (200 mg/d)

- **Alternative antidepressants**: Bupropion: adjunct to SSRI: 150 mg q hs or an alternative? Mirtazapine: 15 mg/d as alternative or adjunct; risk of serotonin syndrome if used with SSRI
- **Drugs with possible aphrodisiac properties**: ginseng root, yohimbine (Yocon; not recommended for rx of organic erectile dysfunction); recreational drugs (long-term risks)
- **Dopaminergic drugs**: ↑ libido and ↑ sex function (L-dopa, bromocriptine, selegiline an MAOI-B); Ropinirole (Requip: used in Parkinson disease): 0.25 mg/d, titrated across 4 wk to 2–4 mg/d (caution if bradycardia, dyskinesias, hallucinations, renal or hepatic insufficiency, hypotension)
- **Hormone rx: androgens** (↑ sex drive in ♂ and ♀; risk of virilization in ♀, HTN, prostatic enlargement); **estrogens** in ♀ (↓ libido, but ↑ vaginal lubrication; vaginal tablets and rings do not ↑ circulating levels); **antiandrogens** (estrogens and progesterone; treat compulsive sexual behavior in ♂ and sexual offenders) and **antiestrogens** (clomiphene/*Clomid*; and tamoxifen/*Novaldex* → ↑ gonadotropin-releasing hormone secretion, ↑ testosterone concentrations, ↑ libido)

- **Mechanical rx**: vacuum pumps to attain erection in ♂ with vascular disease and ring placed around the base of the penis; in ♀, use of a device called EROS to draw blood into the clitoris used to treat ♀ arousal disorder; vibrators used to treat anorgasmia

- **Surgical rx**: male prostheses (semi-rigid rod prostheses → permanent erection and an inflatable type)

SEXUAL DISORDER NOS AND PARAPHILIAS

Paraphilias: abnormal expressions of sexuality, from normal behaviors (goal is creating bonding, mutual pleasure, love between 2 people and possibly procreate) to destructive behaviors (aggression, victimization, one-sidedness); rare or compulsive urges.

TABLE 21.4. General Features in Paraphilias

- Presence of a pathognomonic and fixed fantasy of unusual sexual material
- Intense urge to act it out
- Arousal + orgasm depend on the mental images and the behavioral application
- Ritualized and stereotyped sexual activity
- Sexual object is degraded and dehumanized
- Over a period of at least 6 months
- Must cause distress or interpersonal difficulty

- **Epidemiology**: mostly ♂; 50% onset < 18 yo; frequent *x* paraphilias in the same pt; peak between ages 15 and 25 and ↓; among reported cases: pedophilia (10–20% of all children have been molested before 18) > exhibitionism, voyeurism (20% of adult ♀) > frotteurism > sexual masochism, transvestic fetishism, sexual sadism > fetishism > zoophilia

- **Etiology**:
  - **Psychologic factors** (unresolved oedipal crisis → improper identification with the opposite-sex parent and choice of object for libido cathexis); exhibitionism, voyeurism may be used to ↓ castration anxiety; fetishism to ↓ anxiety by displacing sexual impulses to inappropriate objects; in pedophilia, sexual sadism: need to control the victim as a compensation for feelings of powerlessness during oedipal crisis and narcissism involved in choosing a child as a love object; the masochist directs the harm toward self to overcome fear of injury or sense of powerlessness; past physical or sexual abuse: possibility of an eroticized child; sexual behaviors with paraphiliac fantasies are conditioned
  - **Biologic factors (?)**: abnormal hormone level, soft neurologic signs, chromosome abnormalities, seizures, dyslexia, abnormal EEG, mental disorders, MR

- **Types**:
  - **Exhibitionism**: recurrent urge to expose own genitals to strangers; men to assert their masculinity and watching reactions of fright, surprise, or disgust
  - **Fetishism**: sexual focus is on objects (shoes, gloves, pantyhose, stockings, etc.), linked to someone close or traumatizing to the pt in childhood; in ♂: the fetish symbolizes the phallus
  - **Frotteurism**: crowded spaces, unsuspecting victims; rubbing of the penis against a fully clothed ♀; isolated and passive ♂
  - **Pedophilia**: the **predator is >16 of age and must be 5 years older than the child victim involved** (age 13 or younger); mostly fondling and oral sex (except cases of incest); 60% of the touched victims are boys (opposed to 99% of cases for voyeurism); 90% of predators are heterosexual ♂ and 50% had excess alcohol prior to the act; incest: immature child as a sex object, some coercion, special nature of the adult–child liaison
  - **Sexual masochism (Leopold Von Sacher-Masoch)**: to experience sexual feelings, needs to be humiliated, made to suffer; ♂ > ♀; 30% also have sadistic feelings

- **Sexual sadism (Marquis de Sade)**: humiliation and suffering of the nonconsenting victim is exciting to the pt; ♂ mostly; related to rape; factors: genetic, hormonal, pathologic relationships, past abuse, mental disorders
- **Voyeurism (scopophilia)**: observing persons engaged in grooming, sexual activities, or naked; followed by masturbation
- **Transvestic fetishism (cross-dressing)**: urge to dress in opposite gender clothing for arousal; mostly ♂; from solitary, guilt-ridden to ego-syntonic of a transvestite subculture; may have some gender dysphoria
- **Paraphilia NOS**
  - **Telephone and computer scatologia**: obscene phone or computer messages, chat-rooms, cybersex, sending video images, calls to unsuspecting partners; with masturbation; online contacts developing into offline liaisons (risk poor relationships, child molestations, rapes, homicides)
  - **Necrophilia**: sexual gratification from cadavers; psychosis
  - **Partialism**: sexual activity concentrated on one part of the body to the exclusion of all others
  - **Zoophilia**: sex with animals
  - **Coprophilia**: anal stage fixation; need to defecate on a partner, to be defecated on, to compulsively say obscene words or to eat feces for sexual pleasure
  - **Klismaphilia**: use of enemas for sexual pleasure
  - **Urophilia**: desire to urinate on a partner or be urinated on for sexual pleasure; insertion of foreign objects into the urethra
  - **Masturbation**: normal activity in all stages of life; the person achieves sexual pleasure by autostimulation, resulting in orgasm; 3–4×/wk for an adolescent, 1–2×/wk for an adult, 1×/month for married couples; becomes abnormal if it is the only and preferred type of sex in adults who can have a partner, if compulsive
  - **Hydroxyphilia**: desire to have an altered state of consciousness due to hypoxia for achieving orgasm
- **Differential diagnosis**: experiential vs recurrent and compulsive; R/O: mental disorders, brain diseases
- **Course and prognosis**: poor (early age of onset, ↑ frequency, no guilt or shame, substance abuse, legal charges); good (only 1 paraphilia, normal intelligence, no substance abuse, no antisocial traits, good adult attachment)
- **Treatment**:
  - **External control (jail)**: for sexual crimes, no treatment
  - ↓ **Sex drives**: antiandrogens (medroxyprogesrerone acetate: *Depo-Provera*); limited success with fluoxetine (*Prozac*)
  - **Rx of comorbidity**: depression, schizophrenia, anxiety
  - **Cognitive-behavioral rx**: social skills training, sex education, cognitive rx (confronting the rationalizations supporting victimization of others), development of victim empathy; desensitization, relaxation techniques, learning about triggers of the impulse, modified aversive behavior rehearsal; individual and group rx
  - **Insight-oriented psychotherapy**: understanding dynamics, causative events, feelings of rejection, dealing with stresses, relating to a sexual partner, ↑ self-esteem
  - **Sex therapy**

Sexual disorder NOS:

- **Postcoital dysphoria**: depression, irritability, agitation; mostly ♂ (poor attitude about sex, partner, adulterous sex, contact with prostitute, fear of AIDS)
- **Difference in the partners' sexual needs**: night vs morning, frequency
- **Unconsummated marriage**: duration of the problem does not affect the prognosis; causes: lack of sex education, sexual prohibitions, oedipal pathology, immaturity of both partners, overdependence on families of origin, problems in sexual identification, religious orthodoxy (sex = sin, uncleanliness), distorted concepts about genitals); rx is dual-sex rx, conjoint rx, marital rx, individual rx.
- **Body image problems**: R/O body dysmorphic disorder
- **Sex addiction and compulsivity**: implies psychologic and physical dependence, presence of withdrawal sx if the behavior is frustrated; entire life revolves around sex-seeking behavior and activities, inability to stop; long-standing pattern; possible guilt and remorse; need to ↑ amount, ↑ with stress; produces distress, interferes with normal functioning; frequent with paraphilias, other major mental disorders,

schizophrenia, antisocial, borderline personality disorders; Don Juanism (or sex addiction or satyriasis): need for some ♂ to have x sexual encounters (to mask inferiority feelings or homosexual impulses); nymphomania: pathologic need for coitus in ♀ (to satisfy dependency needs), often associated with orgasmic disorder; comorbidities; rx: self-help groups (Sexaholics Anonymous [SA], Sex and Love Addicts Anonymous [SLAA], Sex Addicts Anonymous [SAA]). Referral to NA or AA meetings if substance abuse. Psychotherapy (insight oriented, supportive, CBT, marital). Treat psychiatric disorders; to ↓ sex drives: SSRIs used for compulsive masturbation, medroxyprogesterone acetate to ↓ libido in men

- **Persistent and marked distress about sexual orientation**: dissatisfaction with homosexual arousal patterns; prognostic factors in favor of heterosexual reorientation are: <35 yo, experience with heterosexual arousal, high motivation; gay counseling centers

GENDER IDENTITY DISORDERS (GIDs)

National organization:

    Intersex Society of North America: http://www.isna.org/

Diagnosis:

Strong, persistent cross-gender identification and persistent discomfort about one's assigned sex or a sense of inappropriateness in the gender role of that sex; not happening with physical intersex condition; causing significant distress, impairment in x areas of functioning.

Definitions:

- Gender identity: sense of being a male or a female
- Gender role: external behaviors reflecting a person's inner sense of gender identity
- Biologic sex: anatomic and physiologic characteristics indicating that a person is a male or a female
- Sexual orientation: a person's erotic-response tendencies (homo or heterosexual or bisexual)

Epidemiology: M > F, prevalence is unclear. Onset age for boys is usually <4.

Etiology:

- **Biology**: role of chromosome Y (the fetus is initially female and only androgens set off by the Y chromosome will produce a male), role of fetal and perinatal androgens and later sex steroids in mature ♂ and ♀; role of testosterone on the masculinization of the brain
- **Psychosocial factors**: culturally learned gender roles; oedipal conflicts (Freud), mother–child relationship (being valued for being boys or girls); mother's death, absence, depression; role of fathers (helping the separation–individuation process, model for male identification)

Clinical features:

- **Children**: continuum of GID in which boys are preoccupied with stereotypically female activities, want to dress in girls' clothes, play with dolls and with ♀ playmates, have feminine gestures, and say they want to become ♀, would want to have no penis, and so on; in which girls want to be boys, act tomboyish, may refuse to sit to urinate, want to have a penis, do not want to grow up like a ♀, have no interest in girls' games.
- **Adolescents and adults**: may request procedures to get rid of primary and secondary sex characteristics and acquire those of the opposite sex

Prognosis: *few children with GIDs become transsexuals and want to change their sex.* People with GID may be sexually attracted to men, or women, or both. The object of the sexual attraction needs to be specified in the diagnosis. *Transsexualism is defined if lasting >2 yr,* not associated with another mental disorder, or intersex, genetic, or sex chromosome abnormality. *Childhood GID must appear before puberty.* Homosexuality develops in 1/3 to 2/3 of cases (more in boys); transsexualism appears in <10% of cases; ↑ depression.

Gender identity disorder NOS:

- **Intersex conditions**: Turner syndrome (XO), Klinefelter syndrome (XXY), congenital virilizing adrenal hyperplasia (adrenogenital syndrome), pseudo-hermaphroditism (XY or XX), true hermaphroditism is very rare (presence of 2 testes and 2 ovaries in the same person), androgen insensitivity syndrome (congenital X-linked recessive trait disorder)
- **Cross-dressing (transvestism)**: *is a GID if related to stress and is transient; if not, it is a paraphilia* (called transvestic fetishism, produces sexual excitement), *may coexist with paraphilias* such as sexual sadism, sexual masochism, pedophilia; *no desire to get rid of sex characteristics* and acquire the opposite sex characteristics
- **Preoccupation with castration**: may have no sexual interest, possible *psychosis to R/O*

Treatment: complex, specialized, psychotherapy parental counseling, group rx for individuals and families; if necessary in adulthood, exploration of possible sex-reassignment surgery in evaluating indications and contraindications.

- **Sex-reassignment surgery**: trial of cross-gender living for at least 3 months or up to 1 yr; hormone rx. 50% of transsexuals will get surgery with variable outcomes. Poor results seen if preexisting mental disorder. 2% suicide following sex-reassignment surgery; very controversial procedure

- **Hormonal rx**:
  - Estrogens used in biologically ♂: ↑ sense of relaxation, ↓ erections and sexual drive. Monitor BP, glucose, liver function tests, and coagulation tests
  - Androgens for biologically ♀: ↑ sexual drives and muscle mass, hair changes, amenorrhea; monitor coagulation, liver functions, lipid profile

- **Intersex conditions**: present at birth, medical emergencies to make an agreed upon sex assignment and how to raise the child (use a *panel of specialists* to determine the sex of rearing on the basis of clinical examination, urological studies, buccal smears, chromosomal analyses, and parents' wishes. *Ethical questions* due to the fact that an infant cannot consent

- **Treatment of cross-dressing**: address stress factors, psychotherapy; Pharmacotherapy for anxiety, depression, and impulse control problems, behavior rx

Personality: permanent style of behavior characteristic of each individual.

Personality disorders: *rigid, stable, maladaptive personality characteristics* (behaviors and inner experience) that deviate from cultural norms and produce significant impairment in life functioning. Their **sx are alloplastic** (adaptable to the environment or able to change it) **and "ego-syntonic"** (feeling natural to the particular individual). They develop in childhood and become fixed in young adulthood.

Classification: can be diagnosed even in children (except for antisocial personality disorder) if the pattern is stable, clear, and incompatible with an Axis I diagnosis of childhood disorder.

- **Personality Disorders**

TABLE 22.1.   Personality Disorder Clusters

● **Cluster A**: paranoid, schizoid, schizotypal personality disorders
● **Cluster B**: antisocial, borderline, histrionic, narcissistic personality disorders
● **Cluster C**: avoidant, obsessive-compulsive personality disorders, personality disorders NOS (passive-aggressive and depressive personality disorders)

- **Personality Disorder NOS**

Etiology:
- **Genetic**: ↑ for schizotypal (↑ in families of pts with schizophrenia) and borderline personality disorders (↑ in families of pts with mood disorders)
- **Biologic factors**: hormones? (androgens → aggression? sexual hormones → impulsivity? neurotransmitters? (↓ levels of 5-HIAA, a metabolite of serotonine in pts with impulsivity, aggressivity, and suicidal attempts)
- **Psychoanalytic factors**: *fixation at a particular psychosexual stage of development?* (passive-dependent at the oral stage, obsessive-compulsive at the anal stage), *defenses against internal drives and anxiety* (cluster of dominant defenses recognized in each type of personality disorder): projection in paranoid personality disorder, fantasy and withdrawal in schizoid personality disorder, dissociation and denial in histrionic personality disorder, splitting in borderline personality disorder, sadomasochism in passive-aggressive personality disorder). If the defenses are effective, the pt will not recognize any anxiety and may not engage in rx. *Internal self-representations and object-representations also play a role* in the development of personalities with abnormal patterns of interpersonal relations.

Personality change due to medical conditions: R/O dementia (global deterioration in cognition and behavior), delirium (more acute, nonclear sensorium), other mental illnesses (schizophrenia, mood disorders, impulse control disorders). Treat the underlying condition.

- **Neurologic diseases**: head trauma, cerebrovascular diseases, epilepsy (mostly temporal lobe and frontal lobe), brain tumors, multiple sclerosis, neurosyphilis, AIDS, Huntington disease, encephalitis
- **Medical disorders**: heavy metal poisoning (lead, manganese, mercury), endocrine disorders, anabolic steroids abuse, drug rx (levodopa for Parkinson disease)

PERSONALITY DISORDERS

(1) **Cluster A**

- **Paranoid personality disorder**:

    Definition: characterized by suspiciousness, mistrust of others, aloofness, coldness, hostility, anger, hypersensitivity to slights, jealousy, fear of intimacy, sarcasm, litigiousness, inability to take responsibility, grandiosity

    Epidemiology: 0.5–2.5% of the population, higher in ♂, higher *in families of pts with schizophrenia.* May be a premorbid stage prior to the onset of schizophrenia in some cases

    Differential diagnosis: delusional disorder (fixed delusions), paranoid schizophrenia (hallucinations, formal thought disorder), other personality disorders

    Course and prognosis: lifelong problems in relationships

    Treatment: psychotherapy (in individual rx: be straightforward and open to explanations and apologies if needed; group rx might be threatening). Use firm limits as needed. Do not tolerate any threats. Antipsychotic drugs: used for agitation or delusional thoughts

- **Schizoid personality disorder**:

    Definition: characterized by social withdrawal, little capacity or wish to form interpersonal relations, lack of humor, lack of competitiveness, introversion, limited emotional range, detachment, little pleasure from social, sexual contacts, or activities, poor eye contact, aloofness, little spontaneous conversation, lack of close friends, inability to express anger directly

Epidemiology: 7.5% of the population, M : F is 2 : 1, prefers solitary jobs (night jobs). *Do not have schizophrenic relatives*

Differential diagnosis: schizophrenia (thought disorder, delusional thinking), paranoid personality disorder (more social, more aggressive, projection of feelings onto others), schizotypal personality disorder (more odd)

Course and prognosis: onset in early childhood, long lasting, might be rarely a precursor of schizophrenia?

Treatment: psychotherapy (like in paranoid personality disorder)

- **Schizotypal personality disorder**:

  Definition: characterized by strangeness, peculiarity, and schizoid (aloof, isolated, anhedonia) features. May have odd, magical beliefs, strange speech (vague, stereotyped, with metaphors), ideas of reference, some suspiciousness, social anxiety, and unusual appearance

  Epidemiology: 3% of the general population. ↑ *relatives with schizophrenia* (is it part of the schizophrenic spectrum?)

  Differential diagnosis: schizophrenia (psychotic process; if psychotic sx appear in schizotypal personality disorder, they are usually brief), paranoid personality disorder (no odd behaviors)

  Course and prognosis: ↑ suicide. Might be in some cases the premorbid personality of pts with schizophrenia. ↑ involvement in cults, strange religious practices, the occult

  Treatment: psychotherapy, antipsychotics if ideas of reference, antidepressants if depression

(2) **Cluster B**

- **Antisocial personality disorder**:

  Definition: characterized by aggressiveness, fighting, lying, theft, truancy, running away, impulsivity, reckless behaviors, violation of other people's rights, irresponsible behaviors, lack of remorse, sexual promiscuity, substances abuse, illegal activities, underlying hostility and rage. May present as charming, seductive (con men), or manipulative, demanding. Testing may show an abnormal MMPI profile (4–9). Synonymous to sociopathy, psychopathy

  Epidemiology: starts <15 yo; ↑ in late adolescence, ↓ in the 30s. 3% of the population. M : F is 3–5 : 1; ↑ severity and earlier in ♂; >50% in prison population. Familial pattern; frequent soft neurologic sx, ADHD, and abnormal EEG. Possible poor rearing practices (rejection, neglect, poverty, inconsistent discipline, unwanted child, criminal, alcoholic, unemployed fathers). Possible genetic component

  Differential diagnosis: substance abuse (antisocial activities are secondary), adult illegal behavior (simple criminality with loyalty, responsibility, sympathy in other areas of life), explosive disorders, impulse control disorders (pathologic gambling, kleptomania, pyromania), dementia and MR (pt unaware of the illegal nature of the act), mania (normal premorbid personality), personality change (frontal lobe disinhibition)

  Course and prognosis: varies. May ↓ in older age (burn out by 40 yr). ↑ Somatization disorder, depression, substance abuse. Imprisonment, violent deaths common

  Treatment: psychotherapy (firm limits, confrontation of interpersonal behaviors, group rx), substance abuse rx, ADHD. Impulsive behavior; anticonvulsants (carbamazepine, valproate). β-adrenergic receptor antagonists may ↓ aggressivity

- **Borderline personality disorder**:

  Definition: characterized by a combination of poor anger control, sarcasm, anxieties, intense mood reactivity, brief disturbances in consciousness, chronic boredom, sense of emptiness, nontolerance of being alone, identity confusion, ambivalence, unstable and tumultuous relationships (seeing people as being good or bad), impulsive, unpredictable behaviors, high sensitivity to abandonment (real or imagined), self-damaging behaviors (suicidal gestures, promiscuity, substance abuse, BN, self-mutilating behaviors), transient stress-related psychotic or dissociative sx. Primitive mechanisms of defense (projection, projective-identification, splitting). Was called ambulatory schizophrenia, pseudo-neurotic schizophrenia, as-if personality, psychotic character disorder. Was described as being at the border of neurosis and psychosis

  Epidemiology: 1–2% of the population. F : M is 2 : 1. Families have ↑ substance and alcohol abuse, MDD; frequent hx of early childhood abuse, abandonment

  Differential diagnosis: schizophrenia (prolonged psychotic sx), schizotypal personality disorder (more odd), paranoid personality disorder (extreme suspiciousness), organic states (mild delirium, psychomotor epilepsy, drug use), dysthymia (depressed, no emptiness feelings), cyclothymia (elevated mood, no emptiness feelings)

  Course and prognosis: no change over time. ↑ Major depressive episodes. Suicide in 10%

TABLE 22.2.   Risk Factors for Suicidal Behavior in Borderline Personality Disorders

Behavioral factors: past suicide attempts, impulsivity, aggression, poor social adjustment, poor problem-solving skills
Cognitive-emotional factors: affective instability, hopelessness
Comorbidity: MDD, antisocial personality, substance abuse disorders
Past hx: past physical or sexual abuse, past hospitalizations

TABLE 22.3.   Clinical Tips to Manage Safety in BPD Patients

- Work with pt to remove lethal means from possession
- Create a detailed safety plan in a suicidal crisis
- Assess suicidal risk in every session
- Involve family and friends if possible
- **Create a "hope" kit**: instruct pt to fill a box with reminders of reasons to live (photos of loved ones) and cues to use coping skills (relaxation tape, a comic book, music, positive written statements). Make this box easily available and use it as a training tool for possible suicidal crisis
- Consider hospitalization if imminent danger
- Consult with other clinicians about safety management issues
- Prepare phone numbers of emergency services available 24 hr a day (911, suicide hotlines, therapist's phone number)

   Treatment:

      Psychotherapy

         Difficult: due to probable episodes of regression, − and + transferences, countertransference issues, splitting, impulsive acts

         Need for firm limits, holding environment; may need a special setting for control and safety (day program, short-term hospitalization, sometimes long term)

         Necessity of reality-oriented therapy, active, directive with a flexible, empathic therapist able to set limits

         Use of individual and/or group rx

         Dialectic-behavioral therapy (DBT) is used if frequent self-injurious behaviors.

       Pharmacotherapy: for anger control and brief psychotic episodes (antipsychotics), depression (SSRI), anxiety (short rx with alprazolam, risk of disinhibition). Anticonvulsants might be helpful. *Give the minimum number of pills at each visit (risk of self-injurious behaviors).*

- **Histrionic personality disorder:**

      Definition: characterized by need for attention, suggestibility, excitability, unstable emotions, shallowness, immaturity, dramatic behaviors (exaggeration of feelings, temper tantrums, tears, flirtatiousness, theatricality), need for reassurance, self-absorption, poor reality testing under stress, superficial relationships

      Epidemiology: 2% of the population, F > M. Onset around puberty

      Differential diagnosis: borderline personality disorder (more identity diffusion, suicide attempts, psychotic episodes)

      Course and prognosis: flamboyant behaviors, ↓ with age. Associated with depression, substance abuse, somatization disorder, suicidal gestures

      Treatment: Psychotherapy. Pharmacotherapy for depression, anxiety

- **Narcissistic personality disorder:**

      Definition: characterized by constant need for admiration, unrealistic self-expectations, grandiose feelings about one's value, high sense of entitlement, feelings of envy, dissatisfaction with others, lack of empathy, exploitative interpersonal relationships. Frequently mixed with other personality disorders

      Epidemiology: 1% of the population. ↑ Rate. M > F

      Differential diagnosis: other personality disorders (*histrionics are more theatrical, antisocials exploit for material gain, narcissists exploit for admiration*)

      Course and prognosis: chronic, vulnerable to mid-life crisis. Risk of depression

      Treatment: Psychotherapy (individual, group), pharmacotherapy for mood swings or depression

(3) **Cluster C**

- **Avoidant personality disorder:**

      Definition: characterized by shyness, social withdrawal, hypersensitivity to rejection, low self-esteem, desire for interpersonal involvement, anxieties

- **Epidemiology**: 1–10% of the population. M : F is 1 : 1.
- **Differential diagnosis**: schizoid personality disorder (wish to be alone), borderline personality disorder (more irritable, demanding, unpredictable), dependent personality disorder (more fear of being abandoned), generalized social phobia (no generalized sense of personal inadequacy)
- **Course and prognosis**: functions well in a protected environment. ↑ risk for depression, anxiety disorders. *May represent a very early onset of generalized social phobia*
- **Treatment**: psychotherapy (individual, group), assertive training, social skills training, pharmacotherapy for complications (depression, anxiety)

- **Dependent personality disorder**:
  - **Definition**: characterized by lack of confidence, passivity, hypersensitivity to criticism, discomfort in being alone, suggestibility, need for reassurance from others, submission, referring to others for assuming responsibilities
  - **Epidemiology**: 2.5% of the population. Onset in childhood or early adolescence. Familial?
  - **Differential diagnosis**: other personality disorders where dependency might exist but here there is usually a long-term relationship with one person
  - **Course and prognosis**: chronic, impaired functioning, ↑ depression
  - **Treatment**: psychotherapy (insight oriented, behavioral, assertive training, group, family), pharmacotherapy for anxiety or depression

- **Obsessive-compulsive personality disorder**:
  - **Definition**: characterized by stubbornness, orderliness, indecisiveness, perfectionism, inflexibility, inability to delegate tasks to others, lack of sense of humor, lack of spontaneity, need to be in control
  - **Epidemiology**: M > F. Lifetime prevalence: 1%. Familial? (> in firstborn)
  - **Differential diagnosis**: OCD (presence of obsessions and compulsions, ego-dystonic)
  - **Course and prognosis**: may develop obsessions and compulsions (→ OCD). *Pts with obsessive-compulsive disorder may not be more likely to have an obsessive-compulsive personality than any other personality disorder.* May ↓ on its own, *may reveal later on a schizophrenic spectrum disorder. Risk of depression*
  - **Treatment**: psychotherapy (individual, group), pharmacotherapy only if extreme sx of anxiety (see OCD rx)

PERSONALITY DISORDER NOS

- **Passive-aggressive personality disorder**:
  - **Definition**: characterized by procrastination, stubbornness, passivity, negativism, resentment, envy, pessimism
  - **Epidemiology**: unknown
  - **Differential diagnosis**: other personality disorders (histrionic, borderline, paranoid)
  - **Course and prognosis**: chronic, risk of substance abuse, depression, suicidal attempts, somatic complaints
  - **Treatment**: supportive rx, limit setting, pharmacotherapy for complications (depression, anxiety)

- **Depressive personality disorder**:
  - **Definition**: characterized by pessimism, anhedonia, self-doubt
  - **Epidemiology**: seems common, M : F is 1 : 1. Familial?
  - **Differential diagnosis**: dysthymic disorder, stressors
  - **Course and prognosis**: dysthymia, depression
  - **Treatment**: psychotherapy (insight-oriented rx, cognitive rx, group), pharmacotherapy if depression, anxiety

- **Sadomasochistic personality disorder, sadistic personality disorder**: characterized by sadism and/or masochism. Rx is insight-oriented psychotherapy.

PSYCHIATRIC ASSESSMENT OF THE ELDER

Mental disorders in the elderly differ clinically and do not always match the categories of *DSM-IV-TR*: coexisting medical diseases, use of multiple medications, possible cognitive impairments; 25% of elderly have significant psychiatric sx.

Psychiatric assessment of the elderly: needs an independent hx from a caretaker; needs privacy.

(1) **Psychiatric hx** includes:

- **Same as those of younger people for psychiatric hx and mental status examination**
- **Review of all medications taken**: including over-the-counter, current, and past
- **Minor memory impairments**: frequent, not significant
- **Childhood and adolescent hx**: to learn about personality organization, coping skills, defense mechanisms, hx of learning disabilities or minimal cerebral dysfunction
- **Occupational hx, friends, hobbies, sports, retirement hx, plans for the future**
- **Family hx**:
  - **Parents**: adaptation to old age, cause of deaths, Alzheimer disease, depression, alcohol abuse
  - **Children**: relationship, financial help
  - **Caretakers**: related or not
- **Marital hx**: presence of a spouse, being a widow
- **Sexual hx**: sexual activity, orientation, libido, masturbation, extramarital affairs, impotence, anorgasmia

(2) **Mental status examination**:

- **General description**: motor disturbances (involuntary movements, sx of Parkinson disease, slowness in depression); speech, tearfulness (depression, frustrations), hearing aid, glasses; attitude toward the examiner (transference reactions)
- **Functional assessment**: capacity to be independent, perform daily life activities
- **Mood, feelings, affect**: risk for suicide (loneliness, depression, alcohol abuse, recent death of a spouse, physical illness, somatic pain), anxiety, euphoric mood (mania or dementia), frontal lobe dysfunction (inappropriate jokes), abnormal affect, dysprosody (inability to express emotions through speech intonation)
- **Perceptual disturbances**: ↓ sensory acuity → transitory hallucinations or illusions; **confusion about time and place** directs to an organic condition as well as **agnosia** (the inability to recognize and interpret sensory impressions; different types: **anosognosia** or denial of illness; **atopognosia** or denial of body part; **visual agnosia** or inability to recognize objects; **prosopagnosia** or inability to recognize faces).
- **Language output**: disorders of language related to organic lesions of the brain
  - **Broca's aphasia or nonfluent aphasia**: normal understanding, impaired ability to speak
  - **Wernicke's aphasia or fluent aphasia**: fluent but meaningless speech, severe impairment in the ability to understand spoken or written words
  - **Global aphasia**: a mixture of both
  - **Ideomotor apraxia**: inability to demonstrate the use of simple objects
- **Visuospatial functioning**: pt is asked to copy figures or a drawing (e.g., clock drawing test)
- **Thought**: process (neologisms, word salad, tangentiality, loose associations, blocking, flight of ideas, loss of abstract thinking); content (phobias, compulsions, delusions, suicidal or homicidal ideas)
- **Sensorium**: functioning of the special senses
- **Cognition** (information processing and intellect):
  - **Consciousness**: alteration in brain dysfunction (fluctuation in awareness, lethargy)
  - **Orientation**: difficulty recognizing people is more significant than orientation to place and time
- **Memory**:
  - **Immediate** (6 digits to repeat forward and backward), **recent** (3 items early in the interview to recall later or brief story to recall or current events), **remote** (place, date of birth; names and birthdays of children, etc.)

- **Recent memory deteriorates first**: look for confabulation
- **Retrograde amnesia**: *the loss of memory before an event*
- **Anterograde amnesia**: *the loss of memory after an event*
- **Intellectual tasks, information, intelligence**: use counting, calculation; fund of knowledge, educational level, socioeconomic status, life experiences
- **Reading and writing**: right or left handedness, ability to write and read
- **Judgment**: capacity to act appropriately in various situations

(3) **Neuropsychologic assessment**:

- **MMSE (mini-mental state examination)** for orientation, attention, calculation, immediate and short-term memory, ability to follow simple commands (max score is 30). Used to detect impairments, follow course of illness, and monitor response to rx
- **Wechsler Adult Intelligence Scale–Revised (WAIS-R)** gives verbal, performance (more sensitive indicator of brain damage), and full-scale intelligence quotient scores
- **Visuospatial functions**:
  - **Bender-Gestalt Test**
  - **Halstead-Reitan Battery** (complex tests for information processing and cognition)

(4) **Medical hx**:

- Past medical problems, surgeries, traumas, hospitalizations, and rx
- Underlying medical illness may be manifested by psychiatric sx first (infections, metabolic syndromes, electrolytes disturbances, CV disorders, strokes)
- Depression and psychosis may be the first manifestations of Parkinson disease.
- Somatic sx (malnutrition) may be due to psychiatric disorders.
- Need to review all medications and their SE, possibility of substance abuse, misuse of the medication (errors, quantities), vitamin deficiencies

MENTAL DISORDERS OF OLD AGE

Risks:

TABLE 23.1.   High-Risk Mental Disorders in Old Age

- **Cognitive disorders**: look for reversible causes of delirium and dementia
- **Depression**: high risk of suicide
- **Phobias**
- **Alcohol use disorders**
- **Medications-induced** psychiatric sx

TABLE 23.2.   Risk Factors

- Loss of social roles
- Loss of autonomy
- Deaths of friends and relatives
- Declining health
- Isolation
- Financial problems
- Decrease in cognitive functions

Dementing disorders: (see dementia in Chapter 9) gradual loss of cognition, memory, language, visuospatial functions, and appearance of behavioral problems (agitation, wandering, rage, violence, sexual disinhibition, sleep disturbances, delusions, hallucinations); usually caused by primary degenerative CNS disorders and vascular disease, but frequently mixed causes; **10–15% are treatable**. Neuroimaging: CT and MRI show smaller brain volume (atrophy in medial and lateral temporal lobe structures) and larger CSF volumes (progressive ventricular enlargement); in predementia stage: evidence of hippocampal atrophy, then progression with neuronal loss.

TABLE 23.3.   Two Major Types

● **Subcortical dementia**	● Huntington disease, Parkinson disease, normal pressure hydrocephalus, multi-infarct dementia, Wilson disease	● Movement disorders, gait apraxia, psychomotor retardation, apathy, akinetic mutism
● **Cortical dementia**	● Alzheimer disease, Creutzfeldt–Jakob disease, Pick disease	● Aphasia, agnosia, apraxia

- **Dementia of Alzheimer type**: *most common* (50–60% of dementias); F > M; 50% of pts in nursing homes; survival range is 1–20 yr; insidious onset, progressive ↓ in cognitive functions; neurofibrillary tangles, senile plaques, tau proteins

- **Vascular dementia**: *second most common* dementia; same cognitive deficits as Alzheimer disease *associated with neurological signs* (focal neurologic signs, ↑ DTRs, Babinski sign, pseudobulbar palsy, gait abnormalities, weakness of extremities); *acute onset, known risk factors* (high BP, diabetes, smoking, arrhythmias)

- **Dementia due to Pick disease**: slow, progressive dementia, associated with focal cortical lesions (frontal lobe → aphasia, agnosia, apraxia), difficult to distinguish clinically from Alzheimer disease; Pick's bodies inclusions in neurons

- **Dementia due to Creutzfeldt–Jakob disease (CJD)**: slow-growing infectious virus, diffuse degenerative disease affecting pyramidal and extrapyramidal systems; not associated with aging; one variant is due to bovine prions (bovine spongioform encephalopathy [BSE]); behavioral and psychiatric abnormalities associated with cerebellar or cognitive impairments

- **Dementia due to Huntington disease**: hereditary (autosomal dominant/chromosome 4); progressive degeneration of basal ganglia and the cerebral cortex (progressive dementia, muscular hypertonicity, choreiform movements)

- **Dementia due to normal pressure hydrocephalus**: *gait disturbances* (*unstable, shuffling gait*) *with urinary incontinence, and dementia*; enlargement of the ventricles with ↑ CSF pressure

- **Dementia due to Parkinson disease**: *motor dysfunction with possible cognitive disturbances* (frontal lobe sx and memory deficits); frequent depression, anxiety; possible risks for psychosis and delirium due to medications (levodopa, amantadine, bromocriptine)

Depressive disorders: recurrent, ↑ if becomes a widower and has a chronic illness; ↑ **somatic complaints**, ↑ **melancholic features** (depression, hypochondriasis, feelings of worthlessness, self-accusatory trends, paranoid and suicidal ideations); **pseudo-dementia** *due to depression*; think about medications causing depression +++

TABLE 23.4.   Signs of Pseudo-Dementia (Compared to True Dementia)

- Less confabulations and less language impairment
- Deficits in attention and concentration are variable
- Pseudo-dementia occurs in 15% of depressed older pts
- 25–50% of demented patients are depressed

Bipolar I disorder: a first episode of mania after age 65 may be due to an *organic cause* (SE of a drug, early dementia) with presence of cognitive impairment, disorientation, fluctuating levels of awareness; may be similar to younger pts' disease; ↑ *lithium toxicity* in the elderly.

Schizophrenia: rare first episode after age 65; late-onset: F > M, more paranoid type. If early onset: sx become less marked with age; the residual type occurs in 30% (emotional blunting, social withdrawal, eccentric behaviors, illogical thinking, inability for self- care); antipsychotics are used at lower dosages.

Delusional disorders: age of onset 40–55 and geriatric period; different forms (persecutory, somatic); may be associated with other disorders (Alzheimer disease, alcohol use disorders, schizophrenia, MDD, bipolar I disorder, brain tumors, medication use); good prognosis with medications and psychotherapy; a variant: **paraphrenia**: late-onset delusional disorder not associated with dementia (↑ in families with schizophrenia).

Anxiety disorders: some appear after 65 (phobias: 4–8%, less severe than in younger pts; panic disorder: 1%); reaction to PTSD in elder pts is greater than in younger pts; OCD may start late in life.

Somatoform disorders: hypochondriasis is common; avoid risky medical procedures.

Alcohol and other substance use disorders: alcohol dependence (20% nursing home pts); also other substances: hypnotics, anxiolytics, narcotics; sx: confusion, poor hygiene, depression, malnutrition, falls, sudden delirium (think of alcohol withdrawal); frequent misuse of nicotine, caffeine, over-the-counter analgesics, laxatives.

Sleep disorders: daytime sleepiness, napping, use of hypnotic drugs, breathing-related sleep disorder, medication-induced movement disorders; interfering with sleep: pain, dysuria, dyspnea, heartburn, lack of daily structure, alcohol (sleep fragmentation); monitor SE of sedative-hypnotics (cognition, memory impairment, one sedation, rebound insomnia, daytime withdrawal, unsteady gait); **sundowning associated with dementia** (↑ confusion and agitation after nightfall).

TABLE 23.5.   Change in Sleep Structure in the Elderly

- REM:
  - Redistribution of REM sleep throughout the night
  - ↑ Number of REM episodes
  - ↓ Length of REM episodes
  - ↓ Total REM sleep
- NREM:
  - ↓ Amplitude of δ waves
  - ↓ % of stages 3 and 4 sleep
  - ↑ % of stages 1 and 2 sleep

Psychiatric symptoms in the medically ill elder

TABLE 23.6.   Psychiatric Symptoms Associated with Specific Medical Disorders Common in the Elderly

● Cerebrovascular disease	● **Depression**: common after a CV accident
	● **Manic episodes or apathy**: seen after right hemisphere strokes
	● **Subcortical dementia**:
	  - Seen in subcortical ischemic disease and parkinsonism
	  - Sx: psychomotor slowing, depression, inattentiveness, poor memory, motor impairment
	● **Acute confusional states**: after a stroke (basal ganglia, other subcortical infarcts)
	● **Psychosis**: in focal brain injuries (lesions of limbic, cortical, and subcortical structures)
	● **Personality changes**: after strokes, in men with severe dementia

● Cardiovascular disease	● **Confusional states**: cerebral hypoperfusion, rx complications (CV drugs, diuretics, repeated resuscitations for ventricular arrhythmias) ● **Depression**: after MI, heart failure (rx of MDD improves prognosis of heart disease) ● **Anxiety**
● Chronic diseases of the lungs, kidneys, liver	● **Acute and chronic encephalopathies**: hypoxemia, hypercapnia, CNS effects of drugs (bronchodilators, steroids, cough suppressants, benzodiazepines); effects of renal and hepatic diseases on nutrition, drug metabolism, hemodialysis (past dementia due to accumulation of aluminum in the brain when aluminum was allowed in the dialysis solution) ● **Depression, anxiety (panic attacks), rare psychosis**
● Arthritis	● **Mood disorder**: if severe disability ● **Others**: complications of use of NSAIDs and prednisone
● Thyroid disease, malnutrition, anemia	● **Possible lethargy** ● **Confusion** ● **Behavioral changes**

Other disorders of old age

- **Vertigo**: fear of falling, dizziness; causes: anemia, low BP, cardiac arrhythmias, CV diseases, basilar artery insufficiency, acoustic neuroma, Meniere disease, use of anxiolytics; rx: meclizine (Antivert: 25–100 mg/d).
- **Syncope**: sudden loss of consciousness; causes: epilepsy, cerebral diseases (ischemia, vertebral-basilar insufficiency) cardiac diseases (arrhythmias, valvular disease, conduction problems), anemia, hypoglycemia.
- **Elder abuse**: *10% of people >65*; physical or sexual, psychologic, financial, medical abuse (withholding or improper administration of medical rx, withholding of false teeth, glasses, hearing aids), neglect (malnutrition, poor hygiene); interventions: legal services, housing, medical, psychiatric, social services.

PSYCHOPHARMACOLOGIC TREATMENT OF GERIATRIC DISORDERS

The most widely used consensus criteria for safe medication use in older adults is **the Beers criteria** (http://www.tahsa.org/files/DDF/medbeer1.pdf).

- Medications to avoid or use within specified dose and duration ranges in elderly patients
- Medications to avoid in elderly patients with specific concomitant diseases
- Refer to the Web site: http://www.tahsa.org/files/DDF/medbeer1.pdf

TABLE 23.7. Principles: Use the Lowest Possible Dose; Know Drug Interactions

- Change of drug dosage may be needed:
  - If renal disease: ↓ renal clearance of drugs
  - If liver disease: ↓ ability to metabolize drugs
  - If CV disease: ↓ cardiac output affects renal and liver drug clearance
  - If GI disease: ↓ gastric acid secretion and changes in drug absorption
- Changes in ratio lean (↓) to fat (↑) body mass: lipid-soluble vs water soluble medications
- Changes in end-organ or receptor-site sensitivity
- Changes in functioning of BP regulating systems

TABLE 23.8. Guidelines

- Pretreatment medical evaluation with ECG, BP, pulse
- Avoid side effects such as daytime sleepiness
- Reassess frequently the need for maintenance on the medications
- Know all medications in use (including over-the-counter medications, herbs)

ANTIDEPRESSANTS

More frequent and severe SE; always do ECG.

- **Tricyclic drugs**: use drugs with less anticholinergic, less orthostatic, less sedative SE; monitor cognition, BP, ECG; **avoid if prostatic hypertrophy, narrow-angle glaucoma; risk of second-degree block in 10% cases if given to pts with right or left bundle branch block; avoid if ischemic heart disease (because of type 1A antiarrhythmic properties of the tricyclics)**. Preferably use:
  - Desipramine (*Norpramin*): 1.5–2 mg/kg of body weight; plasma conc. >115 ng/mL
  - Nortriptyline (*Aventyl, Pamelor*): 1–1.2 mg/kg of body weight; may be used in pts with CHF; plasma conc. 60–150 ng/mL; pts may have higher plasma levels of the metabolite 10-hydroxynortriptyline (may contribute to cardiac conduction problems); better than desipramine if pretreatment systolic orthostatic hypotension (better response?)
- **MAOIs**: good if depression and panic attacks; use low dosages: phenelzine (*Nardil*) 30–45 mg/d or tranylcypromine (*Parnate*) 20–30 mg/d; risks: **orthostatic hypotension (falls, fractures)**, ↑ weight, insomnia, ↓ energy, daytime somnolence, ↑ sweating (with Parnate), peripheral neuropathy (responds to pyridoxine); many **drug interactions and dietary restrictions make them difficult to use.**
- **SSRIs**: effective; ↑ doses gradually; starting doses (fluoxetine: 5–10 mg; paroxetine: 5–10 mg; sertraline: 25 mg; citalopram: 10 mg); average doses (fluoxetine: 20 mg; paroxetine: 20 mg; sertraline: 75 mg; citalopram: 20–30 mg); *less cardiac adverse effects than tricyclics*; frequent SE: insomnia, akathisia, nausea, anorexia, pseudo-parkinsonism, hyponatremia (↑ secretion of antidiuretic hormone); *frequent DDI in the elderly*

TABLE 23.9 Some Drug Interactions of SSRIs

- **Fluoxetine and paroxetine** (by inhibition of CYP 2D6): may ↑ levels of TCAs, antipsychotics, antiarrhythmics type 1A (encainide, flecainide), β-adrenergic receptor antagonists (β-blockers), and verapamil
- **Sertraline** inhibits CYP 2D6 less and citalopram almost not: **less drug interaction with citalopram**
- **Fluvoxamine**: (by inhibition of CYP 3A4): may ↑ levels of alprazolam (*Xanax*), triazolam (*Halcion*), carbamazepine (*Tegretol*), quinidine (*Cardioquin*), erythromycin, terfenadine (*Seldane*), astemizole (*Hismanal*); (by inhibition of CYP 1D12): may ↑↑ levels of theophylline

- **Other antidepressants**:
  - **Venlafaxine**: in resistant depression, in depressed pts with chronic pain
  - **Bupropion (*Wellbutrin*)**: *safe in elderly cardiac patients*; monitor BP (↑); not to be prescribed with MAOIs
  - **Drug augmentation**: Lithium (given at ½ or ⅓ of adult dose) + TCA; TCA+ SSRI; an antidepressant + thyroid hormones; or an antidepressant + psychostimulant; or SSRI (or TCA) + bupropion; or SSRI (or TCA) + pindolol.

PSYCHOSTIMULANTS

Controversial, but may be used if depressive sx + a chronic medical illness.

- **Dextroamphetamine (*Dexedrine*)**: 2.5–10 mg/d; may ↑ analgesia
- **Methylphenidate (*Ritalin*)**: 2.5–20 mg/d

ANTIMANICS

- **Lithium carbonate (*Eskalith*)**: dose 750–900 mg/d; ↑ risk of toxicity in the elderly; adjust if concomitant use of thiazide diuretics; monitor levels; assess cardiac, thyroid, renal functions prior to rx
- **Carbamazepine (*Tegretol*)**; doses 200–1,200 mg/d
- **Valproate, divalproex (*Depakene, Depakote*)**: doses 250–1,000 mg/d

ANTIPSYCHOTICS: BLACK BOX WARNING+++

- **Elderly respond to lower doses** than younger pts; more sensitive to SE (EPS: pts stop speaking, ambulating, swallowing); **start low, go slow.**
- **Risks**: akathisia, acute dyskinesias, and TD; if with anticholinergic SE: may produce confusion, mydriasis, blurred vision; if with adrenergic properties: may produce miosis; risk of fall, fractures. No need to administer prophylactic antiparkinsonian agents (↑ confusion, memory impairment).
- **Geriatric doses**: Chlorpromazine (*Thorazine*): 30–300 mg/d; Perphenazine (*Trilafon*): 8–32 mg/d; Trifluoperazine (*Stelazine*): 1–15 mg/d; Fluphenazine (*Prolixin*): 1–10 mg/d; Mesoridazine (*Serentil*): 50–400 mg/d; Thiothixene (*Navane*): 2–20 mg/d; Loxapine (*Loxitane*): 50–250 mg/d; Molindone (*Moban*): 50–225 mg/d; Haloperidol (*Haldol*): 2–20 mg/d; risperidone (*Risperdal*): 2–4 mg/d.

ANXIOLYTICS AND SEDATIVE-HYPNOTICS: FREQUENT USE IN THE ELDERLY

- **Benzodiazepines**: use a lot of caution with the elderly (fall risk)
  - **Controlled substances**: long-term use is controversial (abuse) → use those with short or intermediate half-lives (long-acting DRUGS such as *Valium* accumulate in the adipose tissue → ataxia, insomnia, confusion)
  - **Geriatric doses**: Alprazolam (*Xanax*): 0.5–6 mg/d; chlordiazepoxide (*Librium*): 15–100 mg/d; clorazepate (*Tranxene*): 7.5–60 mg/d; diazepam (*Valium*): 2–60 mg/d; lorazepam (*Ativan*): 2–6 mg/d; temazepam (*Restoril*): 15–30 mg/d; triazolam (*Halcion*): 0.125–0.25 mg/d
- **Barbiturates**: very rarely prescribed (SE + addictive properties)
  - **Risks**: paradoxical dysphoria, confusion; high abuse potential; controlled substances
  - **Geriatric doses**: Secobarbital (*Seconal*): 50–300 mg/d
- **Others**:
  - Buspirone (*Buspar*): 5–60 mg/d; no potential for abuse, long-onset of action (up to 3 wk), not sedative
  - Chloral hydrate (*Noctec*): 500–1,000 mg/d. May induce sleep at dose of 1 g nightly (elderly may be more sensitive and may need lower dose; not to be given to pts receiving warfarin-type anticoagulants as it may ↑ PTT by displacing the anticoagulant from plasma protein-binding sites)
  - Zolpidem (*Ambien*): 2.5–5 mg/d
  - β-Blockers: Propanolol (*Inderal*): 40–160 mg/d; Atenolol (*Tenormin*): 25–100 mg/d

MANAGEMENT OF AGITATION AND AGGRESSION IN DEMENTIA

- Buspirone
- Trazodone (*Desyrel*): caution for priapism
- β-blockers are used
- **Antipsychotics (risk of EPS, strokes): black box: conventional and atypical antipsychotics are associated with an increased risk of mortality in elderly patients treated for dementia-related psychosis, and antipsychotics are not indicated for the treatment of dementia-related psychosis.+++**
- Benzodiazepines (risk of cognitive impairment, sedation, worsening of behavior)

ECT: may be the most effective, with the least complications in frail elderly with medical comorbidity; early response; used if severe malnutrition, agitation, high risk for suicide.

Psychotherapy:

- Standard psychotherapeutic interventions (insight oriented, supportive, cognitive, group, family rx).
- **Supportive psychotherapy**: to ↑ self-esteem, ↑ sense of control and of safety with weekly short visits.
- **Reminiscence rx**: meaning of life, past conflicts resolution; reunions with family and friends, writing a biography
- **CBT**: focus on here-and-now issues
- **Brief psychodynamic psychotherapy**: psychodynamic understanding of the pt and the pt's transference

- **Insight-oriented psychotherapy**: focused on loss, sexual and physical ↓, trauma, fear of pain, disability, ↓ self-esteem, ↑ dependency; need for more flexible rx (intrusion of real-life problems into the therapeutic process)
- **Integrated rx**: integration of multiple modalities as needed

Institutional care of geriatric patients: 8% of the total health care costs of the United States; 4% of elderly live in nursing homes; will triple by 2040; in 1986 the Institute of Medicine published a report to ↑ the quality of care in nursing homes (concerns: rights violation, inappropriate use of physical, chemical restraints); a reform was enacted in 1987 (Omnibus Budget Reconciliation Act [OBRA]), modified in 1990, required preadmission screening and annual resident review (PASARR):

- **Restraints**: cannot be given to discipline an elderly, for the convenience of nursing staff, and if not required to treat the medical sx; antipsychotics not to be used unless necessary to treat a specific condition (diagnosed and documented); in pts using antipsychotics, there must be attempts to ↓ gradually the dose, to receive behavioral rx in an effort to DC the drugs unless clinically contraindicated. Pts must be free from unnecessary drugs (used without appropriate indication, in excessive dosage, for excessive duration, without adequate monitoring, or if adverse consequences).
- **Quality of life**: attention to dignity, individuality, self-determination, participation in groups, in family, social, religious, community activities, expertise on medical and psychiatric disorders availability; environment demands must match the resident's capabilities.

24 ■ PROBLEMS RELATED TO ABUSE OR NEGLECT

CHILD ABUSE AND NEGLECT

Associated with *x* emotional and psychiatric problems (anxiety, aggressivity, paranoia, PTSD, suicidal behaviors).

National organizations:

Department of social services (NYS: 1-800-342-3720)

Administration for children and families: http://www.acf.hhs.gov/programs/cb/

Epidemiology: each year 150,000 to 200,000 new cases of sexual abuse are reported; abuse + neglect produce 2,000 to 4,000 deaths each year in the United States; sexual assault by age 18: ¼ girls and 1/7 boys.

x unreported cases (fear of retaliation, abandonment, family secrets); rate of physical abuse of children (32% <5 yo, 54% age 5–14 yo, 14% >14 yo); abusers are parents (75%), relatives (15%), or unrelated care takers (10%); young sexual offenders ↑.

Etiology: abusive parents (with past abuse, poor coping skills, poor parenting skills, identification with the aggressor); stressful living conditions (overcrowding, poverty, substance abuse, social isolation, unemployment, mental disorders); child's characteristics (prematurity, MR, physical disabilities, difficult to please child, ADHD); men perpetrators of sexual abuse (in 95% of girls and 80% of boys) may have been victims of past physical or sexual abuse or may be pedophiles.

Diagnosis and clinical features:

- **Physical abuse**:
  - **Any bruise or injury on a child** must be appropriately explained and compatible with the hx given by the care taker.
  - **Suspicion if**: symmetrical injuries, of the shape of an object (belt buckle, cord, cigarette burn, burns from immersion in boiling water, old and new evidence of traumas), internal injuries, *x* fractures, retinal hemorrhage of an infant, repeated ER visits for traumas
  - Think **Munchausen's syndrome by proxy** (a parent repeatedly inflicts injury to the child or makes the child sick in order to seek medical attention and obtains the secondary gains of being seen as a caring parent)
  - Abused children may try to cover up the abuse.

- **Sexual abuse**:
  - **Sexual activity**: coitus (15–25%), oral sex (3–12%), touching genitals (10–35%)
  - **Risk factors**: single-parent homes, marital problems, physical abuse
  - **Frequently nonreported** (sense of guilt, shame, fear; physicians' nonrecognition of the abuse and reluctance to report; fears of family's dissolution)
  - **Physical evidence may be**: genital bruises, pain, bleeding, STDs
  - **Behavioral changes**: sexualized behaviors (too much knowledge for age, initiation of sexual play in peers)
  - **Difficulties in the diagnosis**: 2–8% of false allegations, incomplete cognitive and language development in preschool-age children, *x* contradictions and retraction in the reports
  - **Sequelae**: varies with type of abuse, chronicity, child age, relationship between abuser and child; may be: depression, PTSD, poor impulse control, suicidality, dissociative disorders, paranoia, borderline personality disorder, substance abuse, promiscuity, delinquency
  - **Incest**: sex between close blood relatives or people who are in a formal or informal kinship bond (father, stepfather, uncle, older brother with ♀ child; very rarely mother–son); association: alcohol abuse, crowded environments, rural isolation, mental disorders in the family, mother in denial or with a personality disorder; rare homosexual incests (usually violent, alcoholic, antisocial fathers)
  - **Statutory rape**: if a ♂ is >16 yo and the ♀ is under the age of consent, which varies on the jurisdiction, and may be from 14 to 21 yo (even if the ♀ is consenting). The age difference varies also on the jurisdiction (it may be 2–5 yr)

- **Neglect**: failure to thrive, psychosocial dwarfism, malnutrition, poor hygiene, withdrawal or indiscriminate affection to strangers, running away behaviors, disturbed social relationships, and bizarre eating behaviors

- **Female genital mutilation (female circumcision)**: 2 millions of girls worldwide each yr; age 4–10 yo; ceremonial induction into adulthood in some cultures (clitoridectomy or more mutilations)

Differential diagnosis: severe parental conflicts may make it difficult to assess the possibility of any abuse (false allegations for custody purpose, child being brainwashed, denial of the possibility of abuse by one parent, lies, contradictions, retractions). **Any suspicion of abuse must be reported to the authorities (+++).**

Course and prognosis:

- **Poor outcome**: vulnerable child (MR, PDD, physical disabilities, ADHD); chronic abuse; mental disorder (depression, anxiety, PTSD, dissociative disorder, substance abuse)
- **Better outcome**: normal cognition, brief episode, family supportive of rx

Treatment:

- **Reporting**: +++ (it is the law) call child protective services of your state or call 1-800-4-A-CHILD (1–800–422–4453)/Child Help National Child Abuse Hotline or the police (911)
- **Ensure safety of the child after disclosure**
- **Psychiatric and physical evaluation of the child**
- **Evaluation of**: parenting skills, parental psychopathology, other children involved, understanding of the situation by all family members, motivation of each individual to participate in rx, availability of resources, risk of further abuse if the child remains in the home, removal of the abuser? Family rx.
- **Help with social and environmental stresses**: in-home support, education, psychological and psychiatric help
- **Prevention**: identify families at risk, provide education, report early, prevent separation of family members as much as possible but keeping in mind the safety issues and the willingness to participate in rx.

PHYSICAL ABUSE OF ADULT

National organizations:

> **National Coalition Against Domestic Violence**: http://www.ncadv.org/resources/StateCoalition List_73.ht
>
> **Domestic Violence Hotline number: in English**: 1-800-942-6906; **in Spanish**: 1-800-942-6908
>
> **The National Domestic Violence Hotline number**: 1-800-799-7233

Spouse abuse: More if substance abuse (alcohol, crack); abusing ♂ (inadequacy feelings; coming from violent backgrounds); self-reinforcing behavior; dynamics are: identification with the aggressor, need to feel powerful, dehumanization of women (seen as a piece of property), dependant and isolated ♀; often during pregnancy; may be severe; ♀ who leave their abusers are at a *high risk of being killed*; *cycles of violence exist*; rx involves separation, the ♀ becoming psychologically and financially independent and family rx; abuse of husbands exists.

Elder abuse: any act (physical, psychological, financial, sexual) or omission (withholding food, clothes, medicines) that results in the harming of an elderly person.

SEXUAL ABUSE OF ADULT

National organizations:

> **The National sexual Assault Hotline number**: 1-800-656-4673
>
> **The National Teen Dating Abuse Hotline number**: 1-866-331-9474

Rape is an act of violence+++

- **Rape of women**: ♂ rapists are: sexual sadists, exploitive predators, inadequate ♂, or ♂ who use women to express aggression originally directed toward others; often associated with other criminal acts; between 25 and 45 yo; often alcohol is involved; often unreported; mostly premeditated, possible use of weapons; 50% are done by strangers; 10%: >1 attacker; reactions: shock, panic, fear of dying, later PTSD, vaginismus; depending on the violence of the attack, vulnerability of the ♀, support system. Rape crisis center, hot lines, supportive individual and group rx, legal prosecution
- **Date rape**: the victim often blames herself; frequent in college population
- **Rape of men**: same dynamic; anal penetration or fellatio; ♂ victims may develop a fear of becoming a homosexual

Sexual coercion: one person forces another to perform a sexual act

Stalking: pattern of harassing and threatening behaviors; needs to be reported to the police

Sexual harassment: sexual advances, verbal or physical invitations of a sexual nature, sexual jokes, unwelcomed by the victim; usually ♂ toward ♀ or ♂; workplace procedures to deal with the problem: need to investigate complaints and respond to them

25 ■ ETHICS IN PSYCHIATRY: PRINCIPLES OF CONDUCT GOVERNING THE BEHAVIOR OF PSYCHIATRISTS AND MENTAL HEALTH PROFESSIONALS

Professional codes: consensus about gl standards of appropriate conduct. See manual: *The principles of medical ethics with annotations especially applicable to psychiatry.* (1995). (Washington, DC: American Psychiatric Association). Retrieved September 2, 2010, from http://www.psych.org/MainMenu/PsychiatricPractice/Ethics/ResourcesStandards/PrinciplesofMedicalEthics.aspx. (*The principles*). 2009 Edition Revised.

Physician Charter of Professionalism: work by leaders in the ABIM Foundation, the ACP–ASIM Foundation, and the European Federation of Internal Medicine (http://www.annals.org/cgi/content/full/136/3/243); the principles are primacy of pt welfare, pt autonomy, and social justice. The commitments are professional competence, honesty with the pt, pt confidentiality, maintaining appropriate relations with the pt, improving quality of care and access to care, just distribution of finite resources, scientific knowledge, maintaining trust by managing conflicts of interest, and professional responsibilities.

CORE ETHICAL PRINCIPLES

- **Autonomy of the patient**: a pt makes an autonomous choice by giving informed consent (intentional choice, free of undue outside influence, made with rational understanding)
- **Nonmaleficence**: *primum non nocere* or "first do no harm"
- **Beneficence**: to prevent, remove harm and promote well-being. Beneficence may overrule the pt's autonomy if a "paternalistic act" is needed to provide safety
- **Justice**: a psychiatrist will respect the law

SPECIFIC ISSUES

- **Sexual boundary violations**: "once a patient, always a patient." Parents or parents-surrogates of a child in rx are also "patients."
- **Nonsexual boundary violation**: boundary crossing that is exploitative, gratifying the doctor's need at the expense of the pt; may be business relationship, ideological issues about rx, social issues (friendship should be avoided during rx unless in an emergency), financial (how to deal with fees must be dealt upfront and as needed during rx)
- **Confidentiality**: applies to psychiatry; survives the death of a pt and is owned by the executor; informed consent must be signed by the pt to release information
- **Dealing with the press**: a psychiatrist may comment on mental illness generally but not offer opinions about pts or other people
- **Ethics in managed care**: provided in *The principles*
- **Impaired physicians**: must be reported to an appropriate authority, following the hospital, state, and legal procedures: monitoring must be done by an independent physician or group of physicians with no conflicts of interest. Professional misconduct must be reported.
- **Physicians in training**: must have adequate supervision from an attending physician.

26 ■ FORENSIC PSYCHIATRY

Deals with Mental Disorders as Related to Legal Principles

Organizations

The Legal Center for People with Disabilities and Older People: www.thelegalcenter.org

LawHelp: www.lawhelp.org

Parent/Professional Advocacy League: www.ppal.net

Laws can differ markedly from state to state and may change with time. Be familiar with the laws that apply to your area.

Forensic psychiatry adopts an adversarial position; psychiatrists may act as witness of fact or expert witness.

(1) **Witness of fact (ordinary witness)**: like any witness; may be asked to read a medical record.

(2) **Expert witness**: has expertise in a specific area; decided upon direct and cross-examination (education, publications, certifications questioned); renders opinions after drawing conclusions from data, may determine the standard of care in the court; possible "battle of experts" with different opinions and testimonies:

- **Direct examination**: first questioning of a witness by the attorney for the party on whose behalf the witness is called (friendly, rehearsed prior to trial. Open-ended questions)

- **Cross-examination**: questioning of a witness by the attorney for the opposing party (long, leading questions that demand a yes or no for an answer): listen closely to the question, pause before answering, give time for the other side to object, answer only the question asked, remember the limits of the field, do not make predictions by answering "always or never," do not answer "yes or no" if the question is too complex, answer "I don't know" if it is the case, be prepared prior to going to court, know the literature; you may ask the judge to clarify a question, ask if the material asked for is privileged, you have a right to complete your answer, to refer to written records.

- **Court-mandated evaluations**: a judge asks a clinician to be a consultant to the court; ethically inform the pts at the time of the examination that it is not a confidential situation

- **Evaluation of witnesses' credibility**: it is the judge's decision to determine if a psychiatric examination is necessary.

(1) **Hospitalizations and civil commitments**: when pts are a danger to themselves or others (in some states, also if pts are unable to care for themselves).

Parens patriae: state may act as a surrogate parent for mentally ill pts or minors unable to care for or may harm themselves.

Commitment laws: statutes and regulations allowing forced hospitalization (personal examination by a clinician, a report of danger, seclusion of the pt according to local regulations); civil commitment; see involuntary admissions.

TABLE 26.1. Four Procedures of Admission to Psychiatric Facilities: +++ (Check Local Regulations)

Informal admission	Pt is admitted to the psychiatric unit of a hospital the same way as to a medical or surgical unit, free to enter or to leave even against medical advice—AMA
Voluntary admission	Pt applies in writing on their own wish, if the examination reveals the need for hospitalization
Temporary admission	For senile or confused pts who need hospitalization but cannot make their own decisions or pts on an emergency basis; needs a written recommendation by one physician and another by a psychiatrist; is usually valid up to 15 days
Involuntary admission (is a legal process)	If there is a **danger to self or others**; an **application** must be done by a relative or a friend or a hospital administrator; **the pt must be examined by 2 physicians** confirming the need for admission; these 3 papers will be sent to a local **judge who will allow the involuntary admission**. Next of kin must receive a written notification; pts must have access to legal counsel. A judge may order the pt's release if he thinks the pt should not be in the hospital; usually valid up to 60 days; the case is reviewed regularly in a specialized court system; pts have the right to file a petition for a writ of **habeas corpus** (proclaimed if someone believes he has been illegally deprived of liberty) and the case will be heard immediately (hospitals are obligated to submit the petitions to the court immediately)

Civil rights of patients:

- **Least restrictive alternative**: right to receive the least restrictive means of rx (if can be treated as an out-pt, hospitalization should not be done)
- **Visitation rights**: pts are allowed to receive visitors at customary hospital visiting hours and other hours if necessary (pt's attorney, clergy, private physician/privacy allowed); pts' needs come first and have to be documented if there is a change.
- **Communication rights**: pts have free communication with the outside world through telephone or mail; may be modified if criminal activities are involved.
- **Private rights**: confidentiality, private bathroom, shower space, secure storage for belongings, adequate living space, right to wear own clothes and carry their money
- **Economic rights**: pts may manage their own money and must be paid if they work in the institution (cleaning, gardening, preparing food).

(2) **Seclusion and restraints**: **have complex legal issues,** only to **be used if danger to self or others and there is no less restrictive alternative available;** APA has developed guidelines.

   (**Case of *Youngberg v. Romeo***: challenged the rx practices and helped with guidelines.)

TABLE 26.2.   Risks of Seclusion and Restraints

Asphyxiation	Avoid restraining in prone position Watch for aspiration if restrained in supine position Free airway
Strangulation	Watch geriatric pts in vest restraints Avoid unprotected side-rails Pts with deformities are at higher risks due to improper placement of restraints
Cardiac arrest	Assess pt's medical status: pregnancy, asthma, hx of spinal injury or head trauma, fracture, surgery, seizure disorder, hx of abuse, hx of smoking Remain alert for cardiac arrest
Fire	Prevent access to lighters or matches Continuous observation Search pt and room for hidden items

TABLE 26.3.   Rules: JCAH Regulations Must be Followed for Restraints

- Are safety interventions of last resort to be used only if there is imminent danger to safety?
- May be ordered only by a physician or an independent practitioner licensed to deliver medical services without oversight
- Orders must be time limited: 4 hr max for adults, 2 hr max for adolescents 9–17, and 1 hr for children <9. The intervention must be ended as soon as it is safe to do so
- Certain risky practices ("basket holds" or applying back pressure to a person in a prone position) are prohibited
- A physician or a licensed independent practitioner must conduct a face-to-face assessment in less than 1 hr
- Appropriately trained staff must continuously assess, monitor, and reevaluate the pt in restraint or secluded
- Any extension of the original order must be reviewed and authorized
- Debriefings with the pt and the staff must occur as soon as possible after each restraint or seclusion
- Proper documentation must be done

See: Revised Restraints Regulations December, 2006 (Federal Register: December 8, 2006, Volume 71, Number 236, Part IV, Department of Health and Human Services Centers for Medicare & Medicaid Services 42 CFR Part 482, Medicare and Medicaid Programs; Hospital Conditions of Participation: Patients' Rights; Final Rule).

TABLE 26.4.   Indications for Seclusion and Restraints

1. To prevent imminent harm to self or others and no less restrictive alternative is available
2. Assist in rx as a part of ongoing behavior rx
3. At a pt's voluntary request if appropriate
4. To decrease sensory overstimulation (only with seclusion)

TABLE 26.5.   Contraindications for Seclusion and Restraints

- Very unstable medical or psychiatric conditions
- Delirious or demented pts
- Overtly suicidal pts
- Pts under the influence of substances or with drug reactions needing close medical monitoring
- Use for punishment or convenience

(3) **The right to treatment and the right to refuse treatment**: pts have the right to standard quality of care. *Involuntary commitment is not prima facie evidence that the pt is incompetent to decide what rx he or she is to receive* +++

In *Rouse v. Cameron* (1966): the purpose of involuntary hospitalization is rx (absence of rx is unconstitutional confinement); if alternative rx that infringes less on personal liberty is available, hospitalization cannot take place.

In *Wyatt v. Stickney* (1972): right for individualized rx with minimum staffing, specified physical facilities, nutritional standards. Are added now; right to be free from excessive or unnecessary medications, the right to privacy and dignity, the right to the least restrictive environment, unrestricted visits by attorneys, clergy, and private physicians, the right not to be submitted to lobotomies or ECT without fully informed consent, the right to not be forced to work without payment, **the right to refuse treatment (except in emergencies requiring immediate rx to prevent death or serious harm to the pt or other or to prevent deterioration of the pt's clinical state). Medication or ECT cannot be forcibly given without a court approval.**

In *O'Connor v. Donaldson* (1974): harmless mentally ill pts cannot be confined against their will without rx if they can survive outside.

In *Rennie v. Klein* (1979): pts have the right to refuse rx and to use an appeal process.

In *Roger v. Oken* (1981): pts have an absolute right to refuse rx but a guardian may authorize rx. The judge must make the rx decision.

(4) **Abandonment**: refusing to treat a willing pt may be seen as abandonment.

TABLE 26.6.   Documentation of Interruption of Care

- The reasons for stopping seeing the pt
- Attempts to transfer the pt to another therapist or institution if the pt is willing
- Efforts to minimize risks for the pt
- Arrange to care for the pt "in extremis" until the clinical situation has stabilized

(5) **Competence**: it can be to evaluate the competence of a pt to make a will, a contract, medical decision, handle finances, and testify in court. **The psychiatrist assesses, the court makes the decision.**

To make a will: pt must know the nature and extent of property, that he or she is making a will, the identities of the natural beneficiaries. Rationality at the time of the will must be attested (use of a forensic psychiatrist, videotaping during the signing with a lawyer).

Competence is task specific and determined on the pt's abilities: to weigh, reason and make reasonable decisions, to be able to ask about risks and benefits

A pt is not incompetent until the court decides. Incompetence means being deprived of certain rights (cannot make contracts, marry/divorce, drive, handle their own property, and practice their own profession). The court appoints a guardian to serve the pt's best interests. Another court hearing may be necessary to declare a pt competent again. *Commitment in a mental hospital does not mean incompetence* +++.

Durable power of attorney: a document permitting the advance selection of a substitute decision maker who can act when the pt becomes incompetent.

CRIMINAL LAWS

(1) **Competency to stand trial**:

A mentally incompetent person cannot stand trial.

Case of *Dusky v. United States*: approved a test of competence to ascertain whether a criminal defendant is able to consult with his lawyer with a reasonable degree of rational understanding, and if he has a rational and factual understanding of the proceedings against him.

13 areas of functioning to be determined (McGarry instrument):

TABLE 26.7.   Guidelines for Competency Appraisal

1. Appraisal of available legal defenses
2. Unmanageable behavior
3. Quality of relating to attorney
4. Planning of strategy including plea
5. Appraisal of participant roles
6. Understanding of court procedure
7. Appreciation of charges
8. Appreciation of penalties
9. Appraisal of likely outcome
10. Capacity to disclose facts
11. Capacity to realistically challenge witnesses
12. Capacity to testify relevantly
13. Self-defeating/self-serving motivation

Adapted from McGarry, A. L., Curran, W. J., Lipsitt, P. D., Lelos, D., et al. (1973). *Competency to Stand Trial and Mental Illness.* Rockville, MD: National Institute of Mental Health.

Clinicians offer opinions, the judge rules.

(2) **Criminal responsibility**: to be responsible for a criminal act, two components must be present: *voluntary conduct* (actus reus) *and evil intent* (mens rea). The insanity defense is used rarely: the system requires two psychiatrists' opinions to help the judge to decide.

In *M'Naghten case* (1843): whether the defendant was under such a defect of reason, from a disease of the mind, as not to know the nature + quality of the act he was doing, or if he did, he did not know that what he was doing was wrong.

In *Durham v. United States* (1954): an accused is not criminally responsible if his unlawful act was the product of a mental disease or a mental defect.

In *United States v. Brawner* (1972): Durham rule was thrown out, replaced by the model penal code.

The model penal code: persons are not responsible for criminal conduct if, at the time, as a result of mental disease or defect, they lacked capacity to appreciate the criminality (wrongfulness) of their conduct, or the capacity to conform their conduct to the requirement of the law. Repeated criminal or antisocial conduct is not, of itself, to be taken as mental disease or defect.

Test of criminal responsibility refers to the time of the offense.

Test of competence to stand trial refers to the time of the trial.

Concept of plea of guilty but mentally ill: in some jurisdictions this is used for the defense of ↓ capacity (the defendant suffered impairment sufficient to interfere with the ability to have fore-thoughts of the particular crime).

(3) **Competence to be executed**: the person must be aware of what is happening (the punishment); able to make whatever peace with his world; able, until the execution, to recall a forgotten detail of the crime that may prove exonerating.

PERSONAL ISSUES

(1) **Malpractice**: describes professional negligence; **the 4Ds of malpractice**: **dereliction** (negligent performance or omission) of a **duty** that **directly** led to **damages** (a standard of care must exist; a duty must have been owed by the defendant to the plaintiff, a breach of the duty must be the legal cause of the damages); the plaintiff must provide the evidence of the damages; expert testimony is usually needed; the most frequent malpractice suits are: faulty diagnosis, improper civil commitments, suicide, negative consequences from ECT and drugs, confidentiality, sexual intimacy with pts, false memories recovery.

Respondeat superior: a person occupying a high position in the hierarchy of responsibility is liable for the actions of a person in a lower position (like a psychiatrist supervising a resident); a consultant is an adviser and not a superior; the term responsibility must be precise (what responsibilities are involved?); a psychiatrist should only bear responsibility if he or she can control the rx (may need a vicarious liability insurance).

Suicide by patients: 50% of suicides lead to malpractice action (negligence over the pt's rx that caused injury when the behavior was predictable)

Misdiagnosis: failure to see pt's suicidal or homicidal intent, a concomitant medical condition, a drug SE

Negligent treatment: "overtreatment, undertreatment, or wrong rx." The standard is the information available at the time of the alleged negligence. Document evidence of informed consent in the records (medication risks and before starting any rx).

Preventing liability:

TABLE 26.8.   Tips to Prevent Liability

Provide care you are qualified for
Treat pts with respect
Do not overstretch your abilities
Take good care of yourself
Good documentation includes
• the decision-making process
• the rationale for treatment
• evaluation of costs and benefits
Use a consultant if necessary

(2) **Privilege**:

Is the right to maintain secrecy and confidentiality in the face of a subpoena

The right to privilege belongs to the patient who may waive it

Many exceptions: does not exist in purely federal cases, in military courts, proceedings for hospitalization; pts waive their privilege if they make their mental condition an element of their claim; child custody and child-protection issues are done with the best interest of the child in mind; privilege does not apply to actions between a therapist and a pt.

(3) **Confidentiality**: physicians are bind to hold secret all information given by the pt; other staff members treating the patient, clinical supervisors, consultants share the same obligation and do not need to receive permission from the pt. Permission to release information (done in writing or if not, must be documented) is not an obligation to do so (if the information may be destructive).

Third-party payers: insurance carrier must be able to receive information to administrate and reimburse pts, employers to give benefits; government agencies for welfare benefits

Supervision: quality control of care needs some pt information; supervisors and trainees share information

Discussions about pts: psychiatrists must obtain informed consent to disclose their pts' information in their teaching, conferences, and writings. **Federal Privacy Act: permits release of records without consent in compelling circumstances affecting the health and safety of the pt**

Child abuse: anyone who believes that a child is the victim of physical or sexual abuse *must report* it to the appropriate agency; to report: http://www.childwelfare.gov/systemwide/laws_policies/state/index.cfm

TABLE 26.9.   Child Abuse Hotlines: Where to Call to Get Help or Report Abuse

- If you suspect a child is in immediate danger, contact law enforcement as soon as possible: 911
- To get help in the United States, call:
  1-800-4-A-CHILD (1-800-422-4453)—Child Help National Child Abuse Hotline
- To get help for child sexual abuse, call: 1-888-Prevent (1-888-773-8368)—Stop It Now
  1-800-656-HOPE-Rape, Abuse & Incest National Network (RAINN)

(4) **Informed consent**:

Documenting aspects of the informed consent dialogue such as including information related to the disclosed information and the patient's response to the information; three components: voluntariness (patient must make rx-related choices of his own free will, without coercion), disclosure (information is needed to make a rational decision to accept or reject rx), and capacity (ability to understand).

The typical requirements of disclosure are

- Diagnosis if known
- Nature and purpose of the proposed tx
- Risks and benefits of the proposed rx
- Alternatives to rx and their risks and benefits
- Risks and benefits of no treatment

Exceptions to informed consent: emergencies, incompetence, waivers, therapeutic privilege

Better the alliance, less the risk of liability.

(5) **Managed care**

National Practitioner Data Bank: tracks disciplinary actions, malpractice judgments, settlements against health care professionals; disciplinary actions taken against providers >30 days must be reported. http://www.npdb-hipdb.hrsa.gov/

Negligent Prescription practices: dosages of medications > recommended dosage, unreasonable mixing of drugs, nonnecessary prescriptions, not disclosing medications SE, not obtaining informed consent each time a medication is changed or added, not frequent enough follow-up visits, failure to treat SE, failure to monitor compliance, not following levels, prescribing addictive drugs, not referring to a specialist when needed.

Split treatment: the **psychiatrist retains the full responsibility** for the pt's care in a split rx situation and must remain informed about the pt's clinical status, the nature, the quality of the rx received from the nonmedical therapist; good communication between the providers is primordial.

HIGH-RISK CLINICAL SITUATIONS

TABLE 26.10.   Six Categories of Pt's Safety: SAFE MD

- **S**: suicide
- **A**: aggressivity
- **F**: falls
- **E**: elopement
- **M**: medical comorbidities
- **D**: drug/medications errors

(1) **Suicidal patients**: see Chapter 10, section on Suicidal patient

   No professional standards exist for predicting when and whether a pt will commit suicide.

   Standards exist for assessing suicide risks, but its degree can only be judged clinically after careful psychiatric assessment.

   The law assumes that a suicide is preventable if foreseeable.

(2) **Homicidal patients**: see Chapter 10, section on Violent patient

   The psychiatrist must protect the pts and endangered third parties (professional, moral, and legal obligations).

   Consider the Tarasoff duty as the national standard of care (only in cases of violence)

   Tarasoff I: (case of *Tarasoff v. Regents* of University of California: 1976) "duty to warn": confidentiality may be broken if a pt will probably commit murder or suicide and the act can be stopped only by the psychiatrist notifying the police. A therapist may notify the intended victim of the danger or others likely to notify the victim or to take whatever steps reasonably necessary. The Tarasoff I: no requirement to report a pt's fantasies.

   Tarasoff II: (case of *Tarasoff v. Regents* of University of California: 1982): broadened the earlier ruling to include: **"duty to protect."**

TABLE 26.11.   Options to Warn and Protect

- Voluntary and involuntary hospitalizations
- Warning the intended victim of the threat
- Notifying the police
- Adjusting medications
- Seeing the patient frequently

(3) **Tardive dyskinesia (TD)**: *10–50% of pts treated with neuroleptics >1 yr will probably have TD*; negligence cases (failure to evaluate pts, failure to obtain informed consent, misdiagnosis, failure to monitor rx, to intervene at the beginning of TD, the use of multiple drugs)

OTHER AREAS OF FORENSIC PSYCHIATRY

(1) **Emotional damage and distress**: physical injury or severe stress

(2) **Workers' compensation**: in job-related disabilities or to receive disability retirement benefits

(3) **Civil liability**: sexual exploitation of pts can bring civil and criminal actions + ethical and professional **sanctions.**

(4) **Recovered memories**: ↑ litigations

TABLE 26.12. Some Guidelines in the Treatment of Repressed Memories

● Maintain neutrality (do not suggest abuse); guard against leading questions; be mindful of suggestive influence of therapy
● Focus on treatment of clinical sx
● Be aware of own bias toward belief in recovered memories
● Keep abreast of state/federal laws regarding abuse disclosure, privileged records, and release of information—document carefully the memory recovery process
● Deal with countertransference, boundary management; guard against self-disclosure
● Avoid mixing the roles of therapist and expert witness, clarify this with family
● Avoid special techniques (hypnosis, sodium amytal) unless absolutely indicated and trained in these methods
● Use witness during such procedures

Adapted from Sadock, B. J., & Sadock, V. A. (2002). *Kaplan and Sadock's Synopsis of Psychiatry: Behavioral Sciences/Clinical Psychiatry* (9th ed). Baltimore, MD: Lippincott Williams & Wilkins.

(5) **Child custody**: state juvenile and family courts; may remove the child from parental custody; the welfare department supervises care and custody of the neglected or abused child; disputes are predicated on the **"child's best interests."**

Religious and spiritual problem: loss of faith, conversion; may need pastoral counseling.

Cults:

- Intensely held belief system and ideology imposed on members, mostly young people influenced by charismatic leaders, encouraged to recruit new members, to break up with family or friends; risk of psychiatric sx in followers including committing suicide. Brain washing: deliberate creation of cultural shock by isolating, alienating, intimidating the person (mental + physical coercion). Readjustment to a normal life may need deprogramming with supportive psychotherapy, education, rx of any mental disorder (depression, PTSD).

- **Resource organizations**
  - **Cult Awareness Network:** http://www.cultawarenessnetwork.org/ : **1-800-556-3055 (United States).**
  - **The International Cultic Studies Association (ICSA):** http://www.icsahome.com/

Acculturation problem: cultural transition, culture shock.

Culture bound syndromes: **amok** (dissociative episode: brooding then outburst of violence after a perceived insult, mostly in men, often with persecutory idea, may occur with psychotic process/original reports from Malaysia); **ataque de nervios** (sense of being out of control from stress, resembles panic attack with no acute fear or apprehension/seen among Latinos); **dhat** (severe anxiety or hypochondriasis associated with the discharge of semen, feeling of weakness/reports from India); **hwa-byung** (attributed to the suppression of anger, with palpitations, aches, and pains, fear of impending death, insomnia/reported from Korea); **koro** (sudden, severe anxiety that the penis will recede into the body causing death/seen in South Asia); **latah** (sudden fear followed by echopraxia, echolalia, trance-like behavior, command obedience/middle-aged ♀ from Malaysia); **mal de ojo** ("the evil eye," children with poor sleep, crying without cause, N/V, fever/Mediterranean cultures); **nervios** (sx stress related: somatic complaints, nervousness, poor concentration, irritability, dizziness/Latinos); **piblokto** (abrupt dissociative episode with excitement, frequently followed by seizure, coma up to 12 hours; possible tearing off of clothing, shouting of obscenities, eating feces, amnesia for the attack/seen in Eskimo communities); **rootwork** (pt's illness is considered to be due to witchcraft, sorcery, or an evil influence; fear of voodoo death; the root, spell, or hex must be taken off by a healer/seen in African American, European American, and Caribbean societies); **susto** (fright believed to cause the soul to leave the body resulting in somatic sx with sx of depression/seen in many parts of the world); **zar** (possession by spirits; dissociative episodes with agitation or apathy; not considered pathological locally/seen in Africa and Middle Eastern societies); many others have been described.

Interest in cultural barriers to rx as well as in ethnic differences in responding to rx (pharmacogenetics, adverse effects from medications, differences in metabolism, herbal medicines) is increasing.

28 ■ PSYCHOTHERAPEUTIC MEDICATIONS

Refer to the How to Use Chapter 28: Psychotherapeutic Medications section on page viii for notes on symbols used here.

ALZHEIMER DISEASE—CHOLINESTERASE INHIBITORS

NOTE: Avoid concurrent use of anticholinergic agents; caution in asthma/COPD; may be coadministered with memantine.

Donepezil (*Aricept*) ▶LK ♀C▶? $$$$

ADULT: Alzheimer disease: start 5 mg po q hs; may ↑ to 10 mg po q hs in 4–6 wk; severe disease (MMSE ≤ 10), dose is 10 mg/d.

PEDS: Not approved in children.

UNAPPROVED ADULT: Dementia in Parkinson disease: 5–10 mg/d.

FORMS: Trade only: tabs 5, 10 mg; orally disintegrating tabs 5, 10 mg.

NOTES: May start with 5 mg po qd to ↓ GI side effects. Half-life 70 hr.

DRUG INTERACTIONS: Avoid with beta-blockers to ↓ risk of bradycardia or syncope.

Galantamine (*Razadyne, Razadyne ER, ♣Reminyl*) ▶LK♀ B▶? $$$$

ADULT: Alzheimer disease: extended release: start 8 mg po q AM with food; ↑ to 16 mg q AM after 4 wk. May ↑ to 24 mg q AM after another 4 wk. Immediate release: start 4 mg po bid with food; ↑ to 8 mg bid after 4 wk; may ↑ to 12 mg po bid after another 4 wk.

PEDS: Not approved in children.

UNAPPROVED ADULT: Dementia in Parkinson disease: 4–8 mg po bid (immediate release).

FORMS: Trade only: Tabs (Razadyne) 4, 8, 12 mg; oral solution 4 mg/mL. Extended-release caps (Razadyne ER) 8, 16, 24 mg. Prior to April 2005, it was called Reminyl.

NOTES: Max 16 mg/d if renal, hepatic impairment. Avoid abrupt discontinuation. If interruption of rx for several days or more, restart at the lowest dose. Half-life 7 hr.

DRUG INTERACTIONS: Caution with CYP3A4 and CYP2D6 inhibitors: ↓ galantamine clearance: for example, cimetidine, ranitidine, ketoconazole (2D6, 3A4), erythromycin, paroxetine (2D6), nefazodone (3A4). No significant effect on digoxin levels or PTT (in pts receiving warfarin).

Rivastigmine (*Exelon, Exelon Patch*) ▶K ♀ B▶? $$$$

ADULT: Alzheimer disease: start 1.5 mg po bid with food. ↑ to 3 mg bid after 2 wk. Usual effective dose is 6–12 mg/d. Max 12 mg/d. Patch: start 4.6 mg/24 hr once daily; may ↑ after ≥1 month to max 9.5 mg/24 hr. Dementia associated with Parkinson disease: start 1.5 mg bid with food; ↑ by 3 mg/d at intervals >4 wk to max 12 mg/d. Patch: start 4.6 mg/24 hr once daily; may ↑ after ≥1 month to max 9.5 mg/24 hr.

PEDS: Not approved in children.

FORMS: Trade: caps 1.5, 3, 4.5, 6 mg. Oral solution 2 mg/mL (120 mL). Transdermal: 4.6 mg/24 hr (9 mg/patch), 9.5 mg/24 hr (18 mg/patch).

NOTES: Restart rx with the lowest daily dose (i.e., 1.5 mg po bid) if discontinued for *x* days to ↓ risk of severe vomiting. Use solution if difficulty swallowing (give with food to ↓ GI side effects). From po to patch, pts taking <6 mg/d can be placed on 4.6 mg/24 hr patch. For those taking 6–12 mg/d, start with 9.5 mg/24 hr patch. Have pt start the day after stopping oral dosing. Rotate application sites; do not apply to same spot for 14 days. Half-life: 1.5 hr.

DRUG INTERACTIONS: Minimal effect with regard to cytochrome P450 enzymes.

Tacrine (Cognex) ▶L ♀C▶? $$$$

WARNING: Can be hepatotoxic: rarely used. Not first line; monitor LFT every 2 wk for the first 4 months of rx: if elevation is 3× normal, ↓ the dose. Discontinue if elevation of more than 5× normal or bilirubin >3 mg/dL or hypersensitivity or jaundice.

ADULT: Alzheimer disease (mild–moderate dementia): start 10 mg qid; after 4 wk ↑ to 20 mg qid. Daily dose is ↑ in 40 mg increments q 4 wk up to 120–160 mg/d.

PEDS: Not approved in children.

FORMS: Trade: caps 10, 20, 30, 40 mg.

NOTES: Give at least 1 hr before meals; risk of bradycardia/heart block. Women develop blood levels 50% higher than men. Half-life: 2–4 hr.

DRUG INTERACTIONS: Smoking ↓ tacrine levels (induction of 1A2 isoenzyme).

ALZHEIMER DISEASE: NMDA RECEPTOR ANTAGONISTS

Memantine (*Namenda, ♣ Ebixa*) ▶KL ♀B ▶? $$$$

ADULT: Alzheimer disease (moderate–severe): start 5 mg po/d; ↑ by 5 mg/d q wk to max 20 mg/d. Doses >5 mg/d should be divided bid.

PEDS: Not approved in children.

FORMS: Trade only: tabs 5, 10 mg. Oral solution 2 mg/mL.

NOTES: Reduce target dose to 5 mg po bid in severe renal impairment (CrCl 5–29 mL/min). No adjustment needed for mild–moderate renal impairment; half-life 60–80 hr. No active metabolites; is excreted unchanged in the urine; ↓ glutamate-mediated excitotoxicity. Modest cognitive improvement alone: used in conjunction with acetylcholinesterase inhibitor.

DRUG INTERACTIONS: little metabolism via the cytochrome P450 enzyme. Levels of memantine may increase if coadministration of cimetidine, ranitidine, procainamide, quinidine, nicotine. Avoid coadministration of NMDA antagonists such as amantadine, ketamine, dextromethorphan (risk of psychosis); may enhance dopaminergic agonists and anticholinergic agents.

ANTICONVULSANTS ALSO USED IN PSYCHIATRIC DISORDERS

> NOTE: Avoid rapid discontinuation of anticonvulsants (can precipitate seizures or other withdrawal sx). **In case of pregnancy: antiepileptic drugs (AEDs) Registry: 1–888-233–2334. http://aedpregnancy. org/**(Folic acid supplementation needed). Monitor all patients for notable changes that could indicate the emergence or worsening of **suicidal thoughts or behavior or depression.**

Carbamazepine (*Tegretol, Tegretol XR, Carbatrol, Epitol, Equetro*) ▶LK ♀ D ▶+ $$

WARNING: Risk of aplastic anemia and agranulocytosis, thrombocytopenia; contraindicated if prior marrow depression; CBC at baseline and periodically; associated with spinal cord and craniofacial defects in the newborn.

ADULT: Epilepsy: start 200 mg po bid. ↑ by 200 mg/d at weekly intervals divided tid–qid (regular release), bid (extended release), or qid (suspension) to max 1,600 mg/d. Trigeminal neuralgia: start 100 mg po bid or 50 mg po qid (suspension); ↑ by 200 mg/d until pain relief; max 1,200 mg/d. Bipolar disorder, acute manic/mixed episodes (Equetro): start 200 mg po bid; ↑ by 200 mg/d to max 1,600 mg/d; see "unapproved adult" section for alternative bipolar dosing.

PEDS: Epilepsy, age >12 yo: start 200 mg po bid or 100 mg po qid (suspension); ↑ by 200 mg/d at weekly intervals divided tid–qid (regular release), bid (extended release), or qid (suspension) to max 1,000 mg/d (age 12–15 yo) or 1,200 mg/d (age >15 yo). Epilepsy, age 6–12 yo: start 100 mg po bid or 50 mg po qid (suspension); ↑ by 100 mg/d at weekly intervals divided tid–qid (regular release), bid (extended release), or qid (suspension) to max 1,000 mg/d. Epilepsy, age <6 yo: start 10–20 mg/kg/d po divided bid–tid or qid (suspension). ↑ weekly prn; manic episodes of manic depressive illness, maintenance treatment for manic depressive pts with a history of mania; max 35 mg/kg/d.

UNAPPROVED ADULT: Neuropathic pain: start 100 mg po bid; usual effective dose is 200 mg po bid–qid. Max 1,200 mg/d. Bipolar disorder: start: 100–200 mg po bid, incr. 200 mg/d q 3–4 days; max 1,600 mg/d; rare pts may require up to 2,400 mg/d; info: screen pts of genetically at-risk ancestry (see pkg insert) for HLA-B*1502 allele before initiating rx; div dose qid for susp; give w/food.

UNAPPROVED PEDS: Bipolar disorder (manic or mixed phase): start 100–200 mg po/d or bid; titrate to usual therapeutic level. Usual effective dose is 200–600 mg/d for children and up to 1,200 mg/d for adolescents

FORMS: Generic/trade: tabs 200 mg, chew tabs 100 mg, susp 100 mg/5 mL. Generic only: tabs 100, 300, 400 mg, chew tabs 200 mg. Trade only: extended-release tabs (Tegretol XR given bid): 100, 200, 400 mg. Extended-release caps (Carbatrol given qd or bid and Equetro given bid): 100, 200, 300 mg.

NOTES: Usual therapeutic range = 4–12 mcg/mL. Toxic levels: >12 mcg/mL; timing: just before morning dose; time to steady state: >1 mo; info: induces own metabolism. Monitor: CBC (discontinue if WBC <3,000 mm^3, absolute neutrophil count <1,500 mm^3 or platelet <100,000 cells/mm^3), LFTs. Cr (peds), platelets, reticulocytes, iron at baseline; BUN, urinalysis, ophthal. exams at baseline, then periodically; lipid panel; serum drug levels; s/sx depression, behavior changes, suicidality, Stevens–Johnson syndrome, hepatitis, aplastic anemia, and hyponatremia may occur; should not be used for absence or atypical absence seizures. Not to be given in pregnancy (risk of congenital spina bifida, low birth weight, neonatal vitamin K deficiency and risk of neonatal hemorrhage). Half-life: 25–65 hr (initial doses), 12–17 hr (repeated dosing); info: variable half-life due to autoinduction. Possibly fatal reactions with the HLA-B 1502 allele (most common in people of Asian and Indian ancestry: screen new pts for this allele prior to starting therapy).

DRUG INTERACTIONS: +++

- Drugs increasing carbamazepine levels: verapamil and diltiazem, danazol, erythromycin, fluoxetine, cimetidine (transient effect, not seen with ranitidine or famotidine), isoniazid, ketoconazole, loratadine, propoxyphene, some calcium channel blockers.

- Drugs decreasing carbamazepine levels: rifampin, cisplatin, phenobarbital, phenytoin. Felbamate may decrease carbamazepine levels but increase its active metabolites resulting in toxicity.

- Carbamazepine decreasing other drugs levels: phenytoin, ethosuximide, acetaminophen, clozapine and haloperidol (↓ 50%), olanzapine (↓ 40%), benzodiazepines (alprazolam, triazolam), oral contraceptives, corticosteroids, cyclosporine, doxycycline, mebendazole, methadone, theophylline (which can decrease carbamazepine levels), thyroid medicines (may mask compensatory increases in TSH), valproate, warfarin.

- Carbamazepine increasing other drugs levels: clomipramine, primidone, phenytoin, and may ↑ the neurotoxicity of lithium.

- Lamotrigine and valproate may increase the active metabolites and may produce toxicity with normal carbamazepine levels.

- Use caution with diuretics (hyponatremia with carbamazepine alone possible as well).

- Discontinue at least 14 days before using MAOIs.

Gabapentin (*Neurontin*) ▶K ♀C▷? $$$$

ADULT: Partial seizures, adjunctive rx: start 300 mg po q hs. ↑ gradually to usual dose of 300–600 mg po tid; max 3,600 mg/d. Postherpetic neuralgia: start 300 mg po on day 1. ↑ to 300 mg bid on day 2 and to 300 mg tid on day 3. Max 1,800 mg/d divided tid.

PEDS: Partial seizures, adjunctive rx, 3–12 yo: start 10–15 mg/kg/d po divided tid. Titrate over 3 days to usual dose of 25–40 mg/kg/d divided tid; max 50 mg/kg/d. Age >12 yo: use adult dosing.

UNAPPROVED ADULT: Partial seizures, initial monotherapy: titrate as above. Usual effective dose is 900–1,800 mg/d. Neuropathic pain: 300 mg po tid, max 3,600 mg/d in 3–4 divided doses. Migraine prophylaxis: start 300 mg/d, gradually ↑ to 1,200–2,400 mg/d in 3–4 divided doses. Restless legs syndrome: start 300 mg po q hs. Max 3,600 mg/d divided tid. Hot flashes: 300 mg po tid.

UNAPPROVED PEDS: Neuropathic pain: start 5 mg/kg po at bedtime. Increase to 5 mg/kg bid on day 2 and 5 mg/kg tid on day 3. Titrate to usual range of 8–35 mg/kg/24 hr.

FORMS: Generic only: tabs 100, 300, 400 mg. Generic/trade: caps 100, 300, 400 mg. Tabs 600, 800 mg (scored). Solution 50 mg/mL.

NOTES: ↓ dose in renal impairment (CrCl < 60 mL/min); table in package insert. Discontinue gradually over ≥1 wk; half-life 5–7 hr. Monitor: Cr at baseline; s/sx depression, behavior changes, suicidality; has induced hypomania, withdrawal sx. Efficacy varies among the anxiety disorders (social anxiety disorders respond better to gabapentin than panic).

DRUG INTERACTIONS: No interactions with other anticonvulsants; antacids reduce its absorption.

Lamotrigine (*Lamictal, Lamictal CD, Lamictal ODT*) ▶LK ♀ C (see notes) ▶- $$$$

WARNING: Potentially life-threatening rashes (e.g., Stevens–Johnson syndrome) in 0.3% of adults and 0.8% of children, usually within 2–8 wk of initiation; discontinue at first sign of rash. Drug interaction with valproate—see adjusted dosing guidelines.

ADULT: (A) *Bipolar disorder (maintenance)*: start 25 mg po daily, 50 mg po if on carbamazepine or other enzyme-inducing drugs, or 25 mg po qod if on valproate. Increase for wk 3–4 to 50 mg/d, 50 mg bid if on enzyme-inducing drugs, or 25 mg/d if on valproate, then adjust over wk 5–7 to target doses of 200 mg/d, 400 mg/d divided bid if on enzyme-inducing drugs, or 100 mg/d if on valproate.

(B) *Seizure disorders*: Partial seizures, Lennox–Gastaut syndrome, or generalized tonic-clonic seizures, adjunctive rx with an enzyme-inducing anticonvulsant (age >12 yo): start 50 mg po daily × 2 wk, then 50 mg po bid × 2 wk. ↑ by 100 mg/d q 1–2 wk to maintenance dose of 150–250 mg po bid. Partial seizures, conversion to monotherapy from adjunctive rx with a single enzyme-inducing anticonvulsant (age ≥16 yo): use above guidelines to gradually ↑ the dose to 250 mg po bid; then taper the enzyme-inducing anticonvulsant by 20% a wk over 4 wk. Partial seizures, Lennox–Gastaut syndrome, or generalized tonic-clonic seizures, adjunctive rx with valproate (age >12 yo): start 25 mg po qod × 2 wk, then 25 mg po daily × 2 wk. Increase by 25–50 mg/d q 1–2 wk to usual maintenance dose of 100–400 mg/d (lamotrigine + valproate and other anticonvulsants) or 100–200 mg/d if used with valproate alone given once daily or divided bid. Partial seizures, conversion to monotherapy from adjunctive therapy with valproate (age ≥16 yo): use above guidelines to gradually ↑ the dose to 200 mg/d po given daily or divided bid; then ↓ valproate wkly by

≤500 mg/d to an initial goal of 500 mg/d. After 1 wk at these doses, ↑ lamotrigine to 300 mg/d and ↓ valproate to 250 mg/d divided bid. A week later, discontinue valproate; then ↑ lamotrigine weekly by 100 mg/d to usual maintenance dose of 500 mg/d. Partial seizures, Lennox–Gastaut syndrome, or generalized tonic-clonic seizures, adjunctive rx with other anticonvulsants (not valproate or enzyme inducers) (>12 yo): start 25 mg po daily × 2 wk, the 50 mg po daily × 2 wk. Increase by 50 mg/d q 1–2 wk to usual maintenance dose of 225–375 mg/d divided bid.

PEDS: Partial seizures, Lennox–Gastaut syndrome or generalized tonic-clonic seizures, adjunctive rx with an enzyme-inducing anticonvulsant, age 2–12 yo: start 0.6 mg/kg/d po divided bid × 2 wk, then 1.2 mg/kg/d po divided bid × 2 wk; ↑ q 1–2 wk by 1.2 mg/kg/d (rounded down to the nearest whole tablet) to usual maintenance dose of 5–15 mg/kg/d; max 400 mg/d. Partial seizures, Lennox–Gastaut syndrome, or generalized tonic-clonic seizures, adjunctive rx with valproate, age 2–12 yo: start 0.15 mg/kg/d po (given daily or divided bid) × 2 wk, then 0.3 mg/kg/d po (given daily or divided bid) × 2 wk; ↑ q 1–2 wk by 0.3 mg/kg/d (rounded down to the nearest whole tablet) to usual maintenance dose of 1–5 mg/ kg/d (lamotrigine + valproate and other anticonvulsants) or 1–3 mg/kg/d if used with valproate alone; max 200 mg/d. Partial seizures, Lennox–Gastaut syndrome, or generalized tonic-clonic seizures, adjunctive rx with other anticonvulsants (not valproate or enzyme inducers), age 2–12 yo: start 0.3 mg/kg/d (given daily or divided bid) × 2 wk, then 0.6 mg/kg/d × 2 wk; ↑ q 1–2 wk by 0.6 mg/kg/d (rounded down to the nearest whole tablet) to usual maintenance dose of 4.5–7.5 mg/kg/d; max 300 mg/d. Age >12 yo: use adult dosing for all of the above indications.

UNAPPROVED ADULT: Initial monotherapy for partial seizures: start 25 mg po daily. Usual maintenance dose is 100–300 mg/d divided bid; max 500 mg/d.

UNAPPROVED PEDS: Not approved in children for bipolar disorder. Initial monotherapy for partial seizures: start 0.5 mg/kg/d given daily or divided bid; max 10 mg/kg/d. Newly diagnosed absence seizures: titrate as above. Usual effective dose is 2–15 mg/kg/d.

FORMS: Generic/trade: chewable dispersible tabs 2, 5, 25 mg. Trade only: tabs 25, 100, 150, 200 mg. Chewable dispersible tabs (Lamictal CD) 2 mg not available in pharmacies; obtain through manufacturer representative, or by calling 1-888-825-5249. Lamotrigine ODT (orally disintegrating tablets) is available in 25, 50, 100, and 200 mg doses.

NOTES: ♀ on estrogen-containing oral contraceptives without an enzyme-inducing anticonvulsant will generally require an ↑ of the lamotrigine dose by up to twofold. Consider ↑ the lamotrigine dose when the contraceptive is started; taper lamotrigine by ≤25% of daily dose q wk over a 2 wk period if the contraceptive is stopped. Preliminary evidence suggests that exposure during the first trimester of pregnancy is associated with a risk of cleft palate and/or cleft lip. Report all fetal exposure to the Lamotrigine Pregnancy Registry (800-336-2176) and the North American Antiepileptic Drug Pregnancy Registry (888-233-2334). Monitor: Cr at baseline; ophthal. exams if prolonged rx; sx suicidality, clinical worsening if bipolar disorder, and/ or unusual behavior changes. Half-life: 25, 14 hr (w/enzyme-inducing anticonvulsants), 59 hr (w/valproic acid), 28 hr (w/enzyme-inducing anticonvulsants and valproic acid).

DRUG INTERACTIONS: May increase carbamazepine toxicity. Carbamazepine, Phenobarbital, phenytoin will lower lamotrigine levels. DDI with primidone; Valproate will increase lamotrigine levels (up to twice the level) and ↑ rash risk. Lamotrigine will decrease valproate levels (25%). No interaction with lithium. Alcohol will increase lamotrigine SE. Lamotrigine can be used with MAOIs. Lamotrigine increases sertraline level.

Oxcarbazepine (*Trileptal*) ▶LK ♀C ▶- $$$$$

WARNING: Serious multiorgan hypersensitivity reactions and life-threatening rashes (e.g., Stevens–Johnson syndrome, toxic epidermal necrolysis) have occurred, with some fatalities. Consider discontinuation if skin reactions.

ADULT: Partial seizures, monotherapy: start 300 mg po bid; ↑ by 300 mg/d q 3 days to usual effective dose of 1,200 mg/d; max 2,400 mg/d. Partial seizures, adjunctive: start 300 mg po bid; ↑ by ≤600 mg/d at wkly intervals to usual effective dose of 1,200 mg/d; max 2,400 mg/d.

PEDS: Partial seizures, adjunctive, age 2–16 yo: start 8–10 mg/kg/d po divided bid (max starting dose 600 mg/d). Titrate to max 60 mg/kg/d (age 2 to <4 yo), or to target dose of 900 mg/d (20–29 kg), 1,200 mg/d (29.1–39 kg), or 1,800 mg/d (>39 kg). May consider using a starting dose of 16–20 mg/kg for children aged 2 to <4 yo who weigh <20 kg (higher clearance). Partial seizures, initial monotherapy, 4–16 yo: start 8–10 mg/kg/ d divided bid; ↑ by 5 mg/kg/d q 3 days to recommended dose (in mg/d) of: 600–900 if ~20 kg; 900–1,200 if ~25–30 kg; 900–1,500 if ~35–40 kg; 1,200–1,500 if ~45 kg; 1,200–1,800 if ~50–55 kg; 1,200–2,100 if ~60–65 kg; 1,500–2,100 if ~70 kg. Partial seizures, conversion to monotherapy, age 4–16 yo: start 8–10 mg/kg/d divided bid; ↑ at weekly intervals by ≤10 mg/kg/d to target dose listed for initial monotherapy.

FORMS: Trade only: tabs (scored) 150, 300, 600 mg; oral suspension 300 mg/5 mL.

NOTES: Monitor Na+; ↓ initial dose by one-half in renal dysfunction (CrCl <30 mL/min). Half-life: 2 hr, 9 hr (metabolite), 19 hr (metabolite, CrCl <30).

DRUG INTERACTIONS: Inhibits CYP 2C19 and induces CYP 3A4/5. Interactions with other antiepileptic drugs, oral contraceptives, and dihydropyridine calcium channel blockers (e.g., Carden, Adalat, Procardia). Fewer drug interactions than carbamazepine (less hematologic, dermatologic, hepatic toxicity) and is not associated with neutropenia. Patients switched from carbamazepine typically require 1.5× dose of oxcarbazepine. CYP450 inducers (Phenobarbital, carbamazepine) decrease oxcarbazepine levels.

Pregabalin (*Lyrica*) ►K ♀C ▶? ©V $$$$

ADULT: Painful diabetic peripheral neuropathy: start 50 mg po tid; may ↑ within 1 wk to max 100 mg po tid. Postherpetic neuralgia: start 150 mg/d po divided bid–tid; may ↑ within 1 wk to 300 mg/d divided bid–tid; max 600 mg/d. Partial seizures (adjunctive): start 150 mg/d po divided bid–tid; may ↑ prn to max 600 mg/d divided bid–tid. Fibromyalgia: start 75 mg po bid; may ↑ to 150 mg bid within 1 wk; max dose 225 mg bid.

PEDS: Not approved in children.

FORMS: Trade only: caps 25, 50, 75, 100, 150, 200, 225, 300 mg.

NOTES: Adjust dose if CrCl <60 mL/min; refer to package insert. Look for changes in visual acuity, muscle pain; may ↑ creatine kinase. Must taper if discontinuing to avoid withdrawal sx; ↑ risk of peripheral edema when used with thiazolidinedione antidiabetic agents. Some abuse liability (FDA Schedule V). Half-life: 6.3 hr.

DRUG INTERACTIONS: Minimal, no protein binding; does not inhibit or induce major CYP 450 enzymes; not hepatically metabolized, increases effect of oxycodone, lorazepam, ethanol on cognition and gross motor function.

Topiramate (*Topamax*) ►K♀ C▶? $$$$$

ADULT: Partial seizures or primary generalized tonic-clonic seizures, monotherapy: start 25 mg po bid (wk 1), 50 mg bid (wk 2), 75 mg bid (wk 3), 100 mg bid (wk 4), 150 mg bid (wk 5), then 200 mg bid as tolerated. Partial seizures, primary generalized tonic-clonic seizures, or Lennox–Gastaut syndrome, adjunctive rx: start 25–50 mg po q hs. ↑ weekly by 25–50 mg/d to usual dose of 200 mg po bid; doses >400 mg/d not shown to be more effective. Migraine prophylaxis: start 25 mg po q hs (wk 1), then 25 mg bid (wk 2), 25 mg q AM and 50 mg q PM (wk 3), then 50 mg bid (wk 4 and thereafter).

PEDS: Partial seizures or primary generalized tonic-clonic seizures, monotherapy (age >10 yo): use adult dosing. Partial seizures, primary generalized tonic-clonic seizures, or Lennox–Gastaut syndrome, adjunctive rx, 2–16 yo: start 1–3 mg/kg (max 25 mg) po q hs. Increase by 1–3 mg/kg/d q 1–2 wk to usual dose of 5–9 mg/kg/d divided bid.

UNAPPROVED PEDS: Not approved for psychiatric use in children.

UNAPPROVED ADULT: Essential tremor: start 25 mg po/d. Increase by 25 mg/d q wk to 100 mg/d; max 400 mg/d. Bipolar disorder: start 25–50 mg/d po; titrate to max 400 mg/d divided bid. Alcohol dependence: start 25 mg/d po; titrate weekly to max 150 mg bid.

FORMS: Trade only: tabs 25, 50, 100, 200 mg. Sprinkle caps 15, 25 mg.

NOTES: Give ½ usual adult dose in renal impairment (CrCl <70 mL/min). Confusion, nephrolithiasis, glaucoma, and weight loss may occur. Risk of oligohidrosis and hyperthermia, particularly in children; use caution in warm ambient temperatures and/or vigorous physical activity. Hyperchloremic, nonanion gap metabolic acidosis may occur; monitor serum bicarbonate and either ↓ dose or taper off entirely if this occurs. Max dose tested was 1,600 mg/d; half-life 21 hr.

DRUG INTERACTIONS: Phenytoin, valproic acid, Phenobarbital, and carbamazepine ↓ topiramate levels; topiramate ↑ valproic acid and phenytoin levels. Acetazolamide ↑ the risk of nephrolithiasis; topiramate may ↓ digoxin levels. Topiramate may ↓ the effectiveness of oral contraceptives.

Valproic acid (*Depakene, Depakote, Depakote ER, Depacon, Divalproex, Stavzor, sodium valproate, ♣Epiject, Epival, Deproic*) ►L ♀D ▶+ $$$$

WARNING: Fatal hepatic failure has occurred, especially in children <2 yo with multiple anticonvulsants and comorbidities. Monitor LFTs frequently during the first 6 months. Life-threatening pancreatitis has been reported after initial or prolonged use. Evaluate for abdominal pain, N/V, and/or anorexia and discontinue if pancreatitis occurs; may be more teratogenic than other anticonvulsants (Carbamazepine, lamotrigine, phenytoin). Hepatic failure and clotting disorders have also occurred when used during pregnancy.

ADULT: Mania: start 250 mg po tid (Depakote) or 25 mg/kg once daily (Depakote ER); titrate to therapeutic level; max 60 mg/kg/d. Epilepsy: 10–15 mg/kg/d po or IV infusion over 60 min (≤20 mg/min) divided bid–qid (standard release, delayed release, or IV) or given once daily (Depakote ER). Increase dose by 5–10 mg/kg/d at weekly intervals to max 60 mg/kg/d. Migraine prophylaxis: start 250 mg po bid (Depakote or Stavzor) or 500 mg po daily (Depakote ER) × 1 wk, then ↑ to max 1,000 mg/d po divided bid (Depakote or Stavzor) or given once daily (Depakote ER).

PEDS: Not approved for mania in children. Seizures >2 yo: 10–15 mg/kg/d po or IV infusion over 60 min (rate ≤20 mg/min). ↑ dose by 5–10 mg/kg/d at weekly intervals to max 60 mg/kg/d. Divide doses >250 mg/d into bid–qid; may give once daily (Depakote ER) if >10 yo. For complex partial seizures Stavzor is for ages ≥ 10 yo.

UNAPPROVED ADULT: Status epilepticus (not first line): load 20–40 mg/kg IV (rate ≤ 6 mg/kg/min), then continue 4–8 mg/kg IV tid to achieve therapeutic level; may use lower loading dose if already on valproate.

UNAPPROVED PEDS: Bipolar disorder, manic or mixed phase (>2 yo): start 125–250 mg po bid or 15 mg/kg/d in divided doses. Titrate to therapeutic blood level of 45–125 mcg/mL, max 60 mg/kg/d. Status epilepticus, age >2 yo (not first line): load 20–40 mg/kg IV over 1–5 min, then 5 mg/kg/hr adjusted to achieve therapeutic level; may use lower loading dose if already on valproate.

FORMS: Generic/trade: Caps 250 mg (Depakene), syrup (Depakene, valproic acid) 250 mg/5 mL. Trade only: (Depakote): caps, sprinkle 125 mg, delayed release tabs 125, 250, 500 mg; extended-release tabs (Depakote ER given q hs) 250, 500 mg; trade only (Stavzor): delayed release caps 125, 250, 500 mg; injectable valproate sodium eq 100 mg base/mL (Depacon: IV use only).

NOTES: Contraindicated in urea cycle disorders or hepatic dysfunction; ↓ dose in the elderly. Therapeutic blood level is 50–125 mcg/mL for Depakote and 85–125 mcg/mL for Depakote ER, though higher levels have been used. Hyperammonemia, GI irritation, or thrombocytopenia may occur. Toxic levels: >175 mcg/mL; timing: just before morning dose; time to steady state: 2–4 days; info: draw free levels if hypoalbuminemia. No significant renal or thyroid effects. Monitor: LFTs at baseline, then frequently, especially during 1st 6 mo; Plt, coagulation tests at baseline, then periodically, also before planned surgery; drug levels; ammonia; s/sx depression, behavior changes, suicidality. Depakote and Depakote ER are not interchangeable. Depakote ER is about 10% less bioavailable than Depakote. Depakote releases divalproex sodium over 8–12 hr (daily–qid dosing) and Depakote ER releases divalproex sodium over 18–24 hr (daily dosing), not to be used in pregnancy or breastfeeding (↑ neural tube and other birth defects, toxicity, withdrawal syndrome). Menstrual disturbances, polycystic ovaries, and hyperandrogenism are often encountered in women taking valproate.

DRUG INTERACTIONS: Aspirin, felbamate, cimetidine, fluoxetine, chlorpromazine, and other antipsychotics increase valproic acid levels. Rifampin decreases valproic acid levels. Valproate increases levels of diazepam, amitriptyline, nortriptyline. Valproate inhibits the metabolism of AZT. Valproate may displace warfarin from protein binding (monitor clotting times → ↑ bleeding time). Interactions with anticonvulsants: Phenobarbital and phenytoin lower valproate levels; valproate increases phenobarbital, ethosuximide, phenytoin, primidone, lamotrigine (also ↑ risk of Stevens–Johnson syndrome) levels and the active metabolite of carbamazepine (risk of toxicity). Carbamazepine ↓ VPA levels; the combination of valproate and clonazepam may cause absence seizures. Reduce bupropion if signs of toxicity occur (due to ↑ hydroxybupropion levels).

PARKINSONIAN AGENTS—ANTICHOLINERGICS

Amandadine (Symmetrel, ♣ Endantadine) ▶LK ♀ C ▶? $

WARNING: Antiviral agent. The CDC does not recommend for rx/prevention of influenza in the United States (high levels of resistance); may cause uncontrollable sexual urges, urges to gamble, and others.

ADULTS: Parkinsonism: 100 mg po bid. Max 400 mg/d divided tid–qid. Drug-induced extrapyramidal disorders: 100 mg po bid. Max 300 mg/d divided tid–qid.

PEDS: Safety and efficacy not established in children.

FORMS: Generic: caps 100 mg. Generic/trade: tab 100 mg, syrup 50 mg/5 mL (120 mL)

NOTES: CNS toxicity, suicide attempts, NMS syndrome with ↓ dosage/withdrawal, anticholinergic effect, orthostatic hypotension. Do not stop abruptly in Parkinson disease. ↓ dosage in adults with renal dysfunction: 200 mg po 1st day, then 100 mg po daily for CrCl 30–50 mL/min 200 mg po 1st day then 100 mg po qod for CrCl 15–29 mL/min 200 mg po q wk for CrCl <15 mL/min or hemodialysis. Half-life: 24 hr (> in elderly).

DRUG INTERACTIONS: Anticholinergic or sympathomimetics may cause potentiation; risk of seizures, irritability, arrhythmias with CNS stimulants; Thiazides may increase amantadine levels.

Benztropine mesylate (Cogentin) ▶LK ♀ C ▶? $

ADULT: Parkinsonism: start 0.5–2 mg/d po/IM/IV. ↑ in 0.5 mg increments q wk to max 6 mg/d; may divide doses daily–qid. Drug-induced extrapyramidal disorders: 1–4 mg po/IM/IV given once daily or divided bid.

PEDS: Not approved in children.

UNAPPROVED PEDS: Parkinsonism (>3 yo): 0.02–0.05 mg/kg/dose once daily or divided bid; risk of anticholinergic effects.

FORMS: Generic only: tabs 0.5, 1, 2 mg. Injectable 1 mg/mL.

NOTES: Contraindicated in narrow-angle glaucoma, prostatic hypertrophy, GI obstructions, myasthenia gravis. Anticholinergic SE ↑ in the elderly (may worsen cognition or cause delirium). Avoid concomitant donepezil, rivastigmine, galantamine, or tacrine. Half-life: 3–6 hr.

DRUG INTERACTIONS: Low-potency neuroleptics, tricyclics, sleeping medicines may ↑ the anticholinergic SE (risk of delirium).

Biperiden (*Akineton*) ▶LK ♀ C▶? $$$

ADULT: Parkinsonism: 2 mg po tid–qid; max 16 mg/d. Drug-induced extrapyramidal disorders: 2 mg po daily–tid to max 8 mg/24 hr.

PEDS: Not approved in children.

FORMS: Trade only: tabs 2 mg.

NOTES: Do not use in narrow-angle glaucoma, bowel obstruction, megacolon. Half-life: 4–6 hr.

DRUG INTERACTIONS: Low-potency neuroleptics, tricyclics, sleeping medicines may increase the anticholinergic SE (risk of delirium).

Trihexyphenidyl (*Artane*) ▶LK♀ C ▶? $

ADULT: Parkinsonism: 1 mg po daily. Increase by 2 mg/d at 3–5 day intervals to usual therapeutic dose of 6–10 mg/d divided tid with meals; max 15 mg/d.

PEDS: Not approved in children.

FORMS: Generic only: tabs 2, 5 mg. Elixir 2 mg/5 mL.

NOTES: Contraindicated in glaucoma, pyloric or duodenal obstruction, BPH, and myasthenia gravis. Half-life: 4–6 hr.

DRUG INTERACTIONS: Low-potency neuroleptics, tricyclics, sleeping medicines may increase the anticholinergic SE (risk of delirium).

PARKINSONIAN AGENTS: COMT INHIBITORS

NOTE: May cause uncontrollable sexual urges, urges to gamble, and other intense urges.

Entacapone (*Comtan*) ▶L♀C▶? $$$$$

ADULT: Parkinson disease, adjunctive: start 200 mg po with each dose of carbidopa/levodopa; max 8 tabs (1,600 mg)/d.

PEDS: Not approved in children.

FORMS: Trade only: tabs 200 mg.

NOTES: Adjunct to end-of-dose "wearing off" with carbidopa/levodopa; no antiparkinsonian effect on its own. Caution in hepatobiliary dysfunction. Avoid rapid withdrawal, which may precipitate neuroleptic malignant syndrome. Half-life: 2.4 hr.

DRUG INTERACTIONS: Avoid concomitant nonselective MAOIs.

Tolcapone (*Tasmar*) ▶L♀C ▶- $$$$$

WARNING: Acute fulminant liver failure; always given concomitantly with levodopa/carbidopa; caution if severe dyskinesia or dystonia; monitor AST/ALT at baseline, q 2–4 wk × 6 mo after start or ↑ dose, then periodically; D/C if AST/ALT >2× ULN or clinical sx of hepatic failure, do not restart due to ↑ hepatic injury risk. Reserve for pts on l-dopa/carbidopa w/sx fluctuations who are not candidates or not responding to alternative adjunct rx.

ADULT: Parkinson disease, adjunct rx: start: 100 mg po tid; max 200 mg po tid; info: not first-line rx; always use as levodopa/carbidopa adjunct; D/C if no benefit after 3 wk.

PEDS: Not approved in children.

FORMS: Trade: tablets 100, 200 mg.

NOTES: Half-life 1–3 hr; if no clinical benefit within 3 wk, discontinue (risk of confusion and hyperpyrexia similar to NMS); pts acknowledgment forms to be obtained from www.Tasmar.com or by calling: 1-800-556-1937.

DRUG INTERACTIONS: Do not use with MAOIs.

PARKINSONIAN AGENTS: DOPAMINERGIC AGENTS AND COMBINATIONS

NOTE: May cause hallucinations, particularly when used in combination; have also been associated with the development of impulse control disorders (compulsive gambling, hypersexuality, hyperphagia). Avoid rapid discontinuation, which may precipitate neuroleptic malignant syndrome.

Apomorphine (*Apokyn*) ▶L ♀C▷? $$$$$

WARNING: Never administer IV (risk of severe SE including pulmonary embolism).

ADULT: Acute, intermittent treatment of hypomobility ("off episodes") in Parkinson disease: start 0.2 mL SC test dose in the presence of medical personnel; may ↑ dose by 0.1 mL every few days as tolerated; max 0.6 mL/dose or 2 mL/d. Monitor for orthostatic hypotension after initial dose and with ↑ dose. Potent emetic—pretreat with trimethobenzamide 300 mg po tid (or domperidone 20 mg po tid) starting 3 days prior to use and continue for ≥2 months before weaning.

PEDS: Not approved in children.

FORMS: Trade: cartridges (for injector pen, 10 mg/mL) 3 mL; ampules (10 mg/mL) 2 mL.

NOTES: Write doses exclusively in mL rather than mg to avoid errors; most effective when administered at (or just prior to) the onset of an "off" episode. Inform patients that the dosing pen is labeled in mL (not mg), and that it is possible to dial in a dose of medication even if the cartridge does not contain sufficient drug. Rotate injection sites. Restart at 0.2 mL/d if rx is interrupted for ≥1 wk. Adjust dosing in hepatic impairment; ↓ starting dose to 0.1 mL in pts with mild or moderate renal failure; contains sulfites. Monitor: Cr at baseline; BP at baseline, then q 20 min × 3 after each test dose; dermatologic exams; s/sx orthostatic hypotension especially during dose titration. Avoid abrupt cessation: taper dose gradually (rapid dose reduction of other antiparkinsonian therapy has resulted in a symptom complex resembling neuroleptic malignant syndrome: ↑ temp, muscle rigidity, altered consciousness, autonomic instability). Half-life: 40 min.

DRUG INTERACTIONS: Avoid concomitant use of 5HT3 antagonists (e.g., ondansetron, granisetron, dolasetron, palonosetron, alosetron), which can precipitate severe hypotension and loss of consciousness.

Bromocriptine (Parlodel) ▶L ♀ B ▷- $$$$$

ADULT: Hyperprolactinemia: start 1.25–2.5 mg po q hs, then increase q 3–7 days to usual effective dose of 2.5–15 mg/d, max 40 mg/d. Acromegaly: effective dose is 20–30 mg/d, max 100 mg/d. Doses >20 mg/d can be divided bid. Also approved for Parkinson disease, but rarely used. Take with food to minimize dizziness and nausea.

PEDS: Not approved in children.

UNAPPROVED ADULT: Neuroleptic malignant syndrome: start: 2.5 mg po tid–qid, ↑ as tolerated; max 20 mg po qid; info: continue for 7–10 days, then taper dose over 3 days. Hyperprolactinemia: 2.5–7.5 mg/d; vaginally if GI intolerance occurs with po dosing.

FORMS: Generic/trade: tabs 2.5 mg. Caps 5 mg.

NOTE: Take with food to ↓ dizziness and nausea. Monitor: pregnancy test at least q 4 wk during amenorrhea, then after menses restored if menstrual periods >3 days late; BUN/Cr, CBC w/ diff, LFTs, cardiovascular eval. if chronic rx; visual fields if macroprolactinoma; BP, especially during rx start. Ergots have been associated with potentially life-threatening fibrotic complications. Seizures, stroke, HTN, arrhythmias, and MI have been reported; should not be used for postpartum lactation suppression; avoid pregnancy: use contraceptive method other than oral contraceptives; contraindicated in Raynaud syndrome. Avoid abrupt cessation: taper dose gradually if Parkinson disease rx (rapid dose reduction has resulted in a symptom complex resembling neuroleptic malignant syndrome). Half-life: biphasic 4–4.5 hr, 15 hr.

DRUG INTERACTION: Avoid concomitant use of other ergot medications (potentially life-threatening fibrotic complication). May worsen psychotic sx; antipsychotics will decrease effects of bromocriptine.

Carbidopa (*Lodosyn*) ▶LK ♀ C▷? $$$

ADULT: Parkinson disease, adjunct to carbidopa/levodopa: start 25 mg po/d with first daily dose of carbidopa/levodopa; may give an additional 12.5–25 mg with each dose of carbidopa/levodopa as needed; max 200 mg/d.

PEDS: Not approved in children.

FORMS: Trade only: tabs 25 mg.

NOTES: Adjunct to carbidopa/levodopa to ↓ peripheral SE such as nausea; also ↑ the CNS availability of levodopa. Monitor for CNS SE such as dyskinesias and hallucinations when initiating rx, and ↓ levodopa dose as necessary.

Carbidopa-levodopa (*Sinemet, Sinemet CR, Parcopa*) ▶L ♀ C ▷- $$$$

ADULT: Parkinsonism: standard release and orally disintegrating tablet: start 1 tab (25/100 mg) po tid. Increase by 1 tab/d q 1–2 days prn. Use 1 tab (25/250 mg) po tid–qid when higher levodopa doses are needed. Sustained release: start 1 tab (50/200 mg) po bid; separate doses by ≥4 hours. Increase as needed at intervals ≥3 days. Typical max dose is 1,600–2,000 mg/d of levodopa, but higher doses have been used. Info: 70–100 mg/d carbidopa needed to saturate periph. dopa decarboxylase and ↓ SE.

PEDS: Not approved in children.

UNAPPROVED ADULT: Restless legs syndrome: start ½ tab (25/100 mg) po qhs; increase q 3–4 d to max 50/200 mg (two 25/100 tabs) q hs. If sx recur during the night, then a combination of standard release (25/100 mg, 1–2 tabs q hs) and sustained release (25/100 or 50/200 mg q hs) tablets may be used.

FORMS: Generic/trade: tabs (carbidopa/levodopa) 10/100, 25/100, 25/250 mg. Tabs, sustained release (Sinemet CR, carbidopa-levodopa ER) 25/100, 50/200 mg. Trade only: orally disintegrating tablet (Parcopa) 10/100, 25/100, 25/250 mg.

NOTES: Motor fluctuations and dyskinesias may occur. The 25/100 mg tablets are preferred as initial rx, since most pts require >70–100 mg/d of carbidopa to ↓ the risk of N/V. The 10/100 mg tabs have limited clinical utility. Extended-release formulations have a lower bioavailability than conventional preparations. Do not use within 2 wk of a nonselective MAOI. When used for restless legs syndrome, may precipitate rebound (recurrence of sx during the night) or augmentation (earlier daily onset of sx). Orally disintegrating tablet is placed on top of the tongue and does not require water or swallowing, but is absorbed through the GI tract (not sublingually). Use caution in pts with undiagnosed skin lesions or a hx of melanoma +++. Monitor: Cr at baseline, then if extended rx cont. periodically; CBC, LFTs if extended rx; IOP if chronic wide angle glaucoma; cardiac fxn if extended rx, also during initial inpatient dose adjustment then periodically thereafter if MI hx w/ arrhythmia; dermatologic exams. Avoid abrupt cessation: taper dose gradually (rapid dose ↓ has resulted in symptoms resembling neuroleptic malignant syndrome). Half-life: 0.75–1.5 hr.

Pramipexole (*Mirapex*) ▶K♀ C▷? $$$$$

ADULT: Parkinson disease: start 0.125 mg po tid × 1 wk, then 0.25 mg × 1 wk; after that, ↑ by 0.75 mg/wk divided tid. Usual dose is 0.5–1.5 mg po tid. Max 4.5 mg/d.

Restless legs syndrome: start 0.125 mg po 2–3 hr prior to bedtime; may ↑ q 4–7 days to 0.25 mg then 0.5 mg if needed.

PEDS: Not approved in children.

FORMS: Trade only: tabs 0.125, 0.25, 0.5, 1, 1.5 mg.

NOTES: ↓ dose in renal impairment. Sleep attacks, syncope, and/or orthostatic hypotension may occur. Titrate slowly. Info: taper dose over 7 days to D/C. Monitor: Cr at baseline; dermatologic exams; s/sx orthostatic hypotension especially during dose titration. Half-life: 8, 12 hr (elderly); may be effective in treating depressive sx of pts with Parkinson disease.

DRUG INTERACTIONS: May decrease dopamine agonist efficacy.

Ropinirole (*Requip, Requip XL*) ▶L♀ C▷? $$$$

ADULT: Parkinson disease: start 0.25 mg po tid. Increase by 0.25 mg/dose at wkly intervals to 1 mg po tid; max 24 mg/d. Restless legs syndrome: start 0.25 mg po 1–3 hr before sleep for 2 days, then ↑ to 0.5 mg/d on days 3–7; ↑ by 0.5 mg/d at wkly intervals prn to max 4 mg/d given 1–3 hr before sleep.

PEDS: Not approved in children.

FORMS: Trade only: tabs 0.25, 0.5, 1, 2, 3, 4, 5 mg. Extended-release tabs (Requip XL): 2, 4, 6, 8, 12 mg.

NOTES: Sleep attacks, impulse control disorders, syncope, and/or orthostatic hypotension may occur. Titrate slowly. Info: give w/food; taper dose over 7 days to D/C. Monitor: dermatologic exams; s/sx orthostatic hypotension especially during dose titration. Half-life: 6 hr.

DRUG INTERACTIONS: Ropinirole: metabolized through CYP 1A2; its clearance will be modified by inducers (omeprazole, smoking) or inhibitors (ciprofloxacine, fluvoxamine); dopamine antagonists (neuroleptics, metoclopramide) may ↓ its effectiveness; interaction with high doses of estrogens.

Rotigotine (*Neupro*) ▶L♀ C▷? $$$$$

ADULT: Parkinson disease: start 2 mg/24 hr patch daily × 1 wk, then ↑ to lowest effective dose of 4 mg/24 hr; may ↑ prn in ≥1 wk to max 6 mg/24 hr.

PEDS: Not approved in children.

FORMS: Trade only: transdermal patch 2, 4, 6 mg/24 hr.

NOTES: Contains sulfites. Monitor BP, syncope, ↑ weight, hallucinations, abrupt falling asleep episodes, skin. Remove prior to MRI or cardioversion to avoid burns. Apply to clean, dry, intact skin; hold in place for 20–30 s. Rotate application sites daily, and wash skin after removal. Avoid abrupt discontinuation: taper by 2 mg/24 hr q other day when discontinuing. Half-life: 5–7 hr.

DRUG INTERACTIONS: Dopamine antagonists (antipsychotics) may ↓ the effectiveness of rotigotine; no major interaction with L dopa/Carbodopa, with digoxin, with warfarin.

Stalevo (carbidopa + levodopa + entacapone) ▶L♀ C▶- $$$$$

ADULT: Parkinson disease (conversion from carbidopa-levodopa ± entacapone): start Stalevo tab that contains the same amount of carbidopa-levodopa as the patient was previously taking, and titrate to desired response; may need to ↓ the dose of levodopa in pts not already taking entacapone; max 1,600 mg/d of entacapone or 1,600–2,000 mg/d of levodopa; may be used to replace immediate release of carbidopa/levodopa (without entacapone) when pt experiences the sx of end-of-dose "wearing-off" (only for pts taking levodopa of ≤600 mg/d and if no dyskinesias).

PEDS: Not approved in children.

FORMS: Trade only: tabs (carbidopa/levodopa/entacapone): Stalevo 50 (12.5/50/200 mg), Stalevo 100 (25/100/200 mg), Stalevo 150 (37.5/150/200 mg).

NOTES: If not currently taking entacapone, consider titrating individual components before conversion to this fixed-dose preparation. Caution in hepatobiliary dysfunction. Motor fluctuations and dyskinesias may occur. Monitor CBC, LFTs if extended rx; IOP if chronic wide angle glaucoma; cardiac fxn if extended rx, also during initial inpatient dose adjustment then periodically thereafter if MI hx w/arrhythmia; dermatologic exams (not to use in pts with undiagnosed skin lesions or a hx of melanoma +++). Avoid abrupt cessation: taper dose gradually (rapid dose reduction has resulted in sx resembling neuroleptic malignant syndrome); risk of depression, psychosis. Half-life: 0.7–4 hr.

DRUG INTERACTIONS: Avoid concomitant use of nonselective MAOIs; caution with drugs metabolized by COMT (isoproterenol, epinephrine, NE, dopamine, alpha-methyldopa, dobutamine, apomorphine, isoetherine, bitolterol).

PARKINSONIAN AGENTS: MONOAMINE OXIDASE INHIBITORS (MAOIs)

NOTE: +++ see also note for antidepressants MAOIs +++ in Chapter 8
- Must be on **tyramine-free diet** throughout rx, and for 2 wk after discontinuation.
- **Numerous drug interactions +++: risk of hypertensive crisis and serotonin syndrome with many medications, including OTC**, allow ≥2 wk wash-out when converting from an MAOI.

Rasagiline (*Azilect*) ▶L♀ C▶? $$$$$

WARNINGS: Is an MAOI.

ADULT: Parkinson disease, monotherapy: 1 mg po q AM. Parkinson disease, adjunctive: 0.5 mg po q AM; max 1 mg/d.

PEDS: Not approved in children.

FORMS: Trade only: tabs 0.5, 1 mg.

NOTES: Requires an MAOI diet. Do not use in moderate or severe liver disease. Half-life: 3 hr.

DRUG INTERACTIONS: *Check all contraindications of MAOIs*. May need to ↓ levodopa dose when used in combination; ↓ dose to 0.5 mg when used with CYP1A2 inhibitors (e.g., ciprofloxacin) and in mild hepatic impairment.

Selegiline (*Eldepryl, Zelapar*) ▶LK♀ C▶? $$$$

WARNINGS: Is an MAOI. Selectivity for MAO-B may not be absolute at the dose of 2.5 mg/d; becomes a nonselective MAOI at higher doses.

ADULT: Parkinsonism (adjunct to levodopa): 5 mg po q AM and q noon; max 10 mg/d. Zelapar ODT: start 1.25 mg SL q AM for >6 wk, then ↑ prn to max 2.5 mg q AM.

PEDS: Not approved in children.

UNAPPROVED ADULT: Parkinsonism (monotherapy): 5 mg po q AM and q noon; max 10 mg/d.

FORMS: Generic/trade: caps 5 mg. Tabs 5 mg. Trade only (Zelapar): oral disintegrating tabs (Zelapar ODT) 1.25 mg.

NOTES: Requires an MAOI diet if doses increase. Zelapar should be taken in the AM before food and without water. Half-life: 1.3–10 hr.

DRUG INTERACTIONS: *Check all contraindications of MAOIs;* risk of nonselective MAO inhibition at high doses.

OTHER NEUROLOGY DRUGS

Baclofen (*Lioresal, Kemstro*) ▶K ♀C ▶+ $$

WARNING: Abrupt discontinuation of intrathecal baclofen has been associated with life-threatening sequelae and/or death.

ADULT: Spasticity related to MS or spinal cord disease/injury: 5 mg po tid × 3 days, 15 mg po tid × 3 days, then 20 mg po tid × 3 days. Max dose: 20 mg po qid. Spasticity related to spinal cord disease/injury, unresponsive to oral therapy: specialized dosing via implantable intrathecal pump.

PEDS: Spasticity related to spinal cord disease/injury: specialized dosing via implantable intrathecal pump.

UNAPPROVED ADULT: Trigeminal neuralgia: 30–80 mg/d po divided tid–qid. Tardive dyskinesia: 40–60 mg/d po divided tid–qid. Intractable hiccups: 15–45 mg po divided tid.

UNAPPROVED PEDS: Spasticity: ≥ 2 yo: 10–15 mg/d po divided q 8 hr. Max doses 40 mg/d for 2–7 yo, 60 mg/d for ≥ 8 yo.

FORMS: Generic: tabs 10, 20 mg; trade only: (Kemstro) tabs—orally disintegrating 10, 20 mg.

NOTES: Hallucinations and seizures with abrupt withdrawal. Caution if impaired renal function. Efficacy not established for rheumatic disorders, stroke, cerebral palsy, or Parkinson disease. Half-life: 5.5 hr.

Dantrolene (Dantrium)▶LK ♀C ▶- $$$$

WARNING: Hepatototoxicity, monitor LFTs. Use the lowest possible effective dose.

ADULT: Chronic spasticity related to spinal cord injury, stroke, cerebral palsy, MS: 25 mg po/d to start, ↑ to 25 mg bid–qid, then by 25 mg up to max of 100 mg bid–qid if necessary. Maintain each dosage level for 4–7 days to determine response. Use the lowest effective dose. Malignant hyperthermia: 2.5 mg/kg rapid IV push q 5–10 min continuing until sx subside or to a max 10 mg/kg/dose. Doses of up to 40 mg/kg have been used. Follow with 4–8 mg/kg/d po divided tid–qid × 1–3 days to prevent recurrence.

PEDS: Chronic spasticity: 0.5 mg/kg po bid to start; ↑ to 0.5 mg/kg tid–qid, then by increments of 0.5 mg/kg up to 3 mg/kg bid–qid. Max dose 100 mg po qid. Malignant hyperthermia: use adult dose.

UNAPPROVED ADULT: Neuroleptic malignant syndrome, heat stroke: 1–3 mg/kg/d po/IV divided qid.

FORMS: Generic/trade: caps 25, 50, 100 mg.

NOTES: Photosensitization may occur. Warfarin may ↓ protein binding of dantrolene and ↑ dantrolene's effect. The following Web site may be useful for malignant hyperthermia: www.mhaus.org. Half-life: 4–8 hr.

Oxybate (*Xyrem, GHB, gamma hydroxybutyrate*) ▶ L ♀B▶? ©III $$$$$

WARNING: Restricted access in the United States: 1-866-997-3688 or www.xyrem.com for more info.

CNS depressant with abuse potential; avoid alcohol or sedative use.

ADULT: Narcolepsy-associated cataplexy or excessive daytime sleepiness: 2.25 g po q hs. Repeat in 2.5–4 hr; may ↑ by 1.5 g/d at >2 wk intervals to max 9 g/d. Dilute each dose in 60 mL water.

PEDS: Not approved in children.

FORMS: Trade only: solution 180 mL (500 mg/mL) supplied with measuring device and child-proof dosing cups.

NOTES: Only through the Xyrem Success Program centralized pharmacy (1–866-997–3688). Adjust dose in hepatic dysfunction. Prepare doses just prior to bedtime, and use within 24 hr; may need an alarm to signal second dose. Half-life: 30–60 min.

ANTIDEPRESSANTS: HETEROCYCLIC COMPOUNDS

NOTE
- Prevent withdrawal sx by gradually tapering, when discontinuing (abrupt cessation of TCAs may cause N/V, diarrhea, headache, sleep disturbances, dizziness, malaise, hyperthermia, irritability, akathisia). Seizures, orthostatic hypotension, arrhythmias, and anticholinergic SE may occur.
- Antidepressants ↑ the risk of suicide thinking and behavior in children, adolescents, and young adults; carefully weigh the risks and benefits before starting and monitor closely.
- Drug interactions:
  - Don't use with MAOIs: MAOIs ↑ TCA effect but ↑ or ↓ BP.
  - SSRIs (fluoxetine, paroxetine) may ↑ heterocyclic antidepressant levels.
  - Oral contraceptives, nicotine may ↓ levels of heterocyclics.
  - Heterocyclics may block the effects of antihypertensive agents such as clonidine and propanolol.
  - Sympathomimetics (epinephrine, NE): risk of hypertension, arrhythmias.
  - Stimulants: ↑ antidepressant effect, risk of agitation, and psychosis.
  - Anticonvulsants: anticonvulsants may ↓ effect of TCA. TCA may produce seizures.
  - Alcohol, barbiturates, chloral hydrate may ↓ TCA level.
  - Antipsychotics may ↑ TCA effect, confusion, delirium, risk of anticholinergic toxicity.
  - Antiarrhythmic drugs: additive quinidine-like effects, myocardial depression, dysrhythmias.

Amitriptyline (*Elavil*) ▶L ♀D ▶- $$

ADULT: Depression: start 25–100 mg po q hs; gradually ↑ to usual dose of 50–300 mg/d.

PEDS: Depression, adolescents: use adult dosing. Not approved in children <12 yo.

UNAPPROVED ADULT: Migraine prophylaxis and/or chronic pain: 10–100 mg/d. Fibromyalgia: 25–50 mg/d; useful for insomnia at a dosage of 25–100 mg q hs.

UNAPPROVED PEDS: Depression, <12 yo: start 1 mg/kg/d po divided tid × 3 days, then ↑ to 1.5 mg/kg/d; max 5 mg/kg/d.

FORMS: Generic: tabs 10, 25, 50, 75, 100, 150 mg. Elavil brand name no longer available; retained here for name recognition only.

NOTES: Tricyclic, tertiary amine—primarily inhibits serotonin reuptake; demethylated to nortriptyline, which primarily inhibits norepinephrine reuptake. Usual therapeutic range is 150–300 ng/mL (amitriptyline + nortriptyline). Half-life: 10–50 hr. Strong anticholinergic effects.

Amoxapine (*Asendin*) ▶L ♀C ▶- $$$

ADULT: Rarely used; depression: start 25–50 mg po bid–tid; ↑ by 50–100 mg bid–tid after 1 wk. Usual dose is 150–400 mg/d. Max 600 mg/d.

PEDS: Not approved in children <16 yo.

FORMS: Generic: tabs 25, 50, 100, 150 mg. Asendin brand name no longer available: retained here for name recognition only.

NOTES: Tetracyclic—primarily inhibits norepinephrine reuptake; dose: <300 mg/d may be given once daily at bedtime. Usual therapeutic range is 100–250 ng/mL; is related to the antipsychotic loxapine (blockade of dopamine receptors may produce EPS, hyperprolactinemia, TD); higher rates of seizures, arrhythmia, fatality in overdose than with other antidepressants; useful in the rx of MDD with psychotic features. Half-life: 8 hr (amoxapine), 30 hr (8-hydroxyamoxapine).

Clomipramine (*Anafranil*) ▶L ♀C ▶+ $$$

ADULT: OCD: start 25 mg po q hs; gradually ↑ over 2 wk to usual dose of 150–250 mg/d. Max 250 mg/d.

PEDS: OCD, ≥10 yo: start 25 mg po q hs, then ↑ gradually over 2 wk to 3 mg/kg/d or 100 mg/d, max 200 mg/d. Not approved for <10 yo.

UNAPPROVED ADULT: Depression: 100–250 mg/d. Panic disorder: 12.5–150 mg/d. Chronic pain: 100–250 mg/d.

FORMS: Generic/trade: caps 25, 50, 75 mg.

NOTES: Tricyclic, tertiary amine—primarily inhibits serotonin reuptake. Usual therapeutic range is 150–300 ng/mL. Half-life: 20–50 hr. Useful in depressed patients with obsessional features, SE: sedation, anticholinergic effects, higher risk of seizures than other TCAs.

Desipramine (*Norpramin*) ▶L ♀C +▶ $$

ADULT: Depression: start 25–100 mg po given once/d or in divided doses. Gradually ↑ to usual effective dose of 100–200 mg/d, max 300 mg/d.

PEDS: Adolescents: 25–100 mg/d. Not approved in children.

FORMS: Generic/trade: tabs 10, 25, 50, 75, 100, 150 mg.

NOTES: Tricyclic, secondary amine; primarily inhibits norepinephrine reuptake. Usual therapeutic range is 125–300 ng/mL; *causes fewer anticholinergic SE* than tertiary amines and is the *least sedating of TCAs*; lower doses in adolescents or elderly (first-line heterocyclic agent in elderly). Some pts may need AM dosing due to mild CNS activation. Half-life: 12–24 hr.

Doxepin (*Sinequan*) ▶L ♀C ▶- $$

ADULT: Depression and/or anxiety: start 75 mg po q hs. Gradually ↑ to usual effective dose of 75–150 mg/d, max 300 mg/d.

PEDS: Adolescents: use adult dosing. Not approved in children <12 yo.

UNAPPROVED ADULT: Chronic pain: 50–300 mg/d. Pruritus: start 10–25 mg at bedtime. Usual effective dose is 10–100 mg/d.

FORMS: Generic/trade: caps 10, 25, 50, 75, 100, 150 mg. Oral concentrate 10 mg/mL.

NOTES: Tricyclic, tertiary amine—primarily inhibits norepinephrine reuptake. Do not mix oral concentrate with carbonated beverages. Pts with mild sx may respond with 25–50 mg/d. It is one of the most sedating TCAs (strong antihistamine properties); for insomnia: 25–150 mg q hs. Half-life: 8–24 hr.

Imipramine (*Tofranil, Tofranil PM*) ▶L ♀D ▶- $$$

ADULT: Depression: start 75–100 mg po q hs or in divided doses; gradually ↑ to max 300 mg/d.

PEDS: Not approved for depression if <12 yo. Enuresis ≥6 yo: 10–25 mg/d po given 1 hr before bedtime, then ↑ in increments of 10–25 mg at 1–2 wk intervals, not to exceed 50 mg/d in 6–12 yo children or 75 mg/d if >12 yo. Do not exceed 2.5 mg/kg/d.

UNAPPROVED ADULT: Panic disorder: start 10 mg po q hs, titrate to usual dose of 50–300 mg/d. Enuresis: 25–75 mg po q hs.

UNAPPROVED PEDS: Depression, children: start 1.5 mg/kg/d po divided tid; ↑ by 1–1.5 mg/kg/d q 3–4 days to max 5 mg/kg/d.

FORMS: Generic/trade: tabs 10, 25, 50 mg. Trade only: caps 75, 100, 125, 150 mg (as pamoate salt/PM, may be taken once/d at bedtime)

NOTES: Tricyclic, tertiary amine—inhibits serotonin and norepinephrine reuptake; demethylated to desipramine, which primarily inhibits norepinephrine reuptake. Half-life: 5–25 hr; Usual therapeutic range is 150–300 ng/mL (imipramine + desipramine).

Maprotiline (*Ludiomil*) ▶L ♀B ▶+ $$$

ADULT: Depression: start 25 mg po q hs; gradually ↑ by 25 mg q 3–7 days to usual dose of 75–150 mg/d. At 75 mg/d, after 2 wk, ↑ dose gradually by 25 mg/d. Max dose generally 225 mg/d.

PEDS: Not recommended under age 18. Max dose for children and adolescents is 75 mg/d.

FORMS: Generic only: tabs 25, 50, 75 mg. Ludiomil brand name no longer available: retained only for name recognition.

NOTES: Tetracyclic, predominantly a norepinephrine/noradrenaline reuptake inhibitor; associated with ↑ seizures, arrhythmia, and fatality in overdose; do not use if there is a hx of seizures. Half-life: 21–25 hr; rarely used.

Nortriptyline (*Aventyl, Pamelor*) ▶L ♀D ▶+ $$$

ADULT: Depression: start 25 mg po given once/d or divided bid–qid. Gradually ↑ to 75–100 mg/d, max 150 mg/d.

PEDS: Not approved in children.

UNAPPROVED ADULT: Panic disorder: start 25 mg po q hs, titrate to usual dose of 50–150 mg/d. Smoking cessation: start 25 mg po daily 14 days prior to quit date; ↑ to 75 mg/d as tolerated. Continue for >6 wk after quit date.

UNAPPROVED PEDS: Depression 6–12 yo: 1–3 mg/kg/d po divided tid–qid or 10–20 mg/d po divided tid–qid.

FORMS: Generic/trade: caps 10, 25, 50, 75 mg. Oral solution 10 mg/5mL.

NOTES: Tricyclic, secondary amine—primarily inhibits norepinephrine reuptake. Usual therapeutic range is 50–150 ng/mL; may cause fewer anticholinergic SE than tertiary amines. Is one of the least likely TCAs to cause orthostatic hypotension and a *good choice for the elderly* who requires a TCA; may be used in combination with nicotine replacement for smoking cessation. Half-life: 18–44 hr.

Protriptyline (*Vivactil*) ▶L ♀C ▶+ $$$$

ADULT: Depression: 15–40 mg/d po divided tid–qid. Max dose is 60 mg/d.

PEDS: Not approved in children.

FORMS: Trade only: tabs 5, 10 mg.

NOTES: Tricyclic, secondary amine—primarily inhibits norepinephrine reuptake; may cause fewer anticholinergic SE than tertiary amines. Dose increases should be in the AM. Half-life: 50–200 hr. Usual therapeutic range is 75–200 ng/mL; is *the most activating TCA*. Not commonly used.

Trimipramine (*Surmontil*) ▶L ♀D ▶- $$$

ADULT: Depression: start 25 mg q hs; then ↑ over 1–4 wk period. Average dosage: 150–200 mg/d; max 300 mg/d (elderly: 25–50 mg q hs; max 200 mg/d)

PEDS: Not approved in children.

FORMS: Capsules 25, 50, 100 mg.

NOTES: No advantages over other TCAs; half-life: 9–11 hr.

ANTIDEPRESSANTS: MONOAMINE OXIDASE INHIBITORS (MAOIs)

> **NOTE**
> - May interfere with sleep; avoid q hs dosing.
> - Must be on **tyramine-free diet** +++ throughout rx, and for 2 wk after discontinuation (see Chapter 8 on Mood disorders, section MAOIs).
> - **Numerous drug interactions:** risk of hypertensive crisis and serotonin syndrome with many medications, including OTC, allow ≥2 wk wash-out when converting from an MAOI to an SSRI (6 wk after fluoxetine), TCA, or other antidepressant. Contraindicated with carbamazepine or oxcarbazepine (risk of hypertensive crisis), bupropion (hypertensive crisis), mirtazapine. Opiates analgesics especially *meperidone may lead to delirium and death* (**MAOI-Meperidine** *reaction: agitation, restlessness, headache, rigidity, hyperpyrexia, changes in BP, convulsions, comatose, death*). Sympathomimetics may lead to hypertensive crisis (amphetamines, cocaine, epinephrine, norepinephrine, dopamine, isoproterenol, St. John's wort, methylphenidate, oxymetazoline, phenylephrine, metaraminol). Antihypertensive agents may ↑ the risk of hypotension. MAOIs may ↓ blood glucose if combined with oral hypoglycemics. MAOIs should be discontinued 14 days prior to general anesthesia or local anesthesia containing sympathomimetic vasoconstrictors. Psychosis described with dextromethorphan. Antibacterial agent linezolid (Zyvox) is also a nonselective MAOI.
> - Antidepressants ↑ the risk of suicidal thinking and behavior in children, adolescents, and young adults; weigh the risks and benefits before starting and monitor closely.
> - MAOIs have been associated with a few cases of teratogenicity.
> - **Treatment of hypertensive crisis:** chloropromazine 50 mg po. If pt presents to the ER, may be given: phentolamine: 5 mg IV, followed by 0.25–0.5 mg IM q 4–6 hr as indicated. At this point FDA is not recommending previous rx with dose of 10 mg of nifedipine PO or sublingual for rapid relief prior to ER visit (risk of hypotension, tachycardia, cerebral ischemia/infarction, MI, death). Oral medications used are clonidine (0.2 mg po initial, then 0.1 mg po q 1 hr, max 0.8 mg), captopril (6.25–50 mg po or SL), labetalol (100–300 mg po q 2–3 hr or 200–400 mg q 2–3 hr).

Isocarboxazid (*Marplan*) ▶L ♀C ▶ ? $$$

ADULT: Depression: start 10 mg po bid; increase by 10 mg q 2–4 days. Usual dose is 20–40 mg/d. Max 60 mg/d divided bid–qid.

PEDS: Not approved in children <16 yo.

FORMS: Trade only: tabs 10 mg.

NOTES: Requires MAOI diet. Monitor: BP; LFTs; sx suicidality, clinical worsening, and/or unusual behavior changes, especially during initial rx or after dose changes. Half-life: unknown.

DRUG INTERACTIONS: see MAOIs drug interactions.

Moclobemide (♣ *Manerix*) ▶L ♀C ▶- $$

ADULT: Canada only; depression: start 300 mg/d po divided bid after meal; may ↑ after 1 wk to max 600 mg/d.

PEDS: Not approved in children.

FORMS: Generic/trade: tabs 150, 300 mg. Generic only: tabs 100 mg.

NOTES: No dietary restrictions; ↓ dose in severe hepatic dysfunction.

DRUG INTERACTIONS: Don't use with TCA; caution with conventional MAOIs, other antidepressants, epineph-rine, thioridazine, sympathomimetics, dextromethorphan, meperidine, and other opiates.

Phenelzine (*Nardil*) ▶L ♀C ▶ ? $$$

ADULT: Depression: start 15 mg po bid. Increase 15 mg/d each wk. Usual dose 30–90 mg/d in divided doses.

PEDS: Not approved in children <16 yo.

FORMS: Trade only: tabs 15 mg.

NOTES: Requires MAOI diet; may ↑ insulin sensitivity; higher incidence of ↑ weight, drowsiness, dry mouth, and sexual dysfunction than tranylcypromine. Half-life: 11.6 hr.

DRUG INTERACTIONS: Don't use with meperidine; see MAOIs drug interactions.

Selegiline Transdermal (*EMSAM*) ▶L ♀C▶? $$$$$

ADULT: Depression: start 6 mg/24 hr patch q 24 hr; adjust in ≥ 2 wk intervals by 3 mg/24 hr increments to max 12 mg/d.

PEDS: Not approved in children.

FORMS: Trade only: Transdermal patch 6 mg/24 hr, 9 mg/24 hr, 12 mg/24 hr.

NOTES: MAOI diet if ≥ 9 mg/24 hr; antidepressant activity requires inhibition of MAO-A and MAO-B in the brain. At the 6 mg/24 hr dose, the patch does not significantly inhibit MAO-A in the GI tract but inhibits MAO-A and MAO-B in the brain and does not require the dietary restrictions which are necessary if dose ≥ 9 mg/24 hr; some skin irritation. Half-life: 18–25 hr.

DRUG INTERACTIONS: See MAOIs drug interactions.

Tranylcypromine (*Parnate*) ▶L ♀C ▶ - $$

ADULT: Depression: start 10 mg po q AM; increase by 10 mg/d at 1–3 wk intervals to effective dose of 10–40 mg/d divided bid; max 60 mg/d.

PEDS: Not approved in children.

FORMS: Generic/trade: tabs 10 mg.

NOTES: Requires MAOI diet; may cause more insomnia than phenelzine. Half-life: 2.5 hr.

ANTIDEPRESSANTS: SELECTIVE SEROTONIN REUPTAKE INHIBITORS (SSRIs)

NOTE
- Prevent withdrawal sx by gradually tapering, when discontinuing.
- Observe for worsening depression or emergence of suicidality, anxiety, agitation, panic attacks, insomnia, irritability, hostility, impulsivity, akathisia, mania, or hypomania, particularly early in rx or after ↑ in dose.
- Antidepressants ↑ the risk of suicidal thinking and behavior in children, adolescents, and young adults; weigh the risks and benefits before starting rx and then monitor closely.
- Use during the third trimester of pregnancy: associated with low birth weight, neonatal complications including respiratory (including persistent pulmonary hypertension), GI and feeding problems, seizures, and withdrawal sx. Balance these risks against those of withdrawal and depression for the mother. Paroxetine should be avoided throughout the pregnancy (major and cardiovascular malformations).
- Hyponatremia and syndrome of inappropriate secretion of antidiuretic hormone possible with SSRIs. Common SE: sexual dysfunction, headache, nausea, anxiety, mild sedation, insomnia.
- Drug interactions: don't use sibutramine with SSRIs; ↑ risk of GI bleeding; caution when combined with NSAIDs or aspirin, observe closely for serotonin syndrome if SSRI is used with a triptan. If used with TCAs: ↑ TCA levels (may lead to hypotension, sedation, cardiac abnormalities) and risk of serotonin syndrome (mental status changes, myoclonus). Avoid with MAOIs (serotonin syndrome); ↑ seizures with tramadol.

Citalopram (*Celexa*) ▶LK ♀C but in 3rd trimester ▶ - $$$

ADULT: Depression: start 20 mg po/d; increase by 20 mg/d at >1 wk intervals; Effective dose is 20–40 mg/d, max 60 mg/d.

PEDS: Not approved in children.

FORMS: Generic/trade: tabs 10, 20, 40 mg. Oral solution 10 mg/5 mL. Generic only: oral disintegrating tab 10, 20, 40 mg.

NOTES: Don't use with MAOIs or tryptophan. Half-life: 35 hr. Minimal sedation or activation.

DRUG INTERACTIONS: Low overall effects on P450 enzymes compared to other SSRIs; may lead to mild elevations of TCAs and antiarrhythmics.

Escitalopram (*Lexapro, ♣Cipralex*) ▶LK ♀C but in 3rd trimester ▶ - $$$

ADULT: Depression, generalized anxiety disorder: start 10 mg po/d; may ↑ to max 20 mg po/d after >1 wk.

PEDS: Approved in children from 12 to 17 yo for depression.

UNAPPROVED ADULT: Social anxiety disorder: 5–20 mg po daily.

FORMS: Trade only: tabs 5, 10, 20 mg (10 and 20 mg scored); oral solution 1 mg/mL.

NOTES: Don't use with MAOIs. Doses >20 mg/d are not superior to 10 mg/d. Escitalopram is the active isomer of citalopram. Half-life: 30 hr. Minimal sedation or activation.

DRUG INTERACTIONS: Low overall effects on P450 enzymes compared to other SSRIs; may lead to mild elevations of TCAs and antiarrhythmics.

Fluoxetine (*Prozac, Prozac weekly, Sarafem*) ▶LK ♀C but in 3rd trimester ▶ - $$$

ADULT: Depression, OCD: start 20 mg po q AM; may ↑ after several weeks to usual dose of 20–40 mg/d, max 80 mg/d; depression, maintenance rx: 20–40 mg/d (standard release) or 90 mg po once wkly (Prozac weekly) starting 7 days after last standard-release dose; bulimia: 60 mg po q AM; may need to ↑ to this dose slowly over several days; panic disorder: start 10 mg po q AM, titrate to 20 mg/d after 1 wk, max 60 mg/d. Premenstrual dysphoric disorder (Sarafem): 20 mg po/d given continuously throughout the menstrual cycle (continuous dosing) or 20 mg po/d for 14 days prior to menses (intermittent dosing); max 80 mg/d. Doses >20 mg/d can be divided bid (q AM and q noon).

PEDS: Depression 7–17 yo: 10–20 mg po q AM (10 mg for smaller children), max 20 mg/d. OCD: start 10 mg po q AM; max 60 mg/d (30 mg/d for smaller children).

UNAPPROVED ADULT: Hot flashes: 20 mg/d. PTSD: 20–80 mg po/d. Social anxiety disorder: 10–60 mg po/d.

FORMS: Generic/trade: tabs 10 mg. Caps 10, 20, 40 mg. Oral solution 20/5 mL. Trade only: caps (Sarafem) 10, 15, 20 mg. Caps, delayed release (Prozac weekly) 90 mg. Generic only: tabs 20, 40 mg.

NOTES: Half-life of parent is 2–5 days and for active metabolite norfluoxetine is 6–14 days (permits daily dosing, ↓ withdrawal sx following abrupt discontinuation, relatively safe in overdose). Pregnancy exposure: associated with premature delivery, low birth weight, and ↓ Apgar scores (discontinue 2 months before pregnancy); ↓ dose with liver disease; ↑ risk of mania with bipolar disorder. If a dose > 40 mg/d is required, give bid (AM and noon).

DRUG INTERACTIONS: Potent inhibitor of CYP2D6; may lead to mild elevations of TCAs, antiarrhythmics, and of many neuroleptic agents (risk of dystonias, akathisias, or other EPS sx), ↑ of some benzodiazepines, of carbamazepine, phenytoin levels. Pts on fluoxetine have less pain relief from codeine, hydrocodone, and oxycodone. Don't use with thioridazine, MAOIs, cisapride, sibutramine, or tryptophan; caution with lithium, phenytoin, TCAs, NSAIDs, aspirin, and warfarin. Wait at least 5 wk after discontinuation before starting an MAOI, and several weeks before starting nefazodone (fluoxetine impairs the metabolism of nefazodone, and will produce anxiety).

Fluvoxamine (*Luvox, Luvox CR*) ▶LK ♀C but in 3rd trimester ▶- $$$$

ADULT: OCD: start 50 mg po q hs, then ↑ by 50 mg/d q 4–7 days to effective dose of 100–300 mg/d divided bid. Max 300 mg/d. Luvox CR: start with 100 mg po q hs, ↑ by 50 mg increments up to 300 mg/d (do not crush).

PEDS: OCD (>/8 yo): start 25 mg po q hs; ↑ by 25 mg/d q 4–7 days to usual effective dose of 50–200 mg/d divided bid. Max 200 mg/d (8–11 yo) or 300 mg/d (>11 yo). Therapeutic effect may be seen with lower doses in girls.

FORMS: Generic only: tabs 25, 50, 100 mg. Trade only: caps extended release (Luvox CR) 100, 150 mg.

NOTES: Don't use with thioridazine, pimozide, alosetron, cisapride, tizanidine, tryptophan, or MAOIs; use caution with benzodiazepines, theophylline, TCAs, and warfarin. Half-life: 16–20 hr. Give bid if dose >100–200 mg/d.

DRUG INTERACTIONS: Drug interactions with cytochrome P450 metabolized medications (inhibits CYP1A2); may ↑ the levels of theophylline, clozapine (risk of seizures and hypotension), benzodiazepines (alprazolam), propanolol, calcium channel blockers (diltiazem), methadone, carbamazepine. If used with clozapone or olanzapine; may ↑ antipsychotic level (risk of hypotension, sedation, confusion).

Paroxetine (*Paxil, Paxil CR, Pexeva*) ▶ LK ♀D but in 3rd trimester ▶ ? $$$

ADULT: Depression: start 20 mg po q AM; increase by 10 mg/d at intervals ≥1 wk to usual dose of 20–50 mg/d, max 50 mg/d. Depression, controlled-release tabs: start 25 mg po q AM; may ↑ by 12.5 mg/d at intervals ≥ 1 wk to usual dose of 25–62.5 mg/d. OCD: start 20 mg po q AM; ↑ by 10 mg/d at intervals ≥1 wk to recommended dose of 40 mg/d; max 60 mg/d. Panic disorder: start 10 mg po q AM; increase by 10 mg/d at intervals ≥1 wk to target dose of 40 mg/d; max 60 mg/d. Panic disorder, controlled-release tabs: start 12.5 mg/d; increase by 12.5 mg/d at intervals ≥1 wk to usual effective dose of 12.5–75 mg/d; max 75 mg/d. Social anxiety disorder: start 20 mg po q AM (usual effective dose); max 50 mg/d. PTSD: start 20 mg po q AM; usual dose is 20–40 mg/d; max 50 mg/d. Premenstrual dysphoric disorder (PMDD), continuous dosing: start 12.5 mg po q AM (controlled-release tabs); may ↑ dose after 1 wk to max 25 mg q AM. PMDD, intermittent dosing (given for 2 wk prior to menses): start 12.5 mg po q AM (controlled-release tabs), max 25 mg/d.

PEDS: Not recommended for use in children or adolescents due to ↑ risk of suicidality.

UNAPPROVED ADULT: Hot flashes related to menopause or breast cancer: 20 mg po/d (controlled-release tabs).

FORMS: Generic/trade: tabs 10, 20, 30, 40 mg. Oral suspension 10 mg/5 mL. Controlled-release tabs 12.5, 25 mg. Trade: (Paxil CR) 37.5 mg.

NOTES: Start at 10 mg/d and do not exceed 40 mg/d in elderly, debilitated, those with renal or hepatic impairment. *Taper gradually after long-term use*; ↓ by 10 mg/d q wk to 20 mg/d; continue for 1 wk at this dose, and then stop. If withdrawal sx develop, then restart at prior dose and taper more slowly. Pexeva is paroxetine mesylate, a generic equivalent for paroxetine HCL. Half-life: 15–20 hr (short half-life → high incidence of discontinuation syndrome; anticholinergic activity will give an anticholinergic rebound after discontinuation). *Paroxetine is less activating than fluoxetine and more sedating than fluoxetine or sertraline.* Give q hs due to sedating effects. Give bid dosing if dosages >40 mg/d. Paxil CR 37.5 mg is bioequivalent to 30 mg of immediate-release and may have less SE. Use in the first trimester of pregnancy ↑ the risk of cardiac birth defects.

DRUG INTERACTIONS: Paroxetine is an inhibitor of CYP2D6 and is contraindicated with thioridazine, pimozide, MAOIs, and tryptophan; caution with barbiturates, cimetidine, phenytoin, theophylline, TCAs, antiarrhythmics, risperidone, atomoxetine, and warfarin. It may ↓ the pain relief from codeine, hydrocodone, and oxycodone.

Sertraline (*Zoloft*) ▶LK ♀C but in 3rd trimester▶+ $$$

ADULT: Depression, OCD: start 50 mg po/d; may ↑ after 1 wk. Usual dose is 50–200 mg/d, max 200 mg/d. Panic disorder, PTSD, social anxiety disorder: start 25 mg po/d; may ↑ after 1 wk to 50 mg daily. Usual effective dose is 50–200 mg/d; max 200 mg/d. Premenstrual dysmorphic disorder (PMDD), continuous dosing: start 50 mg po/d; max 150 mg/d; PMDD, intermittent dosing (given 14 days prior to menses): start 50 mg po/d × 3 days, then increase to max 100 mg/d.

PEDS: OCD, 6–12 yo: start 25 mg po/d, max 200 mg/d. OCD ≥ 13 yo: adult dosing.

UNAPPROVED PEDS: Major depressive disorder: start 25 mg po/d; usual dose is 50–200 mg/d.

FORMS: Generic/trade: tabs 25, 50, 100 mg. Oral concentrate 20 mg/mL.

NOTES: Don't use with cisapride, tryptophan, or MAOIs; caution with cimetidine, warfarin, pimozide, or TCAs; dilute oral concentrate before administration. Administration during pregnancy: associated with premature delivery, ↓ birth weight, and ↓ Apgar scores. Half-life: 24 hr for sertraline and 2–4 days for its metabolite desmethylsertraline. Is less sedating than paroxetine or fluvoxamine; minimal activation.

DRUG INTERACTIONS: Low overall P450 enzyme effects; may lead to mild increase of TCAs and antiarrhythmics.

ANTIDEPRESSANTS: SEROTONIN-NOREPINEPHRINE REUPTAKE INHIBITORS (SNRIs)

NOTE
- Monitor for anxiety, agitation, panic attacks, insomnia, irritability, hostility, impulsivity, akathisia, mania, or hypomania, and for ↑ of depression or the emergence of suicidality, particularly early in rx or after ↑ dose.
- Antidepressants ↑ the risk of suicidal thinking and behavior in children, adolescents, and young adults; weigh the risks and benefits before starting rx and then monitor closely.
- Exposure during 3rd trimester of pregnancy may cause a self-limited neonatal behavioral syndrome (respiratory, GI, feeding problems, seizures, and withdrawal sx); balance these risks vs those of withdrawal or depression for the mother.
- Hyponatremia, syndrome of inappropriate secretion of antidiuretic hormone possible with SNRIs.
- ↑ Seizures with tramadol.
- Drug interactions: don't give with MAOIs; monitor for serotonin syndrome if used with triptans
- Monitor BP

Desvenlafaxine (*Pristiq*) ▶LK ♀C but in 3rd trimester▶? $$$$

ADULT: Depression: 50 mg po/d; Max 400 mg/d. No clear evidence of additional benefit if > 50 mg/d.

PEDS: Not approved in children; may ↑ the risk of suicidality in children and teenagers.

FORMS: Trade only: extended-released tabs 50, 100 mg (each tablet contains 76 or 152 mg of desvenlafaxine succinate equivalent to 50 or 100 mg of desvenlafaxine).

NOTES: Monitor for ↑ in BP, lipids; not approved in bipolar depression. Adjust dose if pts with severe renal impairment (give q other day); gradually taper when discontinuing to avoid withdrawal sx after prolonged use. Caution in pts with seizure disorder, glaucoma. Exposure during the third trimester of pregnancy: associated with neonatal complications (respiratory, GI and feeding problems as well as seizures and withdrawal sx). Half-life: 10 hr.

DRUG INTERACTIONS: Don't give with MAOIs; caution with cimetidine, haloperidol; monitor for serotonin syndrome if used with triptans.

Association with aspirin, NSAIDs, warfarin, other anticoagulants may increase bleeding risk.

Duloxetine (*Cymbalta*) ▶L ♀C▶? $$$$

ADULT: Depression: 20 mg po bid; max 60 mg/d given once/d or divided bid. Generalized anxiety disorder: start 30–60 mg/d, max 120 mg/d. Diabetic peripheral neuropathic pain: 60 mg po/d, max 60 mg/d. Fibromyalgia: start 30–60 mg po daily, max 60 mg/d.

PEDS: Not approved in children.

FORMS: Trade only: caps 20, 30, 60 mg (delayed-release enteric-coated pellets, resist acidic pH of stomach).

NOTES: Avoid in renal insufficiency (CrCl <30 mL/min), hepatic insufficiency (↑ liver enzymes), or substantial alcohol use; small BP increases.

(2 mm Hg systolic, 0.5 mm Hg diastolic) have been observed. Exposure during the third trimester of pregnancy: associated with neonatal complications (respiratory, GI and feeding problems as well as seizures and withdrawal sx). Half-life: 12 hr.

DRUG INTERACTIONS: Don't use with thioridazine, MAOIs, or potent inhibitors of CYP1A2; caution with inhibitors of CYP2D6 which will ↑ the duloxetine levels.

Venlafaxine (*Effexor, Effexor XR*) ▶LK ♀C but in 3rd trimester▶? $$$$

ADULT: Depression: start 37.5–75 mg po/d with food (Effexor XR) or 75 mg/d divided bid–tid (Effexor); ↑ in 75 mg increments q 4 days to usual dose of 150–225 mg/d, max 225 mg/d (Effexor XR) or 375 mg/d (Effexor); Generalized anxiety disorder or social anxiety disorder: start 37.5–75 mg po/d (Effexor XR); ↑ in 75 mg increments q 4 days to max 225 mg/d. Panic disorder: start 37.5/d (Effexor XR) may ↑ by 75 mg/d q wk to max 225 mg/d .

PEDS: Not approved in children; may ↑ the risk of suicidality in children and teenagers.

UNAPPROVED ADULT: Hot flashes (primarily in cancer pts): 37.5–75 mg/d of the extended-release form.

FORMS: Trade only: caps, extended release 37.5, 75, 150 mg. Generic/trade: tabs 25, 37.5, 50, 75, 100 mg (scored immediate-release tabs).

NOTES: Noncyclic, serotonin-norepinephrine reuptake inhibitor; ↓ dose in renal or hepatic impairment; monitor for ↑ in BP (for both immediate-release and the XR form); seizures in 0.3% of pts; sexual dysfunction in 10% of pts; frequent nausea and headaches; gradually taper when discontinuing to avoid withdrawal sx after prolonged use; hostility, suicidal ideation, and self-harm reported in children. Exposure during the third trimester of pregnancy: associated with neonatal complications (respiratory, GI and feeding problems as well as seizures and withdrawal sx). Mydriasis and ↑ intraocular pressure can occur: caution in glaucoma; half-life is: 5 hr for venlafaxine and 10 hr for metabolite O-desmethylvenlafaxine.

DRUG INTERACTIONS: Don't give with MAOIs; caution with cimetidine, haloperidol. Monitor for serotonin syndrome if used with triptans; minimal or no inhibition of hepatic enzymes.

ANTIDEPRESSANTS—OTHERS

NOTE
- Monitor for anxiety, agitation, panic attacks, insomnia, irritability, hostility, impulsivity, akathisia, mania, or hypomania, worsening of depression, or suicidality, particularly early in rx or after ↑ in dose.
- Antidepressants ↑ the risk of suicidal thinking and behavior in children, adolescents, and young adults; weigh the risks and benefits before starting rx and monitor closely.
- ↑ Seizures with tramadol.

Bupropion (*Wellbutrin, Wellbutrin SR, Wellbutrin XL, Zyban, Buproban*) ▶LK ♀C ▶- $$$$

ADULT: Depression: start 100 mg po bid (immediate-release tabs); can increase to 100 mg tid after 4–7 days. Usual dose is 300–450 mg/d, max 150 mg/dose and 450 mg/d. Depression, sustained-release tabs (Wellbutrin SR): start 150 mg po q AM; may ↑ to 150 mg bid after 4–7 days, max 400 mg/d. Give the last dose no later than 5 PM. Depression, extended-release tabs (Wellbutrin XL): start 150 mg po q AM; may ↑ to 300 mg q AM after 4 days, max 450 mg q AM; seasonal affective disorder, extended-release tabs (Wellbutrin XL): start 150 mg po q AM in autumn; may ↑ after 1 wk to target dose of 300 mg q AM, max 300 mg/d. In the spring, ↓ to 150 mg/d for 2 wk and then discontinue. Smoking cessation (Zyban, Buproban): start 150 mg po q AM × 3 days, then ↑ to 150 mg po bid × 7–12 wk. Allow 8 hr between doses, with the last dose given no later than 5 PM. Max 150 mg po bid. Target quit date should be after >1 wk of rx. Stop if there is no progress toward abstinence by the 7th wk. Write "dispense behavioral modification kit" on first script. Sustained-release Bupropion: approved for smoking cessation (use with smoking cessation program). Efficacy compared to nicotine patches or gum is unknown.

PEDS: Not approved in children.

UNAPPROVED ADULT: ADHD: 150–450 mg/d po.

UNAPPROVED PEDS: ADHD: 1.4–5.7 mg/kg/d po.

FORMS: Generic/trade (for depression): tabs 75, 100 mg. Sustained-release tabs 100, 150, 200 mg (Wellbutrin SR). Extended-release tabs 150, 300 mg (Wellbutrin XL). Generic/trade (smoking cessation): sustained-release tabs 150 mg (Zyban, Buproban).

NOTES: Weak inhibitor of DA reuptake and inhibition of NE reuptake. Don't use with MAOIs (serotonergic syndrome with severe toxicity). Seizures occur in 0.4% taking 300–450 mg/d; *contraindicated in seizure or eating disorders* or with abrupt alcohol/sedative withdrawal. Little psychosexual inhibition (less than SSRIs: *good choice if sexual side effects from other agents*). Wellbutrin SR, Zyban, and Buproban are all the same formulation. Half-life: 4–24 hr.

DRUG INTERACTIONS: Enzyme inducers (carbamazepine, Phenobarbital, phenytoin) ↓ levels of bupropion; cimetidine ↑ levels of bupropion; bupropion is a CYP2D6 inhibitor and can cause a twofold ↑ in max conc. of CYP2D6 substrates (such as desipramine, TCAs, type 1C antiarrhythmics, beta-blockers, quinidine, oxycodone). Levodopa may cause confusion or dyskinesias. Combination with an MAOI may lead to serotonergic syndrome. Cimetidine may lead to increased bupropion levels.

Mirtazapine (*Remeron, Remeron SolTab*)▶ LK ♀C ▶? $$

ADULT: Depression: start 15 mg po q hs, increase after 1–2 wk to usual effective dose of 15–45 mg/d.

PEDS: Not approved in children.

FORMS: Generic/trade: tabs 15, 30, 45 mg. Tabs, orally disintegrating (SolTab) 15, 30, 45 mg. Generic: tabs 7.5 mg.

NOTES: 0.1% risk of agranulocytosis; may cause drowsiness, ↑ appetite, and ↑ weight; don't use with MAOIs. Half-life: 20–40 hr.

DRUG INTERACTIONS: Low liability for drug interactions.

Nefazodone (*Serzone*)▶L ♀C ▶? $$$

WARNING: *Rare life-threatening liver failure* (↑ risk in 1st 6 months of rx). Discontinue if liver dysfunction. *Serzone brand name product was withdrawn from the market in the United States and Canada: retained only for name recognition.*

ADULT: Depression: start 100 mg po bid. ↑ by 100–200 mg/d at ≥ 1 wk intervals to effective dose of 150–300 mg po bid, max 600 mg/d. Start 50 mg po bid in elderly or debilitated patients.

PEDS: Not approved in children.

FORMS: Generic only: tabs 50, 100, 150, 200, 250 mg. 100 and 150 mg tabs are scored.

NOTES: Half-life: 2–18 hr; does not suppress REM sleep; no adverse effect on sexual functioning.

DRUG INTERACTIONS: Don't use with cisapride, MAOIs (risk of serotonergic syndrome), pimozide; many other drug interactions: may ↑ levels of triazolam, alprazolam, and digoxin. If switching from paroxetine: a washout period of 3–4 days is recommended. If switching from fluoxetine: wait several weeks before starting nefazodone.

Trazodone (*Desyrel, Olepro*)▶L ♀C ▶- $$$$

ADULT: Depression: start 50–150 mg/d po in divided doses, ↑ by 50 mg/d q 3–4 days. Usual dose is 400–600 mg/d.

PEDS: Not approved in children.

UNAPPROVED ADULT: Insomnia: 50–100 mg q hs max 150 mg/d.

UNAPPROVED PEDS: Depression, 6–18 yo: start 1.5–2 mg/kg/d po divided bid–tid; may ↑ q 3–4 days to max 6 mg/kg/d.

FORMS: Generic only: tabs 50, 100, 150, 300 mg. Desyrel brand name was discontinued, retained only for name recognition. Trade only: ER tabs (Olepro) 150, 300 mg (given once a day)

NOTES: May cause priapism (one case for 2,000–4,000 exposures), orthostatic hypotension; rarely used as monotherapy for depression; highly sedating, often used as a sleep aid and adjunct to another antidepressant. Half-life: 4–9 hr.

DRUG INTERACTIONS: Caution with CYP3A4 inhibitors or inducers. Avoid with MAOIs (serotonergic syndrome); potentiate the effects of other sedating drugs; fluoxetine may ↑ trazodone levels but combination is safe for rx of insomnia due to fluoxetine; trazodone may ↑ levels of digoxin and phenytoin; may alter prothrombin time in pts on warfarin.

Tryptophan (♣*Tryptan*)▶K ♀? ▶? $$

ADULT: Canada only. Adjunct to antidepressant rx for affective disorders: 8–12 g/d in 3–4 divided doses.

PEDS: Not approved in children.

FORMS: Trade only: L-Tryptophan tabs 250, 500, 750, 1,000 mg.

NOTES: Caution in diabetics; may worsen glycemic control.

ANTIMANIC (BIPOLAR) AGENTS

See also Anticonvulsants used in psychiatric disorders discussed above (see p. 276).

Lithium (*Eskalith, Eskalith CR, Lithobid, ♣ Lithane*) ►K ♀D ▶-$

WARNING: Lithium toxicity (diarrhea, vomiting, tremor, weakness, ataxia, drowsiness) can occur at therapeutic levels; risk of nephrogenic diabetes insipidus, with polyuria, polydipsia, changes in renal function, hypothyroidism, hyperparathyroidism, EKG changes, encephalopathic syndrome (characterized by weakness, lethargy, fever, tremulousness, extrapyramidal sx, leukocytosis, ↑ serum enzymes, BUN, FBS or similar to NMS) particularly in pts also treated with a neuroleptic; may cause cardiac fetal harm when given to a pregnant woman (Ebstein's anomaly); rare cases of pseudotumor cerebri.

ADULT: Acute mania: start 300–600 mg po bid–tid; usual dose is 900–1,800 mg/d. Bipolar maintenance is usually 900–1,200 mg/d titrated to therapeutic blood level of 0.6–1.2 mEq/L.

PEDS: Adolescents ≥ 12 yo: use adult dosing.

UNAPPROVED PEDS: Mania (<12 yo): start 15–60 mg/kg/d po divided tid–qid. Adjust wkly to achieve therapeutic levels.

FORMS: Generic/trade: caps 300, extended-release tabs 300, 450 mg. Generic only: caps 150, 600 mg, tabs 300 mg, syrup: 300 mg/5 mL.

NOTES: Steady-state levels occur in 5 days (later in elderly, renally impaired pts). Usual therapeutic blood levels are 1–1.5 mEq/L (acute mania) or 0.6–1.2 mEq/L (maintenance), **300 mg = 8 mEq or mmol. A dose increase of 300 mg/d will ↑ the level by approx 0.2 mEq/L. Signs of toxicity may appear early on if levels >1.2 mEq/L or less.** Monitor electrolytes, renal, thyroid functions; avoid dehydration, or salt restriction, watch for polydipsia or polyuria. Dose-related SE (e.g., tremor, GI upset) may improve by dividing doses tid–qid or using extended-release tabs. Lithobid half-life: 24 hr.

DRUG INTERACTIONS: Diuretics, ACE inhibitors (such as enalapril/Vasotec, Vaseretic), angiotensin receptor blockers, calcium channel blockers, metronidazole, COX-2 inhibitors (such as valdecoxib/Bextra) and NSAIDs may ↑ lithium levels to toxicity (ASA, acetaminophen, and sulindac are OK); risk of encephalopathic syndrome with neuroleptics (haloperidol). Lithium combined with SSRIs may produce diarrhea, confusion, tremor, ataxia, agitation. Acetazolamide, sodium bicarbonate may decrease lithium levels; interaction with phenytoin, methyldopa; Carbamazepine ↑ lithium toxicity; Metronidazole ↑ lithium toxicity. Marijuana ↑ lithium concentration; Tetracyclins ↑ lithium levels; Methyldopa: risk of lithium toxicity; hydroxyzine with lithium may produce cardiac conduction disturbance. Neuroleptics may ↑ neurologic toxicity.

ANTIPSYCHOTICS

GENERAL NOTES
- Antipsychotic potency is determined by D2 receptor affinity.
- Extrapyramidal side effects (EPS) including tardive dyskinesia may occur. High potency agents are more likely to cause EPS and hyperprolactinemia, but have less sedative, hypotensive, anticholinergic SE. Can be given in qhs doses, but may be divided initially to ↓ daytime sedation.
- Antipsychotics have been associated with a ↑ risk of venous thromboembolism, especially early in rx.
- Off-label use for dementia-related psychosis in the elderly: associated with ↑ mortality (cardiovascular or infectious events), assess for other risk factors and monitor carefully.
- Use sun lotion to prevent photosensibility.
- Food interactions (antacids, tea, coffee, milk, fruit juice) may decrease phenothiazine effects.
- Drug interactions:
  - Antacids and cimetidine: inhibit absorption of antipsychotics.
  - Anticholinergics, antihistamines, antiadrenergics have additive effects.
  - Antihypertensives: potentiate hypotension.
  - Anticonvulsants ↓ levels of antipsychotics; phenothiazines may ↑ level of phenytoin.
  - Antidepressants may ↑ levels of antipsychotics; antipsychotics may ↑ levels of TCAs.
  - Barbiturates may ↓ levels of antipsychotics. Phenothiazines ↑ risk of respiratory depression.
  - Bromocriptine may ↑ psychotic sx; antipsychotics may ↓ effect of bromocriptine.
  - Nicotine may ↓ levels of antipsychotics.
  - CNS depressants (benzodiazepines, narcotics, alcohol) ↑ sedative effects of antipsychotics.
  - Digoxin absorption may ↑.
  - INH may ↑ liver toxicity of some antipsychotics.
  - L-Dopa: dopamine antagonists block effects of L-Dopa.
  - Lithium: possible neurotoxicity (neuroleptic-induced encephalopathy).
  - MAOIs: potentiate hypotension due to neuroleptics.
  - Metrizamide ↓ seizure threshold.
  - Oral contraceptives may ↑ levels of antipsychotics.
  - Stimulants: may ↑ psychotic sx; antipsychotics may decrease effects of stimulants.
  - Warfarin; may change antipsychotic levels; antipsychotics may ↓ warfarin levels; more frequent PT/INR monitoring is advisable.

TABLE 28.1. Antipsychotic Relative Adverse Effects*

Antipsychotic	Anticholinergic	Sedation	Hypotension	EPS	Weight gain	DM/↑ glucose	Dyslipidemia
First generation (A)							
Chlorpromazine	+++	+++	++	++	++	?	?
Fluphenazine	++	+	+	++++	++	?	?
Haloperidol	+	+	+	++++	++	0	?
Loxapine	++	+	+	++	+	?	?
Molindone	++	++	+	++	+	?	?
Perphenazine	++	++	+	++	+	+/?	?
Pimozide	+	+	+	+++	?	?	?
Thioridazine	++++	+++	+++	+	+++	+/?	?
Thiothixene	+	++	++	+++	++	?	?
Trifluoperazine	++	+	+	+++	++	?	?
Second generation (B)							
Aripiprazole†	++	+	0	0	0/+	0	0
Asenapine	?	++	++	+	+	+	+
Iloperidone	+	++	++	?	+	+	?
Clozapine	++++	+++	+++	0	+++	+	+
Olanzapine	+++	++	+	0‡	+++	+	+
Risperidone	+	++	+	+‡	++	?	?
Paliperidone	+	++	+	+‡	++	?	?
Quetiapine	+	+++	++	0	++	?	?
Ziprasidone	+	+	0	0	0/+	0	0

*Risk: 0 (absent) to ++++ (high). ? = Limited or inconsistent comparative data. DM= diabetes. Goodman & Gilman (11 ed., p. 461–500); *Applied therapeutics* (8th ed., p. 78); APA schizophrenia practice guideline, *Psychiatry Quarterly* [2002], *73*, 297; *Diabetes Care* [2004], *27*, 596.

†Limited comparative data to other second-generation antipsychotics.

‡EPS (extrapyramidal symptoms) are dose related and are more likely for risperidone >6–8 mg/d/olanzapine >20 mg/d. Akathisia risk remains unclear and may not be reflected in these ratings.

A, antipsychotics—first generation (typical).

B, antipsychotics—second generation (atypical).

Sources: Brunton, L. L., Lazo, J. S., Parker, K. L. (2005). *Goodman & Gilman's The Pharmacological Basis of Therapeutics* (11th ed.). New York: McGraw-Hill Professional. p. 461–500. *Applied Therapeutics* (8th ed.). p. 78. *Psychiatry Quarterly, 73*, 297. American Diabetes Association, American Psychiatric Association, American Association of Clinical Endocrinologists, North American Association for the Study of Obesity. (2004). Consensus development conference on antipsychotic drugs and obesity and diabetes. *Diabetes Care, 27*(2), 596–601. APA Schizophrenia Practice Guideline, (2002).

NOTE

- Extrapyramidal side effects (EPS) including tardive dyskinesia may occur. High potency agents are more likely to cause EPS and hyperprolactinemia, but have less sedative, hypotensive, anticholinergic SE. Can be given in qhs doses, but may be divided initially to ↓ daytime sedation.
- Low potency antipsychotics SE: potentiation of anticholinergic, antihistaminic, antiadrenergic agents and higher risk for ECG changes (including T-wave changes), jaundice, ↓ libido, retrograde ejaculation, ↑ sedation. *High potency agents are:* fluphenazine, haloperidol pimozide, thiothixene, trifluoperazine. *Mid-potency agents are:* loxapine, molindone, perphenazine. *Low potency agents are:* chlorpromazine, mesoridazine, thioridazine.
- Drug interactions: see general note for antipsychotics and specific drugs.

Chlorpromazine (*Thorazine*) ▶LK ♀C ▶-$$$

ADULT: Psychotic disorders: 10–50 mg po bid–qid or 25–50 mg IM, can repeat in 1 hr. Severe cases may require 400 mg IM q 4–6 hr up to max of 2,000 mg/d IM. Hiccups: 25–50 mg po/IM tid–qid. Persistent hiccups may require 25–50 mg in 0.5–1 L NS by slow IV infusion. Can be used for N/V (10–25 mg po qid; 25 mg IM qid; 100 mg suppository tid; to avoid use in pregnancy (especially in first trimester).

PEDS: Severe behavioral problems/psychotic disorders age 6 months–12 yo: 0.5 mg/kg po q 4–6 hr prn or 1 mg/kg PR q 6–8 hr prn or 0.5 mg/kg IM q 6–8 hr prn.

FORMS: Generic only: tabs 10, 25, 50, 100, 200 mg. Generic/trade: oral concentrate 30, 100 mg/mL. Trade only: syrup 10 mg/5 mL. Suppositories 25, 100 mg; parenteral injection: 25 mg/mL (IM).

NOTES: Low potency drug. Monitor for hypotension if IM/IV use; higher risk for seizure, cholestatic jaundice, photosensibility, skin discoloration, granular deposits in lens and cornea, anticholinergic SE, agranulocytosis. Caution in patients with cardiovascular, liver, or renal disease. Half-life: 23–37 hr (chlorpromazine), 10–40 hr (7-hydroxychlorpromazine).

Flupenthixol (*♣Fluanxol, Fluanxol Depot*) ▶? ♀? ▶-$$

ADULT: Canada only. Schizophrenia/psychosis: tabs: start 3 mg po/d in divided doses, maintenance 3–12 mg/d in divided doses. IM: initial dose 5–20 mg IM q 2–4 wk, maintenance 20–40 mg q 2–4 wk. Higher doses may be necessary in some pts.

PEDS: Not approved for children.

FORMS: Trade only: tabs 0.5, 3 mg.

NOTES: Relatively nonsedating antipsychotic.

Fluphenazine (*Prolixin, Fluphenazine decanoate, ♣ Modecate, Modeten*) ▶ L K ♀ C▶? $$$

ADULT: Psychotic disorders: start 0.5–10 mg/d divided q 6–8 hr. Usual effective dose is 1–20 mg/d. Max dose is 40 mg/d po or 1.25–10 mg/d IM divided q 6–8 hr. Max dose is 10 mg/d IM. May use long-acting formulations (enanthate/decanoate) when pts are stabilized on a fixed daily dose. **Approximate conversion ratio: 12.5–25 mg IM (depot) q 3 wk = 10–20 mg/d po.**

PEDS: Not approved in children.

FORMS: Generic/trade: tabs 1, 2.5, 5, 10 mg. Elixir 2.5 mg/5 mL. Oral concentrate 5 mg/mL. Parental solution (IM): 2.5 mg/mL; decanoate formulation (long-acting generic: fluphenazine decanoate): 25 mg/mL.

NOTES: High potency drug. Do not mix oral concentrate with coffee, tea, cola, or apple juice; CBC w/diff; LFTs; BUN/Cr; ophthalmologic exams if prolonged rx. Half-life: 14.7–15.3 hr (6–10 days decanoate).

Haloperidol (*Haldol, Haldol decanoate*)▶LK ♀C▶- $$

ADULT: Psychotic disorders/Tourette syndrome: 0.5–5 mg po bid–tid. Usual dose is 6–20 mg/d, max dose = 100 mg/d IM. Agitation q 1–8 hr prn; May use long-acting (depot) formulation when stabilized on a fixed daily dose. **Approximate conversion ratio: 100–200 mg IM (depot) q 4 wk = 10 mg/d po haloperidol.**

PEDS: Psychotic disorders, 3–12 yo: 0.05–0.15 mg/kg/d po divided bid–tid. Tourette or nonpsychotic behavior disorders, 3–12 yo: 0.05–0.075 mg/kg/d po divided bid–tid; ↑ by 0.5 mg q wk to max dose of 6 mg/d. Not approved for IM route in children.

UNAPPROVED ADULT: Acute psychoses and combative behavior: 5–10 mg IV/IM, repeat prn in 10–30 min.

UNAPPROVED PEDS: Psychosis 6–12 yo: 1–3 mg/dose IM q 4–8 hr, max 0.15 mg/kg/d.

FORMS: Generic only: tabs 0.5, 1, 2, 5, 10, 20 mg; oral concentrate 2 mg/mL IM Injectable (Haldol injectable) 5 mg/mL. IM long-acting injectable (Haldol decanoate): 50 and 100 mg/mL.

NOTES: High potency drug; half-life 21–24 hr and 21 days for decanoate; Monitor CBC w/diff; ophthalmologic exams if prolonged rx, ECG (↑ QTc, torsade de pointes); therapeutic range is 2–15 ng/mL.

Loxapine (*Loxitane, ♣Loxapac*) ▶LK ♀C▶- $$$$

ADULT: Psychotic disorders: start 10 mg po bid, usual effective dose is 60–100 mg/d divided bid–qid. Max dose is 250 mg/d.

PEDS: Not approved in children.

FORMS: Generic/trade: caps 5, 10, 25, 50 mg.

NOTE: Mid-potency drug; half-life: 3–4 hr (oral). Monitor CBC w/diff; LFTs; ophthalmologic exams if prolonged rx.

Methotrimeprazine (*♣Nozinan*) ▶L ♀? ▶? $

ADULT: Canada only; anxiety/analgesia: 6–25 mg po/d given tid. Sedation: 10–25 mg hs. Psychoses/intense pain: start 50–75 mg po/d given in 2–3 doses, max 1,000 mg/d. Postoperative pain: 20–40 mg po or 10–25 mg IM q 8 hr. Anesthesia premedication: 10–25 mg IM or 20–40 mg po q 8 hr with last dose of 25–50 mg IM 1 hr before surgery. Limit therapy to ≤ 30 days.

PEDS: Canada only; 0.25 mg/kg/d given in 2–3 doses, max 40 mg/d for child <12 yo.

FORMS: Canada only; generic/trade: tabs 2, 5, 25, 50 mg.

Molindone (*Moban*) ▶LK ♀C▶? $$$$$

ADULT: Psychotic disorders: start 50–75 mg/d po divided tid–qid, usual dose is 50–100 mg/d. Max dose is 225 mg/d.

PEDS: >12 yo: adult dosing.

FORMS: Trade only: tabs 5, 10, 25, 50 mg.

NOTE: Mid-potency drug; monitor CBC w/diff; LFTs; ophthalmologic exams if prolonged rx. Half-life: 12 hr.

Perphenazine (*Trilafon*)▶LK ♀C ▶? $$$

WARNING: Trilafon brand name was discontinued: retained only for name recognition.

ADULT: Psychotic disorders: start 4–8 mg po tid or 8–16 mg po bid–qid (hospitalized pts), max po dose is 64 mg/d. Can give 5–10 mg IM q 6 hr, max IM dose is 30 mg/d.

PEDS: Not approved in children <12 yo.

FORMS: Generic only: tabs 2, 4, 8, 16 mg. Oral concentrate 16 mg/5 mL.

NOTES: Mid-potency drug; do not mix oral concentrate with coffee, tea, cola, or apple juice. Monitor CBC w/diff; LFTs; ophthalmologic exams if prolonged rx. Half-life: 9–12 hr.

Pimozide (*Orap*) ▶L ♀C ▶- $$$

ADULT: Tourette syndrome: start 1–2 mg/d po in divided doses, ↑ q 2 days to usual dose of 1–10 mg/d. Max dose is 0.2 mg/kg/d up to 10 mg/d.

PEDS: Tourette's age >12 yo: 0.05 mg/kg po q hs, ↑ q 3 days to max of 0.2 mg/kg/d up to 10 mg/d.

FORMS: Trade only: tabs 1, 2 mg.

NOTES: High potency drug; ↑ QT may occur; monitor ECG at baseline and periodically throughout therapy, K+, CBC w/diff. Half-life: 55 hr

DRUG INTERACTIONS: Contraindicated with macrolide antibiotics (erythromycin, clarithromycin are CYP3A4 inhibitors and ↑ levels of pimozide; azithromycine or dirithromycin have less inhibitory effect on CYP3A4), nefazodone, and sertraline; contraindicated in pts receiving Citalopram or Escitalopram (QTc prolongation).

Thioridazine (*Mellaril*, ♣*Rideril*) ▶LK ♀C▶? $$

WARNING: Can cause QTc prolongation, torsade de pointes, and sudden death (dose related).

ADULT: Psychotic disorders: start 50–100 mg po tid, usual effective dose is 200–800 mg/d divided bid–qid. Max dose is 800 mg/d.

PEDS: Behavioral disorders 2–12 yo: 10–25 mg po bid–tid, max dose is 3 mg/kg/d.

FORMS: Generic: tabs 10, 15, 25, 50, 100, 150, 200 mg. Oral concentrate 30, 100 mg/mL.

NOTES: Low potency drug. Not recommended as first-line therapy; contraindicated with a hx of cardiac arrhythmias, congenital long QT syndrome; only use for pts with schizophrenia not responding to other antipsychotics; monitor baseline ECG and K+; pigmentary retinopathy with doses >800 mg/d. Half-life: 24 hr.

DRUG INTERACTIONS: Do not use with amiodarone, quinidine (↑ QTc), fluvoxamine, propanolol, pindolol, drugs that inhibit CYP 2D6 (e.g., fluoxetine, paroxetine).

Thiothixene (*Navane*) ▶LK ♀ C ▶ ? $$$

ADULT: Psychotic disorders: start 2 mg po tid. Usual effective dose is 20–30 mg/d; max dose is 60 mg/d po.

PEDS: >12 yo: adult dosing.

FORMS: Generic/trade: caps 1, 2, 5, 10 mg. Oral concentrate 5 mg/mL. Trade only: caps 20 mg.

NOTES: High potency drug. Half-life: 34 hr.

Trifluoperazine (*Stelazine*) ▶LK ♀C ▶- $$$

ADULT: Psychotic disorders: start 2–5 mg po bid. Usual effective dose is 15–20 mg/d, some may require ≥40 mg/d. Anxiety: 1–2 mg po bid for up to 12 wk, max dose is 6 mg/d.

PEDS: Psychotic disorders 6–12 yo: 1 mg po daily–bid, gradually ↑ to a max dose of 15 mg/d.

FORMS: Generic/trade: tabs 1, 2, 5, 10 mg. Trade only: oral concentrate 10 mg/mL.

NOTES: High potency drug. Dilute oral concentrate 10 mg/mL. Monitor CBC w/diff; ophthalmologic exams if prolonged tx. Half-life: 18 hr.

Zuclopenthixol (♣*Clopixol, Clopixol Accuphase, Clopixol Depot*) ▶L ♀? ▶? $$$$

ADULT: Canada only. Tabs: start 10–50 mg po/d, maintenance 20–60 mg/d. Injectable: accuphase (acetate) 50–150 mg IM q 2–3 days, Depot (decanoate) 150–300 mg IM q 2–4 wk.

PEDS: Not approved in children.

FORMS: Trade, Canada only: tab 10, 20 mg (Clopixol).

ANTIPSYCHOTICS—SECOND GENERATION (ATYPICAL)

NOTE
- Tardive dyskinesia, neuroleptic malignant syndrome, drug-induced parkinsonism, and other extrapyramidal SE may occur.
- Associated with weight gain, dyslipidemia, hyperglycemia, and diabetes mellitus; monitor closely.
- Off-label use for dementia-related psychosis in the elderly has been associated with ↑ mortality.
- Antipsychotics have been associated with a ↑ risk of venous thromboembolism, particularly early in rx; assess for other risk factors and monitor.
- Agranulocytosis is most common with clozapine.
- ↑ Risk of suicidality in children, adolescents, and young adults w/major depressive or other psychiatric disorders esp. during the first months of rx w/antidepressants. Drug interactions: see general note for antipsychotics and specific drugs.

Aripiprazole (*Abilify, Abilify Discmelt*) ▶ L ♀C ▶? $$$$$

ADULT: Schizophrenia: start 10–15 mg po/d; max 30 mg/d. Bipolar disorder (acute and maintenance for manic or mixed episodes, monotherapy, or adjunctive to lithium or valproate): start 15 mg po/d; ↑ dose to 30 mg/d based on response and tolerability. Agitation associated with schizophrenia or bipolar disorder: 9.75 mg IM recommended. Consider 5.25–15 mg if indicated. May repeat in >2 hr up to max 30 mg/d. depression, adjunctive therapy: start 2–5 mg po daily. Increase by 5 mg/d at intervals ≥ 1 wk to max of 15 mg/d.

PEDS: Schizophrenia, 13–17 yo: start 2 mg po daily. May increase to 5 mg/d at ≥ 2 days, and to target dose of 0 mg/d after 2 more days. Max 30 mg/d. Bipolar disorder (acute and maintenance for manic or mixed episodes, monotherapy, or adjunctive to lithium or valproate), 10–17 yo: start 2 mg po daily. May increase to 5 mg/d at ≥ 2 days, and to target dose of 10 mg/d after 2 more days. Increase by 5 mg/d to max 30 mg/d.

FORMS: Trade only: tabs 2, 5, 10, 15, 20, 30 mg. Oral solution 1 mg/mL (150 mL). Orally disintegrating tabs (Discmelt) 10, 15, 20, 30 mg.

NOTES: Low EPS and tardive dyskinesia risk. Half-life: 75–140 hr.

DRUG INTERACTIONS: ↓ usual dose by at least half when used with CYP3A4 (ketoconazole) or CYP2D6 inhibitors such as quinidine, fluoxetine, or paroxetine; ↑ dose by one-half to 20–30 mg/d when used with CYP3A4 inducers such as carbamazepine; ↓ when inducer is stopped.

Asenapine (*Saphris*) ▶ L ♀C ▶ - $$$$$

ADULT: Acute treatment of schizophrenia in adults: starting and target dose of 5 mg sublingually twice daily; acute treatment of manic or mixed episodes associated with bipolar I disorder in adults: starting dose 10 mg sublingually twice daily; dose may be decreased to 5 mg twice daily if there are side effects.

PEDS: Not approved in children.

FORMS: Trade: sublingual tablet: 5, 10 mg.

DRUG INTERACTIONS: caution with Fluvoxamine (strong CYP1A2 inhibitor) and Paroxetine (CYP2D6 substrate and inhibitor).

NOTE: **Do not swallow tablet.** SAPHRIS sublingual tablets should be placed under the tongue and left to dissolve completely. The tablet will dissolve in saliva within seconds. *Eating and drinking should be avoided for 10 min after administration. Increases QT interval.*

Clozapine (*Clozaril, FazaClo ODT*) ▶ L ♀B ▶ - $$$$$

WARNING: **Agranulocytosis risk** *1–2%*, monitor WBC and ANC q wk × 6 months, then q 2 wk thereafter, and wkly for 4 wk after discontinuation; contraindicated if WBC <3,500 or ANC <2,000/mm³. See package insert for more details; risk of myocarditis (particularly during the first month), seizures (incidence incr. w/dose) orthostatic hypotension (more likely during initial rx w/rapid dose incr.; if off rx >2 days restart 12.5 mg q 12–24 hr), and cardiopulmonary arrest.

ADULT: Severe, medically refractory schizophrenia or schizoaffective disorder with suicidality: start 12.5 mg po/d or bid; ↑ by 25–50 mg/d to usual dose of 300–450 mg/d, max 900 mg/d. Retitrate if stopped for >3–4 days.

PEDS: Not approved in children.

FORMS: Generic/trade: tabs 25, 100 mg. Generic only: tabs 12.5, 50, 200 mg. Trade only: orally disintegrating tabs (Fazaclo ODT) 12.5, 25, 100 mg (scored).

NOTES: Pts rechallenged after an episode of leucopenia are at ↑ risk of agranulocytosis and must undergo weekly monitoring × 12 months. Register all occurrences of leucopenia, discontinuation, and/or rechallenge to *the* **Clozaril National Registry at 1-800-448-5938.** Much lower risk of EPS and tardive dyskinesia than other neuroleptics; may be effective for rx-resistant pts who have not responded to conventional agents; may cause significant ↑ weight, dyslipidemia, hyperglycemia, or new onset diabetes. Monitor weight, fasting blood glucose, and triglycerides before initiation and at regular intervals during rx. If an orally disintegrating tab is split, discard the remaining portion. Taper when discontinuing (risk of cholinergic rebound); half-life: 4–66 hr.

DRUG INTERACTIONS: Cimetidine may ↑ clozapine levels (use Ranitidine instead); Fluvoxamine may double clozapine levels; TCAs increase risk for seizures, sedation, cardiac changes; caution if start clozapine w/benzodiazepine or any other psychotropic since collapse, resp. arrest and cardiac arrest have occurred w/combo tx; smoking ↓ clozapine levels.

Iloperidone (*Fanapt*) ▶L ♀C ▶- $$$$$

WARNING: **Prolongs QT interval,** risk of torsade de pointes-type arrhythmia; not to use if hepatic impairment.

ADULT: Schizophrenia: low starting dose of 1 mg bid (to **avoid orthostatic hypotension),** moving to 2, 4, 6, 8, 10, and 12 mg bid on days 2, 3, 4, 5, 6, and 7, respectively, to reach the 12 mg/d to 24 mg/d dose range; max 12 mg bid.

PEDS: Not approved in children.

FORMS: Trade: tabs 1, 2, 4, 6, 8, 10, 12 mg.

NOTES: SE: dizziness, dry mouth, fatigue, nasal congestion, orthostatic hypotension, somnolence, tachycardia, and ↑ weight; titration needed delaying rx response. Check K+, Mg++, ECG; half-life 18–31 hr; administered without regard to meals.

DRUG INTERACTIONS: ↓ *dosage by half if taken with* strong CYP3A4 inhibitors such as ketoconazole, clarithomycin, drugs that prolong QTc including Class 1A (e.g., quinidine, procainamide) or Class III (e.g., amiodarone, sotalol) antiarrhythmic medications, antipsychotics (e.g., chlorpromazine, thioridazine), antibiotics (e.g., gatifloxacin, moxifloxacin), or medications prolonging QTc (e.g., pentamidine, levomethadyl acetate, methadone). Avoid in patients with congenital long QT syndrome or hx of cardiac arrhythmias. Discontinue if QTc ≥ 500 ms. Risk of toxicity if taken with CYP2D6 inhibitors (fluoxetine, paroxetine): ↓ dosage by half.

Olanzapine (*Zyprexa, Zyprexa Zydis*) ▶L ♀C ▶- $$$$$

WARNING: **New long-acting form (Zyprexa Relprevv)** with risk of **postinjection delirium/sedation syndrome (PDSS):** pt must be observed in a registered facility for at least 3 hr after the injection (pt, health care provider, health care facility, and pharmacy must be enrolled in the Zyprexa Zyprevv Patient Care Program), 877–772-9390.

ADULT: Psychotic disorders: start 5–10 mg po/d. ↑ weekly to usual dose of 10–15 mg/d, max 20 mg/d. Bipolar disorder, maintenance rx, or monotherapy for acute manic or mixed episodes: start 10–15 mg po/d; ↑ by 5 mg/d at intervals ≥ 24 hr. Efficacy seen at doses of 5–20 mg/d, max 20 mg/d. Bipolar disorder, adjunctive rx for acute mixed/manic episodes: start 10 mg/d; usual effective dose is 5–20 mg/d, max 20 mg/d. Agitation in schizophrenia or bipolar disorder: 10 mg IM, may repeat 2 hr after initial dose ×1 prn, may repeat 4 hr after 2nd dose ×1 prn to max 30 mg/d; may use 2.5–7.5 mg/dose if clinically warranted; use 2.5–5 mg/dose in elderly; use 2.5 mg/dose if debilitated pt; switch to po ASAP.

PEDS: Not approved in children.

UNAPPROVED ADULT: Augmentation of SSRI rx for OCD: start 2.5–5 mg po/d, max 20 mg/d. PTSD, adjunctive rx: start 5 mg po/d, max 20 mg/d.

UNAPPROVED PEDS: Bipolar disorder, manic/mixed phase: start 2.5 mg po/d; ↑ by 2.5 mg/d every 3 days to max 20 mg/d.

FORMS: Trade only: tabs 2.5, 5, 7.5, 10, 15, 20 mg. Tabs, orally disintegrating (Zyprexa Zydis) 5, 10, 15, 20 mg. Injectable (short-acting) IM 10 mg/vial. Long-acting **(Zyprexa Relprevv)** IM gluteal injection q 2–4 wk eq 210 mg base/vial; eq 300 mg base/vial; eq 405 mg base/vial (see full prescribing information +++)

NOTES: Use for short-term (3–4 wk) acute manic episodes associated with bipolar disorder. May cause significant weight ↑, dyslipidemia, hyperglycemia, or new onset diabetes; monitor weight, blood glucose, and triglycerides before initiation and at regular interval; low EPS, monitor for orthostatic hypotension, particularly when given IM (also risk of bradycardia and hypoventilation if used with other drugs with these effects); ↓ dose in elderly. Olanzapine levels tend to be higher in females. Half-life: 21–54 hr. Use caution with benzodiazepines.

DRUG INTERACTIONS: Use caution with benzodiazepines; nicotine and carbamazepine ↓ olanzapine levels; fluvoxamine ↑ olanzapine levels.

Paliperidone (*Invega, Invega Sustenna* ▶KL ♀C ▶- $$$$$

ADULT: Schizophrenia (alone for acute rx or maintenance rx) and schizoaffective disorders (for acute rx: alone or as an adjunct with mood stabilizers or antidepressant): start 6 mg po q AM. 3 mg/d may be sufficient; max 12 mg/d. Long-acting (Invega Sustenna): R/O first any sensitivity to Risperdal or Invega; reduce dose if renal impairment, initiation dosing: (day 1: 234 mg in deltoid; 1 wk later: 156 mg in deltoid) then 1 month after second initiation dose: 117 mg in deltoid/gluteal and continue q month. Does not need any oral supplementation.

If missed dose: 4–6 wk late: resume monthly dosing; > 6 wk–6 months late: dosing at previously stabilized dose with a first injection in deltoid and same dose 1 wk later, then one month later after the 2nd dose (if pt was stabilized on 234 mg, the first 2 doses should be 156 mg each); > 6 months late: restart as an initiation dosing for the two first injections at 1 wk interval and then resume to previous stabilized dose.

PEDS: Not approved in children.

FORMS: Trade only: extended-release (OROS technology) tabs 3, 6, 9, 12 mg. Extended-release injectable suspension: Invega Sustenna (paliperidone palmitate): given once/month 234, 156, 117, 78, 39 mg.

NOTES: Active metabolite of risperidone. Maximum 3 mg/d if CrCl is 10–49 mL/min. Half-life: 23 hr.

DRUG INTERACTIONS: Carbamazepine may ↓ paliperidone levels; caution with other CNS acting drugs and alcohol. No clinical significant interactions with drugs that are metabolized by CYT P450 isoenzymes. Caution in renal impaired pts.

Quetiapine (Seroquel, Seroquel XR) ▶LK ♀C ▶- $$$$$

WARNING: Antidepressants including quetiapine when used for bipolar depression ↑ the risk of suicidal thinking and behavior in children, adolescents, and young adults; weigh the risks and benefits before starting rx, and monitor closely.

ADULT: Schizophrenia: start 25 mg po bid (regular tabs); increase by 25–50 mg bid–tid on day 2 and 3, and then to target dose of 300–400 mg/d divided bid–tid on day 4. Usual effective dose is 150–750 mg/d, max 800 mg/d. Schizophrenia, extended-release tabs: start 300 mg po daily in evening, ↑ by up to 300 mg/d at intervals of >1 d to range of 400–800 mg/d. Acute bipolar mania monotherapy or adjunct: start 50 mg po bid on day 1, then ↑ to no higher than 100 mg bid on day 2, 150 mg bid on day 3, and 200 mg bid on day 4. May ↑ prn to 300 mg bid on day 5 and 400 mg bid thereafter. Usual dose is 400–800 mg/d. Acute bipolar mania monotherapy or adjunct, extended-release tabs: day 1 (300mg), day 2 (600 mg), day 3 (between 400 and 800 mg), recommended dose (400–800 mg/d). Bipolar depression: 50 mg po at hs on day 1,100 mg at hs on day 2, 200 mg at hs day 3, and 300 mg at hs day 4; may ↑ prn to 400 mg at hs on day 5 and 600 mg at hs on day 8. Bipolar depression, extended-release tabs: day 1 (50 mg), day 2 (100 mg), day 3 (200 mg), day 4 (300 mg), recommended dose (300 mg/d). Bipolar maintenance: continue dose required to maintain symptom remission. Bipolar I disorder—maintenance treatment as an adjunct to lithium or divalproex: 400–800 mg/d. Major depressive disorder, adjunctive therapy with antidepressant: day 1 and 2 (50 mg/d) and day 3 and 4 (150 mg/d), recommended dose (150–300 mg/d).

PEDS: Not approved in children.

UNAPPROVED ADULT: Augmentation of SSRI rx for OCD: start 25 mg po bid, max 300 mg/d. Adjunctive for PTSD: start 25 mg daily, max 300 mg/d.

UNAPPROVED PEDS: Bipolar disorder (manic or mixed phase): start 12.5 mg po bid (children) or 25 mg po bid (adolescents); max 150 mg po tid.

FORMS: Trade: tabs 25, 50, 100, 200, 300, 400 mg. Extended-release tabs 50, 200, 300, 400 mg.

NOTES: Eye exam for cataracts q 6 months; low risk of EPS and tardive dyskinesia. May cause significant weight ↑, dyslipidemia, hyperglycemia, or new onset diabetes; monitor weight, blood glucose, and triglycerides before initiation and regularly during rx. Use lower doses and slower the titration in elderly pts or if hepatic dysfunction. Extended-release tabs: take without food or after light meals; possible postural dizziness. No anticholinergic effect; low incidence of EPS; no sustained ↑ of prolactin. Half-life: 6 hr.

DRUG INTERACTIONS: Low potential for drug interactions. Diphenylhydantoin can lower levels.

Risperidone (Risperdal, Risperdal Consta) ▶LK ♀C ▶- $$$$$

ADULT: Psychotic disorders: start 1 mg po bid; ↑ by 1 mg bid on the second and third day, and then at intervals ≥1 wk. Start 0.5 mg/dose and titrate by ≤ 0.5 mg bid in the elderly, debilitated, hypotensive, renally or hepatically impaired. Usual dose is 4–8 mg/d given 1×/d or divided bid; max 16 mg/d. Long-acting injection (Consta) for schizophrenia: start 25 mg IM q 2 wk while continuing oral dose × 3 wk; may ↑ q 4 wk to max 50 mg q 2 wk (no evidence to ↑ beyond 50 mg). Bipolar mania: start 2–3 mg/d; may adjust by 1 mg/d at 24 hr intervals to max 6 mg/d.

PEDS: Autistic disorder irritability for children 5–16 yr: start 0.25 mg (<20 kg) or 0.5 mg (≥20 kg) po/d. May increase after ≥4 days to 0.5 mg/d (<20 kg) or 1 mg/d (≥20 kg). Maintain ≥14 days. May then ↑ at ≥14 day intervals by increments of 0.25 mg/d (<20 kg) or 0.5 mg/d (≥20 kg) to max 1 mg/d (<20 kg), 2.5 mg/d (20–44 kg) or 3 mg/d (>45 kg). FDA approved for schizophrenia age 13–17 yr: start 0.5 mg/d, ↑ 0.5–1 mg/d, target dose 3 mg/d, effective dose 3–6 mg/d. FDA approved for short-term rx of bipolar I disorder (acute manic or mixed episodes) for children and adolescents age 10–17 yr: start 0.5 mg/d, ↑ 0.5–1 mg daily, at intervals ≥24 h, target dose 2.5 mg/d, effective dose 0.5–6 mg/d, max dose: 6 mg/d.

UNAPPROVED ADULT: Augmentation of SSRI rx for OCD: start 1 mg/d po, max 6 mg/d. Adjunctive rx for PTSD: start 0.5 mg po q hs, max 3 mg/d.

UNAPPROVED PEDS: Aggression: 0.5–1.5 mg/d po.

FORMS: Trade only: tabs 0.25, 0.5, 1, 2, 3, 4, mg (1 mg tab is scored). Orally disintegrating tabs (M-TAB) 0.5, 1, 2, 3, 4 mg. Oral solution. 1 mg/mL. Long-acting IM formulation (Consta) 25, 37.5 mg and 50 mg vials (for gluteal injection use 2-inch needles; for deltoid injection use the 1-inch needle).

NOTES: Greater tendency to produce extrapyramidal SE (EPS) than other atypicals. EPS reported in neonates following use in the third trimester of pregnancy; may cause ↑ weight, hyperglycemia, or new onset diabetes. Monitor closely. Patients with Parkinson disease and dementia have ↑ sensitivity to SE such as EPS, confusion, falls, and neuroleptic malignant syndrome. Solution is compatible with water, coffee, orange juice, and low-fat milk but is NOT compatible with tea or cola. Place orally disintegrating tablets on tongue, do not chew. Establish tolerability with oral form before starting long-acting injection; alternate injections between buttocks. Half-life: 20 hr (po); 3–6 days (IM, drug effects may persist 7–8 wk after last dose); lower dose for elderly.

DRUG INTERACTIONS: Fluoxetine and paroxetine ↑ risperidone levels; risperidone may antagonize the effects of levodopa and dopamine and may potentiate the effects of hypotensive drugs; clozapine may decrease the clearance of risperidone; carbamazepine and other enzyme inducers (phenytoin, rifampin, phenobarbital) may decrease levels of risperidone; risperidone ↑ levels of valproate.

Ziprasidone (*Geodon*) ▶L ♀C ▶- $$$$$

WARNING: May prolong QTc. Avoid with drugs that prolong QTc or in those with long QT syndrome or cardiac arrhythmias. Monitor K+, Mg++, glucose, ECG.

ADULT: Schizophrenia: start 20 mg po bid with food; may ↑ at >2-day intervals to max 80 mg po bid. Acute agitation in schizophrenia: 10–20 mg IM, May repeat 10 mg dose q 2 hr or 20 mg dose q 4 hr to max 40 mg/d, switch to po ASAP. Bipolar mania: start 40 mg po bid with food; may ↑ to 60–80 mg bid on day 2. Usual dose is 40–80 mg bid.

PEDS: Not approved in children.

FORMS: Trade only: Caps 20, 40, 60, 80 mg. Susp 10 mg/mL. IM formulation (acute use): 20 mg/mL single-dose vial.

NOTES: Half-life 4–7 hr. *Should be taken with food (doubles bioavailability).*

DRUG INTERACTIONS: May antagonize effects of levodopa and dopamine agonists; do not use with drugs that prolong QTc; may enhance hypotensive effects of antihypertensive drugs; little interaction with lithium, dextromethorphan, contraceptives, benzotropine, propanolol, lorazepam, cimetidine, Maalox. Interactions with carbamazepine and ketoconazole.

ANXIOLYTICS/HYPNOTICS: BENZODIAZEPINES

GENERAL NOTE:

- Associated with abuse, dependence, withdrawal reactions, oversedation, cognitive and motor impairment. To avoid withdrawal, gradually taper when discontinuing after prolonged use. All benzodiazepines are **Schedule IV controlled drugs (US DEA)**

- Use cautiously in the elderly; may accumulate and lead to SE. Sedative-hypnotics have been associated with severe allergic reactions and complex sleep behaviors including sleep driving, sedation, ↑ the risk of respiratory depression. Alcohol use should be limited

- Drug interactions: Most are metabolized via CYP 3A4: most other drugs metabolized through this pathway may ↑ the level of the benzodiazepine (except lorazepam, oxazepam, and temazepam which are less affected by severe hepatic disease). Other agents that ↑ benzodiazepine levels include: cimetidine, floxetine, ketoconazole, metoprolol, propanolol, estrogens, alcohol, erythromycin, disulfiram, valproic acid, nefazodone, and isoniazid. Benzodiazepine level may be decreased by carbamazepine, rifampin, and antacids

- Increased risk of congenital malformations (cleft palate, CNS disorders)

TABLE 28.2.   Classification of Benzodiazepines

Overview		
	High potency	**Low potency**
Short acting	Alprazolam (*Xanax*), lorazepam (*Ativan*), triazolam (*Halcion*)	Oxazepam (*Serax*), Temazepam (*Restoril*)
Long acting	Clonazepam (*Klonopin*), estazolam (*ProSom*)	Diazepam (*Valium*), clorazepate (*Tranxene*), quazepam (*Doral*), flurazepam (*Dalmane*), chlordiazepoxide (*Librium*)

A. LONG HALF-LIFE (25–100 HR)

Bromazepam (*Lectopam*)►L ♀D ▶ - $

ADULT: Canada only. 6–18 mg/d po in equally divided doses.

PEDS: Not approved in children.

FORMS: Generic/trade: tabs 1.5, 3, 6 mg.

NOTES: Do not exceed 3 mg/d initially in the elderly or debilitated; gradually taper when discontinuing after prolonged use; half-life ~20 hr in adults but ↑ in elderly. Cimetidine may prolong elimination.

Chlordiazepoxide (*Librium*) ►LK ♀D▶ - ©IV $$

ADULT: Anxiety: 5–25 mg po tid–qid or 25–50 mg IM/IV tid–qid (acute/severe anxiety). Acute alcohol withdrawal: 50–100 mg po/IM/IV, repeat q 3–4 hr prn up to 300 mg/d.

PEDS: Anxiety and > 6 yo: 5–10 mg po bid–qid.

FORMS: Generic/trade: caps 5, 10, 25 mg.

NOTES: Half-life: 5–30 hr (chlordiazepoxide), 3–200 hr (active metabolites); will accumulate with x dosing. Slower onset of action than valium. In anxiety: once-a-day dosing possible.

Clonazepam (*Klonopin, Klonopin Wafer, ♣Rivotril, Clonapam*) ►LK ♀D▶ - ©IV $

ADULT: Panic disorder: 0.25 mg po bid, increase by 0.125–0.25 mg q 3 days to max of 4 mg/d. Akinetic or myoclonic seizures: start 0.5 mg po tid. ↑ by 0.5–1 mg q 3 days prn; max 20 mg/d.

PEDS: Akinetic or myoclonic seizures, Lennox–Gastaut syndrome (petit mal variant), or absence seizures (≤10 yo or ≤30 kg): 0.01–0.03 mg/kg/d po divided bid–tid; ↑ by 0.25–0.5 mg q 3 days prn. Max 0.1–0.2 mg/kg/d divided tid.

UNAPPROVED ADULT: Neuralgias: 2–4 mg po/d. Restless legs syndrome: start 0.25 mg po qhs; max 2 mg q hs. REM sleep behavior disorder: 1–2 mg po q hs.

FORMS: Generic/trade: Tabs 0.5, 1, 2 mg. Orally disintegrating tabs (approved for panic disorder only) 0.125, 0.25, 0.5, 1, 2 mg.

NOTES: Half-life 18–50 hr. No active metabolites; Contraindicated in hepatic failure or acute narrow angle glaucoma; rapid onset for anxiety relief. Long half-life allows for once/d dosing. Usual therapeutic range = 20–80 ng/mL.

Clorazepate (*Tranxene, Tranxene SD*) ►LK ♀D▶ - ©IV $$

ADULT: Anxiety: Start 7.5–15 mg po qhs or bid–tid, usual effective dose 15–60 mg/d. Acute alcohol withdrawal: 60–90 mg/d on first day divided bid–tid, gradually ↓dose to 7.5–15 mg/d over 5 days. Max dose is 90 mg/d; May transfer pts to single-dose tabs (Tranxene- SD) when stabilized.

PEDS: Not approved in children < 9 yo.

FORMS: Generic/trade: tabs 3.75, 7.5, 15 mg. Trade only (Tranxene-SD): extended-release tabs 11.25, 22.5 mg.

NOTES: Half-life 40–50 hr. Will accumulate with x dosing. May be used once/d for anxiety; metabolized by P450 isoenzymes. Avoid in elderly and patients with hepatic dysfunction (slowed metabolism).

Diazepam (*Valium, Diastat AcuDial, ♣Vivol, E Pam, Diazemuls*) ►LK ♀D▶ - ©IV $

ADULT: Status epilepticus: 5–10 mg IV. Repeat q 10–15 min prn to max 30 mg. Epilepsy, adjunctive rx: 2–10 mg po bid–qid. Increased seizure activity: 0.2–0.5 mg/kg (rectal gel) to max 20 mg/d. Skeletal muscle spasm, spasticity related to cerebral palsy, paraplegia, athetosis, stiff man syndrome: 2–10 mg po/PR tid–qid, 5–10 mg IM/IV initially, then 5–10 mg q 3–4 hr prn; ↓ dose in elderly. Anxiety: 2–10 mg po bid–qid or 2–20 mg IM/IV, repeat dose in 3–4 hr prn. Alcohol withdrawal: 10 mg po tid–qid × 24 hr then 5 mg po tid–qid prn.

PEDS: Skeletal muscle spasm: 0.1–0.8 mg/kg/d po/PR divided tid–qid; 0.04–0.2 mg/kg/dose IV/IM q 2–4 hr. Max dose 0.6 mg/kg within 8 hr. Status epilepticus, age 1 month to 5 yo: 0.2–0.5 mg IV slowly q 2–5 min to max 5 mg. Status epilepticus, >5 yo: 1 mg IV slowly q 2–5 min to max 10 mg. Repeat q 2–4 hr prn. Epilepsy, adjunctive rx, age >6 months: 1–2.5 mg po tid–qid; gradually ↑ to max 30 mg/d; ↑ seizure activity: (rectal gel, age >2 yo): 0.5 mg/kg PR (2–5 yo), 0.3 mg/kg PR (6–11 yo), or 0.2 mg/kg PR (>12 yo). Max 20 mg. May repeat in 4–12 hr prn.

UNAPPROVED ADULT: Loading dose strategy for alcohol withdrawal: 10–20 mg po or 10 mg slow IV in closely monitored setting, then repeat similar or lower dose q 1–2 hr prn until sedated. Further doses should be unnecessary due to long half-life. Restless legs syndrome: 0.5–4 mg po q hs.

FORMS: Generic/trade: tabs 2, 5, 10 mg. Generic only: oral solution 5 mg/5 mL. Oral concentrate (Intensol) 5 mg/mL. Trade only: rectal gel (Diastat) 2.5 mg/0.5 mL, 5 mg/mL, 10 mg/2 mL, 15 mg/3 mL, 20 mg/4 mL. Rectal gel (Diastat AcuDial) 10 mg/2 mL, 20 mg/4 mL.

NOTES: Half-life: 30–60 hr (diazepam), 30–100 hr (desmethyldiazepam), respiratory and CNS depression may occur. Caution in liver disease; abuse potential. Long half-life may ↑ the risk of adverse effects in the elderly.

DRUG INTERACTIONS: Cimetidine, oral contraceptives, disulfiram, fluoxetine, isoniazid, ketoconazole, metoprolol, propoxyphene, propranolol, and valproic acid may ↑ diazepam conc. Diazepam may ↑ digoxin and phenytoin conc. Rifampin may ↑ diazepam metabolism; avoid (or ↓ diazepam dose) with protease inhibitors. Diastat AcuDial is for home use and allows dosing from 5 to 20 mg in 2.5 mg increments.

Flurazepam (*Dalmane*) ▶LK ♀X ▶ - ©IV $

ADULT: Insomnia: 15–30 mg po q hs.

PEDS: Not approved in children <15 yo.

FORMS: Generic/trade: caps 15, 30 mg.

NOTES: Half-life: 2–3 hr (flurazepam); 40–100 hr (active metabolite); for short-term tx of insomnia; monitor CBC, LFTs if prolonged tx; taper dose gradually to D/C.

B. MEDIUM HALF-LIFE (10–15 HR)

Estazolam (*ProSom*) ▶LK ♀X ▶ - ©IV $$

ADULT: Insomnia: 1–2 mg po qhs for up to 12 wk. Reduce dose to 0.5 mg in elderly, small, or debilitated pts.

PEDS: Not approved in children.

FORMS: Generic/trade: tabs 1, 2 mg.

NOTES: For short-term rx of insomnia. Monitor CBC, LFTs, urinalysis, blood chemistries if prolonged rx; taper dose gradually to D/C.

DRUG INTERACTIONS: Avoid with ketoconazole or itraconazole; caution with less potent inhibitors of CYP3A4.

Lorazepam (*Ativan*) ▶LK ♀D ▶ - ©IV $

ADULT: Anxiety: start 0.5–1 mg po bid–tid, usual dose is 2–6 mg/d. Max dose 10 mg/d po. Anxiolytic/sedation: 0.04–0.05 mg/kg IV/IM; usual dose 2 mg, max 4 mg. Insomnia: 2–4 mg po q hs. Status epilepticus: 4 mg IV over 2 min; may repeat in 10–15 min.

PEDS: Not approved in children.

UNAPPROVED ADULT: Alcohol withdrawal: 1–2 mg po/IM/IV q 2–4 hr prn or 2 mg po/IM/IV q 6 hr × 24 hr then 1 mg q 6 hr × 8 doses. Chemotherapy-induced N/V: 1–2 mg po/SL/IV/IM q 6 hr.

UNAPPROVED PEDS: status epilepticus: 0.05–0.1 mg/kg IV over 2–5 min; may repeat 0.05 mg/kg × 1 in 10–15 min. Do not exceed 4 mg as single dose. Anxiolytic/sedation: 0.05 mg/kg/dose q 4–8 h po/IV, max 2 mg/dose. Chemotherapy-induced N/V: 0.05 mg/kg po/IV q 8–12 hr prn, max 3 mg/dose; or 0.02–0.05 mg/kg IV q 6 hr prn, max 2 mg/dose.

FORMS: Generic/trade: tabs 0.5, 1, 2 mg. Generic only: oral concentrate 2 mg/mL. Injectable form: 4 mg/mL solution (IV, IM).

NOTES: Half-life 10–20 hr. No active metabolites; for short-term rx of insomnia. Best choice in pts with serious or x medical problems; metabolism is not significantly affected by age (elderly may be more susceptible to SE). IM form is the only available benzodiazepine with rapid, complete, predictable absorption.

Nitrazepam (♣*Mogadon*) ▶L ♀C ▶ - $

ADULT: Canada. Insomnia: 5–10 mg po q hs.

PEDS: Canada only. Myoclonic seizures: 0.3–1 mg/kg/d in 3 divided doses.

FORMS: Generic/trade: tabs 5, 10 mg.

NOTES: Use lower doses in elderly/debilitated.

Temazepam (*Restoril*) ▶LK ♀X ▶ - ©IV $

ADULT: Insomnia: 7.5–30 mg po q hs ×7–10 day.

PEDS: Not approved in children.

FORMS: Generic/trade: caps 15, 30 mg. Trade only: caps 7.5, 22.5 mg.

NOTES: Half-life 8–25 hr; short-term rx of insomnia. Monitor CBC, LFTs, U/A, blood chemistries if prolonged rx; taper dose gradually to D/C.

C. SHORT HALF-LIFE (<12 HR)

Alprazolam (*Xanax, Xanax XR, Niravam*) ▶LK ♀D ▶- ©IV $

ADULT: Anxiety: start 0.25–0.5 mg po tid; may ↑ q 3–4 days to a max dose of 4 mg/d. Use 0.25 mg po bid in elderly or debilitated pts. Panic disorder: start 0.5 mg po tid (or 0.5–1 mg po/d of Xanax XR), may ↑ by up to 1 mg/d q 3–4 days to usual effective dose of 5–6 mg/d (3–6 mg/d for Xanax XR), max dose is 10 mg/d.

PEDS: Not approved in children.

FORMS: Trade only: orally disintegrating tab (Niravam) 0.25, 0.5, 1, 2 mg. Generic/trade: tabs 0.25, 0.5, 1, 2 mg. Extended-release tabs: 0.5, 1, 2, 3 mg. Generic only: oral concentrate (Intensol) 1 mg/mL.

NOTES: Half-life 12 hr, but need to give tid; fast onset for anxiety relief but high incidence of interdose anxiety (divide administration time evenly during waking hours). Dependence and withdrawal are serious problems (is no longer a first-line drug for treatment of anxiety.

DRUG INTERACTIONS: Don't give with antifungals (i.e., ketoconazole, itraconazole); caution with macrolides, propoxyphene, oral contraceptives, TCAs, cimetidine, antidepressants, anticonvulsants, paroxetine, sertraline, and others that inhibit CYP 3A4.

Oxazepam (*Serax*) ▶LK ♀D ▶- ©IV $$$

ADULT: Anxiety: 10–30 mg po tid–qid. Acute alcohol withdrawal: 15–30 mg po tid–qid.

PEDS: Not approved in children <6 yo.

UNAPPROVED ADULT: Restless legs syndrome: start 10 mg po q hs; max 40 mg qhs.

FORMS: Generic/trade: caps 10, 15, 30 mg. Trade only: tabs 15 mg.

NOTES: Half-life 8 hr.

Triazolam (*Halcion*) ▶LK ♀ X ▶- ©IV $

ADULT: Hypnotic: 0.125–0.25 mg po q hs ×7–10 days, max dose is 0.5 mg/d. Start 0.125 mg/d in elderly or debilitated pts.

PEDS: Not approved in children.

UNAPPROVED ADULT: Start 0.125 mg po q hs for restless legs syndrome; max 0.5 mg q hs.

FORMS: Generic/trade: tabs 0.125, 0.25 mg.

NOTES: Half-life: 1.5–5.5 hr anterograde amnesia may occur; taper dose gradually to D/C.

DRUG INTERACTIONS: Don't use with protease inhibitors, ketoconazole, itraconazole, or nefazodone; caution with macrolides, cimetidine, and other CYP 3A4 inhibitors.

ANXIOLYTICS/HYPNOTICS: OTHER

NOTE: Sedative-hypnotics: associated with severe allergic reactions, complex sleep behaviors (also sleep driving). Use caution; discuss with pts.

Buspirone (*BuSpar, Vanspar*) ▶K ♀B ▶- $$$

ADULT: Anxiety: start 15 mg/d (7.5 mg po bid), ↑ by 5 mg/d q 2–3 days to usual dose of 30 mg/d, maximum dose is 60 mg/d.

PEDS: Not approved in children.

FORMS: Generic/trade: tabs 5, 10, 15 mg. Trade only: dividose tab 15, 30 mg (scored, easily bisected or tri-sected). Generic: tabs 7.5 mg.

NOTES: Slower onset than benzodiazepines; optimum effect requires 3–4 wk of rx (pt may be started on benzodiazepine and buspirone for 2 wk, then slow tapering of the benzodiazepine); less effective if pt has taken benzodiazepines in the past; lacks sedation and dependence associated with benzodiazepines. Half-life: 2–11 hr. No active metabolites.

DRUG INTERACTIONS: Don't use with MAOIs; caution with itraconazole, cimetidine, nefazodone, erythromycin, and other CYP 3A4 inhibitors. Avoid grapefruit juice.

Chloral hydrate (*Aquachloral Supprettes, Somnote*) ▶LK ♀C ▶+ ©IV $

ADULT: Sedative: 250 mg po/PR tid after meals. Hypnotic: 500–1,000 mg po/PR q hs Acute alcohol withdrawal: 500–1,000 mg po/ PR q 6 hr prn.

PEDS: Sedative: 25 mg/kg/d po/PR divided tid–qid, up to 500 mg tid. Hypnotic: 50 mg/kg po/PR q hs, up to max of 1 g. Preanesthetic: 25–50 mg/kg po/PR before procedure.

UNAPPROVED PEDS: Sedative: higher than approved doses 75–100 mg/kg po/PR.

FORMS: Generic only: syrup 500 mg/5 mL, rectal suppositories 500 mg. Trade only: caps 500 mg; rectal suppositories: 325, 650 mg.

NOTES: Give syrup in ½ glass fruit juice, water. Half-life: 8–10 hr. Tolerance and dependence develop; highly lethal in overdose.

DRUG INTERACTIONS: IV furosemide may cause flushing and labile BP; additive effects with CNS depressants.

Eszopiclone (*Lunesta*) ▶L ♀C ▶? ©IV $$$$

ADULT: Insomnia: 2 mg po q hs prn, max 3 mg. Elderly: 1 mg po q hs prn, max 2 mg.

PEDS: Not approved for children.

FORMS: Trade only: tabs 1, 2, 3 mg.

NOTES: Half-life: 6 hr. Nonbenzodiazepine hypnotic; take immediately before bedtime (rapid onset of action). Longer duration of action than Zolpidem CR (Ambien CR) and zaleplon (Sonata); no dependence or withdrawal.

DRUG INTERACTIONS: Drugs that inhibit CYP 3A4 such as ketoconazole may ↑ eszopiclone levels. Drugs that induce CYP3A4 such as rifampin may decrease eszopiclone levels; potentiates other CNS depressants (such as alcohol).

Ramelteon (*Rozerem*) ▶L ♀C ▶? $$$

ADULT: Insomnia: 8 mg po q hs. Doses >8 mg are not approved but have been used.

PEDS: Not approved for children.

FORMS: Trade only: tabs 8 mg.

NOTES: Is a Melatonin MT1 and MT2 agonist; do not take with/after high-fat meal. No evidence of dependence or abuse liability. Avoid with severe liver disease; may ↓ testosterone and ↑ prolactin levels. Half-life: 1–2.5 hr.

DRUG INTERACTIONS: Inhibitors or CYP 1A2 (such as fluvoxamine, may ↑ blood level 70-fold), 3A4 (such as ketoconazole), and 2C9 may increase serum level and effect. Strong inducers of cytochrome enzymes, such as rifampin, may decrease efficacy of ramelteon; ramelteon may potentiate effect of other CNS depressants (alcohol).

Zaleplon (*Sonata*, ✦*Starnoc*) ▶L ♀C ▶- ©IV $$$

ADULT: Insomnia: 5–10 mg po q hs prn, maximum 20 mg.

PEDS: Not approved in children.

FORMS: Trade only: caps 5, 10 mg.

NOTES: Nonbenzodiazepine hypnotic; half-life: 1 hr; useful if problems with sleep initiation or morning grogginess; for short-term rx of insomnia. Take immediately before bedtime or after going to bed; use 5 mg dose in pts with mild–moderate hepatic impairment, elderly pts. Do not use for benzodiazepine or alcohol withdrawal.

DRUG INTERACTIONS: Rifampin, phenytoin, carbamazepine, and phenobarbital. Cimetidine may ↑ serum level; potentiate other CNS depressants (alcohol).

Zolpidem (*Ambien, Ambien CR*) ▶L ♀C ▶+ ©IV $$$$

ADULT: Hypnotic: 10 mg po q hs (standard tabs) or 12.5 mg po q hs (controlled release tabs). Max dose is 10 mg (regular release) or 12.5 mg (controlled release). Start with 5 mg (regular release) in elderly or debilitated.

PEDS: Not approved in children.

FORMS: Generic/trade: tabs 5, 10 mg. Trade only: controlled release tabs 6.25, 12.5 mg.

NOTES: Half-life: 2.5 hr; CR useful if problems with sleep initiation and maintenance. Ambien regular release is for short-term rx of problems with sleep initiation. Possible anterograde amnesia and morning "hangover" at normal dosages; no dependence or withdrawal; may be used during lactation; do not use for benzodiazepine or alcohol withdrawal.

DRUG INTERACTIONS: Potentiate other CNS depressants.

Zopiclone (✦*Imovane*) ▶L ♀D ▶- $

ADULT: Canada only. Short-term rx of insomnia: 5–7.5 mg po q hs. In elderly or debilitated, use 3.75 mg q hs initially, and ↑ prn to 5–7.5 mg q hs. Max 7.5 mg q hs.

PEDS: Not approved in children.

FORMS: Generic/trade: tabs 5, 7.5 mg. Generic only: tabs 3.75 mg.

NOTES: Rx should usually not exceed 7–10 days without reevaluation.

COMBINATION DRUGS

NOTE
- Monitor for anxiety, agitation, panic attacks, insomnia, irritability, hostility, impulsivity, akathisia, mania, or hypomania and for the worsening of depression or the emergence of suicidality, particularly early in therapy or after increases in dose.
- Antidepressants ↑ the risk of suicidal thinking and behavior in children, adolescents, and young adults; weigh the risks and benefits before starting rx and then monitor closely.
- The use of atypical antipsychotics to treat behavioral problems in pts with dementia has been associated with higher mortality rates.
- Atypical antipsychotics have been associated with weight gain, dyslipidemia, hyperglycemia, and diabetes mellitus: monitor closely.
- Multiple drug interactions.

Limbitrol (chlordiazepoxide + amitriptyline, *Limbitrol DS*) ▶LK ♀D ▶ - ©IV $$$

ADULT: Rarely used; depression/anxiety: 1 tab po tid—qid may ↑ up to 6 tablets/d.

PEDS: Not approved in children <12 yo.

FORMS: Generic/trade: tabs 5/12.5, 10/25 mg chlordiazepoxide/amitriptyline.

Symbyax (olanzapine + fluoxetine) ▶LK ♀C ▶ - $$$$$

WARNING: Observe SSRI pts for worsening depression/emergence of suicidal thoughts (see above note). The use of atypical antipsychotics to treat behavioral problems in dementia has been associated with higher mortality rates.

ADULT: Bipolar depression: start: 6 mg/25 mg po q PM; may start 3 mg/25 mg po q PM in elderly or ♀ pts; max 18 mg/75 mg/d; info: for acute rx; taper dose gradually to D/C.

PEDS: Not approved in children <12 yo.

FORMS: Trade only: caps (olanzapine/fluoxetine) 3/25, 6/25, 6/50, 12/25, 12/50 mg.

NOTES: Efficacy beyond 8 wk not established. Monitor weight, glucose, triglycerides before initiation and during rx. Pregnancy exposure to fluoxetine associated with premature delivery, ↓ birth weight, ↓ Apgar scores; ↓ dose with liver disease.

DRUG INTERACTIONS: Contraindicated with thioridazine, cisapride, tryptophan, or MAOIs; caution with lithium, phenytoin, TCAs, ASA, NSAIDs, warfarin.

DRUG DEPENDENCE THERAPY

Acamprosate (*Campral*) ▶K ♀C ▶? $$$$

ADULT: Maintenance of abstinence from alcohol: 666 mg (2 tabs) po tid. Start after alcohol withdrawal and when pt is abstinent.

PEDS: Not approved in children.

FORMS: Trade: delayed-release tabs 333 mg.

NOTES: ↓ dose to 333 mg if CrCl 30—50 mL/min. Contraindicated if CrCl <30 mL/min. Half-life 20—33 hr. Adverse drug reactions: diarrhea, nausea, headaches, rash, insomnia, anxiety, depression.

DRUG INTERACTIONS: Does not inhibit cytochrome enzymes.

Buprenorphine (*Subutex, Suboxone*) ▶L ♀C ▶ - ©III $$$$$

WARNING: Synthetic opioid; Subutex is buprenorphine; Suboxone is buprenorphine + naloxone (preferred for maintenance); half-life: 37 hr for buprenorphine and 1.1 hr for naloxone; respiratory and CNS depression can occur especially if used IV; Buprenorphine produces opioid dependence. The naloxone in Suboxone can cause marked opioid withdrawal if used IV or SL by opioid-dependent pts; cases of hepatic failure and allergic reactions.

ADULT: Rx of opioid dependence: maintenance: 16 mg SL daily. Can individualize to range of 4—24 mg SL daily; induction: Subutex should be used for induction when sx of withdrawal are present. To avoid precipitating withdrawal, pts may be given 8 mg of Subutex on day 1 and 16 mg of Subutex on day 2. From day 3, give Suboxone: 16 mg/d. For maintenance: use Suboxone and ↑ the dosage by 2—4 mg/d to suppress opioid-withdrawal sx; the range is 4—24 mg/d. Administer Subutex at least 4 hr after use of heroin or other short-acting opioids.

PEDS: Not approved in children.

FORMS: Trade only: Suboxone: SL tabs 2/0.5 mg buprenorphine/naloxone and 8/2 mg buprenorphine/naloxone. Subutex: 2 or 8 mg sublingual tablets of buprenorphine.

NOTES: Suboxone preferred over Subutex (which does not contain naloxone) for unsupervised administration. Titrate in 2–4 mg increments/decrements to maintain rx compliance and prevent withdrawal. Tablets must be placed under the tongue until dissolved (swallowing ↓ bioavailability). Prescribers must complete training and apply for special DEA number. See www.suboxone.com.

DRUG INTERACTIONS: Drug interactions with CYP 3 A4 inhibitors (ketoconazole, erythromycin, protease inhibitors) which ↑ the levels of buprenorphine); CYP 3 A4 inducers (carbamazepine, St. John's wort) may decrease buprenorphine levels; reports of coma and death with benzodiazepines or other sedative-hypnotics (after self-injection of crushed buprenorphine).

Clonidine (*Catapres, Catapres-TTS, ♣Dixarift*) ▶LK ♀C▷? $$

ADULT: HTN: start 0.1 mg po bid, usual maintenance dose 0.2–1.2 mg/d divided bid–tid, max 2.4 mg/d. Transdermal (Catapres-TTS): start 0.1 mg/24 hr patch q wk, titrate to desired effect, max dose 0.6 mg/24 hr (two of 0.3 mg/24 hr patches). Used for opioid withdrawal: oral: day 1: 0.1–0.2 mg po q 4 hr up to 1 mg; day 2–4: 0.1–0.2 mg po q 4 hr up to 1.2 mg; day 5 to completion: reduce 0.2 mg/d; given in divided doses; the night-time dose should be reduced last; or ↓ total dosage by 1/2 q day not to exceed 0.4 mg/d. Patch: Clonidine patch (3 strengths: #1, #2, #3), delivering over one week the equivalent of a daily dose of oral clonidine (e.g., #2 patch = 0.2 mg oral clonidine, daily, etc.). Apply one #2 patch for pts <100 lbs, two #2 patches for pts 100–200 lb, and three #2 patches for pts >200 lb. On day 1 (the day the patch is applied), oral clonidine may be necessary—0.2 mg q 6 hr for 24 hr, then 0.1 mg q 6 hr for the second 24 hr. Remove the patches if systolic pressure <80 mm Hg or diastolic pressure <50 mm Hg. Advantages of patch: pts don't have to take pills x times/d, even blood levels of medication, buildup of withdrawal sx during night is prevented. Monitor BP before and 20 min after each dose of clonidine: risk of low BP (especially in thin pts). Give adequate fluid.

PEDS: HTN: Start 5–7 mcg/kg/d po divided q 6–12 hr, ↑ at 5–7 day intervals to 5–25 mcg/kg/d divided q 6 hr; max 0.9 mg/d. Transdermal not recommended in children.

UNAPPROVED ADULT: HTN urgency: Initially 0.1–0.2 mg po followed by 0.1 mg q 1 hr prn up to a total dose of 0.5–0.7 mg. Menopausal flushing: 0.1–0.4 mg/d po divided bid–tid; transdermal applied wkly 0.1 mg/d. Tourette syndrome: 3–5 mcg/kg/d po divided bid–qid. Opioid withdrawal, adjunct: 0.1–0.3 mg po tid–qid or 0.1–0.2 mg po q 4 hr tapering off over days 4–10. Alcohol withdrawal, adjunct: 0.1–0.2 mg po q 4 hr prn. Smoking cessation: start 0.1 mg po tid, increase 0.1 mg/d at wkly intervals to 0.75 mg/d as tolerated; transdermal (Catapres TTS): 0.1–0.2 mg/24 hr patch q wk for 2–3 wk after cessation. ADHD: 5 mcg/kg/d po x 8 wk; PTSD: start 0.1 mg po hs, max 0.6 mg/d in divided doses.

UNAPPROVED PEDS: ADHD: Start 0.05 mg qhs, ↑ based on response over 8 wk to max 0.2 mg/d (<45 kg) or 0.4 mg/d (>45 kg) in 2–4 divided doses. Tourette syndrome: 3–5 mcg/kg/d po divided bid–qid.

FORMS: Generic/trade: Tabs, nonscored 0.1, 0.2, 0.3 mg. Trade only: transdermal wkly patch 0.1 mg/d (TTS-1), 0.2 mg/d (TTS-2), 0.3 mg/d (TTS-3).

NOTES: Sedation, bradycardia, rebound HTN with abrupt discontinuation of tabs, especially at doses ≥ 0.8 mg/d; taper rx over 4–7 days to avoid rebound HTN. Dispose of patches carefully, keep away from children. Remove patch before MRI to avoid skin burns. SE: hypotension, sedation, dizziness, dry mouth, nausea, constipation, depression, anxiety, ↑ weight, and photophobia. Half-life:12–16 hr.

DRUG INTERACTIONS: ↑ sedation effects of alcohol, barbiturates, sedative/hypnotics; TCAs antidepressants inhibit the hypotensive effects of clonidine; antihypertensive drugs ↑ the hypotensive effects of clonidine.

Disulfiram (*Antabuse*) ▶L ♀C▷? $

WARNING: Never give to the intoxicated; drug interactions; do not give if severe cardiovascular or pulmonary disease, severe liver disease; leads to elevated levels of acetaldehyde with toxic effects.

ADULT: Sobriety: 125–500 mg po/d.

PEDS: Not approved in children.

FORMS: Trade only: tabs 250, 500 mg.

NOTES: Must abstain from any alcohol for ≥12 hr before using. Reactions: flushing, headaches, nausea, vomiting, dyspnea, diaphoresis, hypotension, palpitations, anxiety, blurred vision, confusion (supportive rx needed) and possible severe reactions (respiratory depression, arrhythmias, heart failure, seizures, death). Disulfiram reaction may occur for up to 2 wk after discontinuing disulfiram; hepatotoxicity. Rare complications: peripheral neuropathy, optic neuritis, psychosis; half-life 60–120 hr.

DRUG INTERACTIONS: Metronidazole and alcohol in any form (e.g., cough syrups, tonics) contraindicated. INH may cause ataxia and mental status changes. Disulfiram may ↑ levels of diazepam, paraldehyde, phenytoin, TCAs, anticoagulants, barbiturates, benzodiazepines.

Methadone (*Diskets, Dolophine, Methadose ♣Metadol*) ▶L ♀C▷+ ◎II $

WARNING: Synthetic opioid, opioid-receptor agonist used for detoxification and maintenance rx of opioid addiction; produces tolerance and dependence; can only be prescribed in a federally approved rx center. The drug may be continued if the pt is hospitalized for another reason. High doses (mean: 400 mg/d) have been inconclusively associated with QTc ↑ and arrhythmia (torsade de pointes), esp. if risk factors. Methadone peak resp. depressant effects typically occur later, last longer than peak analgesic effects. Caution in opiate-naïve pts. Elimination half-life (8–59 hr) is far longer than its duration of action (4–8 hr); monitor accordingly. Use caution with ↑ doses. Overdose can lead to respiratory and cardiovascular depression, coma, and death. Pts tolerant to other opioid may be incompletely tolerant to methadone; deaths have occurred from iatrogenic overdose or combination with MAOIs. Women who conceive while on methadone should continue; however, the newborn will require medical care for withdrawal sx. Chronic dosing may induce own metabolism.

ADULT: Severe pain in opioid-tolerant pts: 2.5–10 mg IM/SC/po q 3–4 hr prn. Opioid dependence: 20–100 mg po/d. Rx > 21 days is considered maintenance (40–80 mg/d is usually effective to prevent relapse). Detoxification: for short-term use (max 21 days): give 10–20 mg po on day 1; ↑ by 5–10 mg/d over the next few days, up to 40 mg/d in a single or divided dose. Maintain for 2–5 days and then decrease by 5 mg qd.

PEDS: Not approved in children.

UNAPPROVED PEDS: Pain ≤ 12 yo: 0.7 mg/kg/24 hr divided q 4–6 hr po/SC/IM/IV prn; max 10 mg/dose.

FORMS: Generic/trade: Tabs: 5, 10 mg. Dispersible tabs 40 mg. Oral concentrate: 10 mg/mL generic only; oral solution: 5 and 10 mg/5 mL.

NOTES: ↑ dose as high as necessary to relieve cancer pain or nonmalignant pain where chronic opioids are necessary. Every 8–12 hr dosing may ↓ the risk of accumulation and overdose. Rx for opioid dependency >3 wk is maintenance and only permitted in approved programs certified by SAMSA and approved by designated state authority; certified rx programs dispense methadone in oral form only and according to federal opioid rx standards; monitor: Cr at baseline; s/sx resp. depression especially w/ start, incr. dose, or opioid conversion. Avoid abrupt cessation: taper dose gradually to D/C if at risk for physical dependence (abrupt cessation may cause a withdrawal syndrome including restlessness, irritability, anxiety, insomnia, mydriasis, lacrimation, rhinorrhea, sneezing, yawning, sweating, ↑ body temp, chills, piloerection, myalgia, backache, arthralgia, weakness, abdominal and muscle cramps, muscle twitching, anorexia, N/V, diarrhea, ↑BP, ↑RR, ↑HR).

DRUG INTERACTIONS: leading to ↓ methadone levels with enzyme-inducing HIV drugs (efavirenz, nevirapine) and other potent inducers such as rifampin. Monitor for opiate withdrawal sx and ↑ dose if necessary. Rapid metabolizers require more frequent daily dosing. Potentiates effects of CNS depressants, effects of alcohol, sedative/hypnotics, narcotics, anesthetics, and TCAs; the combination of an MAOI and meperidine and fentanyl have led to deaths; carbamazepine may lower methadone levels; methadone ↑ desipramine levels.

Naltrexone (*ReVia, Depade, Vivitrol*) ▶LK ♀C▷? $$$$

WARNING: Opioid antagonist; hepatotoxicity with higher than approved dose; may precipitate acute opiate withdrawal in addicted pts. Accidental OD may lead to death by respiratory depression.

ADULT: Alcohol dependence: 50 mg po/d. Extended-release injectable suspension: 380 mg IM q 4 wk or monthly. Opioid dependence: start 25 mg po/d, ↑ to 50 mg po/d if no sx of withdrawal.

PEDS: Not approved in children.

FORMS: Generic/trade: Tabs 50 mg. Trade only (Vivitrol): extended-release injectable suspension kits 380 mg.

NOTES: Avoid if recent (past 14 days) ingestion of opioids. Conflicting evidence of efficacy for chronic alcoholism: ↓ euphoria associated with alcohol consumption and craving. Half-life:13 hr (including active metabolite).

DRUG INTERACTIONS: blocks the analgesic effects of opioids (higher doses of analgesics will be needed for pain relief). Do not combine with disulfiram (hepatotoxic effects).

Nicotine gum (*Nicorette, Nicorette DS*) ▶LK ♀X▷- $$$$$

ADULT: Smoking cessation: Gradually taper 1 piece (2 mg) q 1–2 hr × 6 wk, 1 piece (2 mg) q 2–4 hr × 3 wk, then 1 piece (2 mg) q 4–8 hr × 3 wk; max 30 pieces/d of 2 mg gum or 24 pieces/d of 4 mg gum. Use 4 mg pieces (Nicorette DS) for high cigarette use (>24 cigarettes/d).

PEDS: Not approved in children.

FORMS: OTC/generic/trade: gum 2, 4 mg.

NOTES: Chew slowly and park between cheek and gum periodically. May cause N/V, hiccups. Coffee, juices, wine, and soft drinks may ↓ absorption. Avoid eating/drinking × 15 min before/during gum use; available in original, orange, or mint flavor. Do not use beyond 6 months; half-life: 1–2 hr.

Nicotine inhalation system (*Nicotrol Inhaler, ♣Nicorette inhaler*) ▶LK ♀D▷- $$$$$

ADULT: Smoking cessation: 6–16 cartridges/d × 12 wk.

PEDS: Not approved in children.

FORMS: Trade: Oral inhaler 10 mg/cartridge (4 mg nicotine delivered) with 42 cartridges/box.

NOTE: Half-life: 1–2 hr.

Nicotine lozenge (*Commit*) ▶LK ♀D ▶ - $$$$$

ADULT: Smoking cessation: If pts smoke <30 min after waking use 4 mg lozenge; others use 2 mg. Take 1–2 lozenges q 1–2 hr × 6 wk, then q 2–4 hr in wk 7–9, then q 4–8 hr in wk 10–12; length of rx 12 wk.

PEDS: Not approved in children.

FORMS: OTC/generic/trade: lozenge 2, 4 mg in 72, 168-count packages.

NOTES: Allow lozenge to dissolve, do not chew. Do not eat or drink within 15 min before use. Avoid other sources of nicotine. Half-life: 1–2 hr.

Nicotine nasal spray (*Nicotrol NS*) ▶LK ♀D ▶ - $$$$$

ADULT: Smoking cessation: 1–2 doses q hr, with each dose = 2 sprays, one in each nostril (1 spray = 0.5 mg nicotine). Minimum recommended: 8 doses/d, max 40 doses/d.

PEDS: Not approved in children.

FORMS: Trade only: nasal solution 10 mg/mL (0.5 mg/inhalation); 10 mL bottles.

NOTE: Half-life: 1–2 hr.

Nicotine patches (*Habitrol, NicoDerm CQ, Nicotrol, ♣Prostep*) ▶LK ♀D ▶ - $$$$

ADULT: Smoking cessation: start one patch (14–22 mg) daily and taper after 6 wk. Total duration of rx is 12 wk.

PEDS: Not approved in children.

FORMS: OTC/rx/generic/trade: patches 11, 22 mg/24 hr; 7, 14, 21 mg/24 hr (Habitrol and NicoDerm). OTC/trade: 15 mg/16 hr (Nicotrol).

NOTES: Ensure pt has stopped smoking. Dispose of safely; can be toxic to kids, pets. Remove opaque NicoDerm CQ patch prior to MRI procedures to avoid possible burns.

Varenicline (*Chantix*) ▶K C ♀▶? $$$$

WARNING: Has been associated with the development of suicidal ideations, changes in behavior, depressed mood and attempted/completed suicides—both during tx and after withdrawal. Unclear safety in serious psychiatric conditions.

ADULT: Smoking cessation: start 1 wk before smoking quit date; start 0.5 mg po/d for days 1–3, then 0.5 mg bid days 4–7, then 1 mg bid thereafter. Take after meals with full glass of water. Start 1 wk prior to cessation and continue × 12 wk. ↓ dosage if renal impairment.

PEDS: Not approved in children.

FORMS: Trade only: tabs 0.5, 1 mg.

NOTES: In severe renal dysfunction: ↓ max dose to 0.5 mg bid. If hemodialysis: may use 0.5 mg once/d if tolerated. Half-life: 17–24 hr. Does not reduce weight gain associated with smoking cessation.

DRUG INTERACTIONS: Cimetidine ↑ serum level of varenicline by 29%; SE if used with nicotine patches.

STIMULANTS/ADHD/ANOREXIANTS

NOTE: Sudden cardiac death in pts who have heart problems or defects, stroke and heart attacks in adults, ↑ BP and ↑ HR has been reported with stimulants at usual ADHD doses; assess prior to rx and avoid if cardiac conditions or structural abnormalities. Amphetamines are associated with high abuse potential and dependence with prolonged administration. Stimulants may also cause or ↑ underlying psychosis or induce a manic or mixed episode in bipolar disorder. They may produce in children and adolescents new psychotic sx (such as hearing voices, believing things that are not true, are suspicious) or new manic sx. They may produce or ↑ aggressive behavior or hostility. Problems with visual accommodation have also been reported with stimulants.

Amphetamine + dextroamphetamine (*Adderall, Adderall XR*) ▶L♀ C ▶ - ©II $$$$

WARNING: Requires a triplicate prescription; high potential for abuse, tolerance, and dependence. Chronic users may become suicidal upon abrupt cessation. Is contraindicated if HTN, hyperthyroidism, cardiac disease, glaucoma, psychotic pt or pts with substance abuse; risk of premature delivery and ↓ birth rate in infants born to mothers using amphetamines.

ADULT: Narcolepsy, standard release: start 10 mg po q am, ↑ by 10 mg q wk, max dose is 60 mg/d divided bid–tid at 4–6 hr intervals. ADHD, extended-release caps (Adderall XR): 20 mg po/d.

PEDS: ADHD, standard-release tabs: start 2.5 mg (3–5 yo) or 5 mg (≥6 yo) po qd–bid, ↑ by 2.5–5 mg q wk, max 40 mg/d. ADHD, extended-release caps (Adderall XR): If 6–12 yo, then start 5–10 mg po/d to a max of 30 mg/d; if 13–17 yo: start 10 mg po/d to a max of 20 mg/d. Not recommended if <3 yo. Narcolepsy, standard release: 6–12 yo: start 5 mg po/d,↑ by 5 mg q wk. Age >12 yo: start 10 mg po q AM, ↑ by 10 mg q wk, max dose is 60 mg/d, divided bid–tid at 4–6 hr intervals.

FORMS: Generic/trade: tabs 5, 7.5, 10, 12.5, 15, 20, 30 mg. Trade only: caps, extended release (Adderall XR) 5, 10, 15, 20, 25, 30 mg.

NOTES: Capsules may be opened and the beads sprinkled on applesauce; do not chew beads. Adderall XR should be given upon awakening. Avoid PM doses (do not give after 12 PM to avoid sleep problems). Monitor growth and use drug holidays when appropriate. May ↑ pulse and BP. May exacerbate bipolar or psychotic conditions.

DRUD INTERACTIONS: High blood levels of propoxyphene ↑ CNS stimulatory effects of Adderall (risk of seizures and death); Adderall ↑ activity of TCAs and tetracyclics (↑cardiovascular effects). Typical antipsychotics and lithium may inhibit CNS stimulatory effects of stimulants. Do not give with MAOIs (fatal reactions, HTN, seizures). Adderal delays absorption of ethosuximide, phenobarbital, phenytoin. Urinary alkalinizing agents ↑ blood levels and decrease excretion of amphetamines.

Armodafinil (*Nuvigil*) ▶L♀ C ▶? ©IV $$$$$

WARNING: Controlled substance (C-IV): can be abused or lead to dependence; serious rash, including Stevens–Johnson syndrome, of multiorgan hypersensitivity reactions.

ADULT: Obstructive sleep apnea/hypopnea syndrome and narcolepsy: 150–250 mg po q AM; inconsistent evidence for improved efficacy of 250 mg/d dose. Shift work sleep disorder: 150 mg po 1 hr prior to start of shift.

PEDS: Not approved in children.

FORMS: Trade only: tabs 50, 150, 250 mg.

NOTES: Is R-enantiomer of modafinil; ↓ dose with severe liver impairment. Rare cases of mania, delusions, hallucinations, and suicidal ideation.

DRUG INTERACTIONS: Weak inducer for substrates of CYP 3A 4/5 (e.g., carbamazepine, cyclosporine), which may require dose adjustments; may inhibit metabolism of substrates of CYP2C19 (e.g., omeprazole, diazepam, phenytoin). May ↓ efficacy of oral contraceptives; consider alternatives during rx. Do not use with MAOIs.

Atomoxetine (*Strattera*) ▶K♀ C ▶? $$$$$

WARNING: Is not a stimulant and not a controlled substance; severe liver injury and failure reported (discontinue if jaundice or ↑ LFTs), orthostatic hypotension, and syncope. ↑ risk of suicidal thinking and behavior in children and adolescents; weigh risks/benefits before starting, monitor closely for ↑ depression or emergence of suicidality or behaviors esp. early in rx or after ↑ dose. Monitor: anxiety, agitation, panic attacks, insomnia, irritability, hostility, impulsivity, akathisia, mania, and hypomania.

ADULT: ADHD: Start 40 mg po/d, then ↑ after >3 days to target of 80 mg/d divided daily–bid; May ↑ to 100 mg/d after 2–4 wk. Max dose 100 mg/d.

UNAPPROVED ADULT: Adjunct rx in depression and schizophrenia to improve cognition (?)

PEDS: ADHD: Children/adolescents ≤70 kg: start 0.5 mg/kg/d, then ↑ after >3 days to target dose of 1.2 mg/kg/d divided daily–bid. Max dose 1.4 mg/kg or 100 mg/d. If >70 kg use adult dose.

FORMS: Trade only: caps 10, 18, 25, 40, 60, 80, 100 mg.

NOTES: May be stopped without tapering. Monitor growth. Give "Patient Medication Guide" when dispensed; ineffective in depression. Half-life: 4 hr. May be as effective as methylphenidate but has a lower incidence of appetite suppression and insomnia. Caution in pts with tachycardia, HTN, narrow angle glaucoma, CV disease.

DRUG INTERACTIONS: If taking strong CYP2D6 inhibitors (fluoxetine, paroxetine: will have 5× plasma levels and the drug will have a longer half-life of 24 hr): use same starting dose but only ↑ if well tolerated at 4 wk and sx unimproved. Caution when coadministered with albuterol or other beta-2 agonists, as ↑ in heart rate and BP may occur. Not to be used within 2 wk of discontinuation of an MAOI.

Benzphetamine (*Didrex*) ▶K ♀X ▶? ©III $$$

WARNING: Controlled substance. Chronic overuse/abuse can lead to marked tolerance and psychic dependence; caution with prolonged use (risk of depression, psychosis).

ADULT: Short-term rx of obesity: start with 25–50 mg q d in AM and ↑ if needed to 1–3×/d.

PEDS: Not approved for children <12 yo.

FORMS: Generic/trade: tabs 25, 50 mg.

NOTES: Tolerance to anorectic effect develops within weeks and cross-tolerance to other drugs in class is common; contraindicated in pregnancy.

DRUG INTERACTIONS: May ↓efficacy of oral contraceptives; consider alternatives during rx. Do not use with MAOIs. Urinary alkalinizing agents ↑ blood levels and ↓ excretion of amphetamines.

Caffeine (*NoDoz, Vivarin, Caffedrine, Stay Awake, Quick-Pep, Cafcit*) ▶ L ♀B/C ▶? $

ADULT: Fatigue: 100–200 mg po q 3–4 hr prn.

PEDS: Not approved in children <12 yo, except for apnea in premature infants FORMS: OTC/generic/trade: tabs/caps 200 mg. OTC/trade: extended-release tabs 200 mg. Lozenges 75 mg. Oral solution caffeine citrate (Cafcit): 20 mg/mL in 3 mL vials.

NOTES: 2 mg caffeine citrate = 1 mg caffeine base. Half-life: 3–7 hr (adults), 3–4 days (infants <9 mo).

Dexmethylphenidate (*Focalin, Focalin XR*) ▶ LK♀ C ▶? ©II $$$

WARNING: Requires a triplicate prescription; high potential for abuse, tolerance, and dependence; chronic users may become suicidal upon abrupt cessation. Is contraindicated if HTN, hyperthyroidism, cardiac disease, glaucoma, psychosis, or pts with substance abuse.

ADULT: ADHD, not already on stimulants: start 10 mg po q AM (extended release) or 2.5 mg po bid (immediate release); max 20 mg/d for both. If taking racemic methylphenidate: *use conversion of 2.5 mg for each 5 mg of methylphenidate*, max 20 mg/d. Doses should be ≥4 hr apart for immediate release.

PEDS: ADHD and ≥6 yo and not already on stimulants: start 5 mg po q AM (extended release) or 2.5 mg po bid (immediate release), max 20 mg/24 hr. If already on racemic methylphenidate, use conversion of 2.5 mg for each 5 mg of methylphenidate given bid, max 20 mg/d. Doses should be ≥4 hr apart.

FORMS: Generic/trade: immediate-release tabs 2.5, 5, 10 mg. Trade only: extended-release caps (Focalin XR) 5, 10, 15, 20 mg.

NOTES: Avoid PM doses. Monitor growth, use drug holidays when appropriate. May ↑ pulse and BP. 2.5 mg is equivalent to 5 mg racemic methylphenidate. Focalin XR capsules: may open and sprinkle on applesauce; do not chew beads; may ↑ bipolar or psychotic conditions.

DRUG INTERACTIONS: May antagonize effects of antihypertensives; ↑ the levels of TCAs and tetracyclics, warfarin, phenytoin, phenobarbital, primidone, phenylbutazone.

Dextroamphetamine (*Dexedrine, Dextrostat*) ▶ L ♀C ▶ - ©II $$$

WARNINGS: Triplicate prescription; high potential for abuse. Tolerance and dependence develop. Chronic users may become suicidal upon abrupt cessation. Is contraindicated if HTN, hyperthyroidism, cardiac disease, glaucoma, psychosis, or pts with substance abuse; risk of premature delivery and ↓ birth rate in infants born to mothers using amphetamines.

ADULT: Narcolepsy: start 10 mg po q AM, increase by 10 mg q wk, max 60 mg/d divided daily (sustained release) or bid–tid at 4–6 hr intervals.

UNAPPROVED ADULT: Depression in the medically ill: 5–20 mg/d.

PEDS: Narcolepsy: 6–12 yo: start 5 mg po q AM, ↑ by 5 mg q wk. >12 yo: start 10 mg po q AM, ↑ by 10 mg q wk, max 60 mg/d divided daily (sustained release/Dexedrine Spansule) or bid–tid at 4–6 hr intervals. ADHD, 3–5 yo: start 2.5 mg po/d, ↑ by 2.5 mg q wk. ≥6 yo: start 5 mg po daily–bid, ↑ by 5 mg q wk, max 40 mg/d divided daily–tid at 4–6 hr intervals. Not recommended if <3 yo. Extended-release caps not recommended <6 yo.

FORMS: Generic/trade: tabs 5, 10, 15 mg. Extended-release caps 5, 10, 15 mg. Generic only: tabs 5, 10mg. Oral solution 5 mg/5 mL.

NOTES: Avoid PM doses. Monitor growth, use drug holidays when appropriate. Monitor BP and cardiac status. May ↑ bipolar or psychosis; can precipitate tics and Tourette syndrome. Half-life: 8–12 hr.

DRUG INTERACTIONS: High blood levels of propoxyphene ↑ CNS stimulatory effects of Adderall with risk of seizures and death; Adderall ↑ activity of TCAs and tetracyclics (↑ cardiovascular effects). Typical antipsychotics and lithium may inhibit CNS stimulatory effects of stimulants. Do not give with MAOIs (fatal reactions, HTN, seizures). Adderal delays absorption of ethosuximide, phenobarbital, phenytoin. Urinary alkalinizing agents ↑ blood levels and ↓ excretion of amphetamines.

Diethylpropion (*Tenuate, Tenuate Dospan*) ▶ K♀ B ▶? ©IV $

WARNING: Controlled substance; chronic overuse/abuse can lead to marked tolerance and psychic dependence; caution with prolonged use.

ADULT: Short-term rx of obesity: 25 mg po tid 1 hr before meals and mid-evening if needed or 75 mg sustained-release daily at mid-morning.

PEDS: Not approved for <12 yo.

FORMS: Generic/trade: tabs 25 mg, sustained-release tabs 75 mg.

NOTES: Tolerance to anorectic effect develops within weeks and cross-tolerance to other drugs in class common. Monitor: baseline cardiovascular eval.; ECG periodically and after D/C. Half-life: 4–6 hr.

DRUG INTERACTIONS: MAOI, sibutramine, other anorexiants, stimulants.

Lisdexamfetamine (*Vyvanse*) ▶L♀ C ▶- ©II $$$$

WARNING: Triplicate prescription; high potential for abuse; tolerance and dependence develop. Chronic users may become suicidal upon abrupt cessation; contraindicated if HTN, hyperthyroidism, cardiac disease, glaucoma, psychosis, or pts with substance abuse; risk of premature delivery and ↓ birth rate in infants born to mothers using amphetamines.

ADULT: Not approved for use in adults.

PEDS: ADHD ages 6–12 yo: start 30 mg po q AM; may increase wkly by 10–20 mg/d to max 70 mg/d. Adolescents use adult dosing.

FORMS: Trade: caps 20, 30, 40, 50, 60, 70 mg.

NOTES: Is a prodrug of dextroamphetamine; may open capsule and place contents in water for administration. Avoid PM doses. Monitor growth, use drug holidays when appropriate; half-life <1 hr.

DRUG INTERACTIONS: High blood levels of propoxyphene ↑ CNS stimulatory effects of stimulants (risk of seizures and death). May ↑ activity of TCAs and tetracyclics (↑ cardiovascular effects). Typical antipsychotics and lithium may inhibit CNS stimulatory effects of stimulants. Do not give with MAOIs (fatal reactions, HTN, seizures). Urinary alkalinizing agents: ↑ blood levels and ↓ excretion of amphetamines.

Methylphenidate (*Ritalin, Ritalin LA, Ritalin SR, Methylin, Methylin ER, Metadate ER, Metadate CD, Concerta, Daytrana, ♣ Biphentin*) ▶LK♀ C ▶? ©II $$

WARNING: Requires a triplicate prescription; high potential for abuse, tolerance, and dependence. Chronic users may become suicidal upon abrupt cessation; contraindicated if HTN, hyperthyroidism, cardiac disease, glaucoma, psychosis, or pts with substance abuse.

ADULT: Narcolepsy: 10 mg po bid–tid before meals. Usual effective dose is 20–30 mg/d, max 60 mg/d. Use sustained release tabs when the 8-hr dosage corresponds to the titrated 8-hr dosage of the conventional tabs. ADHD (Concerta): start 18–36 mg po q AM, usual dose range 18–72 mg/d.

UNAPPROVED ADULT: Depression in medically ill: 10–20 mg/d; augmentation of antidepressant: 10–40 mg/d.

PEDS: ADHD ≥6 yo: start 5 mg po bid before breakfast and lunch, ↑ gradually by 5–10 mg/d at wkly interval to max 60 mg/d. Sustained and extended release: start 20 mg po/d, max 60 mg/d. Concerta (extended release) start 18 mg po q AM; ↑ in 9–18 mg increments at wkly intervals to max 72 mg/d. Consult product labeling for dose conversion from other methylphenidate regimens. Discontinue after 1 month if no improvement; transdermal patch 6–12 yo: start 10 mg/9 hr; may ↑ at wkly intervals to max 30 mg/9 hr. Apply 2 hr prior to desired onset and remove 9 hr later. Effect may last up to 12 hr after application; must alternate sites daily.

FORMS: Trade only: tabs 5, 10, 20 mg (Ritalin, Methylin, Metadate). Extended-release tabs 10, 20 mg (Methylin ER, Metadate ER). Extended-release tabs 18, 27, 36, 54 mg (Concerta). Extended-release caps 10, 20, 30, 40, 50, 60 mg (Metadate CD). May be sprinkled on food. Sustained-release tabs 20 mg (Ritalin SR). Extended-release caps 10, 20, 30, 40 mg (Ritalin LA); chewable tabs 2.5, 5, 10 mg (Methylin); oral solution 5 mg/5 mL, 10 mg/5 mL (Methylin); transdermal patch (Daytrana) 10 mg/9 hr, 15 mg/9 hr, 20 mg/9 hr, 30 mg/9 hr. Generic only: tabs 5, 10, 20 mg, extended-release tabs 10, 20 mg; sustained-release tabs 20 mg.

NOTES: Avoid PM doses. Monitor growth, use drug holidays when appropriate. May increase pulse and BP. Ritalin LA may be opened and sprinkled on applesauce. Apply transdermal patch to hip below beltline to avoid rubbing it off; may ↑ bipolar or psychotic conditions. Half-life: 3–4 hr; 6–8 hr for sustained release; monitor tics, Tourette syndrome. Leukopenia, anemia, elevated liver enzymes have been reported.

DRUG INTERACTIONS: May antagonize effects of antihypertensives; ↑ the levels of TCAs and tetracyclics, warfarin, phenytoin, Phenobarbital, primidone, phenylbutazone. Sudden death has been reported when methylphenidate used with clonidine.

Modafinil (*Provigil, ♣Alertec*) ▶L ♀C ▶? ©IV $$$$$

WARNING: Controlled substance (C-IV): can be abused or lead to dependence; Serious rashes in adults and children, including Stevens–Johnson syndrome, risk of multiorgan hypersensitivity reactions. Discontinue immediately if unexplained rash.

ADULT: Narcolepsy and sleep apnea/hypopnea: 200 mg po q AM. Max 400 mg/d. Shift work sleep disorder: 200 mg po 1 hr before shift.

UNAPPROVED ADULT: Adjunctive in rx of depression, for negative sx of schizophrenia, for cognitive alertness in dementia (poor data); some effectiveness for ADHD (300 mg po q AM).

PEDS: Not approved in children <16 yo.

FORMS: Trade only: tabs 100, 200 mg.

NOTES: ↓ dose in severe liver impairment and in elderly. Half-life: 15 hr. Absorption is delayed by food; rare cases of mania, delusions, hallucinations, and suicidal ideation.

DRUG INTERACTIONS: May ↑ levels of diazepam, phenytoin, TCAs, warfarin, or propranolol; may ↓ levels of cyclosporine, oral contraceptives, or theophylline. Do not use with MAOIs.

Phendimatrizine (*Bontril, Bontril SR*) ►K♀C▶? ©III $$

WARNING: Controlled substance; chronic overuse/abuse can lead to marked tolerance and psychic dependence; caution with prolonged use.

ADULT: Short-term rx of obesity: start 35 mg 2–3×/d, 1 hr before meals; Sustained-release 105 mg once in AM before breakfast.

PEDS: Not approved in children <12 yo.

FORMS: Generic/trade: tabs/caps 35 mg, sustained-release caps 105 mg.

NOTES: Tolerance to anorectic effect develops within weeks and cross-tolerance to other drugs in class is common. Monitor: consider cardiovascular eval. at baseline; consider ECG periodically and after D/C. Half-life: 1.9 hr, 9.8 hr (ER).

DRUG INTERACTIONS: MAOI, sibutramine, other anorexiants, stimulants.

Phentermine (*Adipex-P, Ionamin, Pro-Fast*) ▶KL ♀C ▶ - ©IV $$

WARNING: Controlled substance; chronic overuse/abuse can lead to marked tolerance and psychic dependence; caution with prolonged use.

ADULT: Obesity: 8 mg po tid before meals or 1–2 hr after meals. May give 15–37.5 mg po q AM or 10–14 hr before bedtime.

PEDS: Not approved in children <16 yo.

FORMS: Generic/trade: caps 15, 18.75, 30, 37.5 mg. Tabs 8, 30, 37.5 mg. Trade only: extended-release caps 15, 30 mg (Ionamin).

NOTES: Indicated for short-term (8–12 wk) use only. Half-life: 19–24 hr. Monitor ECG periodically and after D/C.

DRUG INTERACTIONS: Contraindicated for use during or within 14 days of MAOIs (hypertensive crisis), with sibutramine, sibutramine, other anorexiants, stimulants.

Sibutramine (*Meridia*) ►KL ♀C ▶ - ©IV $$$$

WARNING: Controlled substance; chronic overuse/abuse can lead to marked tolerance and psychic dependence; caution with prolonged use.

ADULT: Obesity: start 10 mg po q AM, may ↑ to 15 mg/d after one month. Max 15 mg/d; reevaluate rx if weight loss <4 lb in first 4 wk.

PEDS: Not approved in children <16 yo.

FORMS: Trade only: caps 5, 10, 15 mg.

NOTES: Indicated for BMI > 30 kg/m^2 or > 27 kg/ m^2 with risk factors for cardiovascular disease or diabetes; monitor pulse, BP; don't use if uncontrolled HTN, heart disease, severe renal impairment. Half-life: 1.1 hr (sibutramine), active metabolites: 14 hr (M1), 16 hr (M2).

DRUG INTERACTIONS: Caution using with SSRIs or other antidepressants, sumatriptan, ergotamine, and other serotonin agents to avoid serotonin syndrome. Contraindicated for use during or within 14 days of MAOIs (hypertensive crisis), with sibutramine, other anorexiants, stimulants.

α2-ADRENERGIC RECEPTOR AGONISTS: SEE ALSO CLONIDINE UNDER SECTION DRUG DEPENDENCE THERAPY ABOVE (SEE P. 307)

Guanfacine (*Tenex, Intuniv*) ►K♀ B▶? $

ADULT: HTN: start 1 mg po qhs, increase to 2–3 mg q hs if needed after 3–4 wk, max 3 mg/d.

PEDS: HTN: ≥12 yo, same as adult; ADHD: 6–17 yo extended-release Intuniv: used once/d.

UNAPPROVED PEDS: ADHD: start 0.5 mg po/d, ↑ by 0.5 mg q 3–4 days as tolerated to 0.5 mg tid.

FORMS: Generic/trade: tabs, nonscored 1, 2 mg. Guanfacine extended-release tabs (Intuniv): tabs, 1, 2, 3, 4 mg.

NOTES: Most of the drug's rx effect is seen at 1 mg/d. Rebound HTN with abrupt discontinuation, but generally BP returns to pretreatment levels slowly without ill effects. Less sedation and hypotension compared to clonidine. Monitor BP; avoid abrupt cessation: taper dose gradually to D/C, taper the dose in decrements of no more than 1 mg every 3 to 7 days (abrupt cessation may cause ↑ plasma catecholamines, rebound HTN, nervousness/anxiety). Half-life: 17 hr.

DRUG INTERACTIONS: CNS depressants ↑ sedative SE of guanfacine; contraindication with MAOIs; may ↑ serum valproic acid concentrations.

β-ADRENERGIC RECEPTOR ANTAGONISTS

NOTE
- Developed as cardiac drugs to rx hypertension, angina, specific cardiac arrhythmias, left ventricular dysfunction. Abrupt discontinuation may precipitate angina, MI, arrhythmias, or rebound HTN in predisposed pts. Discontinue by tapering over 2 wk.
- Used for social phobia (e.g., performance anxiety), lithium-induced postural tremor, control of aggressive behavior, and neuroleptic-induced acute akathisia.
- Sometimes used as adjunctive rx for alcohol withdrawal and other substance-related disorders, for antipsychotic and antidepressant augmentation.
- Avoid using nonselective beta-blockers and use agents with beta-1 selectivity very cautiously in asthma/COPD. Beta-1 selectivity ↓ at high doses. Avoid in decompensated heart failure, sick sinus syndrome, and severe peripheral artery disease.
- May mask hypoglycemic response.
- SE: vasodilatation (dizziness, headache, tachycardia, nausea, dysesthesiaa, peripheral edema), rash, constipation, wheezing, fatigue.
- Cross-sensitivity between beta-blockers can occur.
- Drug interactions: Caution if used with clonidine and need to discontinue both: (discontinue beta-blocker several days before the clonidine to prevent rebound hypertension). Some inhalation anesthetics may ↑ the cardiodepressant effect of beta-blockers; concomitant use of digoxin or nondihydropyridine calcium channel blockers may ↑ risk of bradycardia.

Acebutol (*Sectral,♣ Rhotral*) ▶LK♀ B ▶- $$

ADULT: HTN: start 400 mg po/d or 200 mg po bid, maintenance 400–800 mg/d, max 1200 mg/d. Bid more effective than q day.

PEDS: Not approved in children <12.

UNAPPROVED ADULTS: Angina: start 200 mg po bid, ↑ as needed up to 800 mg/d.

FORMS: Generic/trade: caps, 200, 400 mg.

NOTES: Mild intrinsic sympathomimetic activity (partial β-agonist activity); β-1 receptor selective.

Atenolol (*Tenormin*) ▶L♀ D ▶- $

WARNING: Avoid abrupt cessation in coronary heart disease or HTN.

ADULT: HTN: start 25–50 mg po/d or divided bid, max 100 mg/d; renal impairment, elderly: start 25 mg po/d, ↑ as needed; angina: start 50 mg po/d or divided bid, ↑ as needed to max of 200 mg/d.

PEDS: Not approved in children.

UNAPPROVED ADULT: Atrial fibrillation/flutter: start 25 mg po/d, titrate to desired HR.

UNAPPROVED PEDS: HTN: 1–1.2 mg/kg/dose po daily, max 2 mg/kg/d.

FORMS: Generic/trade: Tabs, nonscored 25, 100; scored, 50 mg.

NOTES: Doses > 100 mg/d usually do not provide further ↓ BP; β-1 receptor selective; risk of hypoglycemia to neonates born to mothers using atenolol at parturition or while breastfeeding; may be less effective for HTN than other β-blockers.

Labetanol (*Normodyne, Trandate*) ▶LK♀ C ▶+ $$$

ADULT: HTN: start 100 mg po bid, usual maintenance dose 200–600 mg bid, max 2,400 mg/d.

PEDS: Not approved in children.

UNAPPROVED PEDS: HTN: 4 mg/kg/d po divided bid, ↑ as needed up to 40 mg/kg/d.

FORMS: Generic/trade: tabs, scored 100, 200, 300 mg.

NOTES: Hypotension; contraindicated in asthma/COPD; α-1, β-1, and β-2 receptor blocker.

Metoprolol (*Lopressor, Toprol-XL, ♣ Betaloc*) ▶L♀ C ▶? $$

WARNING: Avoid abrupt cessation in coronary heart disease or HTN.

ADULT: HTN (immediate release): start 100 mg po/d or in divided doses, ↑ as needed up to 450 mg/d; may require × daily doses to maintain 24-hr BP control. HTN (extended release): start 25–100 mg po/d, ↑ as needed q 1 wk up to 400 mg/d. Heart failure: start 12.5–25 mg (extended release) po/d, double dose every 2 wk; max 200 mg/d. Angina: start 50 mg po bid (immediate release) or 100 mg po/d (extended release), ↑ as needed up to 400 mg/d.

PEDS: HTN ≥ 6 yo: start 1 mg/kg, max 50 mg/d. Not recommended <6 yo.

UNAPPROVED ADULT: Heart failure; atrial tachyarrhythmia, except with Wolff–Parkinson–White syndrome; reentrant PSVT. Reduce perioperative cardiac events (death in high risk pts undergoing noncardiac surgery); rate control of atrial fibrillation/flutter: start 25 mg po daily, titrate to desired heart rate.

FORMS: Generic/trade: tabs, scored 50, 100 mg, extended release 25, 50, 100, 200 mg. Generic only: tabs scored 25 mg.

NOTES: Monitor closely for heart failure and hypotension when titrating dose. Avoid in decompensated heart failure; stabilize dose of digoxin, diuretics, and ACEI before starting metoprolol; β-1 receptor selective; extended-release tabs may be broken in half, but do not chew or crush. Avoid using extended-release tabs with verapamil, diltiazem, or peripheral vascular disease; may need ↓ doses in elderly. Monitor BP with potent CYP 2D6 inhibitors that may ↑ levels (e.g., bupropion, cimetidine, diphenhydramine, fluoxetine, hydroxychloroquine, paroxetine, propafenone, quinidine, thioridazine, ritonavir, terbinafine). Take with food.

Nadolol (*Corgard*) ▶K♀ C ▶- $$

ADULT: HTN: start 20–40 mg po/d, maintenance dose 40–80 mg/d, max 320 mg/d. Renal impairment: start 20 mg po/d, adjust dosage interval based on CrCl: CrCl 31–50 mL/min, q 24–36 hr; CrCl 10–30 mL/min, q 24–48 hr; CrCl <10 mL/min, q 40–60 hr. Angina: start 40 mg po/d, maintenance dose 40–80 mg/d, max 240 mg/d.

PEDS: Not approved in children.

UNAPPROVED ADULT: Prevent rebleeding esophageal varices: 40–160 mg/d po. Titrate dose to reduce HR to 25% below baseline. Ventricular arrhythmia: 10–640 mg/d po.

FORMS: Generic/trade: tabs scored 20, 40, 80, 120, 160 mg.

NOTES: β-1 and β-2 receptor blocker.

Pindolol (♣*Visken*) ▶K♀ B ▶? $$$

ADULT: HTN: start 5 mg po bid, maintenance dose 10–30 mg/d, max 60 mg/d.

PEDS: Not approved in children.

UNAPPROVED ADULT: Angina: 15–40 mg/d po in divided doses tid–qid.

FORMS: Generic only: tabs scored 5, 10 mg.

NOTES: Has intrinsic sympathomimetic activity (partial β-agonist activity); B-1 and β-2 blocker.

DRUG INTERACTIONS: Contraindicated with thoridazine.

Propanolol (*Inderal, Inderal LA, InnoPran XL*) ▶L♀ C ▶+ $$

WARNING: Avoid abrupt cessation in coronary heart disease or HTN.

ADULT: HTN: start 20–40 mg po bid, maintenance 160–480 mg/d, max 640 mg/d; extended release (Inderal LA): start 60–80 mg po/d, maintenance 120–160 mg/d, max 640 mg/d; extended release (InnoPran XL): start 80 mg qhs (10 PM), max 120 mg qhs. Angina: start 10–20 mg po tid–qid, maintenance 160–240 mg/d, max 320 mg/d; extended release (Inderal LA): start 80 mg po/d, same usual dosage range and max for HTN. Migraine prophylaxis: start 40 mg po bid or 80 mg po/d (extended releases) max 240 mg/d. Supraventricular tachycardia or rapid atrial fibrillation/flutter: 10–30 mg po tid–qid. MI: 180–240 mg/d po in divided doses bid–qid. Used also in Pheochromocytoma surgery. Not for use in HTN emergency. Essential tremor: start 40 mg po bid, titrate prn to 120–320 mg/d.

PEDS: HTN: start 1 mg/kg/d po divided bid, maintenance 2–4 mg/kg/d po divided bid, max 16 mg/kg/d.

UNAPPROVED ADULT: Prevent rebleeding esophageal varices: 20–180 mg/d po; titrate dose to ↓ HR to 25% below baseline. Control HR with A-fibr.: 80–240 mg/d once/d or in divided doses.

UNAPPROVED PEDS: Arrhythmia. Manufacturer does not recommend IV propanolol in children.

FORMS: Generic only: tabs, scored 10, 20, 40, 60, 80 mg. Caps, extended release 60, 80, 120, 160 mg. Generic only: solution 20, 40 mg/5 mL. Concentrate 80 mg/mL. Trade only: (InnoPran XL qhs) 80, 120 mg.

NOTES: β-1 and β-2 receptor blocker. Do not substitute extended-release for immediate-release product on mg-for-mg basis. (Dosage titration may be necessary with extended release when converting from immediate-release tabs.) Extended-release caps (Inderal LA) may be opened and the contents may be sprinkled on food. Caps contents should be swallowed whole without crushing or chewing. InnoPran XL is a chronotherapeutic product: give at bedtime to blunt early morning surge in BP.

DRUG INTERACTIONS: Contraindication with thioridazine. Concomitant use of alcohol may ↑ propanolol levels.

ANTIHISTAMINICS

NOTE: Contraindicated in narrow angle glaucoma, prostate enlargement, stenosing peptic ulcer disease, and bladder obstruction. Use half the dose in the elderly. May cause drowsiness and/or sedation, which may be enhanced with alcohol, sedatives, and other CNS depressants. Deaths have occurred in children <2 yo attributed to toxicity from cough and cold medications: use in this age group only with extreme caution.

Diphenhydramine (*Benadryl, Banophen, Allermax, Diphen, Diphenist, Dytan, Siladryl, Sominex, ♣Allerdryl, Nytol***)** ▶LK♀ B▶- $

ADULT: Allergic rhinitis, urticaria, hypersensitivity reactions: 25–50 mg po/IM/IV q 4–6 hr; max 300–400 mg/d. Motion sickness: 25–50 mg po preexposure and q 4–6 hr prn. Drug-induced parkinsonism: 10–50 mg IV/IM. Antitussive: 25 mg po q 4 hr. Max 100 mg/d. EPS: 25–50 mg po tid–qid or 10–50 mg IV/IM tid–qid. Insomnia: 25–50 mg po qhs.

PEDS: Hypersensitivity reactions: ≥12 yo: use adult dose, 6–11 yo: 12.5–25 mg po q 4–6 hr or 5 mg/kg/d po/IV/IM divided qid. Max 150 mg/d. Antitussive (syrup): 6–12 yo:12.5 mg po q 4 hr. Max 50 mg/d. 2–5 yo: 6.25 mg po q 4 hr. Max 25 mg/d. EPS: 12.5–25 mg po tid–qid or 5 mg/kg/d IV/IM divided qid, max 300 mg/d. Insomnia age ≥12 yo: 25–50 mg po qhs.

FORMS: OTC: Trade only: tabs 25, 50 mg, chew tabs 12.5 mg. OTC and rx: generic only: caps 25, 50 mg, softgel cap 25 mg. OTC: generic/trade: solution 6.25 or 12.5 mg/5 mL. Rx: trade only: (Dytan) suspension 25 mg/mL, chew tabs 25 mg.

NOTES: Anticholinergic SE ↑ in the elderly and may worsen dementia or delirium.

DRUG INTERACTIONS: avoid use with donepezil, rivastigmine, galantamine, or tacrine.

Hydroxyzine (*Atarax, Vistaril***)** ▶L♀ C▶- $$

ADULT: Pruritus: 25–100 mg IM/po daily–qid or prn.

PEDS: Pruritus: <6 yo: 50 mg/d po divided qid.≥6 yo: 50–100 mg/d po divided qid.

FORMS: Generic only: tabs 10, 25, 50, 100 mg. Caps 100 mg, syrup 10 mg/5 mL. Generic/trade: caps 25, 50 mg. Suspension 25 mg/5 mL (Vistaril) (caps = Vistaril; tabs = Atarax).

NOTES: Atarax (hydrochloride salt), Vistaril (pamoate salt).

Promethazine (Phenergan) ▶LK♀ C▶- $

WARNING: Contraindicated if < 2yo: risk of fatal respiratory depression; caution if older.

ADULT: N/V: 12.5–25 mg q 4–6 hr po/IM/PR prn. Motion sickness: 25 mg po/PR 30–60 min prior to departure and q 12 hr prn. Hypersensitivity reactions: 25 mg IM/IV, may repeat in 2 hr. Allergic conditions: 12.5 mg po/PR/IM/IV qid or 25 mg po/PR qhs.

PEDS: N/V,≥ 2 yo: 0.25–1 mg/kg/dose po/IM/PR q 4–6 hr prn. Motion sickness: 0.5 mg/kg po 30–60 min prior to departure and q 12 hr prn; max 25 mg/dose. Hypersensitivity reactions >2 yo: 6.25–12.5 mg po/PR/IM/IV q 6 hr prn.

UNAPPROVED ADULT: N/V: 12.5–25 mg IV q 4 hr prn.

UNAPPROVED PEDS: N/V, ≥ 2 yo: 0.25–0.5 mg/kg/dose IV q 4 hr prn.

FORMS: Generic/trade: tab/supp 12.5, 25, 50 mg. Generic only: syrup 6.25 mg/5 mL.

NOTES: May cause sedation, extrapyramidal reactions (esp. with high IV doses), hypotension with rapid IV administration, anticholinergic SE (dry mouth, blurred vision).

Cyproheptadine (Periactine) ▶LK ♀B▶-$

ADULT: Allergic rhinitis/urticaria: start 4 mg po tid, usual effective dose is 12–16 mg/d; max 32 mg/d.

PEDS: Allergic rhinitis/urticaria: 2–6 yo: start 2 mg po bid–tid; max 12 mg/d. 7–14 yo: start 4 mg po bid –tid; max 16 mg/d.

UNAPPROVED ADULT: Appetite stimulant: 2–4 mg po tid 1 hr ac. Prevention of cluster headaches: 4 mg po qid. Treatment of acute serotonin syndrome: 12 mg po/NG followed by 2 mg q 2 hr until sx clear, then 8 mg q 6 hr maintenance while syndrome remains active.

FORMS: Generic only: tabs 4 mg. Syrup 2 mg/5 mL.

BARBITURATES AND SIMILARLY ACTING DRUGS

NOTE
- Rarely used since use of benzodiazepines (the lower therapeutic index and high abuse potential): continued use of barbiturates >3–4 wk is associated with tolerance, dependence, and withdrawal syndrome. To avoid an abstinence syndrome: ↓ gradually upon discontinuation; may use a long half-life benzodiazepine (clonazepam) to ↓ the severity of withdrawal (irritability, anxiety, agitation, dysphoria, confusion, memory deficits, hallucinations, sensory disturbances, paresthesias, psychosis, seizures, insomnia, tremors, muscle twitching, muscle cramps, abdominal cramps, GI disturbances, tachycardia, diaphoresis).
- Induce hepatic microsomal enzymes.
- Not to be used in pregnancy: infants may have respiratory depression at birth and withdrawal sx.
- Contraindicated in pts with porphyria or with hepatic dysfunction (toxicity).
- Drug interactions: reduce effectiveness of anticoagulants, TCAs, propranolol, carbamazepine, estrogens, corticosteroids, quinidine, theophylline; effects on phenytoin are unpredictable; valproic acid ↑ barbiturate levels.

Amobarbital ▶KL ♀D ▶- ©II $$

WARNING: rarely used for psychotic agitation; even for Amytal interview (replaced by lorazepam).

ADULT: sedation: 50–100 mg po or IM; hypnosis: 50–200 mg IV (max 400 mg/d).

PEDS: Not applicable.

FORMS: Tabs: 30, 50, 100 mg. Caps: 65, 200 mg. Injectable solution (IM, IV): 250 mg/5 mL, 500 mg/5 mL.

NOTES: Half-life: 8–42 hr.

DRUG INTERACTIONS: Multiple.

Butabarbital (*Butisol*) ▶KL ♀D ▶? ©II $$$

WARNING: Severe allergic reactions and complex sleep-related behaviors.

ADULT: Sedation 15–30 mg po tid–qid; preoperative sedation: 50–100 mg po ×1, Info: give 60–90 min pre-op; insomnia, short-term tx: 50–100 mg po qhs.

PEDS: Nonapplicable.

FORMS: Tabs: 30, 50 mg, Elixir 30 mg/5 mL.

NOTES: Half-life: 34–42 hr.

DRUG INTERACTIONS: Can make birth control pills less effective, multiple other drug interactions.

Meprobamate: ▶ L ♀ D▶ ? ©II $$$

WARNING: Rarely used.

ADULT: Anxiety: 400 mg po tid–qid, max 2,400 mg/d; info: taper dose gradually over 1–2 wk to D/C.

PEDS: Anxiety 6–12 yo; dose: 100–200 mg; info: taper dose gradually over 1–2 wk to D/C.

FORMS: Generic tabs: 200, 400 mg.

NOTES: Half-life: 10 hr.

DRUG INTERACTIONS: Multiple.

Phenobarbital (*Luminal*) ▶L ♀D ▶- ©IV $

WARNING: Barbiturate. Multiple drug interactions (see above note).

ADULT: Epilepsy: 100–300 mg/d po divided daily–tid. Status epilepticus: 20 mg/kg IV at rate ≤60 mg/min.

PEDS: Epilepsy: 3–5 mg/kg/d po divided bid–tid. Status epilepticus: 20 mg/kg IV at rate ≤60 mg/min.

UNAPPROVED ADULT: Status epilepticus: may give up to a total dose of 30 mg/kg IV.

UNAPPROVED PEDS: Status epilepticus: 15–20 mg/kg IV load; may give additional 5 mg/kg doses q 15–30 min to max total dose of 30 mg/kg.

FORMS: Generic only: tabs 15, 16.2, 30, 32.4, 60, 100 mg. Elixir 20 mg/5 mL. IM, IV.

NOTES: Usual therapeutic range = 15–40 mcg/mL. Monitor cardiopulmonary function closely when administering IV. Decrease dose in renal or hepatic dysfunction. Many drug interactions. Half-life: 79–120 hr.

DRUG INTERACTIONS: additive effects of respiratory depression with other CNS drugs including antipsychotics and antidepressants and alcohol; caution with cardiac drugs and anticonvulsants that are metabolized in the liver; caution with antibiotics, antiarrhythmics, anticoagulants, beta adrenergic receptor antagonists, dopamine receptor antagonists, contraceptives, immunosuppressants.

Secobarbital (*Seconal*) ▶L ♀B ▶? ©II $

WARNING: severe allergic reactions and complex sleep-related behaviors (sleep-driving, with no memory of the event).

ADULT: Insomnia, short-term rx: 100 mg po at hs.

PEDS: Not indicated.

FORMS: Caps 50, 100 mg.

NOTES: Half-life 14–40 hr.

DRUG INTERACTIONS: Multiple.

CALCIUM CHANNEL INHIBITORS

NOTE
- Used as antimanic agents if pt does not respond to first-line agents (lithium, valproic acid, carbamazepine, and other anticonvulsants).
- Used for the control of mania and ultradian bipolar disorder (with mood cycling in less than 24 hr).
- Risk of peripheral edema, esp. with higher doses. Extended/controlled/sustained-release tabs should be swallowed whole; do not crush or chew. Avoid concomitant grapefruit/grapefruit juice, which may enhance effects. Avoid in decompensated heart failure.
- DDIs: may precipitate carbamazepine-induced + lithium neurotoxicity; check other beta-adrenergic antagonists, hypotensive drugs, digoxin, aspirin.
- The drugs are Diltiazem, Nifedipine, Isradipin, Amlodipine. The calcium channel inhibitors sometimes used for psychiatric disorders have been Verapamil, Nimodipine

Verapamil (*Calan, Calan −SR, Isoptin-SR, Covera-HS, Verelan, Verelan-PM, Verapamil, ♣Veramil*) ▶L ♀C ▶+ $$

WARNING: SE: delirium, hyperprolactinemia, hypotension, bradycardia, AV heart block. Elderly are more sensitive. Caution if renal or hepatic impairment.

ADULT: Used in SVT and PSVT/rate control with atrial fibrillation: 240−480 mg/d po divided tid−qid. In angina: start 40−80 mg po tid−qid, max 480 mg/d; sustained-release (Isoptin SR, Calan SR, Verelan): start 120−240 mg po/d, max 480 mg/d (use bid dosing for doses >240 mg/d with Isoptin SR and Calan SR); extended release (Covera HS): start 180 mg po qhs, max 480 mg/d. HTN: same as angina, except (Verelan PM) start 100−200 mg po qhs, max 400 mg/d; (Covera HS) start 180 mg po qhs, max 480 mg/d; avoid immediate-release tabs when treating HTN.

UNAPPROVED ADULTS: In mania and ultradian bipolar disorder: start 40 mg po tid, then ↑ in increments every 4−5 days up to 80−120 mg tid.

PEDS: Immediate release and sustained release not approved in children.

FORMS: Genetic/trade: tabs, immediate release, scored 40, 80, 120 mg; sustained-release tablets nonscored (Calan SR, Isoptin SR): 120, 180, 240 mg; caps, sustained release (Verelan): 120, 180, 200, 240, 360 mg. Trade: tabs, extended release (Covera HS) 180, 240 mg; caps, extended release (Verelan PM) 100, 200, 300 mg. Verapamil hydrochloride injectable 2.5 mg/mL.

NOTES: Half-life: 5−12 hr. Monitor LFTs; BP, HR; ECG contraindicated in severe LV dysfunction, hypotension, sick sinus syndrome, AV block, Wolff−Parkinson−White. Avoid grapefruit juice (enhances effect). Do not chew or crush caps. Sustained-release caps may be open and content mixed with apple sauce (do not chew). Covera-HS and Verelan PM are given at bedtime to blunt early morning surge in BP.

DRUG INTERACTIONS: May precipitate carbamazepine-induced neurotoxicity and lithium neurotoxicity; mixed with aspirin: risk of ↑ bleeding time. See interactions with beta-adrenergic antagonists, hypotensive drugs, and digoxin.

Nimodipine (*Nimotop*) ▶L ♀C ▶- $$$$$

WARNING: SE: skin flushing, sense of chest tightness.

ADULT: Subarachnoid hemorrhage: 60 mg po q 4 hr for 21 days (begin therapy within 96 hr. Give 1 hr before or 2 hr after meals. May give cap contents SL or via NG tube).

UNAPPROVED ADULTS: Has been used at 60 mg q 4 hr for ultrarapid-cycling bipolar disorder and sometimes briefly at up to 630 mg/d. In mania: start 30 mg po tid, usually between 240 and 450 mg/d.

PEDS: Not approved in children.

FORMS: Caps: 30 mg.

NOTE: Decrease dose in hepatic dysfunction. Half-life: 1−2 hr. Caution in the elderly.

DRUG INTERACTIONS: May precipitate lithium neurotoxicity.

Isradipine (*DynaCirc, DynaCirc CR*) ▶L ♀ C ▶? $$$$

ADULT: HTN: start 2.5 mg po bid, maintenance 5−10 mg/d, max 20 mg/d divided bid (max 10 mg/d in elderly). Controlled-release (DynaCirc CR): start 5 mg daily, maintenance 5−10 mg/d, max 20 mg/d.

UNAPPROVED ADULTS: In mania and ultradian bipolar disorder: start 2.5 mg/d, then ↑ to a max of 15 mg/d in divided doses.

PEDS: Not approved in children.

FORMS: Generic/trade: immediate release caps 2.5 mg. Generic: immediate release caps 5 mg. Trade: tabs, controlled release 5, 10 mg.

NOTES: Half-life: 1−2 hr. Caution in the elderly.

DRUG INTERACTIONS: May precipitate lithium neurotoxicity.

Amlodipine (*Norvasc*) ▶L ♀C ▶? $$$

WARNING: Only case reports in mania.

ADULT-HTN: Start 2.5–5 mg po/d, max 10 mg/d. If coronary artery disease: start 5 mg po/d, maintenance dose 10 mg daily.

UNAPPROVED ADULTS: In mania and ultradian bipolar disorder: start 5 mg at hs, then ↑ up to 10–15 mg/d (cases reports).

PEDS: HTN (6–17 yo): 2.5–5 mg po/d.

UNAPPROVED PEDS: HTN start 0.1–0.2 mg/kg/d, max 0.3 mg/kg/d.

FORMS: Generic/trade: tabs, nonscored 2.5, 5, 10 mg.

NOTES: Half-life: 30–50 hr. Caution in the elderly.

DRUG INTERACTIONS: May precipitate lithium neurotoxicity.

THYROID HORMONES

Levothyroxine (*L-thyroxine, Levolet, LevoT, Levothroid, Levoxyl, Novothyrox, Synthroid, Thyro-Tabs, Tirosint, Unithroid, T4, ♣Eltroxin, Euthyrox*) ▶L ♀A ▶+ $

WARNING: Do not use for obesity/weight loss.

ADULT: Hypothyroidism: start 100–200 mcg po/d (healthy adults) or 12.5–50 mcg po/d (elderly or CV disease), ↑ by 12.5–25 mcg/d at 3–8 wk intervals; usual dose 100–200 mcg po/d, max 300 mcg/d.

PEDS: Hypothyroidism: 0–6 months: 8–10 mcg/kg/d po, 6–12 months: 6–8 mcg/kg/d po; 1–5 yo: 5–6 mcg/kg/d po; 6–12 yo: 4–5 mcg/kg/d po; >12 yo: 2–3 mcg/kg/d po, max 300 mcg/d.

UNAPPROVED ADULT: Hypothyroidism: 1.6 mcg/kg/d po; start with lower doses (25 mcg po/d) in elderly and cardiac disease.

FORMS: Generic/trade: tabs 25, 50, 75, 88, 100 112, 125, 137, 150, 175, 200, 300 mcg. Trade only: caps: 25, 50, 75, 100, 125, 150 mcg in 7-day blister packs.

NOTES: May crush tabs for infants and children. May give IV or IM at ½ oral dose in adults and ½–¾ oral dose in children; adjust based on tolerance and rx response. Generics are not necessary bioequivalent to brand products; reevaluate thyroid function when switching.

Liothyronine (*T3, Cytomel, Triostat*) ▶L ♀A ▶? $$

WARNING: Do not use for obesity/weight loss.

ADULT: Mild hypothyroidism: 25 mcg po/d, ↑ by 12.5–25 mcg/d at 1–2 wk intervals to desired response; maintenance dose 25–75 mcg po/d. Goiter: 5 mcg po/d, ↑ by 5–10 mcg/d at 1–2 wk intervals; maintenance dose 75 mcg po/d. Myxedema: 5 mcg po/d, ↑ by 5–10 mcg/d at 1–2 wk intervals; maintenance dose 50–100 mcg/d.

PEDS: Congenital hypothyroidism: 5 mcg po/d; may ↑ by 5 mcg/d, at 3–4 day intervals, up to desired response.

FORMS: Trade only: tabs 5, 25, 50 mcg.

NOTES: Start rx at 5 mcg/d in children and elderly and ↑ by 5 mcg increments only; rapidly absorbed from the GI tract; monitor T3 and TSH. Elderly may need lower doses due to potential decreased renal function.

HERBS, VITAMINS, DIETARY SUPPLEMENTS, OTHER HORMONES, AMINO ACIDS

NOTE: FORMS are not all by prescriptions. Herbal and alternative therapy products are regulated as dietary supplements, not drugs (US Dietary Supplements Health and Education Act [DSHEA] of 1994). Contact http://www.consumerlab.com for information. Premarketing evaluation and FDA approval are not required unless specific therapeutic claims are made. These products are not required to demonstrate efficacy. Considerable variability in content from lot to lot or between products. Many of them have DDIs as well as SEs. See also www.tarascon.com/herbals for the evidence-based efficacy ratings used by the Tarascon editorial staff. Recommended Daily Allowance (RDA).

Bacopa monnieri or Brahmi

UNAPPROVED ADULT: Poor memory; mood disorders (?). Start dose: 225–450 mg bid; max 450 mg bid.

FORMS: Many formulations; cap containing standardized whole plant extract with 20% of bacosides A + B.

NOTES: Ayurvedic *herb to* ↑ *memory*; strong antioxidant.

DRUG INTERACTIONS: Potentiate sedatives and narcotics.

L-Carnitine (*Carnitor*) ▶L ♀ B ▶? $$$

WARNING: Only the L-stereoisomer is safe and available.

ADULTS: FDA approved to treat carnitine deficiency (Reye-like encephalopathy, hypoketotic hypoglycemia, and/ or cardiomyopathy, ESRD on hemodialysis). Associated sx included hypotonia, muscle weakness, and failure to thrive. OTC: starting dose: 500 mg po bid, up to 1,000–2,000 mg po bid; Carnitor: starting dose: 330 mg po tid up to 330–990 mg po bid–tid. Carnitine deficiency: IV 50 mg/kg/d IV div dose q 4–6 hr. Start: 50 mg/ kg IV loading dose if severe metabolic crisis; max 300 mg/kg/d.

PEDS: Carnitine deficiency, oral: 50–100 mg/kg/d po, start: 50 mg/kg/d, ↑ gradually; max 3 g/d; info: div dose q 8–12 hr if using tablets, q 3–4 hr if using sol; admin. w/ or after meals; mix sol w/ juice or other liquid, drink slowly to improve tolerance. Carnitine deficiency, ESRD on HD: 10–20 mg/kg IV after each HD session. Info: dose based on dry body wt; initiate rx/adjust dose based on trough free plasma carnitine levels.

UNAPPROVED ADULTS: ↓ *mortality rates in severe valproate-induced hepatotoxicity* (especially IV route); ↓ valproate-induced hyperammonemia (measure it only if there is a change in the mental status, and use after discontinuation of valproate); used for prevention of ↑ weight from valproate (but trial was negative).

FORMS: OTC: 500 mg. Carnitor: solution: 1 g/10 mL, tabs: 330 mg, injectable: 200 mg/mL IV.

NOTES: N/V, diarrhea, body odor, rare seizures (racemic mixture?). Monitor: blood chemistries, vital signs periodically. Half-life: 17.4 hr.

DRUG INTERACTIONS: No significant interactions known.

Chromium picolinate

WARNING: Mild activation.

ADULTS: RDA: 25–50 mcg/d of elemental chromium.

UNAPPROVED ADULT: Used as *adjunct in refractory mood disorders*; insulin resistance, obesity: start dose 200–400 mcg/d of elemental chromium. Max 1,000 mcg/d.

UNAPPROVED PEDS: Same as above; dose: 50–150 mcg/d.

FORMS: OTC formulations.

NOTES: ↑ dreams; is a trace mineral.

Cyanocobolamin (*Vitamin B_{12}, CaloMist, Nascobal*) ▶K ♀C ▶+ $

ADULT: See also unapproved adult dosing. Maintenance of nutritional deficiency following IM correction: 500 mcg intranasal wkly (Nascobal: 1 spray one nostril q wk) or 50–100 mcg intranasal q/d (CaloMist: 1–2 sprays each nostril daily). Pernicious anemia: 100 mcg IM/SC qd for 6–7 days, then qd for 7 doses, then q 3–4 days for 2–3 wk, then q month. Other patients with vitamin B_{12} deficiency: 30 mcg IM daily for 5–10 days, then 100–200 mcg IM once a month. RDA for adults is 2–4 mcg.

PEDS: Nutritional deficiency: 100 mcg/24 hr deep IM/SC × 10–15 days then at least 60 mcg/month IM/deep SC. Pernicious anemia: 30–50 mcg/24 hr for ≥14 days to total dose of 1,000–5,000 mcg deep IM/SC then 100 mcg/month deep IM/SC. Adequate daily intake for infants: 0.6 mo: 0.4 mcg; 7–11 mo: 0.5 mcg. RDA for children: 1–3 yo: 0.9 mcg; 4–8 yo: 1–2 mcg; 9–13 yo: 1.8 mcg; 14–18 yo: 2–4 mcg.

UNAPPROVED ADULT: Pernicious anemia and nutritional deficiency states: 1,000–2,000 mcg po/d for 1–2 wk, then 1,000 mcg po/d. Prevention and rx of cyanide toxicity associated with nitroprusside. Anecdotal reports of relieving depression when vitamin B_{12} deficiency presented as MDD is treated with B12; used *sometimes as an adjunct in refractory depression.*

UNAPPROVED PEDS: Prevention and rx of cyanide toxicity associated with nitroprusside.

FORMS: OTC generic only: tab 100, 500, 1,000, 5,000 mcg; lozenges 100, 250, 500 mcg. Rx trade: nasal spray 500 mcg/spray (Nascobal 2.3 mL); 25 mcg/spray (CaloMist 18 mL). SC, IM.

NOTES: Prime nasal pump before use per package insert directions. Although official dose for deficiency states is 100–200 mcg IM q month, some give 1,000 mcg IM periodically. Oral supplementation is safe and effective for B_{12} deficiency even when intrinsic factor is not present (if B_{12} given in high dosage >1 mg). Providing folic acid alone may normalize the CBC, and thus mask a B_{12} deficiency. Always use them together!

Monitor B_{12}, folate, iron, K+, platelets, and CBC; aluminum content: toxic levels w/ prolonged rx if renal impairment, especially premature neonates; CNS, bone toxicity may occur (SC/IM form); Benzyl Alcohol content: avoid use in neonates; serious, potentially fatal "gasping syndrome" may occur (SC/IM form). Half-life: 6 days; info: 90% stored in liver.

DRUG INTERACTIONS: Chloramphenicol, omeprazole, colchicine.

Dehydroepiandrosterone (*DHEA, Aslera, Fidelin, Prasterone*) ▶ Peripheral conversion to estrogens and androgens♀-▶- $

UNAPPROVED ADULT: *No evidence that DHEA slows aging or* ↑ *cognition in the elderly.* To ↑ well-being in ♀ with adrenal insufficiency: 50 mg po daily (conflicting clinical trials results). Used by athletes as a substitute for anabolic steroids (no evidence of ↑ athletic performance or ↑ muscle mass; banned by many sports organizations).

UNAPPROVED PEDS: Not for use in children.

FORMS: Multiple formulations, wide range.

NOTES: Chronic use may ↑ risk of hormone-related cancers (prostate, breast, ovarian).

Folic acid (*folate, Folvite*) ▶K ♀A ▶+ $

WARNING: Some prescription B vitamins (FDA approved as medical foods) contain folic acid such as **Metanx** (each tab contains 2.8 mg L-methylfolate, 2 mg B_{12}, and 25 mg B_6; approved for reducing homocysteine levels in CAD); **Cerefolin** (approved for multi-infarct dementia/each tab contains 5.6 mg L-methylfolate, 2 mg B_{12}, and 600 mg N-acetylcysteine); **Deplin** (approved for low folate levels and sometimes used as an augmentation rx with antidepressants/each tab contains 7.5 mg of L-methylfolate). Caution in pts with cancer.

ADULT: Megaloblastic anemia: 1 mg po/IM/IV/SC daily. When sx subside and CBC normalizes: give maintenance dose of 0.4 mg po/d and 0.8 mg po/d in pregnant and lactating ♀. RDA for adults: 0.4, 0.6 mg for pregnant ♀, and 0.5 mg for lactating ♀. Max daily dose 1 mg.

PEDS: Megaloblastic anemia: infants: 0.05 mg po/d, maintenance of 0.04 mg po/d; children: 0.5–1 mg po/d, maintenance of 0.4 mg po/d. Adequate daily intake for infants: 0–6 months: 65 mcg; 7–12 mo: 80 mcg. RDA for children: 1–3 yo: 150 mcg; 4–8 yo: 200 mcg; 9–13 yo: 300 mcg; 14–18 yo: 400 mcg.

UNAPPROVED ADULT: Hyperhomocysteinemia: 0.5–1 mg po/d. *Used as augmentation of antidepressant in unipolar depression; may be used with lithium as an augmentation agent.*

FORMS: OTC generic only: tab 0.4, 0.8 mg. Rx generic 1 mg.

NOTES: Folic acid doses > 0.1 mg/d obscure pernicious anemia. Prior to conception, all ♀ should receive 0.4 mg/d to ↓ the risk of neural tube defects in infants. Consider high dose (up to 4 mg) in ♀ with prior hx of infant with neural tube defect. Use oral route except in cases of severe intestinal absorption. No known toxicity unless high doses (>20 mg); may decrease risk of MI (by ↓ homocysteine level).

Ginger root (*Zingiber officinale*) ▶? ♀? ▶? $

UNAPPROVED ADULT: Prevention of motion sickness (efficacy unclear): 500–1,000 mg powdered rhizome po single dose 1 h before exposure. The American College of Obstetrics and Gynecology considers ginger 250 mg po qid a nonpharmacologic *option for N/V of pregnancy.* Some experts advise pregnant ♀ to limit dose to usual dietary amount (≤1 g/d); conflicting clinical trials for post-op N/V; efficacy unclear for relief of osteoarthritis pain.

UNAPPROVED PEDS: Not for use in children.

NOTES: Increased INR > 10 attributed to ginger in phenprocoumon-treated pt, but study in healthy volunteers found no effect of ginger on INR or pharmacokinetics of warfarin.

Ginkgo biloba (*EGb 761, Ginkgold, Ginkoba, Quanterra Mental Sharpness*) ▶K ♀- ▶- $

UNAPPROVED ADULT: Dementia (modest benefit for mild–moderate disease): 40 mg po tid of standardized extract containing 24% ginko flavone glycosides and 6% terpene lactones. It may take up to 4 wk to be effective; *does not appear to improve memory in elderly* with normal function; does not appear effective for the prevention of acute altitude sickness. Limited benefit in intermittent claudication. The American College of Cardiology found insufficient evidence for rx of peripheral vascular disease. ArginMax (also contains L-arginine and other ingredients) promoted for SSRI-induced sexual dysfunction.

UNAPPROVED PEDS: Not for use in children.

NOTES: Case reports of intracerebral, subdural, and ocular bleeding. Does not appear to increase INR with warfarin, but monitoring for bleeding is advised. Ginkgo seeds contain a neurotoxin. A few reports of seizures may be due to the neurotoxin. Avoid ginko in those with seizures or if taking drugs that ↓ the seizure threshold.

Inositol

WARNING: Risk of hypomania/mania. Used as a filler in illegal drugs. Inositol is a cutting agent in Meth and Cocaine.

PEDS: Not recommended in children. Children with ADHD might do worse on inositol.

UNAPPROVED ADULTS: Promoted for *major depression, OCD, panic disorder.* Start dose: 5 g inositol powder qd–bid. Max 16 g/d.

FORMS: Powder.

NOTES: Natural isomer of glucose, though generally considered to be a member of the B vitamin family. Precursor to second messenger molecule linked to 5-HT2 receptors. Mild lower GI side effects.

DRUG INTERACTIONS: May reverse some Lithium side effects (unproved).

Kava Kava (*Piper methysticum, One-a-day Bedtime and Rest, Sleep-Tite*) ▶K ♀- ▶- $

WARNING: Hepatotoxicity (extract dependent?).

UNAPPROVED ADULT: *Promoted as anxiolytic (possibly effective) or sedative*; Start dose: 100 mg tid (standardized extract). Max 600 mg/d.

UNAPPROVED PEDS: Not for use in children.

NOTES: Reports of severe hepatotoxicity leading to liver transplantation; Reversible yellow skin discoloration with long-term use and thick, scaly skin. Low abuse potential.

DRUG INTERACTIONS: May potentiate CNS effects of benzodiazepines and other sedatives, including alcohol.

Magnesium salts (magnesium chloride/*Slow-Mag*; magnesium gluconate/*Almora, Magtrate, Maganate, ♣ Maglucate*; magnesium oxide/*Mag-200, Mag-Ox 400, magnesium sulfate, magnesium aspartate*) ▶K♀A▶+ $

WARNING: May require concomitant pyridoxine (vitamin B₆); contraindicated in renal failure and cardiac diseases.

ADULT: Dietary supplement. RDA (elem. Mg): adult ♂: 19–30 yo: 400 mg; > 30 yo: 420 mg. Adult ♀: 19–30 yo: 310 mg; >30 yo: 320 mg. Starting dose: 100–200 mg qd–bid of elemental Mg. Target dose: 400–1,000 mg/d in divided doses. Max 1,000 mg/d.

PEDS: Not approved in children.

UNAPPROVED ADULT: *Some studies in bipolar disorders, PMS*: 200–300 mg elemental Mg++ bid–tid.

FORMS: Multiple forms; magnesium chloride: OTC trade: enteric-coated tab 64 mg (64 mg tab Slow-Mag = 64 mg elem. Mg); magnesium gluconate: OTC generic only: tab 500 mg, liquid 54 mg elem. Mg/5 mL; magnesium oxide: OTC generic/trade: cap 140, 250, 400, 420, 500 mg (approximately 60% elem. magnesium).

NOTES: Blocks Ca++ channels and NMDA receptors, inhibits PKC; has sedative and anticonvulsant effects. Magnesium chelates (such as aspartate) give less GI symptoms. Is an essential mineral.

Melatonin (*N-acetyl-5-methoxytryptamine*) ▶L ♀- ▶- $

UNAPPROVED ADULT: To *reduce jet lag* after flights across >5 time zones (possibly effective, especially traveling East; may also help for 2–4 times zones): 0.5–5 mg po qhs (10 PM to midnight) ×3–6 nights starting on day of arrival. Faster onset + better sleep quality with 5 mg vs 0.5 mg, but no greater benefit with >5 mg. No benefit with use before departure or slow-release forms. Do not take earlier in day (may cause drowsiness and delay adaptation to local time); *orphan drug for circadian rhythm-related sleep disorders in blind patients with no light perception; possibly effective for difficulty falling asleep, but not for staying asleep.*

UNAPPROVED PEDS: Not usually for use in children. Sleep-onset insomnia in ADHD, ≥ 6 yo (possibly effective): 3–6 mg po qhs. Orphan drug for circadian rhythm-related sleep disorders in blind patients with no light perception.

NOTES: High melatonin levels linked to nocturnal asthma.

Omega-3 fatty acids (*fish oil, Lovaza, Omacor, Promega, Cardio-Omega 3, Sea-Omega, Marine Lipid Concentrate, MAXEPA, SuperEPA 1200*) ▶L ♀ C ▶? $$

WARNING: Caution in seafood allergy. Fish oil preferred to flaxseed oil at this time.

ADULTS: Lovaza, adjunct to diet to reduce high triglycerides (≥500 mg/dL): 4 capsules po/d or divided bid.

PEDS: Not approved in children.

UNAPPROVED ADULTS: Hypertriglyceridemia: 2–4 g EPA + DHA content daily under physician's care. Secondary prevention of CHD: 1–2 g EPA+DHA content daily. Adjunctive rx in rheumatoid arthritis: 20 g/d po. Psoriasis: 10–15 g/d po. Prevention of early restenosis after coronary angioplasty in combination with dipyridamole and aspirin: 18 g/d; *improves depressive sx in pts with clearly defined depression or bipolar affective disorder; heterogeneous results; either as augmentation or monotherapy. Ceiling effect of 1 g for EPA?*

FORMS: Trade: Lovaza 1 g cap (total 840 mg EPA + DHA). Generic/trade: cap, shown as EPA+DHA mg content, 240 (Promega Pearls), 300 (Cardi-Omega 3, Max EPA), 320 (Sea-Omega), 400 (Promega), 500 (Sea-Omega), 600 (Marine Lipid Concentrate, SuperEPA 1200), 875 mg (SuperEPA 2000).

NOTES: *Lovaza is the only FDA-approved fish oil, previously known as Omacor.* Dose-dependent GI upset (divide the dose, ginger root, Daikon radish), may ↑ LDL-cholesterol, excessive bleeding, hyperglycemia. Marine Lipid Concentrate, Super EPA 1,200 mg cap contains EPA 360 mg + DHA 240 mg, daily dose = 5–8 caps. Rx doses lowers triglycerides by 30–50%. Caps may contain omega-6 fatty acids and/or vitamin E; content varies with product. Monitor sugar in type 2 diabetes. Food ↑ omega-3 absorption; higher content of EPA is desirable. Antioxidants (vitamin C 250–500 mg/d and vitamin E 400–800 IU/d) may prevent in vivo degradation of omega-3s. Possible risks with fish oil: fishy aftertaste (better taste with flax oil), hypervitaminose A (cod liver oil), impaired platelet function (EPA binds reversibly to platelets), exposure to heavy metals or chemical pollutants (mercury, Cd, PCBs/FDA has advised pregnant ♀ and young children to avoid eating fish containing them such as shark, swordfish, king mackerel, tilefish). No omega-3 content in catfish, tilapia, shrimp.

DRUG INTERACTIONS: May potentiate warfarin; caution with xenical (orlistat), high dose NSAID.

Pyridoxine (*Vitamin B₆*) ►K ♀A▶+ $

WARNING: *Is the only B vitamin with toxic potential*; rare peripheral neuropathy at >200 mg/d.

ADULTS: Dietary deficiency: 10–20 mg po/d for 3 wk. Prevention of deficiency due to isoniazid in high-risk pts: 10–25 mg po daily. Rx of neuropathies due to INH: 50–200 mg po/d. INH overdose (>10 g): give an equal amount of pyridoxine: 4 g IV followed by 1 g IM q 30 min. RDA for adults: 19–50 yo: 1.3 mg; >50 yo: 1.7 mg (♂), 1.5 mg (♀). Max 100 mg/d.

PEDS: Not approved in children.

UNAPPROVED ADULTS: PMS dysphoria: 50–500 mg/d po. Hyperoxaluria type I and oxalate kidney stones: 25–300 mg/d po. Prevention of oral contraceptive-induced deficiency: 25–40 mg/d. Hyperemesis of pregnancy: 10–50 mg q 8 hr; has been used in hydralazine poisoning, in augmentation of Mg++, for *antidepressant augmentation (as an adjunct). Rarely used in bipolar disorders. Used in treatment or prevention of tardive dyskinesia: start 100 mg/d, increasing weekly in 100 mg increments to a total of 400 mg/d (some go up to 1,400 mg/d)*

UNAPPROVED PEDS: Dietary deficiency: 5–10 mg po/d for 3 wk. Prevention of deficiency due to isoniazid: 1–2 mg/kg/d po. Rx of neuropathies due to INH: 10–15 mg po/d. Pyridoxine-dependent epilepsy: neonatal: 25–50 mg/dose IV; older infants and children: 100 mg/dose IV for 1 dose then 100 mg po/d.

FORMS: OTC generic only: tab 25, 50, 100 mg, time-released tab 100 mg.

NOTES: Cofactor for many enzymes, poorly understood role in the brain. No adverse effect usually if <200 mg/d. If >200 mg/d: risk of sensory neuropathy. Other SE: GI, breast soreness. Probably safe if <200–400 mg/d. Mg++ salts may improve B₆ efficacy (200–300 mg bid–tid of Mg++; amino acid chelates such as MG++ glycinate produce less GI distress). Half-life: 15–20 days.

DRUG INTERACTIONS: Vitamin B₆ ↓ effects of L-DOPA. B₆ decrease phenytoin levels. Carbamazepine and valproate decrease B₆. Phenelzine and isoniazid decrease B₆. High doses of oral contraceptives decrease B₆. Alcoholism decreases B₆. B₆ may improve the effectiveness of certain tricyclic antidepressants.

S-Adenosylmethionine (*SAMe, sammyl*) ►L ♀? ▶? $$$

WARNING: High dosage associated with hypomania/mania.

UNAPPROVED ADULTS: *Depression* (possibly effective): start: 200–400 mg bid; usual dose: 400–1,600 mg/d po; extreme dosage: 3,000 mg/d. Used also for antidepressant augmentation; osteoarthritis (possibly effective): 400–1,200 mg/d po (onset of response in OA in 2–4 wk); efficacy unclear for alcoholic liver disease; hepatoprotection (↓ retrovirus); fibromyalgia.

UNAPPROVED PEDS: Not for use in children.

FORMS: Caplets containing SAMe salts: 1, 4-butanedisulfonate (BDS) form (from brands such as GNC, Nature Made, Puritan's) or Tosylate form (from brands such as: Natrol, Source): 200, 400 mg.

NOTES: Take on an empty stomach: 30–60 min before meals or 90–120 min after meals; ↑ by 200–400 mg q 3–7 days. Use with B vitamins: folic acid (1–5 mg/d), B₆ (50–100 mg/d), B₁₂ (250–1,000 mcg/d).

DRUG INTERACTIONS: Serotonin syndrome possible with SSRIs. Do not use within 2 wk of an MAOI or in bipolar disorder; Reported interaction w/ oral contraceptive pills. Facilitates monoamine synthesis (5HT, NA, DA) and modification of second messenger systems.

Selenium

WARNING: Small therapeutic index (risk of inadvertent toxicity); vitamin E may enhance toxicity. Toxicity if >700 mcg/d. (Hair, finger nails changes, GI sx, neuropathy, irritability.)

ADULT: RDA: 70 mcg/d (♂), 55 mcg/d (♀).

PEDS: Not recommended for children.

UNAPPROVED ADULT: Possible efficacy in *depression*. Start 50–100 mcg qd; target dose is 100–200 mcg/d; max is 200 mcg/d.

FORMS: Cap: 200 mcg (salts or amino acid chelates).

NOTES: Strong antioxidant, radioprotectant; is an essential trace mineral.

St. John's wort (*Alterra, Hypericum perforatum, Kira, Movana, One-a-Day Tension and Mood, LI-160, St John's wort*) ▶ L ♀- ▶-$

WARNING: Marginally effective in major depression; induction of mania and hypomania possible; contraindicated in pregnancy, lactation, cardiovascular disease, and pheochromocytoma.

UNAPPROVED ADULTS: Short-term rx of mild depression (effective): 300 mg po tid of standardized extract. Max 1,500 mg/d. Conflicting trials for moderate major depression.

UNAPPROVED PEDS: Not for use in children.

FORMS: Standardized products contain 0.3% hypericin (equivalent to 2–4 g of dried herb). Usually cap 300 mg.

NOTES: Adverse effects: GI problems, dry mouth, sedation, hair loss, photosensitivity (if doses >1,800 mg/d); unclear mechanism of action (affects number of systems/NE, 5-HT1A, DA, GABA, MAO enzymes).

DRUG INTERACTIONS: CYP 3A4, 2C9, 2C19, and p-glycoprotein induction may lead to significant interactions, serotonergic SE including serotonin syndrome (with SSRIs, triptans, nefazodone). Possible MAOI activity (caution with foods containing tyramine, serotonergic, and sympathomometic drugs); decrease levels of cyclosporine (risk of rejection of transplanted organs), ↓ levels of nonnucleoside reverse transcriptase inhibitors, digoxin, theophylline, amiodarone, warfarin (decreased INR), methadone, alprazolam, amitriptyline, omeprazole, oral contraceptives, protease inhibitors, statins, voriconazol; may need increased dose of tricyclic antidepressants.

Tocopherol *(vitamin E, ♣ Aquasol E)* ▶ L ♀ A ▶? $

ADULT: RDA is 22 units (natural, d-alpha-tocopherol) or 33 units (synthetic, d l-alpha-tocopherol) or 15 mg (alpha-tocopherol). Max 1,000 mg (alpha-tocopherol); usually 200–400 IU qd.

PEDS: RDA (alpha-tocopherol): infants 0–6 mo: 4 mg; 7–12 mo: 6 mg. RDA for children (alpha-tocopherol): 1–3 yo: 6 mg; 4–8 yo: 7 mg; 9–13 yo: 11 mg; 14–18 yo: 15 mg.

UNAPPROVED ADULT: *Alzheimer disease*: 1,000 units po bid (controversial, limited data, and efficacy). May be effective in *Tardive dyskinesia (high dose: start: 400 IU bid, max dosage: 800 IU bid. May be used at higher doses if used alone (1,200–2,000 IU).*

UNAPPROVED PEDS: Nutritional deficiency: neonates: 25–50 units po/d; children: 1 unit/kg/d. Cystic fibrosis: 5–10 units/kg/d (use water soluble form), max 400 units/d.

FORMS: OTC generic only: tab 200, 400, units, cap 73.5, 100, 147, 165, 200, 330, 400, 500, 600, 1,000 units, drops 50 mg/mL.

NOTES: Natural vitamin E (d-alpha-tocopherol) recommended over synthetic (d l alpha-tocopherol due to higher bioavailability). Do not exceed 1,500 units natural vitamin E per day. Higher doses may ↑ risk of bleeding. Large randomized trials have failed to demonstrate cardioprotective effects (may ↑ cardiac risk); crucial lipid antioxidant; may protect omega-3s from oxidation in vivo.

DRUG INTERACTIONS: Reduces statin efficacy.

L-Tyrosine

WARNING: Risk of mania.

UNAPPROVED ADULTS: Inadequately tested as an *adjunct for antidepressants* and stimulants in depression. Start dose: 500 mg bid. Max 1,500 mg bid.

FORMS: Cap 500, 1,000 mg.

NOTES: Essential precursor for catecholamines. Take on an empty stomach (competes with other amino acids).

L-Tryptophan

WARNING: FDA banned it in the United States in 1989 for eosinophilia-myalgia syndrome (EMS) which was due in fact to the toxic "peak X" and product was reintroduced in 2003 only as a herbal supplement (no regulated standards). Toxicity: sedation, rare cases of serotonin syndrome, EMS sx (myalgias, weakness, vomiting, headaches, death). Always check if tested for "peak X."

UNAPPROVED ADULT: *Insomnia, bipolar disorder, augmentation of antidepressants.* Start dose: 500 mg bid. Max 1,500 mg bid.

FORMS: Cap 500, 1,000 mg.

NOTES: Take on an empty stomach (competes with other amino acids).

DRUG INTERACTIONS: CNS depressants, antidepressants. Do not use with MAOIs.

Valerian (*Valeriana officinalis, Alluna, One-a-day Bedtime and Rest, Sleep-Tite*)▶? ♀-▶-$

WARNING: Liver dysfunction reported (check regularly LFTs, may depend on extract such as valepotriates). Cases of liver toxicity reported with use of herbal product (skullcap). Withdrawal sx after chronic use (delirium).

UNAPPROVED ADULTS: *Sleep disorders*: 200–800 mg/d; generalized anxiety disorder.

UNAPPROVED PEDS: Sleep disorders.

FORMS: Cap of 0.8% valerenic acid, or 1–1.5 % valtrate preferred.

NOTES: SE: nausea, blurred vision, vivid dreams, morning hangover. Tastes like "dirty socks"; low abuse potential.

DRUG INTERACTIONS: Does not seem to inhibit CYP 1A2, 2D6, 2 E1, or 3A4, potentiates effects of CNS depressants.

Vitamin D or 1, 2, 5-dihydroxyvitamin D_3 (*vitamin D_2, ergocalciferol, Calciferol, Drisdol, Osteoforte*) ▶L ♀A (C if exceed RDA) ▶+ $

ADULT: Familial hypophosphatemia (vitamin D resistant rickets): 12,000–500,000 units po daily. Hypoparathyroidism: 50,000–200,000 units po/d. Adequate daily intake adults: 10–50 yo: 5 mcg (200 units); 51–70 yo: 10 mcg (400 units); >70 yo: 15 mcg (600 units). Max daily dose in nondeficiency 50 mcg (2,000 units).

PEDS: Adequate daily intake infants and children: 5 mcg (200 units). Hypoparathyroidism: 1.25–5 mg po daily.

UNAPPROVED ADULT: Osteoporosis prevention: 400–800 units po/d with calcium supplements. Fanconi syndrome: 50,000–200,000 units po/d. Osteomalacia: 1,000–5,000 units po/d. Anticonvulsant-induced osteomalacia: 2,000–50,000 units po/d. Vitamin D deficiency: 50,000 units po q wk to q month. 400–800 IU/d × 5 days significantly improved *winter mood; unclear role in MDD*.

UNAPPROVED PEDS: Familial hypophosphatemia: 400,000–800,000 units po/d, ↑ by 10,000–20,000 units/d q 3–4 months as needed. Hypoparathyroidism: 50,000–200,000 units po daily. Fanconi syndrome: 250–50,000 units po/d.

FORMS: OTC: trade: solution 8,000 units/mL. Rx: trade: cap 50,000 units, inj 500,000 units/mL.

NOTES: 1 mcg ergocalciferol = 40 units vitamin D IM or high-dose oral rx may be necessary if malabsorption exists. Familial hypophosphatemia also requires phosphate supplementation; hypoparathyroidism also requires calcium supplementation. Sunlight required for making active form (D3). Chronic ingestion of >100,000 IU/d of D2 or D3 leads to toxicity (secondary to hypercalcemia; risk of renal damage, kidney stones). Half-life: 19–48 hr; info: stored in fat deposits for prolonged periods. Monitor: alk phos; BUN; Ca q 2 wk or if high-dose rx then frequently; Mg; PO_4 q 2 wk; 24 hr urinary Ca and PO_4; bone x-ray q month until stable.

Zinc sulfate (*Orazinc, Zincate*), Zinc acetate (*Galzin*) and Zinc gluconate ▶ Minimal absorption ♀A▶-$

WARNING: With chronic use, add copper (for every 50 mg zinc, use 5–10 mg copper).

ADULT: RDA (elemental Zn): adult ♂: 11 mg/d. Adult ♀: 8–12 mg/d. Zinc deficiency: 25–50 mg/d (elemental). Max 200 mg.

PEDS: RDA (elemental Zn): Age 7 mo–3 yo: 3 mg/d; 4–8 yo: 5 mg; 9–13 yo: 8 mg; 14–18 yo (males): 8 mg; 14–18 yo (females): 9–14 mg. Zinc deficiency: 0.5–1 mg elemental Zn mg/kg/d divided bid–tid.

UNAPPROVED ADULT: Wound healing in Zn deficiency: 200 mg tid. Start 50 mg/d; target dose 50–200 mg/d; max 200 mg/d.

FORMS: Zinc sulfate: OTC generic/trade: tab 66, 110, 200 mg; rx: cap 220 mg. Zinc acetate (Galzin): Zinc acetate: trade: cap 25, 50 mg elemental zinc.

NOTES: Zinc sulfate is 23% elemental Zn. ↓ absorption of tetracycline and fluoroquinilones. Poorly absorbed; ↑ absorption on empty stomach; however, administration with food ↓ GI upset. Is immunostimulant (may be dangerous if patient has TB or sarcoid). Helps improving taste and smell function in various ENT, nutritional, CNS disorders, *SE of drugs (drugs used to treat anxiety, lithium)*.

APPENDIX: INHIBITORS, INDUCERS, AND SUBSTRATES OF CYTOCHROME P450 ISOZYMES

The cytochrome P450 (CYP) inhibitors and inducers below do not necessarily cause clinically important interactions with substrates listed. Underlined drugs have shown potential for important interactions in human case reports or clinical studies. We exclude in vitro data which can be inaccurate. Refer to the Tarascon Pocket Pharmacopoeia drug interactions database (PDA edition) or other resources for more information if an interaction is suspected based on this chart. A drug that inhibits CYP subfamily activity can block the metabolism of substrates of that enzyme and substrate accumulation and toxicity may result. CYP inhibitors are classified by how much they increase the area-under-the-curve (AUC) of a substrate: weak (1.25ñ2 fold), moderate (2ñ5 fold), or strong (≥5 fold). A drug is considered a sensitive substrate if a CYP inhibitor increases the AUC of that drug by ≥5-fold. While AUC increases of >50% often do not affect patient response, smaller increases can be important if the therapeutic range is narrow (e.g., theophylline, warfarin, cyclosporine). A drug that induces CYP subfamily activity increases substrate metabolism and reduced substrate efficacy may result. This table may be incomplete since new evidence about drug interactions is continually being identified.

CYP 1A2

Inhibitors. *Strong*: fluvoxamine. *Moderate*: ciprofloxacin, mexiletine, propafenone, zileuton. *Weak*: acyclovir, cimetidine, famotidine, norfloxacin, verapamil. *Unclassified*: amiodarone, atazanavir, citalopram, clarithromycin, erythromycin, estradiol, ipriflavone, isoniazid, paroxetine, peginterferon alfa-2a, tacrine, ziprasidone.

Inducers: barbiturates, carbamazepine, charcoal-broiled foods, phenytoin, rifampin, ritonavir, smoking.

Substrates. *Sensitive*: alosetron, duloxetine, tizanidine. *Unclassified*: acetaminophen, amitriptyline, bortezomib, caffeine, cinacalcet, clomipramine, clozapine, cyclobenzaprine, estradiol, fluvoxamine, haloperidol, imipramine, lidocaine, mexiletine, mirtazapine, naproxen, olanzapine, ondansetron, propranolol, ramelteon, rasagiline, riluzole, ropinirole, ropivacaine, R-warfarin, tacrine, theophylline, verapamil, zileuton, zolmitriptan.

CYP 2C8

Inhibitors. *Strong*: gemfibrozil. *Weak*: trimethoprim.

Inducers: barbiturates, carbamazepine, rifabutin, rifampin.

Substrates. *Sensitive*: repaglinide. *Unclassified*: amiodarone, carbamazepine, ibuprofen, isotretinoin, loperamide, paclitaxel, pioglitazone, rosiglitazone, tolbutamide.

CYP 2C9

Inhibitors. *Moderate*: amiodarone, fluconazole, oxandrolone. *Weak*: ketoconazole. *Unclassified*: atazanavir, capecitabine, chloramphenicol, cimetidine, cotrimoxazole, delavirdine, disulfiram, etravirine, fenofibrate, fluorouracil, fluvoxamine, imatinib, isoniazid, leflunomide, metronidazole, sulfamethoxazole, voriconazole, zafirlukast.

Inducers: aprepitant, barbiturates, bosentan, carbamazepine, phenytoin, rifampin, rifapentine, St John's wort.

Substrates. *Sensitive*: Flurbiprofen. *Unclassified*: alosetron, bosentan, celecoxib, chlorpropamide, diclofenac, etravirine, fluoxetine, flurbiprofen, fluvastatin, formoterol, glimepiride, glipizide, glyburide, ibuprofen, irbesartan, isotretinoin, losartan, mefenamic acid, meloxicam, montelukast, naproxen, nateglinide, phenytoin, piroxicam, ramelteon, rasagiline, rosiglitazone, rosuvastatin, sildenafil, tolbutamide, torsemide, valsartan, vardenafil, voriconazole, S-warfarin, zafirlukast, zileuton.

CYP 2C19

Inhibitors. *Strong*: omeprazole. *Weak*: citalopram. *Unclassified*: armodafinil, delavirdine, esomeprazole, etravirine, felbamate, fluconazole, fluoxetine, fluvoxamine, isoniazid, letrozole, modafinil, oxcarbazepine, telmisartan, voriconazole.

Inducers: rifampin, St John's wort.

Substrates. *Sensitive*: omeprazole. *Unclassified*: ambrisentan, amitriptyline, arformoterol, bortezomib, carisoprodol, cilostazol, citalopram, clomipramine, desipramine, diazepam, escitalopram, esomeprazole, etravirine, formoterol, imipramine, lansoprazole, nelfinavir, pantoprazole, phenytoin, progesterone, proguanil, propranolol, rabeprazole, thioridazine, voriconazole, R-warfarin.

CYP 2D6

Inhibitors. *Strong*: cinacalcet, fluoxetine, paroxetine, quinidine. *Moderate*: duloxetine, terbinafine. *Weak*: amiodarone, citalopram, escitalopram, sertraline. *Unclassified*: bupropion, chloroquine, cimetidine, clomipramine, delavirdine, diphenhydramine, fluphenazine, fluvoxamine, haloperidol, hydroxychloroquine, imatinib, perphenazine, propafenone, propoxyphene, ritonavir, tolterodine, thioridazine, venlafaxine.

Inducers: None

Substrates. *Sensitive:* desipramine. *Unclassified:* almotriptan, amitriptyline, arformoterol, aripiprazole, atomoxetine, carvedilol, cevimeline, chlorpheniramine, chlorpromazine, cinacalcet, clomipramine, clozapine, codeine*, darifenacin, delavirdine, dextromethorphan, dihydrocodeine*, dolasetron, donepezil, doxepin, duloxetine, flecainide, fluoxetine, formoterol, galantamine, haloperidol, hydrocodone*, imipramine, loratadine, maprotiline, methadone, methamphetamine, metoprolol, mexiletine, mirtazapine, morphine, nebivolol, nortriptyline, ondansetron, oxycodone, palonosetron, paroxetine, perphenazine, procainamide, promethazine, propafenone, propoxyphene, propranolol, quetiapine, risperidone, ritonavir, tamoxifen, thioridazine, timolol, tolterodine, tramadol*, trazodone, venlafaxine.

CYP 3A4

Inhibitors. *Strong:* atazanavir, clarithromycin, indinavir, itraconazole, ketoconazole, nefazodone, nelfinavir, ritonavir, saquinavir, telithromycin, voriconazole. *Moderate:* amprenavir, aprepitant, diltiazem, erythromycin, fluconazole, fosamprenavir, grapefruit juice (variable), verapamil. *Weak:* cimetidine. *Unclassified:* amiodarone, conivaptan, cyclosporine, danazol, darunavir, delavirdine, ethinyl estradiol, fluoxetine, fluvoxamine, imatinib, miconazole, posaconazole, sertraline, quinupristin/dalfopristin, troleandomycin, zafirlukast.

Inducers: armodafinil, barbiturates, bexarotene, bosentan, carbamazepine, dexamethasone, ♣efavirenz, ethosuximide, etravirine, griseofulvin, modafinil, nafcillin, ♣nevirapine, oxcarbazepine, phenytoin, primidone, rifabutin, ♣rifampin, rifapentine, ritonavir, St Johns wort.

Substrates. *Sensitive:* budesonide, buspirone, conivaptan, eletriptan, eplerenone, felodipine, 7, lovastatin, midazolam, saquinavir, sildenafil, simvastatin, triazolam, vardenafil. *Unclassified:* acetaminophen, alfentanil, alfuzosin, aliskiren, almotriptan, alosetron, alprazolam, amiodarone, amlodipine, amprenavir, aprepitant, argatroban, aripiprazole, atazanavir, atorvastatin, bexarotene, bortezomib, bosentan, bromocriptine, buprenorphine, carbamazepine, cevimeline, cilostazol, cinacalcet, cisapride, citalopram, clarithromycin, clomipramine, clonazepam, clopidogrel, colchicine, clozapine, corticosteroids, cyclophosphamide, cyclosporine, dapsone, darifenacin, darunavir, dasatinib, delavirdine, desogestrel, dexamethasone, diazepam, dihydroergotamine, diltiazem, disopyramide, docetaxel, dofetilide, dolasetron, domperidone, donepezil, doxorubicin, dutasteride, efavirenz, ergotamine, erlotinib, erythromycin†, escitalopram, esomeprazole, eszopiclone, ethinyl estradiol, etoposide, etravirine, fentanyl, finasteride, galantamine, gefitinib, glyburide, haloperidol, hydrocodone, ifosfamide, imatinib, imipramine, indinavir, irinotecan, isotretinoin, isradipine, itraconazole, ixabepilone, ketoconazole, lansoprazole, lapatinib, letrozole, lidocaine, loperamide, lopinavir, loratadine, losartan, maraviroc, methadone, methylergonovine, mifepristone, mirtazapine, modafinil, mometasone, montelukast, nateglinide, nefazodone, nelfinavir, nevirapine, nicardipine, nifedipine, nimodipine, nisoldipine, ondansetron, oxybutynin, oxycodone, paclitaxel, pantoprazole, paricalcitol, pimozide, pioglitazone, praziquantel, quetiapine, quinidine, quinine, ranolazine, repaglinide, rifabutin, risperidone, ritonavir, ropivacaine, sertraline, sibutramine, sirolimus, solifenacin, sorafenib, sufentanil, sunitinib, tacrolimus, tadalafil, tamoxifen, telithromycin, temsirolimus, testosterone, theophylline, tiagabine, tinidazole, tipranavir, tolterodine, toremifene, tramadol, trazodone, venlafaxine, verapamil, vinblastine, vincristine, vinorelbine, voriconazole, R-warfarin, zaleplon, zileuton, ziprasidone, zolpidem, zonisamide.

♣ potent inducer

* Metabolism by CYP2D6 required to convert to active analgesic metabolite; analgesia may be impaired by CYP2D6 inhibitors.

† Risk of sudden death may be increased in patients receiving erythromycin concurrently with CYP 3A4 inhibitors like ketoconazole, itraconazole, fluconazole, diltiazem, verapamil, and troleandomycin (NEJM 2004;351:1089).

SOME PSYCHIATRIC BOOKS AND REFERENCES

BASIC BOOKS

American Psychiatric Association. (2000). *Diagnostic and statistical manual of mental disorders* (4th ed., text revision; *DSM-IV-TR*). Washington, DC: (Corporate Author).

Comment: Complete criteria for each mental illness described in the *DSM-IV-TR* have not been reported here in this book because of space reasons and the expected release of the next edition of the *DSM*: the *DSM-V* manual (scheduled for 2013). The reader will have to refer to this indispensable book for specific criteria and coding.

Cassem, N. H., Stern, T., Rosenbaum, J., Fricchione, G. L., & Jellinek, M. (Eds.). (2010). *Massachusetts General Hospital handbook of general hospital psychiatry* (6th ed.). St. Louis, MO: Mosby.

Comment: Informed, balanced, comprehensive, and practical perspective; very useful for clinical issues in the medical and surgical environment.

Sadock, B. J., Sadock, V. A., & Ruiz, P. (Eds.). (2009). *Kaplan and Sadock's Comprehensive textbook of psychiatry* (9th ed., 2 Vols.). Philadelphia: Lippincott Williams & Wilkins.

Comment: Established as the cornerstone text in the field of psychiatry and mental health; the comprehensive and up to date specialist reference.

Stahl, S. M. (2008). *Essential psychopharmacology: The prescriber's guide* (rev. and updated 3rd ed.). New York: Cambridge University Press.

Comment: Essential clearly presented data for anyone who prescribes psychotropic medication.

OTHER REFERENCES

Agrell, B., & Dehljn, O. (1998). The clock drawing test. *Age and Ageing, 27*, 399–403.

Anthony, J. C., Bassett, S. S., & Folstein, M. F. (1993). Population-based norms for the Mini-Mental State Examination by age and educational levels. *Journal of the American Medical Association, 18*, 2386–2391.

Bradley, M., & Muskin, P. R. (2007). 5-step psychiatric workup of HIV patients. *Current Psychiatry, 6*(12), 11–17.

Brennan, D., Betzelos, S., Reed, R., & Falk, J. (1995). Ethanol elimination rates in an ED population. *American Journal of Emergency Medicine, 13*(3), 276–280.

Charney, D. S., & Nestler, E. J. (2004). *Neurobiology of mental illness* (2nd ed.). New York: Oxford University Press.

Cobert, B., & Biron, P. (2009). *Practical drug safety from A to Z* (p. 285). Sudbury, MA: Jones & Bartlett Learning.

Cook, S. (2004). The metabolic syndrome: Antecedent of adult cardiovascular disease in pediatrics. *Journal of Pediatrics, 145*(4), 439–444.

Dattilo, P. B., Hailpern, S. M., Fearon, K., Sohal, D., Nordin, C., et al. (2008). JC: β-blockers are associated with reduced risk of myocardial infarction after cocaine use. *Annals of Emergency Medicine, 51*, 117–134.

Fairburn, C. G. (1995). *Overcoming binge eating*. New York: Guilford Press.

Garner, D. M., & Garfinkel, P. E. (Eds.). (1997). *Handbook of treatment for eating disorders* (2nd ed.). New York: Guilford Press.

Goldsmith, S. (1983–1984). A strategy for evaluating "psychogenic" symptoms. *International Journal of Psychiatry in Medicine, 13*(2), 167–172.

Halmi, K. A. (2005, May). A complicated process: Diagnosing and treating anorexia nervosa and bulimia. *Psychiatric Times, XXII*(6).

Kaye, N. S. (2005). Is your depressed patient bipolar? *Journal of American Board of Family Practitioners, 18*(4), 271–281.

Kubler-Ross, E. (1997). *On Death and Dying*. New York: Scribner.

Lerner, V., et al. (2001). Vitamin B(6) in the treatment of tardive dyskinesia: A double-blind, placebo-controlled, crossover study. *American Journal of Psychiatry, 158*(9), 1511–1514.

Lock, J., Le Grange, D., Agras, W. S., & Dare, C. (2005). *Treatment manual for anorexia nervosa: A family-based approach*. New York: Guilford Press.

Masters, W. H., & Johnson, V. E. (1974). *The Pleasure Bond*. Toronto: Bantam Books.

Mayo-Smith, M. F., Beecher, L. H., Fischer, T. L., Gorelick, D. A., Guillaume, J. L., Hill, A., et al., Working Group on the Management of Alcohol Withdrawal Delirium, Practice Guidelines Committee, *American Society of Addiction Medicine*. (2004). Management of alcohol withdrawal delirium. An evidence-based practice guideline. *Archives of Internal Medicine, 164*(13), 1405–1412.

McElroy, S. L., Kotwal, R., Guerdjikova, A. I., Welge, J. A., Nelson, E. B., Lake, K. A., et al. (2006). Zonisamide in the treatment of binge eating disorder with obesity: A randomized controlled trial. *Journal of Clinical Psychology, 67*(12), 1897–1906.

McGarry, A. L., Curran, W. J., Lipsitt, P. D., Lelos, D., et al. (1973). *Competency to stand trial and mental illness.* DHEW 73–9105. Washington, DC: Government Printing Office. Thirteen aspects to be considered when making a determination of criminal responsibility.

Moore, D. P. (2006). *The little black book of psychiatry* (3rd ed.). Sudbury, MA: Jones & Bartlett Learning.

Nikoletti, S., Porock, D., Kristjanson, L., et al. (2000). Performance status assessment in home hospice patients using a modified form of the Karnofsky Performance Status Scale. *Journal of Palliative Medicine, 3*, 301–311.

Pajeau, A. K., & Roman, G. C. (June 1992). HIV encephalopathy and dementia. In J. Biller & R. G. Kathol (Eds.), *Psychiatric clinics of North America.* Philadelphia: W.B. Saunders.

Prochaska, J. O., DiClemente, C. C., & Norcross, J. (1992). In search of how people change: Applications to addictive behaviors. *American Psychologist, 47*, 1102–1114.

Ries, R. K., Miller, S. C., Fiellin, D. A., & Saitz, R. (2009*). Principles of addiction medicine source* (4th ed.). Philadelphia: Lippincott Williams & Wilkins.

Sansone, R. A., Levitt, J. L., & Sansone, L. A. (2005). A primer on psychotherapy treatment of anorexia nervosa in adolescents. *Psychiatry, 2*, 40–46.

Sullivan, J. T., Sykora, K., Schneiderman, J., Naranjo, C. A., & Sellers, E. M. (1989). Assessment of alcohol withdrawal: The revised Clinical Institute Withdrawal Assessment for Alcohol Scale (CIWA-Ar). *British Journal of Addiction, 84*(11), 1353–1357.

Tomb, D. A. (1995). *Psychiatry* (5th ed., p. 44). Baltimore, MD: Williams & Wilkins.

Tranter, R., & Healy, D. (1998). Neuroleptic discontinuation syndromes. *Journal of Psychopharmacology, 12*, 401–406.

Vaillant, G. E. (1971). Theoretical hierarchy of adaptive ego mechanisms. *Archives of General Psychiatry, 24*, 107–118.

Yudofsky, S. C., & Hales, R. E. (Eds). (1992). *The American Psychiatric Press textbook of neuropsychiatry* (2nd ed.). Washington, DC: American Psychiatric Press.

Zachary, N., Stowe, M. D., & Newport, D. J. (2007). *The management of bipolar disorder during pregnancy: Treatment options for women with bipolar disorder during pregnancy.* Retrieved August 19, 2010, from http://www.medscape.com/viewarticle/565128_4.

RESOURCES

ONLINE ALGORITHMS

Texas Medication Algorithm Project (TMAP): www.dshs.state.tx.us/mhprograms/TMAPtoc.shtm

Harvard Psychopharmacology Algorithm Project: http://mhc.com/Algorithms

International Psychopharmacology Algorithm Project: IPAP, www.ipap.org

MacArthur Initiative on depression and Primary Care Toolkit: www.depressionprimarycare.org/clinicians/toolkit/full/

GUIDELINES

American Association of Child and Adolescent Psychiatry (AACAP): wwsw.aacap.org/publications/pubcat/guideline.htm and www.jaacap.com

- Practice parameters for the assessment and treatment of children and adolescents with bipolar disorder. *Journal of the American Academy of Child and Adolescent Psychiatry* (January 2007), *46*(1).

American Psychiatric Association (APA): www.psych.org/psych-pract/treatg/pg/prac-guide.cfm and http://ajp.psychiatryonline.org

- Practice guidelines for the treatment of patients with schizophrenia (2004, 2nd ed.). *American Journal of Psychiatry, 161*(Suppl 2), 1–56.
- APA practice guidelines. *Assessment and treatment of patients with suicidal behaviors*, http://www.psychiatryonline.com/pracGuide/pracGuideTopic_14.aspx
- *APA practice guidelines for treatment of patients with acute stress disorder and posttraumatic stress disorder* (November 2004) and Guideline Watch (March 2009).
- *APA practice guidelines for treatment of patients with panic disorders* (January 2009, 2nd ed.).
- Practice guidelines for the treatment of eating disorders, *American Journal of Psychiatry* (2006), *163*(7 suppl), 1–54.
- *Manual: The principles of medical ethics with annotations especially applicable to psychiatry* (1995). Washington, DC: American Psychiatric Association.

National Guideline Clearinghouse: www.guideline.gov

- Park, M., Hsiao-Chen Tang, J., & Ledford, L. (November 2005). *Changing the practice of physical restraint use in acute care* (47 pp.). Iowa City: University of Iowa Gerontological Nursing Interventions Research Center, Research Translation and Dissemination Core.

Veterans Affairs/Department of Defense Guidelines: www.oqp.med.va.gov/cpg/CPG.htm

EVIDENCE-BASED MENTAL HEALTH

National Electronic Library for Mental Health: http://www.nelmh.org

Evidence-Based Mental Health: http://ebmh.bmjjournals.com

Centre for Evidence-Based Mental Health: http://www.cebmh.com

CLINICAL TRIALS

http://clinicaltrials.gov/

INDEX

Note: Page numbers followed by "*t*" refer to tables.

Stay Connected with Tarascon Publishing!

Monthly Dose eNewsletter
—Tarascon's Monthly eNewsletter

Stay up-to-date and subscribe today at: www.tarascon.com

Written specifically with **Tarascon** customers in mind, the Tarascon Monthly Dose will provide you with new drug information, tips and tricks, updates on our print, mobile and online products as well as some extra topics that are interesting and entertaining.

Sign up to receive the Tarascon Monthly Dose Today! Simply register at www.tarascon.com.

You can also stay up-to-date with **Tarascon** news, new product releases, and relevant medical news and information on Facebook, Twitter page, and our Blog.

STAY CONNECTED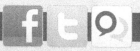

Facebook: www.facebook.com/tarascon
Twitter: @JBL_Medicine
Blog: portfolio.jblearning.com/medicine

CPSIA information can be obtained
at www.ICGtesting.com
Printed in the USA
LVHW081624080419
613372LV00027B/956/P